# www.harcourt-international.com

Bringing you products from all Harcourt Health Sciences companies including Baillière Tindall, Churchill Livingstone, Mosby and W.B. Saunders

- **Browse** f... nals and electronic pr...
- **Search** for information on over 20 000 published titles with full product information including tables of contents and sample chapters
- **Keep up to date** with our extensive publishing programme in your field by registering with eAlert or requesting postal updates
- **Secure online ordering** with prompt delivery, as well as full contact details to order by phone, fax or post
- **News** of special features and promotions

If you are based in the following countries, please visit the country-specific site to receive full details of product availability and local ordering information

USA: www.harcourthealth.com

Canada: www.harcourtcanada.com

Australia: www.harcourt.com.au



Baillière Tindall

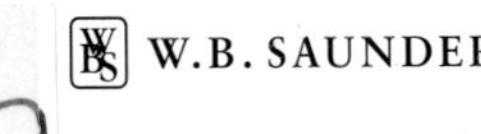

# Anatomy and Physiology for Midwives

*For Mosby:*

*Publishing Manager:* Inta Ozols
*Project Manager*: Gail Murray
*Project Development Manager:* Karen Gilmour
*Designer:* George Ajayi
*Illustrators:* Debbie Maizels and Philip Wilson
*Photograph of sperm on cover:* Dr Kevin Pedley and Dr Susan Hawes

# Anatomy and Physiology for Midwives

**Jane Coad** BSc PhD PGCEA

*Senior Lecturer, European Institute of Health and Medical Sciences, University of Surrey, Guildford, UK*

with

**Melvyn Dunstall** BSc MSc PGCEA RM RGN

*Lecturer/Practitioner in Midwifery, Ashford and St Peter's Hospitals NHS Trust, St Peter's Hospital, Chertsey*

*European Institute of Health and Medical Sciences, University of Surrey, Guildford, UK*

Foreword by

**Meryl Thomas** MA BA DipEdMan MTD ADM RGN RM

*Director of Midwifery Education and Practice, English National Board of Nursing, Midwifery and Health Visiting, Bristol, UK*



**Mosby**

Edinburgh London New York Philadelphia St Louis Sydney Toronto 2001

MOSBY
An imprint of Harcourt Publishers Limited



First published 2001

ISBN 0 7234 2979 0

**British Library Cataloguing in Publication Data**
A catalogue record for this book is available from the British Library

**Library of Congress Cataloging in Publication Data**
A catalog record for this book is available from the Library of Congress

**Note**
Medical knowledge is constantly changing. As new information becomes available, changes in treatment, procedures, equipment and the use of drugs become necessary. The authors and the publishers have taken care to ensure that the information given in this text is accurate and up to date. However, readers are strongly advised to confirm that the information, especially with regard to drug usage, complies with the latest legislation and standards of practice.

The publisher's policy is to use **paper manufactured from sustainable forests**

Printed in Spain

# Contents

# Foreword

A sound knowledge of the biological sciences which are involved in human reproduction and which underpin the art of midwives' care of mothers and babies throughout childbearing is fundamental to safe practice. High-quality, optimal care is, to an even greater extent, dependent on analysis, interpretation and synthesis by midwives of scientific knowledge and evidence, to inform the role of the midwife with women and their families.

Over the last two decades, the importance of sound theoretical underpinning of clinical care has been emphasized. Countries such as Australia, New Zealand and the United Kingdom have established midwifery education within the universities, where it is flourishing as an academic subject with a strong practice focus. In British Columbia, Canada, where midwifery received its statutory recognition in 1993, there has been great care to ensure that the status of midwifery is given recognition by demonstrating the academic underpinning of that regulated role.

There are books, some of them well known medical texts, which contain learned information and scientific knowledge relating to the anatomy and physiology of obstetrics. Other textbooks, written by midwives or through collaborative writing between midwives and doctors, contain selected knowledge of the biological and behavioural sciences as these relate to the aspects of maternity care on which the book is focused. Both these forms of text play their part in the education of midwives.

In 1999, following the International Confederation of Midwives Congress in Manilla, there was an agreement by the participating countries on midwifery competencies. These have as their basis the World Health Organization Definition of the Midwife. The delivery of midwifery programmes of education in all countries which would aspire to enable their midwives to achieve the competencies must include levels of theoretical knowledge which inform their development.

There have been many references to the problems caused by the theory–practice divide, of which students and their mentors become aware during educational programmes. There are fewer references to how the problem can be addressed, or what solutions are emerging in educational processes which reduce the related tensions between those who, on the one hand, manage education and, on the other, manage midwifery care provision.

Increasingly, midwife teachers and their colleagues who work as clinically based midwives will work in multidisciplinary and multiprofessional teams. The expectation of such collaboration is in the best interests of women and their families and should form the basis of educational approaches. Core curricula for education of healthcare professionals, with a common understanding of that knowledge which must underpin each professional contribution to care of patients, is fundamental to achieving shared values and client-focused practice. This may not be achieved in many countries for many decades. However, it helps if, at the least, midwives, obstetricians and all professionals contributing to women's experience during childbearing, with the lasting impact this experience has on their lives, have a sound, common understanding of its scientific basis. Conception, fetal development, maternal changes throughout the time of pregnancy, birth and the postnatal period are complex processes. Optimal care of mothers and their babies will be possible only where a firm grounding in the knowledge of those complex processes is gained, and is utilized effectively to inform sensitive and safe practice. Midwives, more so than any other professionals involved in the care of women in childbearing, have a continuing and influential part to play in achieving woman-centred optimal care and in ensuring that the memory women carry with them beyond their experience of childbirth is of a positive nature.

The production of this book is welcome in that the authors, through collaboration, bring together in a meaningful and applied way the art of midwifery care, and the science of reproduction and birth. The scientific facts are clearly described and made relevant to clinical scenarios in a way which should help readers understand and aid their recall in practice. In the World Health Organization's recent agenda, health for all is a target to be achieved in the early years of the new millennium. In the United Kingdom, there is a current emphasis on reducing health inequality, increasing health awareness and on increasing public empowerment, information and involvement in decisions about care. The midwife in any country can have a significant influence on the health of the current and future generation. As such, midwives should be seen as key players in the development and delivery of effective maternity care. Through a sound and continually developing knowledge base, with understanding of the way this can positively impact on practice, midwives can contribute to the reality of safe motherhood and health for all. This book will be a valuable aid to students preparing to become midwives, and to registered midwives wishing to further their knowledge and understanding wherever, and in whatever culture, they practice.

Meryl Thomas

# Preface

Many of the most magical aspects of physiology are associated with reproduction, from before conception, through fetal development and maternal responses to the growing fetus, to the signalling and progression of labour, continued development of the neonate and the mother's subsequent return to fertility. Reproductive physiology is also a fast-moving field as recent advances in fertility treatment, postnatal care of premature infants and the implications of HIV make evident.

Midwives are expected to understand in depth the science underpinning midwifery practice but have often had little background in this exciting field. Midwives also often find themselves to be bombarded with questions from interested and fascinated parents. This book aims to support students and practising midwives wanting more detailed scientific knowledge that can be applied within the practice setting.

The book provides a thorough review of anatomy and physiology applicable to midwifery from first principles through to current research. It acknowledges the importance of the research basis and aims to integrate theory and practice.

The chapters are organized so learning objectives lead into the body of the chapter. Case studies provide the reader with the opportunity to reflect on the implications for practice. Wherever possible, information is provided as illustrations. At the end of each chapter, key points are provided and the applications of the scientific content to practice are summarized. Each chapter is comprehensively referenced and has a list of annotated recommendations for further reading.

Chapter 1 begins by introducing the reader to the basic unit of structure, the cell, and describes the relationship between cellular structure and function. It provides an introduction to the major tissue types and physiological systems found within the body and focuses on how the regulation and maintenance of homeostatic systems are achieved.

Chapter 2 focuses on the reproductive and urinary systems of the human. The basic anatomy and physiology of the urinary system are explored in the first part of this chapter. The female reproductive tract and the organs associated with it are then described, relating both their structure and function specifically to childbirth. The last part of this chapter focuses on the male reproductive organs and the process of spermatogenesis.

Chapter 3 provides an essential foundation for the overall understanding of how human reproduction is achieved, as described in further chapters, by introducing the principles of endocrinology. It describes the different types of hormones, how and where they are produced, and their modes of action.

Chapter 4 covers the endocrine control and regulation of reproductive cycles. Ovarian function and follicular development lead on to gamete formation within the female and consideration is given to why this is so dramatically different to spermatogenesis within the male. One of the essential roles of reproductive cycles is that the coordination of oogenesis and the cyclical changes within the endometrium occur to optimize fertilization and implantation. Thus the menstrual cycle is described in depth within this chapter.

Chapter 5 integrates the concepts introduced in the first four chapters by focusing on how sexual differentiation is achieved and the biological basis for a difference in reproductive physiology and behaviour. This chapter leads on to the next two chapters. Chapter 6 describes how sexual bimorphism facilitates fertilisation, implantation of the developing zygote and the maternal physiological response towards successful fertilization and implantation. Chapter 7 introduces the science of genetics, highlighting an essential component of the human reproductive strategy: that of how genetic mixing and thus variation within the species is achieved. An introduction to the aetiology and types of genetic disease and how these may be detected within the clinical situation is also included.

Chapter 8 presents the development and function of the placenta and its interaction with maternal physiology. Following this, Chapter 9 provides a comprehensive overview of the development of the embryo and the factors that promote and influence fetal growth.

Chapter 10 brings the reader back to maternal physiology by introducing and giving an overview of immunological issues and principles related to pregnancy. The maternal acceptance of the fetus and its implications are discussed, as are the effects of pregnancy upon the maternal immune system. A section is included on the interaction of the maternal and fetal immune systems, using some clinical conditions as examples of these interactions. The neonate's vulnerability to infection is described in relation to midwifery care. Finally, the specific effects of the HIV virus in pregnancy are considered.

One of the most striking aspects of reproductive physiology is the physiological changes that occur within the pregnant female. Chapter 11 explores why these changes occur and how they are achieved in order to facilitate an optimal outcome of pregnancy. Following on from this, Chapter 12 explores how maternal nutrition and health may also impact upon pregnancy outcomes not only for the mother but also the fetus, both *in utero* and potentially throughout life.

Chapter 13 specifically explores the physiology of parturition and how the maternal physiology changes to facilitate this. Current theories and evidence relating to the timing and initiation of labour in humans are discussed. An overview is provided of pain physiology related to labour and how this is affected by pain-relieving interventions. This chapter includes a section that explores the effects of labour upon the fetal physiology.

Following birth, the physiological changes that occur during pregnancy are dramatically and efficiently reversed and so the puerperium is the subject of Chapter 14. Alongside the maternal postnatal changes, the neonate has to quickly adapt to life outside the womb and so Chapter 15 focuses on the transition to neonatal life.

The final chapter, Chapter 16, highlights the physiology of lactation and how this meets the unique requirements of the neonate not only from a nutritional perspective but from an immunological basis and a developmental basis as well. It is essential that midwives understand the physiological aspects of lactation in order to promote breastfeeding as the evidence is overwhelming that successful breastfeeding can positively influence the health and well-being of the infant for the rest of its life.

The demand for this book came primarily from our students, including pre-registration students, midwives returning to practice and those following post-registration study. Enthusiastic questions, demands for explanation and an evident relish of understanding the theory related to practice stimulated the birth and development of the book. We hope that readers will continue to enquire about and enjoy this exciting field.

Jane Coad
Guildford and Chertsey 2001 Melvyn Dunstall

# Acknowledgements

Over the last three years, if it had not been for the support of our families, we would never have persevered and completed this book and so it is to them that we are particularly indebted. We would also like to thank all of our colleagues, both at the European Institute for Health and Medical Sciences and at Ashford and St Peter's Hospitals NHS Trust, for their help, support and guidance throughout the production of this book. We would especially like to thank our students who asked the questions and demanded answers. Many of these students have used the material in developing their understanding of reproductive physiology in the context of midwifery practice and we have used their feedback in shaping the presentation and layout of the book.

We owe much to the production team at Harcourt Health Sciences, especially Karen Gilmour and Gail Murray for their constant encouragement and patience in enabling us to complete the project.

# List of abbreviations

**A-II** angiotensin-II
**AA** arachidonic acid
**ABP** androgen-binding protein
**ACTH** adrenocorticotrophic hormone (corticotrophin)
**ADH** antidiuretic hormone
**AFP** alpha fetoprotein
**ANP** atrial natriuretic peptide
**APC** antigen-presenting cell
**ARM** artificial rupture of the membranes
**ATP** adenosine triphosphate
**AV** arteriovenous
**BAT** brown adipose tissue
**BMI** body mass index
**BPD** biparietal diameter
**2,3-BPG** 2,3-bisphosphoglycerate
**cAMP** cyclic adenosine monophosphate
**CCT** controlled cord traction
**CD** cluster of differentiation
**CDH** congenital dislocation of the hips
**CMV** cytomegalovirus
**CNS** central nervous system
**COC** combined oral contraceptive
**CRH** corticotrophin-releasing hormone
**CRH-BP** corticotrophin-releasing hormone-binding protein
**CRL** crown–rump length
**CVS** chorionic villus sampling
**D&C** dilatation and curettage
**DHA** docosahexaenoic acid
**DHEAS** dehydroepiandrosterone sulphate
**5α-DHT** 5α-dihydrotestosterone
**DIC** disseminated intravascular coagulation
**DNA** deoxyribonucleic acid
**DOC** deoxycorticosterone
**2,3-DPG** 2,3-diphosphoglycerate
**DVT** deep vein thrombosis
**$E_1$** oestrone
**$E_2$** oestradiol-17β
**$E_3$** oestriol
**ED-PAF** embryo-derived platelet-activating factor
**EDRF** endothelium-derived relaxing factor
**EGF** epidermal growth factor
**EIPS** endogenous inhibitors of prostaglandin synthesis
**EPF** early pregnancy factor
**ER** endoplasmic reticulum
**ERPC** evacuation of retained products of conception
**FBM** fetal breathing movement
**FHR** fetal heart rate
**FHV** fetal heart variability
**FIL** factor inhibiting lactation
**FISH** fluorescent in-situ hybridization
**FSH** follicle-stimulating hormone
**GALT** gut-associated lymphoid tissue
**GFR** glomerular filtration rate
**GH** growth hormone
**GIFT** gamete intrafallopian transfer
**GL** greatest length
**GLUT** glucose-transport protein
**GnRH** gonadotrophin-releasing hormone
**Hb** haemoglobin
**hCG** human chorionic gonadotrophin
**HDL** high-density lipoprotein
**HDNB** haemorrhagic disease of the newborn
**HELLP** haemolysis, elevated liver enzymes and low platelet counts
**HIV** human immunosuppressant virus
**HLA** human leukocyte antigen
**hMG** human menopausal gonadotrophin
**hPL** human placental lactogen
**ICSI** intracytoplasmic sperm injection
**IDDM** insulin-dependent diabetes mellitus
**Ig** immunoglobulin
**IGF** insulin-like growth factor
**IGF-BP** insulin-like growth factor binding protein
**IL** interleukin
**IUGR** intrauterine growth retardation
**IVF** in vitro fertilization
**LDL** low-density lipoprotein
**LH** luteinizing hormone
**LHRH** luteinizing hormone releasing hormone
**LIF** leukaemia-inhibiting factor
**LSCS** lower-segment caesarean section
**LUS** lower uterine segment
**MCV** mean blood cell volume
**MHC** major histocompatibility complex
**MIH** Müllerian-inhibiting hormone

**MLCK** myosin light-chain kinase
**MPF** M-phase-promoting factor
**MRSA** methicillin-resistant *Staphylococcus aureus*
**MSAFP** maternal serum alpha fetoprotein
**MSH** melanocyte-stimulating hormone
**NIDDM** non-insulin-dependent diabetes mellitus
**NK** natural killer
**NO** nitrous oxide
**NPN** non-protein nitrogen
**NPU** net protein utilization
**NPY** neuropeptide Y
**NSAID** non-steroidal anti-inflammatory drug
**NST** non-shivering thermogenesis
**NT** nuchal translucency
**NTD** neural tube defect
**NVP** nausea and vomiting in pregnancy
**17α-OHP** 17α-hydroxyprogesterone
**PAPP-A** pregnancy-associated plasma protein A
**PCOS** polycystic ovary syndrome
**PCR** polymerase chain reaction
**PE** pulmonary embolism
**PG** prostaglandin
**PKU** phenylketonuria
**$PLA_2$** phospholipase $A_2$
**PPH** postpartum haemorrhage
**PRL** prolactin
**PROM** premature rupture of the membranes
**RAS** renin–angiotensin system
**RBC** red blood cell
**RDS** respiratory distress syndrome
**REM** rapid eye movement
**RER** rough endoplasmic reticulum
**m/r/tRNA** messenger/ribosomal/transfer ribonucleic acid
**RSA** recurrent spontaneous abortion
**SAN** sinoatrial node
**SER** smooth endoplasmic reticulum
**SGA** small for gestational age
**SLE** systemic lupus erythematosus
**TBP** thyroid-binding protein
**TNF** tumour necrosis factor
**TSH** thyroid-stimulating hormone
**Tx $A_2$** thromboxane $A_2$
**U-LGL** uterine large granular leukocytes
**UTI** urinary tract infection
**VIP** vasoactive intestinal peptide
**VLDL** very-low-density lipoprotein
**ZIFT** zygote intrafallopian transfer

# 1 Introduction to physiology

**Learning objectives**

- To describe the structure of a typical cell and the role of its organelles.
- To appreciate how cell differentiation and organization permit physiological function.
- To recognize features of different tissue types that facilitate their function and characteristics.
- To describe the control of provision of oxygen and nutrients to cells.
- To identify key features of physiological control mechanisms.
- To describe the principles and components of a homeostatic system.
- To review the physiological systems involved in maintaining homeostasis.

## Introduction

Physiology explores how living organisms are able to function in order to survive and reproduce. This book explores reproductive function and how it is achieved within human beings. This chapter aims to provide an illustrated introduction to, and an overview of, some of the basic physiological concepts referred to and developed in subsequent chapters with specific references to reproduction. (If more detail is required, readers are recommended to look at the list of further reading at the end of the chapter.)

## The cell

The cell is the basic unit of structure within all multicellular organisms. The evolution of multicellular organisms has led to the differentiation of cells, which means that different cells have evolved to perform specific functions and processes that contribute to the well-being of the organism as a whole. Differentiated cells form tissues, which combine with other tissues to form organs, which are linked together in physiological systems (Fig. 1.1). However, although cells can be highly specialized they all share common features of the single cellular organisms from which we evolved. A typical human cell is about 10 μm in diameter. The largest human cell is the oocyte (see Ch. 6); it can just be seen with the naked eye. The follicular cells surrounding it are a more typical human cell size. The sperm cell is one of the smallest human cells. Smaller cells and organelles can be visualized by light and electron microscopy.

### *Cell structure*

Most cells contain cytoplasm and are bound by a plasma membrane. Within them are various structures, called organelles (see Table 1.1), and a specialized part of the cell, called the nucleus (Fig. 1.2). The fluid surrounding the organelles is called cytosol.

## Cells and tissues

Although about 200 types of cells with different structures can be identified within the body, cells can be grouped together in functional categories (Table 1.2). The study of the physical characteristics of cells is called histology (see Box 1.1).

### *Epithelial tissue*

Epithelial cells line the internal and external surfaces of the body organs (Fig. 1.3). They are relatively

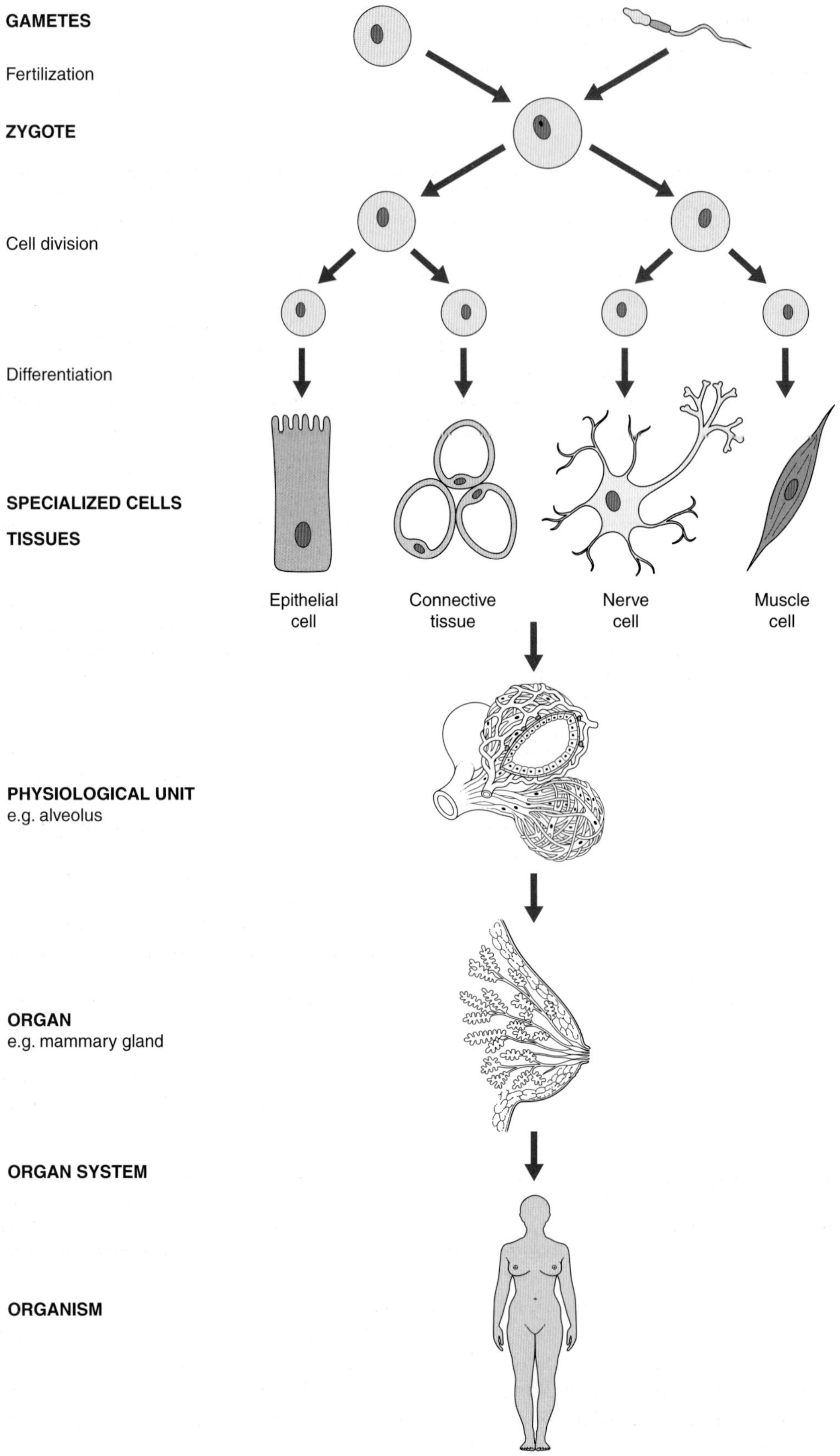

**GAMETES**

Fertilization

**ZYGOTE**

Cell division

Differentiation

**SPECIALIZED CELLS**

**TISSUES**

Epithelial cell

Connective tissue

Nerve cell

Muscle cell

**PHYSIOLOGICAL UNIT**
e.g. alveolus

**ORGAN**
e.g. mammary gland

**ORGAN SYSTEM**

**ORGANISM**

**Fig. 1.1** *Physiological systems: levels of organization of cells, tissues, organs and physiological systems, using breast tissue as an example.*

**Table 1.1** *Cell components*

| Cell component | Structure | Function |
|---|---|---|
| Cell membrane | The cell membrane is composed of a phospholipid bilayer embedded with various protein structures such as hormone receptors, ion channels and antigen markers | The membrane acts as a differential permeable membrane between the cell and its immediate environment |
| The nucleus | The nucleus is bound by a membrane, similar to the plasma membrane of the cell; this contains openings referred to as nuclear pores, which allow the movement of substances in and out of the nucleus | The nucleus contains deoxyribonucleic acid (DNA), the genetic instruction for the organism. Most of the time, the DNA is organized as chromatin threads; these condense into chromosomes prior to cell division. The nucleus stores and replicates DNA, which is expressed to synthesize proteins via a second type of nucleic acid, ribonucleic acid (RNA). These proteins determine the structure and function of the cell |
| Endoplasmic reticulum | This is a system of membranes, enclosing a space, which is continuous with the nuclear membrane. Endoplasmic reticulum (ER) exists as rough (granular) endoplasmic reticulum (RER) and smooth (agranular) endoplasmic reticulum (SER) | RER appears rough because of the attached ribosomes. RER is involved in protein packaging. SER is involved in lipid and steroid synthesis and the regulation of intracellular calcium levels |
| Mitochondria | Spherical or elongated rod-like structures surrounded by a folded inner membrane and a smooth outer membrane. There are more mitochondria in cells that are metabolically active and have a high energy requirement | Chemical processes involved in the formation of adenosine triphosphate (ATP). The cristae (inner membrane folds) are the site of oxidative phosphorylation and the electron transfer chain of aerobic respiration. Krebs' (tricárboxylic acid or TCA) cycle and the oxidation of fatty acids take place within the matrix. Mitochondria contain mitochondrial DNA, which is maternally inherited and contains the genes for mitochondrial proteins |
| Golgi apparatus (complex) | A series of flattened curved membranous sacs | Modifies proteins from the RER and sorts them into secretory vesicles |
| Lysosomes | Spherical or oval organelles enclosed by a single membrane | Enclose acidic fluid containing digestive enzymes which act as a 'cellular stomach' breaking down cellular debris |
| Peroxisomes | Similar structure to lysosomes | Destroy reactive oxygen species and protect cell |
| Cytoskeleton | Filamentous network | Involved in maintaining cell shape and motility |

undifferentiated and tend to undergo frequent mitotic divisions (see Ch. 7). This is because they often are exposed to wear and tear and so replacement epithelial cells are generated from a basal layer where cell division takes place. Epithelial cells form a barrier, which allows secretion and absorption of substances from one compartment to another. The skin is a specialized epithelial layer; the basal layer produces cells that are enriched with the protein keratin. The outer layers of skin cells are dead but the keratinized cells provide the barrier function of the skin.

Fig. 1.2 *A typical cell.*

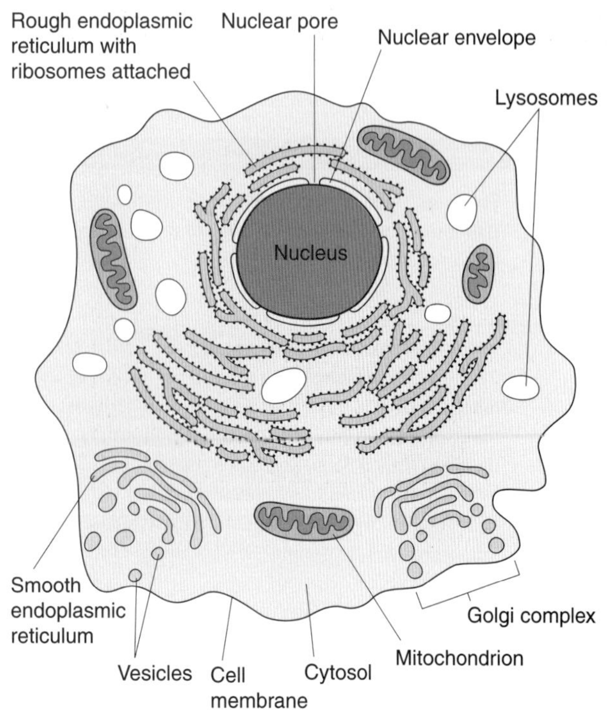


**Box 1.1**

**Histology**

The study of tissue structure is described as histology. The functions of tissues are reflected in the microscopic structure of the cells of which the tissue is composed. For example cells that are metabolically active contain many mitochondria, whereas cells that produce hormones or enzymes, for instance, will contain a large proportion of ER. Specific tissues and cellular structures are often identified by the application of various chemicals that stain particular tissues. Histology is important in diagnosing cancer as the cancerous tissue often has histological characteristics different from those of the tissue in which the cancer has developed. Malignant cancerous tumours have highly differentiated cells, whereas benign tumours have undifferentiated cells, which may closely resemble the cells of the tissue from which they arose.

## *Muscle tissue*

Muscle cells contain contractile elements so the cells can generate the mechanical force required for movement (Fig. 1.4). Skeletal muscle may be attached to bones and controls movement of the skeleton. Skeletal muscle can also be attached to the skin, for instance

Table 1.2 ***Functional classification of cells***

| Cell group | Epithelial cells | Support cells | Contractile cells | Nerve cells | Germ cells | Blood cells | Immune cells | Hormone-secreting cells |
|---|---|---|---|---|---|---|---|---|
| Example | Lining gut and blood vessels Covering skin | Fibrous support tissue, cartilage, bone | Muscle | Brain | Spermatozoa Ova | Circulating 1. red cells 2. white cells 3. platelets | Lymphoid tissues, nodes and spleen | Islets, thyroid, adrenal |
| Function | Barrier; absorption; secretion | Organize and maintain body structure | Movement | Direct cell communication | Reproduction | 1. Oxygen transport 2. Defence | Defence | Indirect cell communication |
| Special features | Tightly bound together by cell junctions | Produce and interact with extracellular matrix material | Contractile proteins | Release chemical messengers directly on to other cells | Haploid (i.e. half-normal chromosome number) | 1. Proteins bind oxygen 2. Proteins destroy bacteria 3. Blood clotting | Recognize and destroy foreign material | Secrete chemical messengers into blood |

**Fig. 1.3** *Types of epithelial cell: A squamous epithelium provides a smooth lining of blood vessels (endothelium, alveoli of lung and glomeruli of kidney); B cuboidal epithelium is often found on absorptive surfaces such as in kidney tubules; C columnar epithelium is often associated with secretory and absorptive tissues and may have microvilli, as in the gut; it may also be ciliated, as in the upper airways. (Reproduced with permission from Brooker 1998.)*

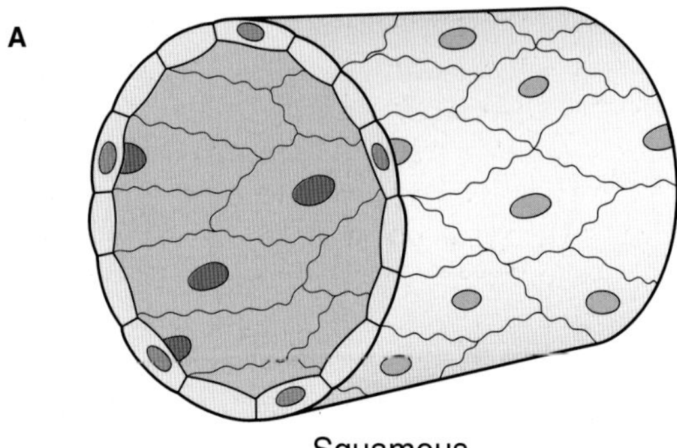


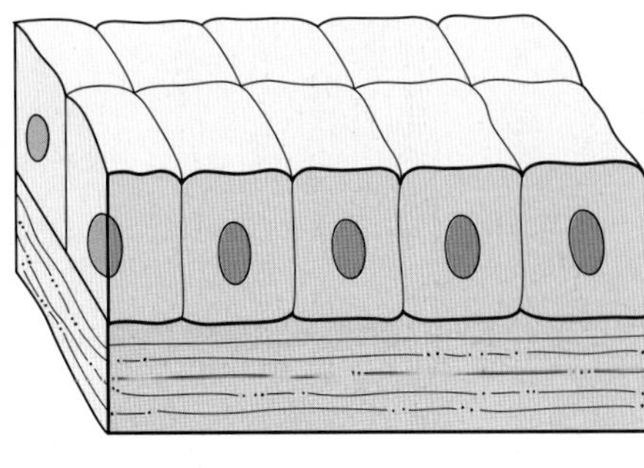


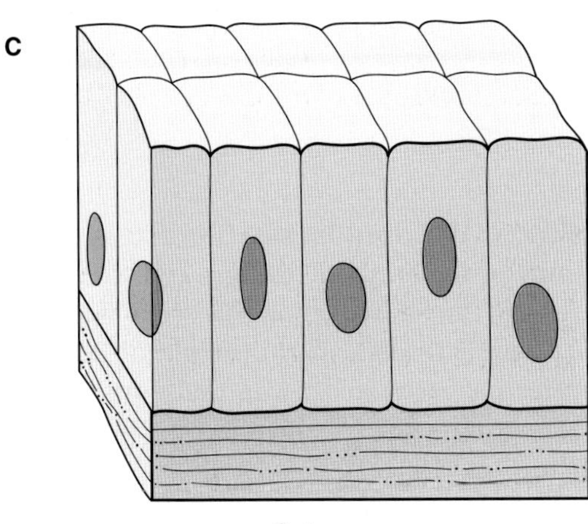


the muscles of the face involved with expression. Contraction of skeletal muscle is frequently under voluntary or conscious control. Skeletal muscle is often described as 'striated' because of the striped appearance of the muscle observed under the light microscope.

Smooth muscle is usually under involuntary control (meaning there is no conscious awareness of the control) and surrounds many of the 'tubes' in the body, maintaining the function of several body systems. Blood pressure is maintained by the contraction of a smooth muscle layer in the walls of the blood

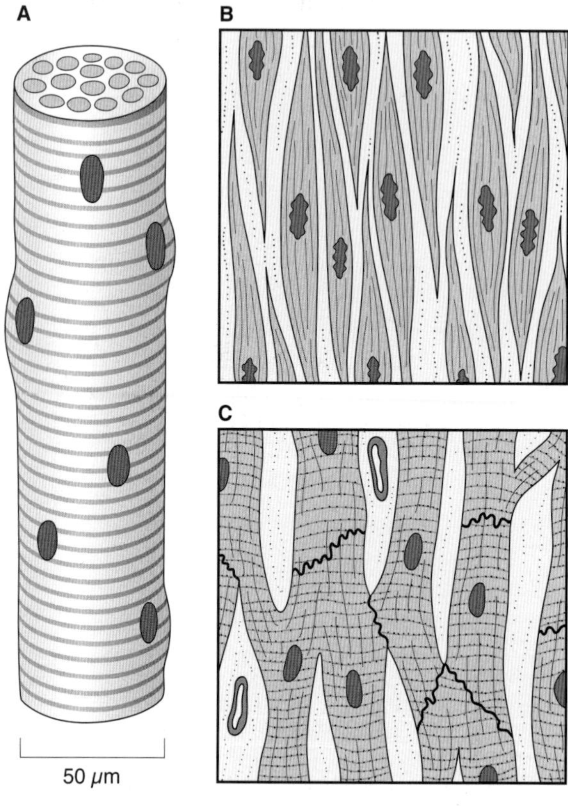


**Fig. 1.4** *Muscle: A skeletal muscle; B smooth muscle; C cardiac muscle. (Adapted with permission from Brooker 1998.)*

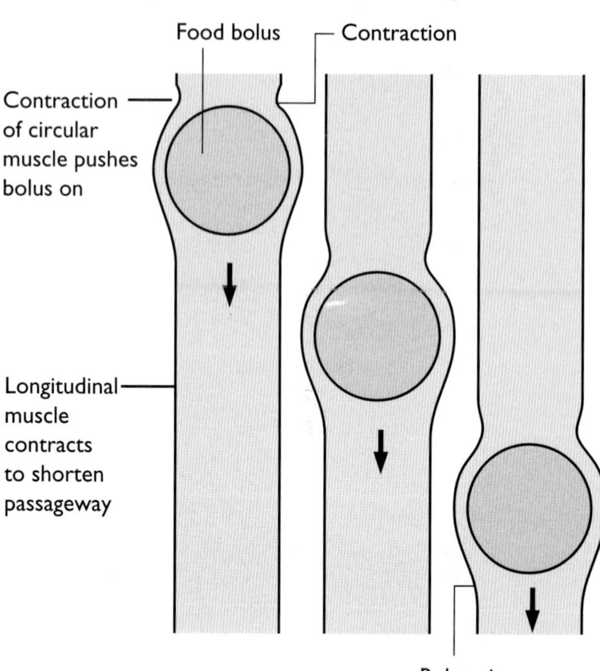


**Fig. 1.5** *Peristaltic waves: peristalsis is achieved through the interaction of both longitudinal and circular smooth muscle fibres found in vessels with patent lumen. The peristaltic waves are responsible for (usually) unidirectional movement of the contents within the lumen. (Reproduced with permission from Brooker 1998.)*

vessels. If the smooth muscle constricts, described as 'vasoconstriction', the internal lumen of the vessel will decrease and blood pressure will increase. 'Vasodilatation' is the opposite condition: the smooth muscle relaxes and the lumen diameter increases so blood pressure falls. Organized synchronized waves of smooth muscle contraction, for instance in the gut, renal system and uterine tubes, generate peristaltic waves; these produce unidirectional movement of the contents within the lumen of the tube (Fig. 1.5).

## Connective tissue

Connective tissue functions to connect, anchor and support body structures (Fig. 1.6). Connective tissue cells often produce an extracellular matrix composed of proteins in a ground substance of sugars, proteins and minerals. Bone is a type of connective tissue, whereas collagen is an example of an extracellular matrix. Adipose tissue is composed of specialized cells that store fat for future energy requirements. Adipose tissue also acts as an insulating layer to conserve body heat loss and so contributes to the maintenance of the homeothermic status of the organism. Fibrous tissue is an example of dense connective tissue. It is a tough tissue that forms ligaments, tendons and protective membranes.

## Neural tissue

Neurons are cells that are specialized to initiate and conduct electrical signals (Fig. 1.7). Neurons require the presence of other cells called glial cells for nourishment and support. As neurons are so highly specialized, they do not undergo further mitotic divisions once developed. Therefore, in the fetal and early neonatal period, the number of neurons produced far exceeds the level required for normal neurological function. Neurons need regular stimulation if they are to survive and function. Throughout life millions of neurons become dysfunctional and die.

**Fig. 1.6** *Connective tissue: A adipose tissue; B fibrous tissue; C compact bone. (Reproduced with permission from Brooker 1998.)*

A

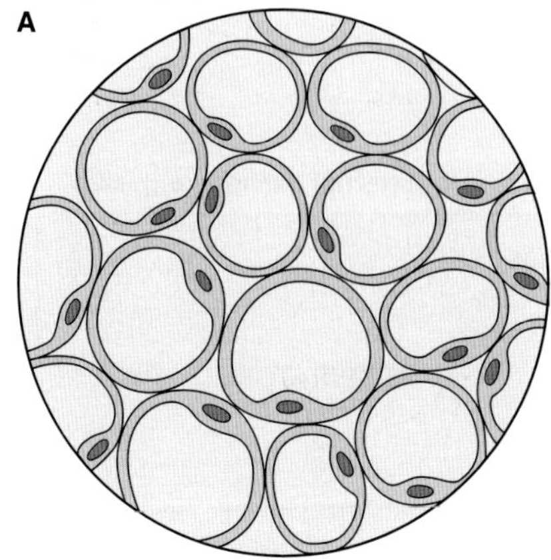

B

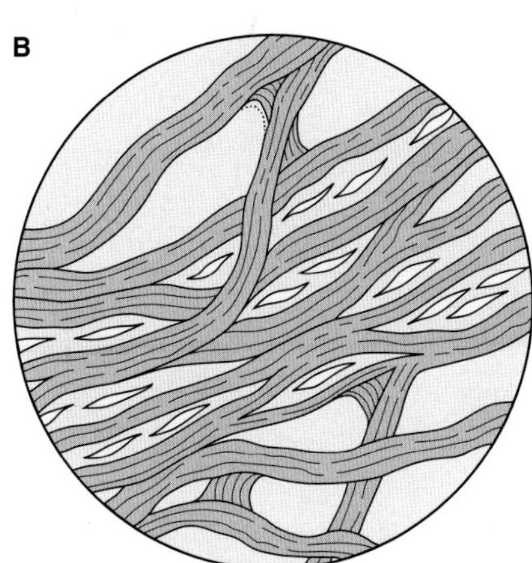

C

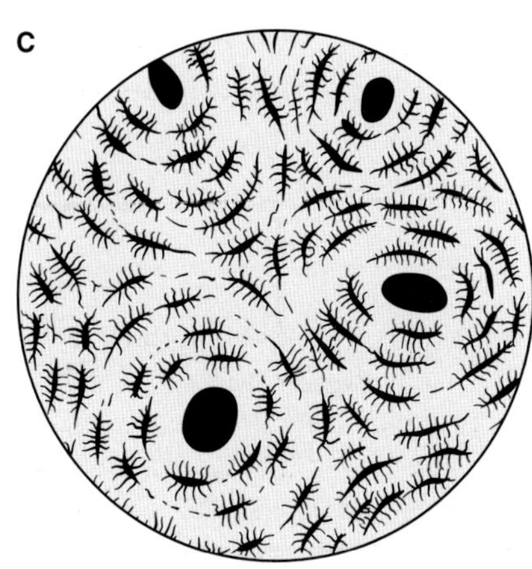

**Fig. 1.7** *Types of neuron: A bipolar; B unipolar; C multipolar.*

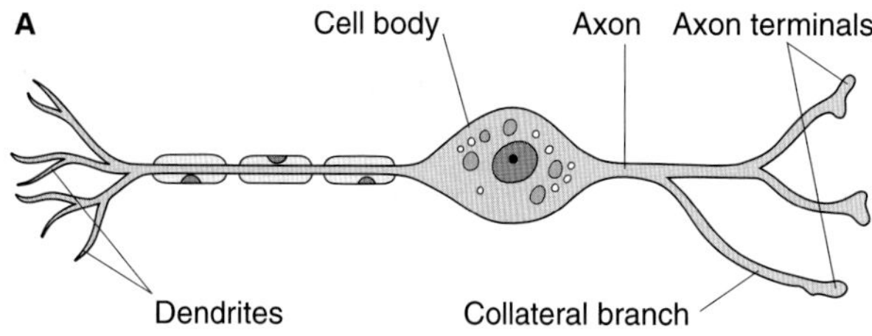


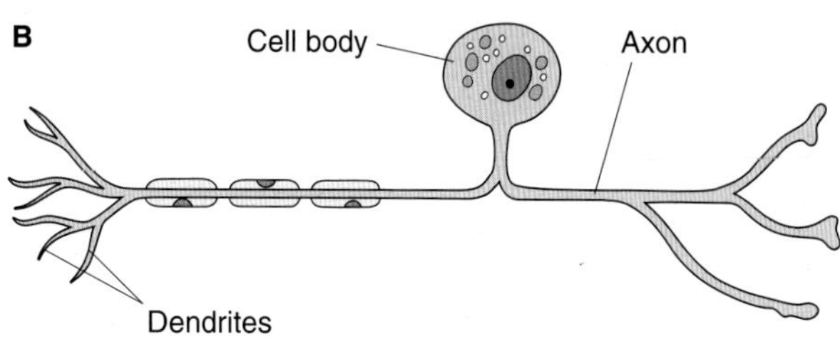


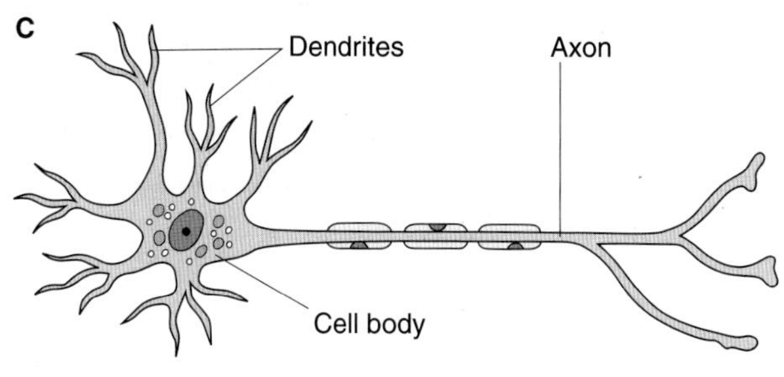


## The organization of the body

The body's organization can be understood by considering each component organ system separately (see below). However, these systems all work together, as a whole. Together the systems provide nutrients and oxygen for the cells and the excretion of waste products (Fig. 1.8). Movement is controlled and the temperature is maintained. Survival until reproduction function is completed has allowed the species to multiply. Cells are bathed in extracellular fluid, which can be divided into the interstitial fluid surrounding the tissue cells and the plasma within the blood vessels.

### *Homeostasis*

Homeostasis is the term used to describe the processes of the various physiological systems that maintain the constancy of the internal environment. Multicellular animals are able to maintain an internal stability that

Fig. 1.8 *Organization of the body.*

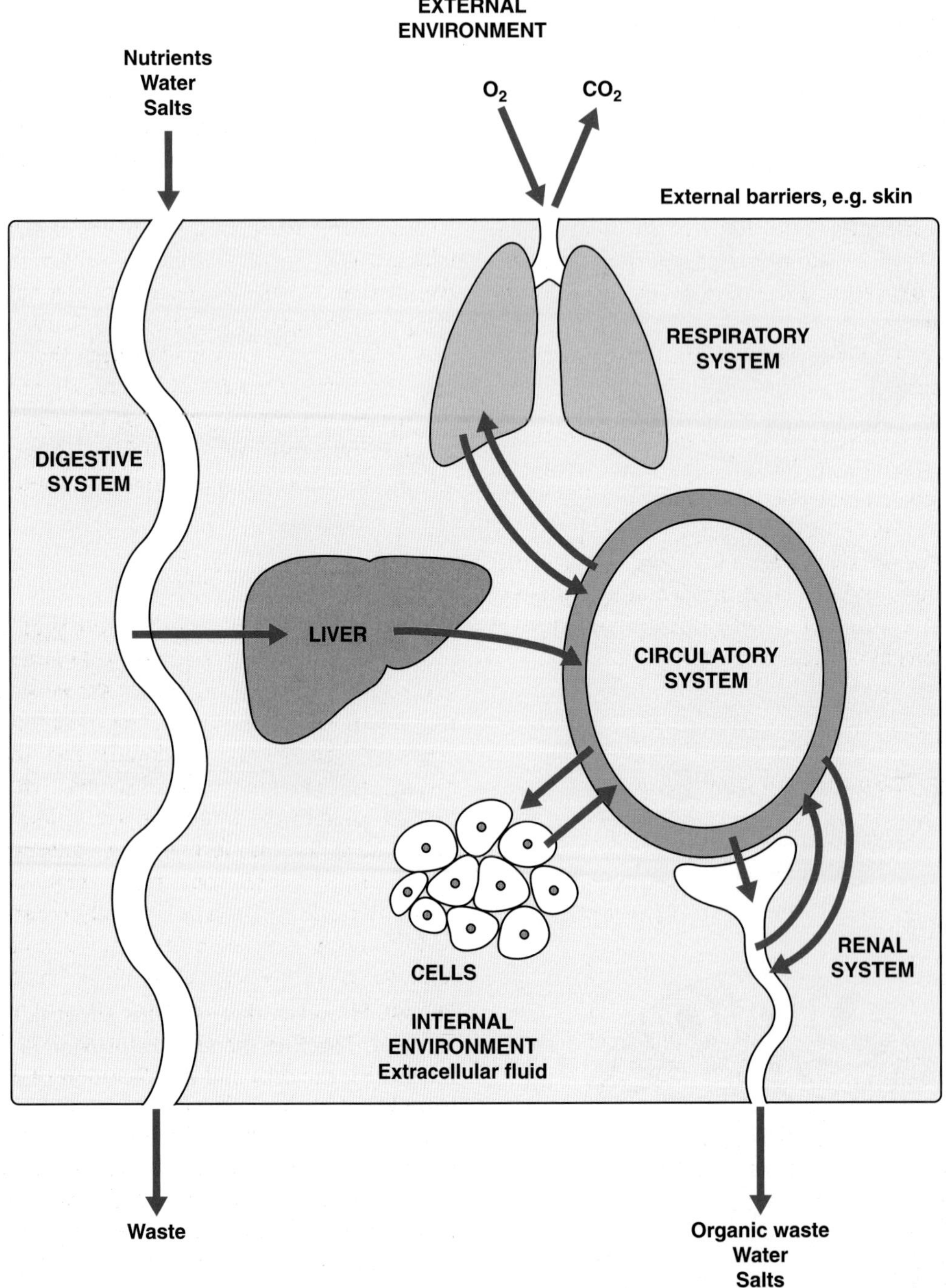


is essential for the optimal functioning of all body systems, whereas simple unicellular organisms tend to inhabit stable environments or have adapted to overcome fluctuations in the environment—for instance by forming spores during dry periods. Unicellular organisms rely on basic nutrients being present in the environment to allow cell growth and reproduction.

The evolution of multicellular organisms and the development of motility meant these animals were able to move within the environment to seek out the conditions that suited them best. Mammals have developed homeostasis to a high degree. Motility, together with the homeostatic challenge of counteracting fluctuations in the external environment, places a huge energy burden upon these individuals. This increased energy requirement is above the basal metabolic rate, which is the rate of energy required to maintain essential functioning only.

Homeostasis can be considered to have three main components:

- chemostasis: the maintenance of electrolytes and pH balance
- haemostasis: the maintenance of an adequate circulatory system facilitating the passage of nutrients and oxygen in and waste products out of the organism
- thermostasis: the maintenance of a constant internal temperature.

Homeostasis is regulated by the nervous system, the endocrine system and behavioural factors that are dependent on conscious or subconscious action by the organism. A homeostatic control system requires the monitoring of a variable, detecting changes and generating responses which will restore the composition of the internal environment (Fig. 1.9). (This type of system, involving a process called negative feedback, is dealt with in more detail under Hormonal regulation in Ch. 3, p. 63.)

**Fig. 1.9** ***The principles of homeostasis.***

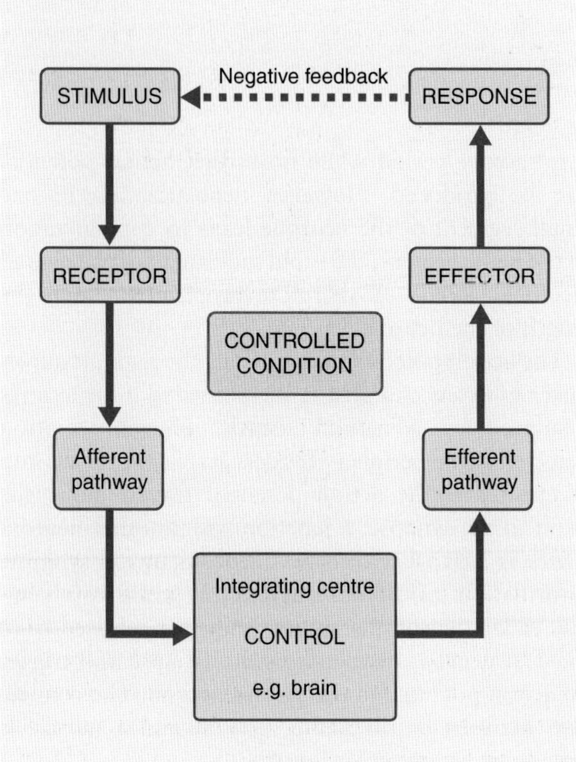


## *Thermoregulation*

Temperature regulation is an example of homeostasis (Fig. 1.10). Enzymes regulating biochemical changes, and physiological functions, have optimal activity within a narrow temperature range. Outside this physiological temperature range, the protein structure of the enzyme begins to denature so the configuration (shape) of the enzyme distorts, which affects its functional activity. A warm-blooded (homeothermic) animal is well prepared to react quickly and efficiently to changes within the environment, unlike a cold-blooded (poikilothermic) animal, which depends upon the ambient temperature of the environment.

## *The nervous system*

The nervous system is an organization of millions of neurons, or nerve cells, and glial cells, which support and regulate the composition of the nervous system. It is composed of the brain, the spinal cord (in the centre of the vertebral column) and the neurons throughout the body. The skull and the vertebral column protect the brain and the spinal cord. The brain and spinal cord form the central nervous system (CNS) and the remainder is the peripheral nervous system (Fig. 1.11). Neurons usually consist of a cell body and dendrites (extensions) and an axon or nerve fibre, which carries information from the cell body to or from the CNS. They are a variety of different sizes; some neurons have axon projections over 1 metre in length. A nerve is a collection of axons running alongside each other over the same distance. A ganglion is a collection of cell bodies of neurons within the peripheral nervous system. Ganglions are located in dorsal (back) or ventral (front) branches of the spinal cord. The spinal cord and spinal nerves are organized on a segmental basis; this corresponds to the embryonic origin of the dermatomes (see Ch. 9). Cranial nerves carry information between the brain and regions of the head. Neurons that carry information towards the brain, entering the dorsal roots of the spinal cord, are sensory or afferent neurons. Neurons carrying information from the CNS to the skeletal muscles, and leaving the spinal cord at the ventral roots, are motor or efferent neurons (Fig. 1.12). Neurons that carry information between a sensory

Fig. 1.10 *Temperature regulation: a homeostatic system in operation.*

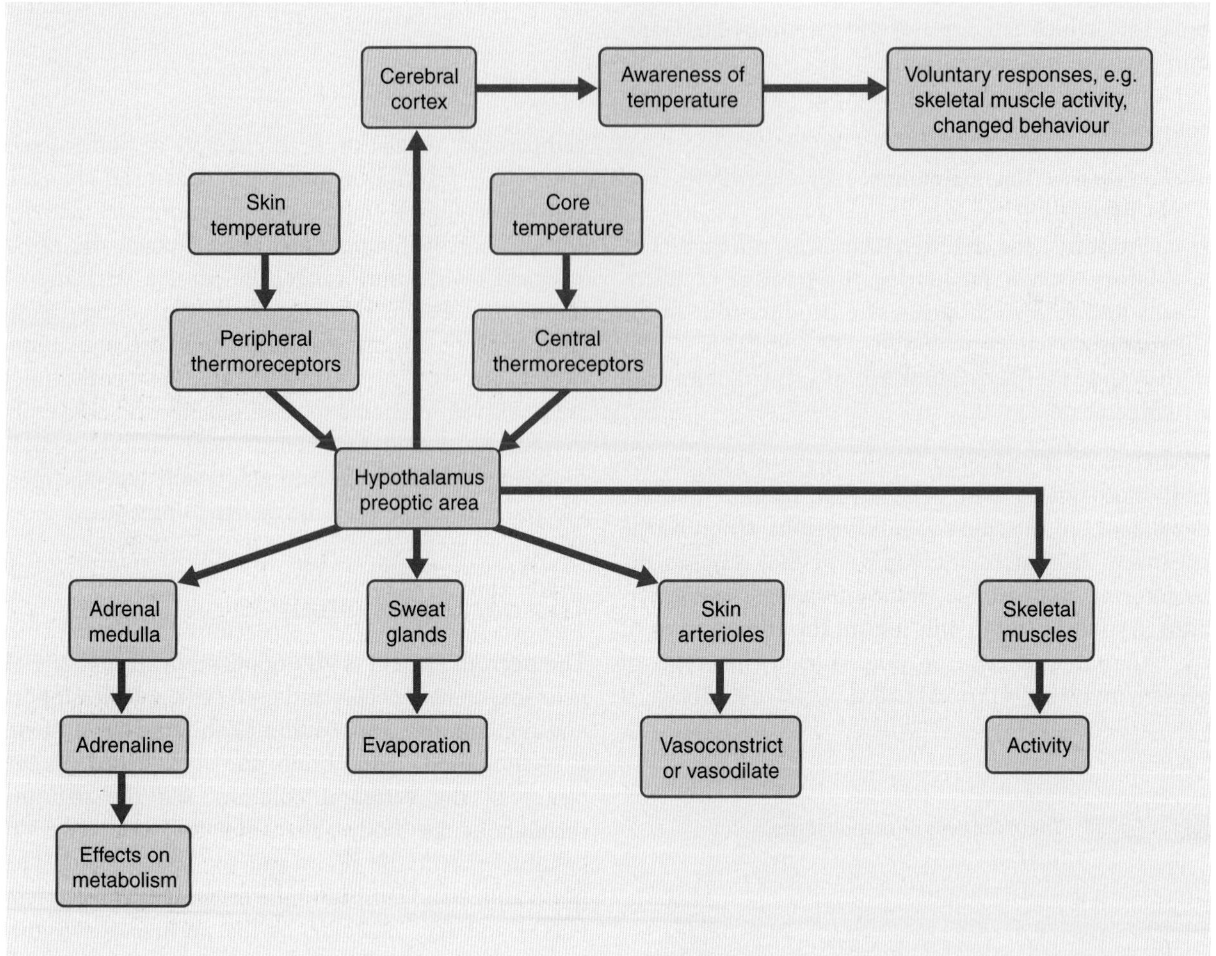


neuron and the CNS (or between the CNS and a motor neuron) are known as interneurons.

## The action potential

Neurons carry information by changing the electrical charge along their length. A change in electrical charge is termed an 'action potential'. When the impulse reaches the axon, specific channels known as 'sodium gates' open allowing the movement of extracellular sodium ions across the concentration gradient into the axon. As the sodium ions carry a positive charge, the inside of the axon becomes electrically positive compared with the outside and the membrane is depolarized. At the height of the action potential (about 1 ms) the sodium channels close and the membrane becomes leaky to potassium ions; these move out of the axon down the electrochemical gradient. The result is restoration of the membrane potential, described as 'repolarization'. That segment of the axon then enters a refractory period when no further action potential can be produced. However, depolarization in one small segment of the neurone leads to depolarization in the next segment; the rapid movement of the altered electrical activity is therefore propagated along the length of the neuron.

The action potential moves along the axon. It moves faster in axons of a greater diameter and if the axon is insulated by a myelin sheath. The information detected at the periphery triggers activity at the neuron receptor and the action potential travels along the axon to the synapse, a junction with another neuron. There is a gap between two neurons at the synapse. Information transmission across this gap is by chemicals called neurotransmitters. These are released from the first neuron, travel across the synapse and trigger an action potential in the second neuron. The connection between a stimulating neuron and a muscle is called a neuromuscular junction.

**Fig. 1.11** *Organization of the nervous system.*

- Nervous system
  - Central nervous system
    - Brain
    - Spinal cord
  - Peripheral nervous system
    - Somatic nervous system (voluntary)
      - Afferent nerves (sensory)
      - Efferent nerves (motor)
    - Enteric nervous system
      - Afferent nerves (gut)
      - Efferent nerves (gut)
    - Visceral nervous system (involuntary)
      - Afferent nerves (sensory)
      - Efferent nerves (motor)
        - Autonomic nervous system
          - Sympathetic
          - Parasympathetic

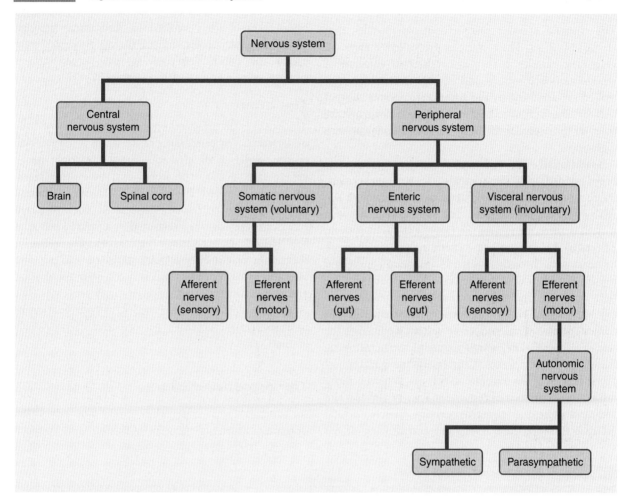

**Fig. 1.12** *Afferent and efferent neurons.*

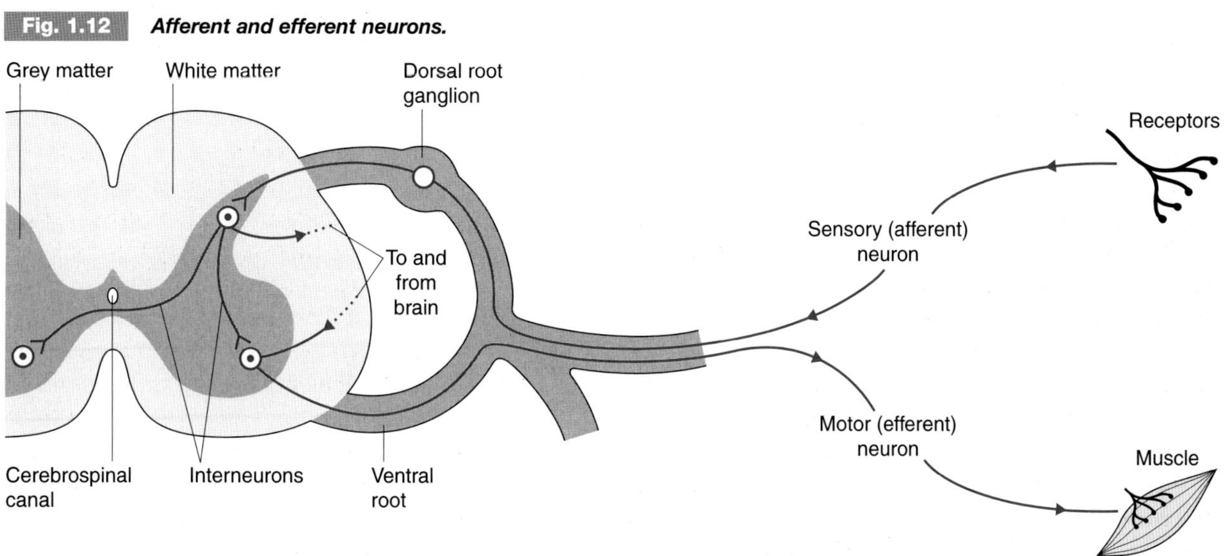

### The somatic and autonomic nervous systems

The somatic nervous system controls muscles that change position. These muscles are called skeletal or voluntary muscles as they are controlled voluntarily, whereas smooth muscle and cardiac muscle are controlled involuntarily by the autonomic nervous system (ANS). The autonomic nervous system controls the internal functions of the body such as circulation and digestion.

Traditionally the autonomic nervous system has been divided into the sympathetic and parasympathetic systems (Table 1.3); these two branches of the ANS exert opposite effects. The sympathetic nervous system is often known as the fear–fight–flight system. Effects of the sympathetic system include an increase in heart rate, bronchial dilation, increase in skeletal muscle blood flow and other responses that facilitate fight or escape and heightened awareness to threatening situations. The sympathetic system operates in conjunction with the endocrine system facilitating the release of adrenaline, which augments the manifesting fear–fight–flight reflexes. Conversely, the parasympathetic branch of the autonomic nervous system is more influential in periods of rest and inactivity and favours rest and increased digestive activity. Effects include increase in blood flow to the gut and slowing of the heart rate. In the autonomic nervous system, two neurons carry information from the CNS to the target organ. These are described as autonomic ganglia. There is a further division of the autonomic system called the enteric nervous system, which affects smooth muscle and secretion in the gut.

### The brain

The brain is the most complex organ and is not fully understood. The outer layer of the brain is the cerebral cortex, which is divided into a left and right hemisphere (Fig. 1.13). The fibres that link these hemispheres are called the corpus callosum. Different regions of the cortex are associated with different functions; they can be illustrated in a figure known as the 'sensory homunculus' (Fig. 1.14). The reticular formation is concerned with states of waking and alertness. The hypothalamus is involved in motivation and regulation and integration of many processes. The cerebellum is mainly concerned with coordination of movement and repetitive performance of previously learned tasks.

## *The digestive system*

As animals grew larger they could not rely upon obtaining nutrients through diffusion and random

**Table 1.3** *The autonomic nervous system*

| | Sympathetic division | Parasympathetic division |
|---|---|---|
| Characteristics | Preganglionic outflow originates in thoracolumbar portion of spinal cord | Preganglionic outflow originates in midbrain, hindbrain and sacral portions of spinal cord |
| | Chain of ganglia | Terminal ganglia near or in effector organs |
| | Postganglionic fibres distributed throughout body | Postganglionic fibres mainly associated with head and viscera |
| | Divergence of pathways so system as a whole is usually stimulated. | Little divergence so limited parts of the system are stimulated |
| | 'Fear, fight and flight' | 'Resting and digesting' |
| Examples of effect | Eye: dilation of pupil | Eye: constriction of pupil |
| | Cardiovascular system: increased heart rate and increased strength of myocardial contraction, vasoconstriction of peripheral vessels and increased blood pressure | Cardiovascular system: decreased heart rate and vasodilation of peripheral vessels and decreased blood pressure |
| | Lungs: dilation of bronchioles | Lungs: constriction of bronchioles |
| | Bladder: increased muscle tone | Bladder: increased contraction |
| | Uterus: contraction in pregnant woman; relaxation in non-pregnant woman | |
| | Penis: ejaculation | Penis: vasodilation and erection |

Fig. 1.13 *The brain: an overview of some of the functional areas.*

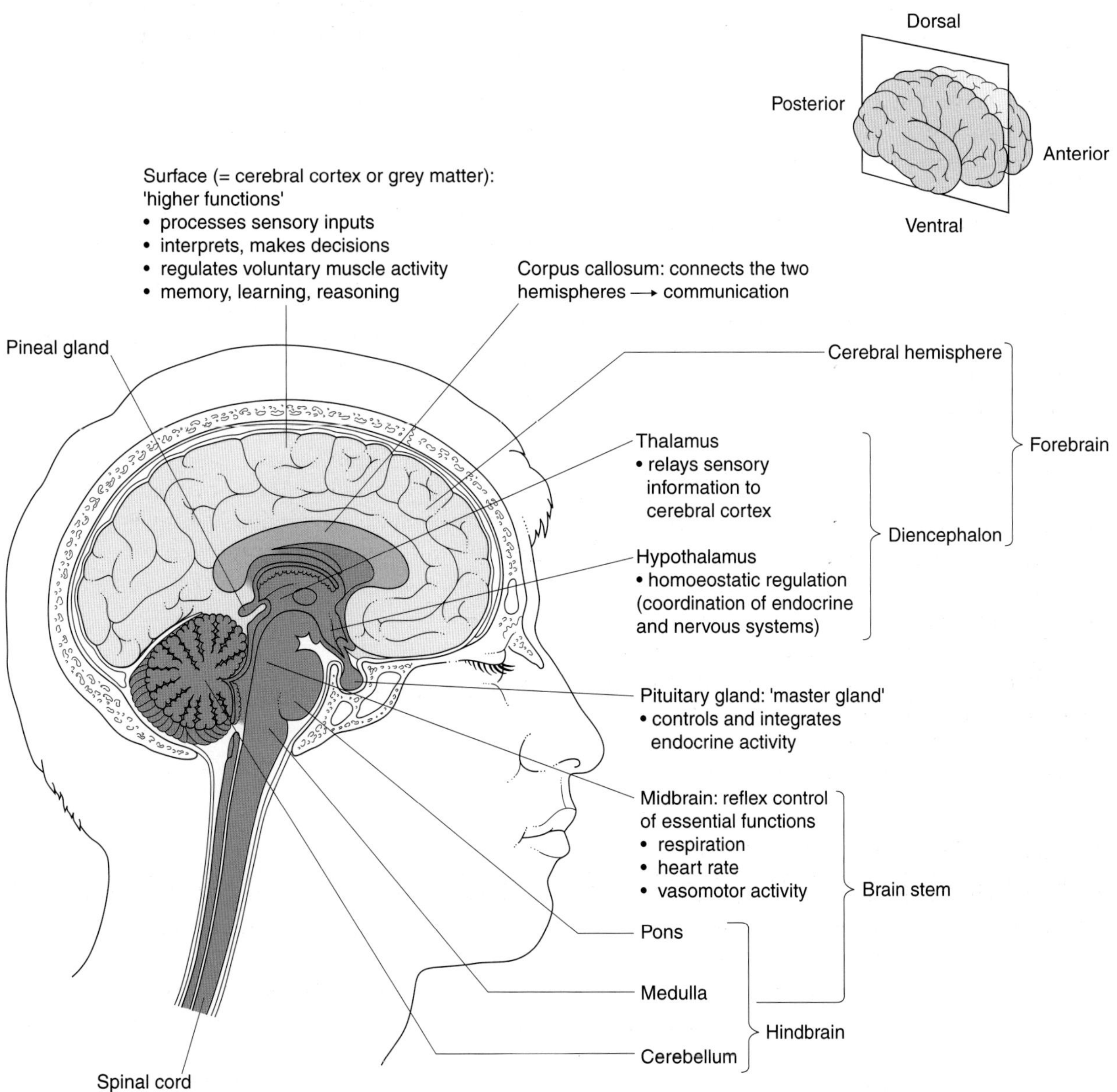


contact with the environment; they became hunters and grazers. As they evolved they became able to feed intermittently. They could do this because they had developed the ability to digest (break down) large organic macromolecules into smaller molecules through the action of digestive enzymes. They were able to store and digest food slowly. Mechanisms for food storage, such as the deposition of fat within adipose tissue, enabled periods of food shortage to be overcome. The ability to synthesize new tissue with energy expenditure is termed anabolism. When tissue is broken down there is a reverse process termed catabolism; this usually results in the production of energy.

The gastrointestinal tract, or gut, is a long tube that runs from mouth to anus (Table 1.4) in which food is digested and absorbed. Food enters the mouth; here it is masticated (mechanically broken down), lubricated and enzymes are added before it is passed through the oesophagus to the stomach. The stomach is a bag-like swollen structure where the first major digestive processes occur. Hydrochloric acid secreted into the

Fig. 1.14 *The 'homunculus': a representation of the (A) motor and (B) sensory areas of the brain illustrating the proportion of brain tissue dedicated to these areas. (Reproduced with permission from Brooker 1998.)*

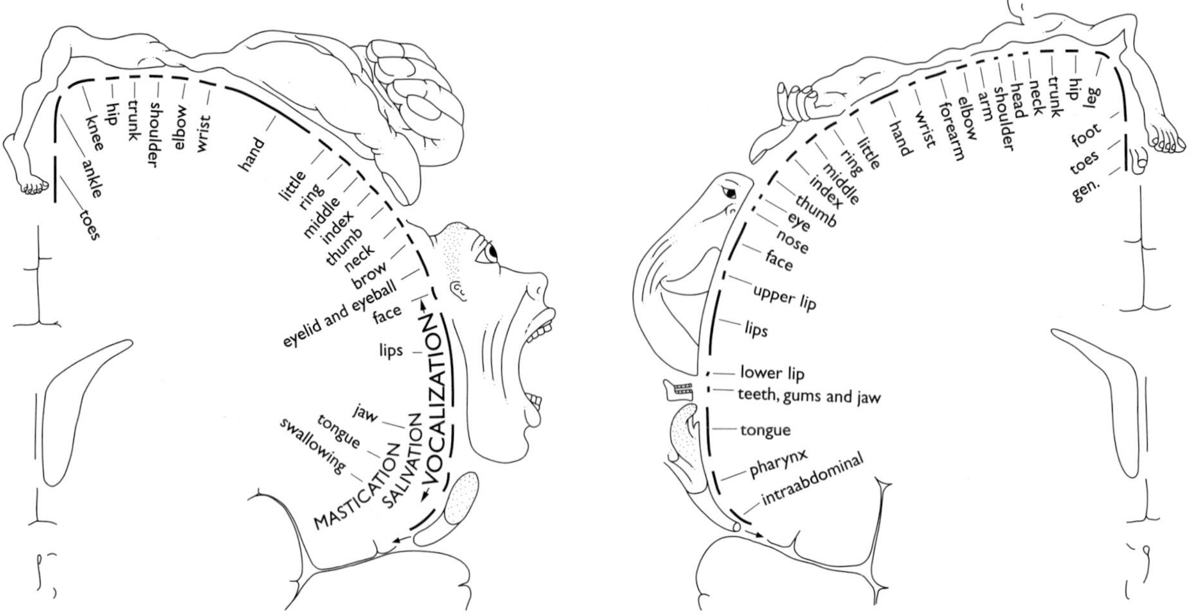


Table 1.4 *The digestive system*

| Region of gastrointestinal system | Main digestive events |
|---|---|
| Mouth | ■ Taste<br>■ Mechanical digestion (chewing, mastication)<br>■ Food moistened and lubricated, to facilitate passage down oesophagus<br>■ Starch digestion (amylase) |
| Oesophagus | ■ Peristalsis enables transfer of food bolus to stomach<br>■ Buccal amylase activity continues |
| Stomach | ■ Stores, mixes, dissolves, releases food<br>■ Hydrochloric acid (HCl)<br>— lowers pH to 2<br>— kills microbes<br>— denatures proteins<br>— converts pepsinogen to pepsin<br>■ Mucus: protects gastric lining<br>■ Pepsin: protein digestion |
| Pancreas | ■ Enzyme production: digestion<br>■ Bicarbonate: neutralizes pH |
| Liver | ■ Bile production |
| Gall bladder | ■ Bile concentration and coordinated release facilitating emulsification of fats |
| Small intestine | ■ Digestion and absorption of most nutrients |
| Large intestine | ■ Passage of undigested matter<br>■ Absorption of water and vitamins<br>■ Provides environment for commensal symbiotic bacteria |
| Rectum | ■ Storage of undigested matter<br>■ Defaecation |

stomach maintains a pH of about 2, which has an important role in destroying microorganisms. There is some protein breakdown in the stomach and the food is mixed well. The mixed food, or chyme, then moves into the duodenum where most of the digestion occurs. Digestive enzymes and bicarbonate ions (which neutralize the acidic pH) are produced from the pancreatic exocrine tissue and secreted into the duodenum. Bile salt secretion is important for the digestion of fats. The small intestine is a major site of absorption and has a very large surface area provided by finger-like projections called villi (Fig. 1.15). Tiny projections or microvilli on the surface of the individual epithelial cells further increase the surface area. The net result is a surface area of about 300 square metres. The epithelial cells lining the absorptive surfaces of the gastrointestinal system have membrane-bound enzymes, for further digestion of the food molecules, and specific transport mechanisms for absorbing different molecules into the bloodstream.

Cells lining the gut have a very rapid turnover; the entire cell lining is renewed every 4 or 5 days. Therefore agents that inhibit cell division such as radiation and chemotherapy drugs compromise the epithelium and total surface area. The absorbed nutrients pass from the capillaries of the small intestine into the hepatic portal vein to the liver. The wall of the gut is lined with smooth muscle, which undergoes synchronous contraction, generating waves of peristaltic movement propelling the food along the gut. The control of the smooth muscle is via the enteric nervous system.

The large intestine is important in the maintenance of fluid and iron balance and the absorption of vitamins. It is colonized and inhabited by bacteria, many of which synthesize vitamins, including vitamin $B_{12}$, vitamin K, thiamin and riboflavin, which can be absorbed across the gut wall. Motility of food through the gut is increased if there are more undigested polysaccharides (fibre) present. Some breakdown of these

**Fig. 1.15** ***Structure of the small intestinal villi: A transverse section through the intestinal wall; B a villus; C detail of the epithelium. (Reproduced with permission from Saffrey & Stewart 1997.)***

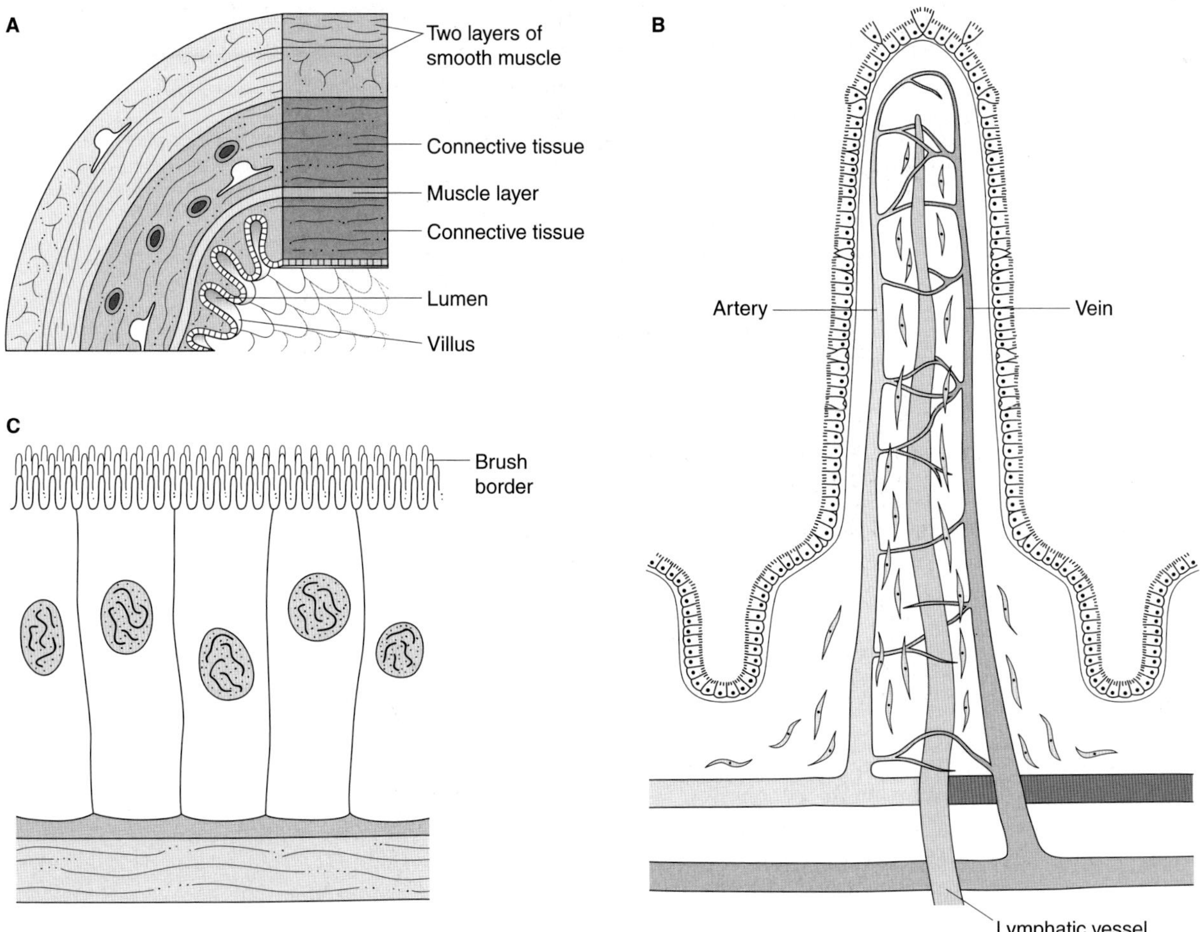

Fig. 1.16 *Phases of hormonal control of the stomach and associated organs.*

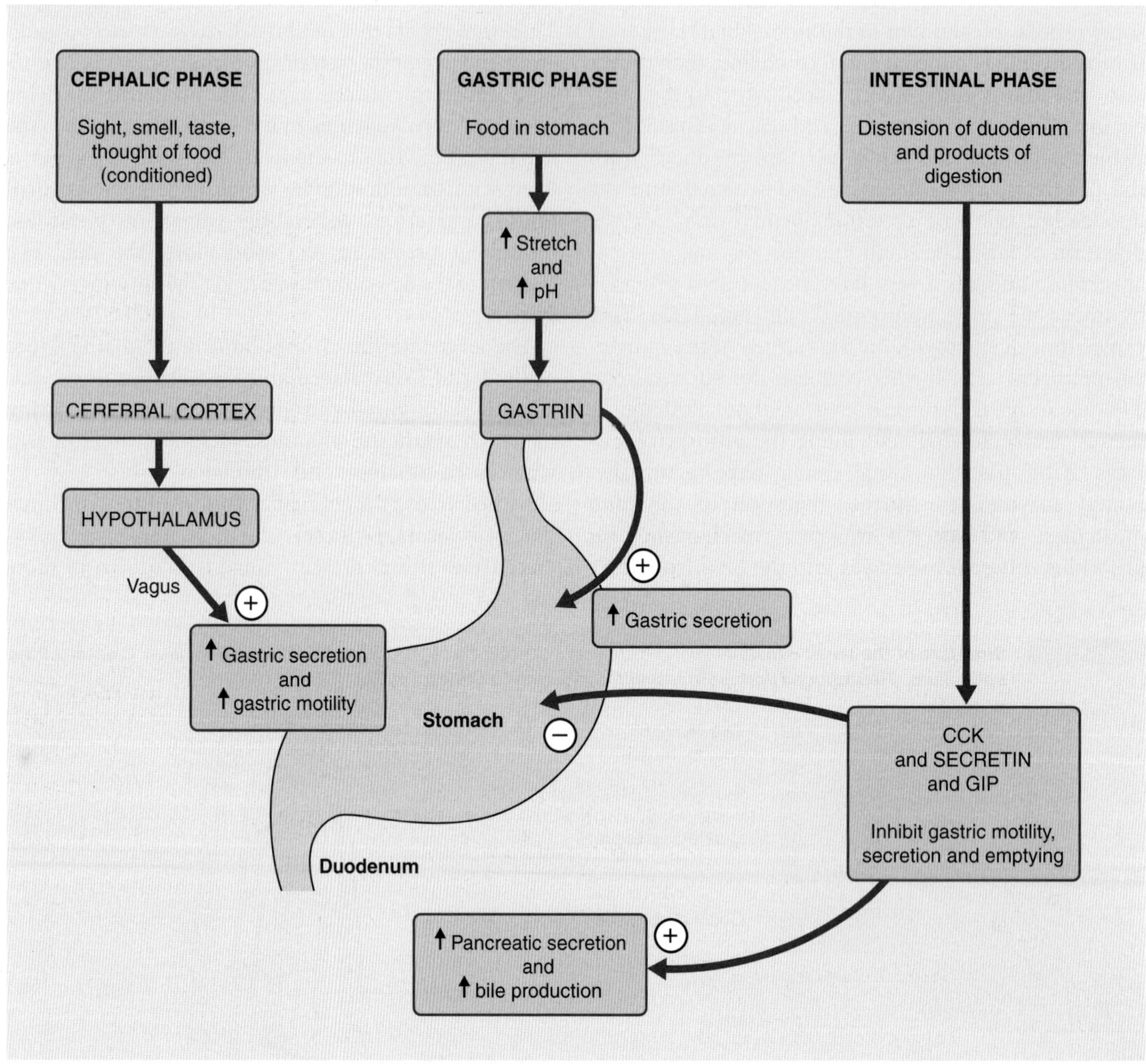


polysaccharides occurs by bacterial action, which can produce gas (flatus), nitrogen, carbon dioxide, hydrogen, methane and hydrogen sulphide.

Secretion and motility of the gut are controlled by nervous stimulation (Fig. 1.16). There are three phases or stages of nervous control. The cephalic phase is stimulated by the smell, taste and sight of food, which increase motility and hydrochloric acid secretion. When food reaches the stomach it causes distension, increased acidity and increased peptide formation, which stimulate the gastric phase of control. The hormone gastrin is released, which stimulates secretion of acid and affects the lower regions of the gut. The third phase of control is the intestinal phase, which is stimulated by food within the intestine. The intestinal phase causes the reflex inhibition of gastric secretion.

## The respiratory system

Respiration is the exchange of gases between the environment and the body. Respiration is essential for the functioning of all living organisms. There are two types: aerobic and anaerobic. In aerobic respiration, organic molecules from the food are oxidized to produce energy (Fig. 1.17). Anaerobic respiration is when energy is produced in the absence of oxygen.

Fig. 1.17 *A summary of metabolism: substrate molecules (such as glucose from food) are oxidized (using respiratory oxygen), producing carbon dioxide (expired) and energy in the form of ATP.*

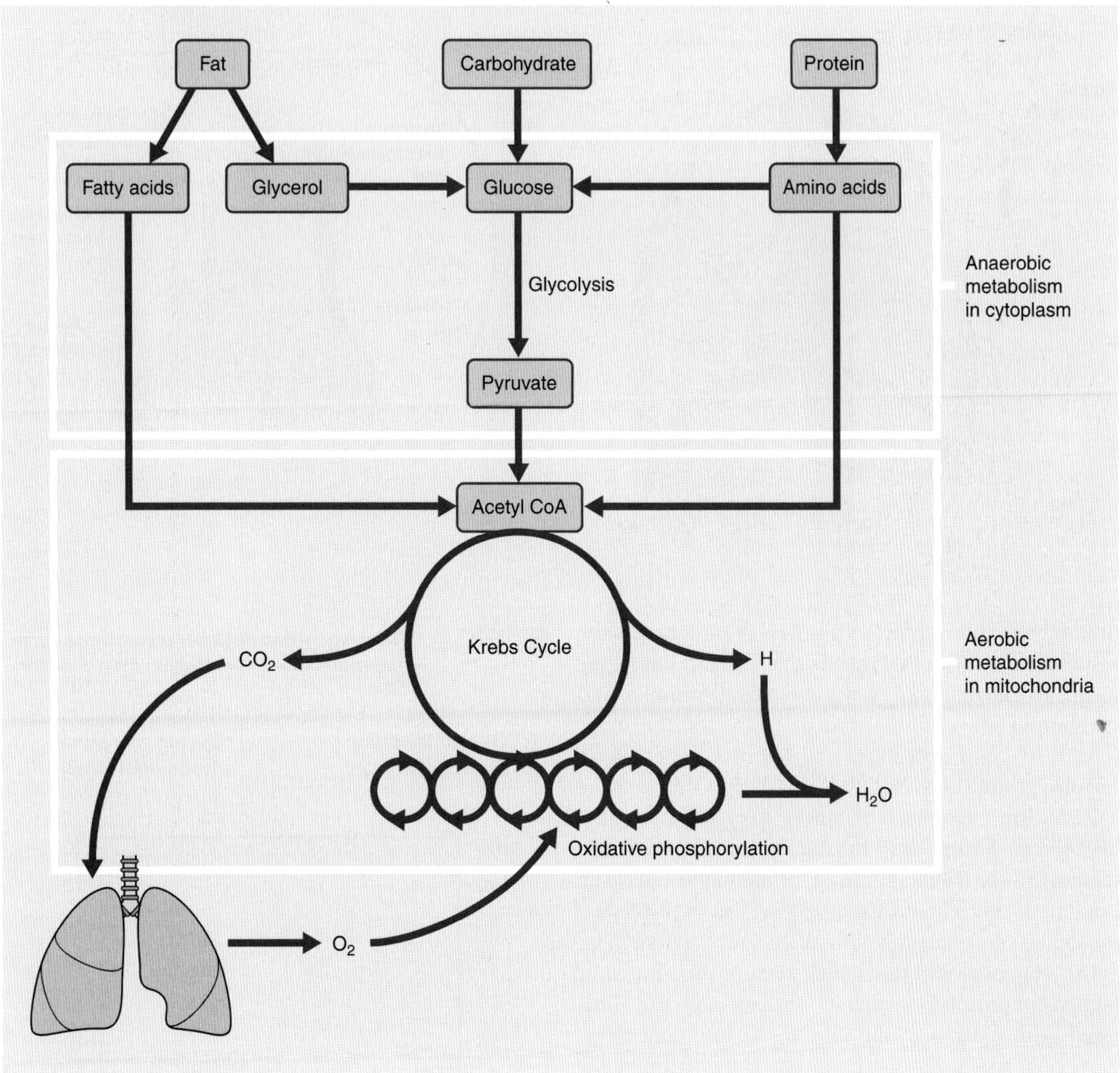


This form of respiration is relatively inefficient compared with aerobic respiration.

Anaerobic respiration is common among single-celled organisms. Large animals, such as humans, can produce some energy anaerobically, for instance in times of acute stress and rapid muscle activity when oxygen demand exceeds oxygen provision. However, anaerobic respiration results in the rapid accumulation of toxic metabolites. In simple organisms, these may simply diffuse out of the cell into the environment but for large animals this rapid excretion cannot be achieved so anaerobic processes are self-limiting. 'Asphyxia' is the term that describes irreversible damage of cells due to the build-up of these toxins.

Aerobic respiration is an extension of anaerobic respiration. The metabolites, produced under anaerobic processes such as glycolysis, are further broken down producing carbon dioxide, water and significantly more energy. Aerobic respiration requires the presence of oxygen and mitochondria, the sites of the enzymes involved in these biochemical pathways. Cells require a continuous source of oxygen for metabolism.

The respiratory system consists of the lungs, the branching airways, the gaseous exchange membranes,

Fig. 1.18 *The respiratory system.*

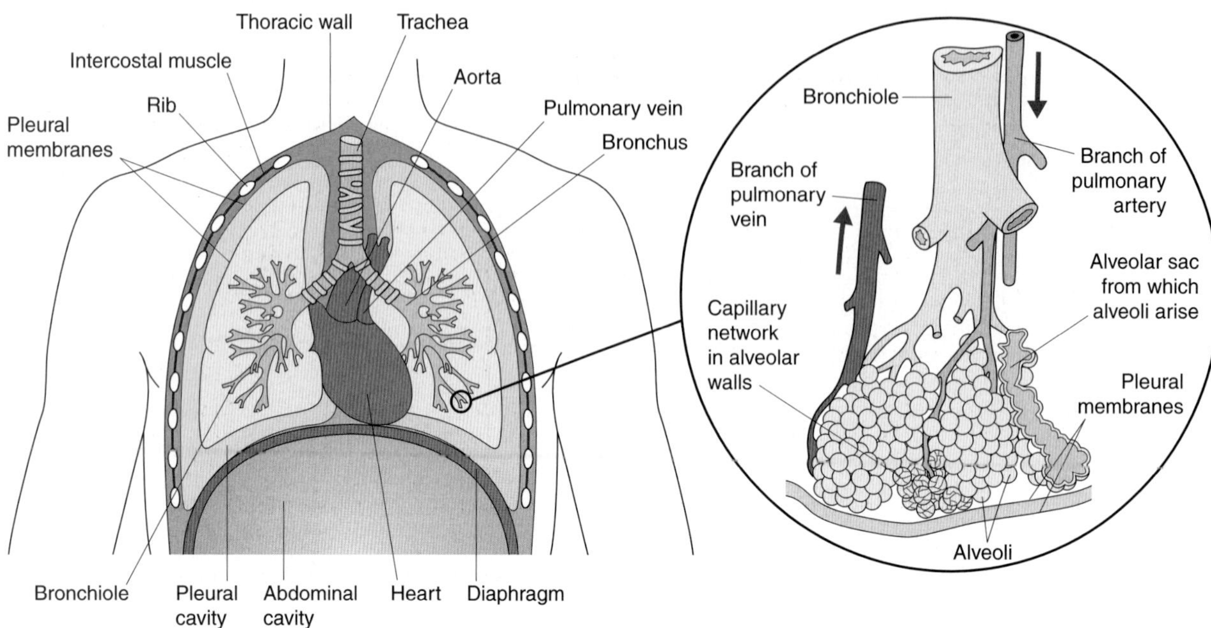


the rib cage and respiratory muscles. Ventilation is the mechanical activity that moves gases in and out of the lungs; the movements of the intercostal muscles and diaphragm allow filling and emptying of the lungs (Fig. 1.18). Gas exchange occurs across the capillary membranes of the alveoli, which are very thin so have a very low diffusion distance. Oxygen from the inspired air diffuses into the capillaries where it binds temporarily to haemoglobin in the red blood cells. The binding of oxygen and haemoglobin can be described by the oxygen–haemoglobin dissociation curve (Fig. 1.19). Haemoglobin has a high affinity for oxygen at higher concentrations and its binding sites are saturated with oxygen in the alveoli. At low concentrations of oxygen, haemoglobin has a low affinity for oxygen so it releases oxygen at the tissues. Binding of oxygen to haemoglobin is altered by carbon dioxide, pH, temperature and the glycolytic intermediate 2,3-bisphosphoglycerate (2,3-BPG, also known as 2,3-diphosphoglycerate or 2,3-DPG). These substances alter the shape of the haemoglobin molecule, which affects its oxygen-binding sites. Substances that reduce haemoglobin–oxygen affinity increase the release of oxygen (so the curve is shifted towards the right).

Carbon dioxide diffuses from the tissues into the capillaries. It is taken up by the red blood cells where it reacts with water to form carbonic acid. This reaction is catalysed by the enzyme carbonic anhydrase in the red blood cell. Carbonic acid is unstable and

Fig. 1.19 ***The oxygen–haemoglobin dissociation curve. (Reproduced with permission from Brooker 1998.)***

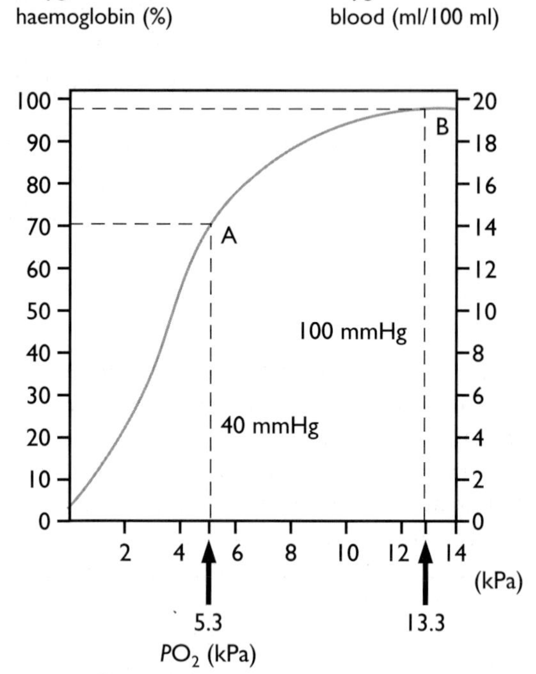


A=Venous blood (at the tissues)
B=Arterial blood (at the lungs)

Fig. 1.20 *Carbon dioxide transport. (Reproduced with permission from Brooker 1998.)*

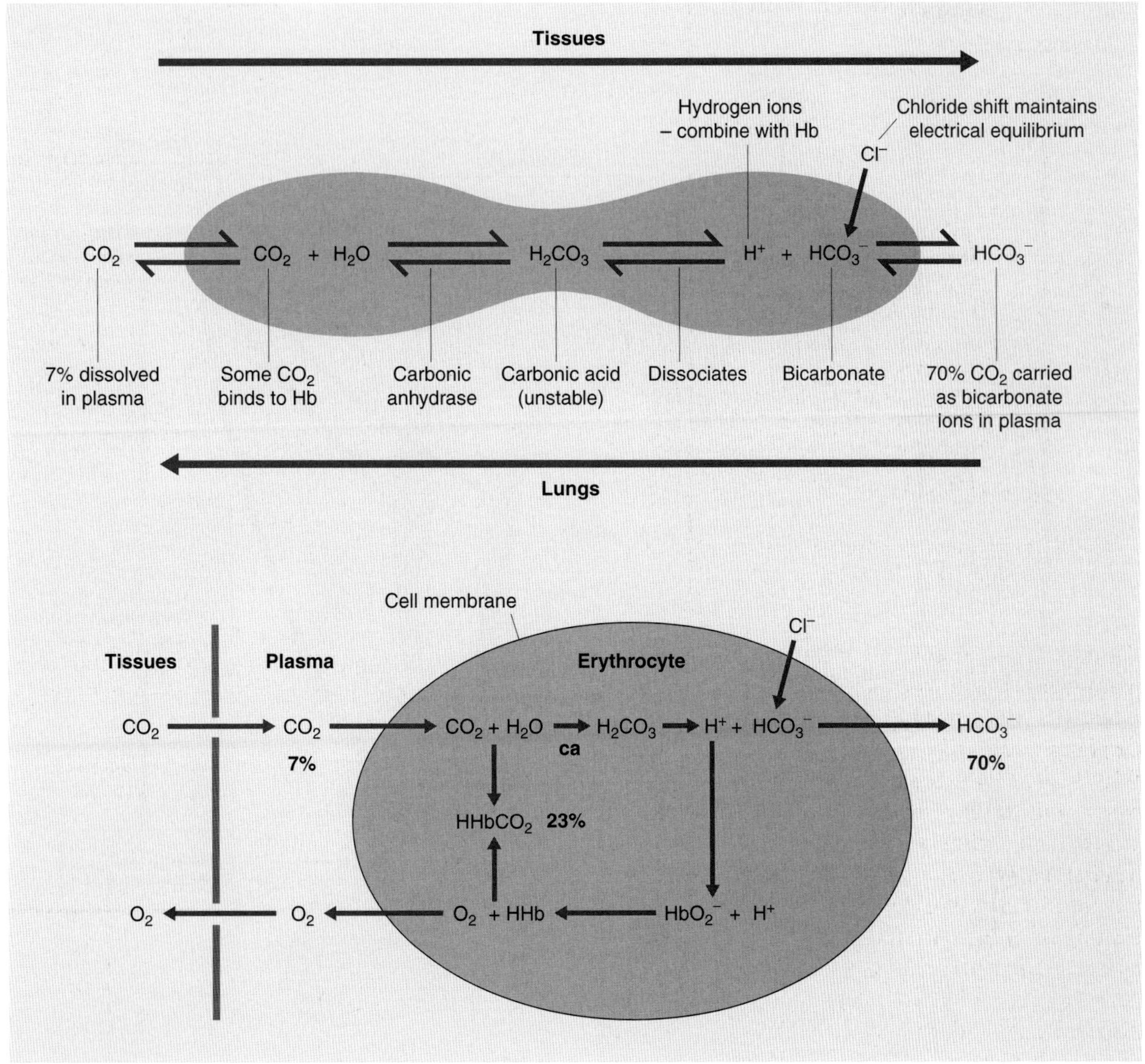


dissociates to bicarbonate and hydrogen ions (Fig. 1.20); the bicarbonate diffuses out of the red blood cell into the plasma.

The respiratory control centre, in the medulla oblongata of the brain-stem, affects the activity of the inspiratory and expiratory neurons that control the respiratory muscles, which contract to allow inspiration and expiration. The respiratory centre receives information from stretch receptors in the lungs and from the peripheral and central chemoreceptors that monitor the pH and oxygen content of the blood (Fig. 1.21).

There is homeostatic regulation of acid–base balance to maintain pH within narrow parameters at around 7.3 (Fig. 1.22). This regulation involves both the respiratory and renal systems (see Ch. 2).

## The cardiovascular system

The cardiovascular system includes the heart, the blood vessels and the blood. The blood is pumped around a network of blood vessels (Fig. 1.23). Arteries transport blood away from the heart and have thick muscular walls. Veins carry blood towards the heart; they function as a capacitance system. Capillaries link the arterial and venous systems and allow exchange of substances between the blood and the tissues.

Fig. 1.21 *Chemoreceptor control of respiration: the regulation of ventilation is achieved via peripheral and central chemoreceptors, which sample the blood, and then via a neuronal pathway influencing the rate and depth of breathing.*

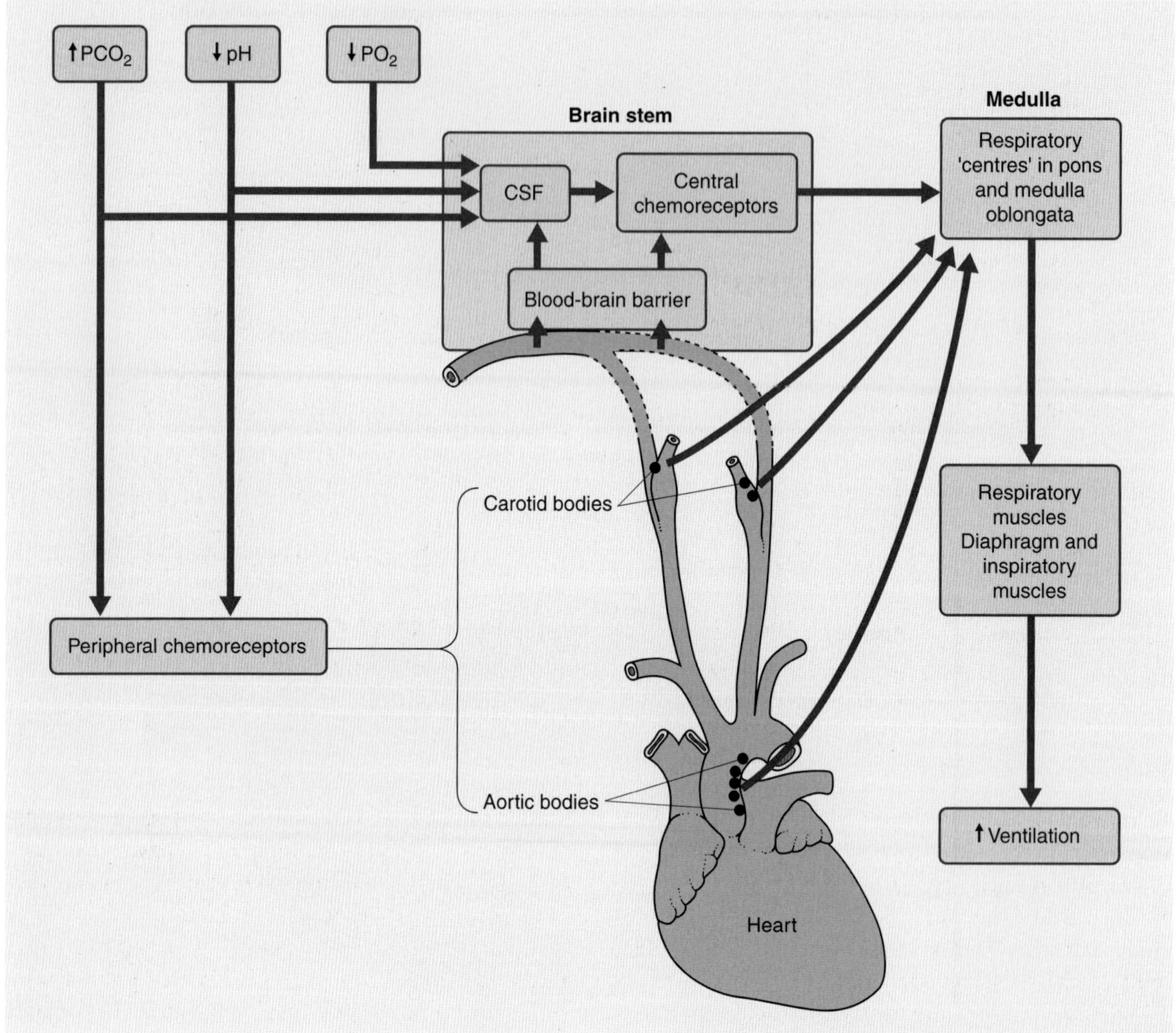


The heart functions as a double pump, pumping blood to the tissues of the body and the lungs (Fig. 1.24). Blood from the right side of the heart enters the pulmonary circulation to the capillaries surrounding the alveoli of the lungs where the blood is oxygenated. Oxygenated blood returns to the left side of the heart in the pulmonary veins. The oxygenated blood is then pumped from the left side of the heart around the body. The pulmonary circulation takes blood from the right side of the heart, to the lungs, and back to the left side of the heart. The systemic circulation is the circulation of blood around the body from the left side of the heart to the tissues and back to the right side of the heart. The coronary circulation is the circulation of blood within the vessels of the heart. Blood flow to the brain is via a circular arrangement of vessels (the circle of Willis); this ensures that there will always be sufficient oxygen and nutrients, albeit at the expense of other parts of the body when the circulatory system is under stress. The blood–brain barrier protects the brain against the entry of some harmful substances, such as toxins.

The heart beats about 70 times a minute at rest, forcing blood from the ventricles into the pulmonary artery and the aorta. The increased volume of blood entering the blood system causes a fluctuating increase in blood pressure. Blood pressure can be measured using a sphygmomanometer to record pressure within

Fig. 1.22 *Acid–base balance.*

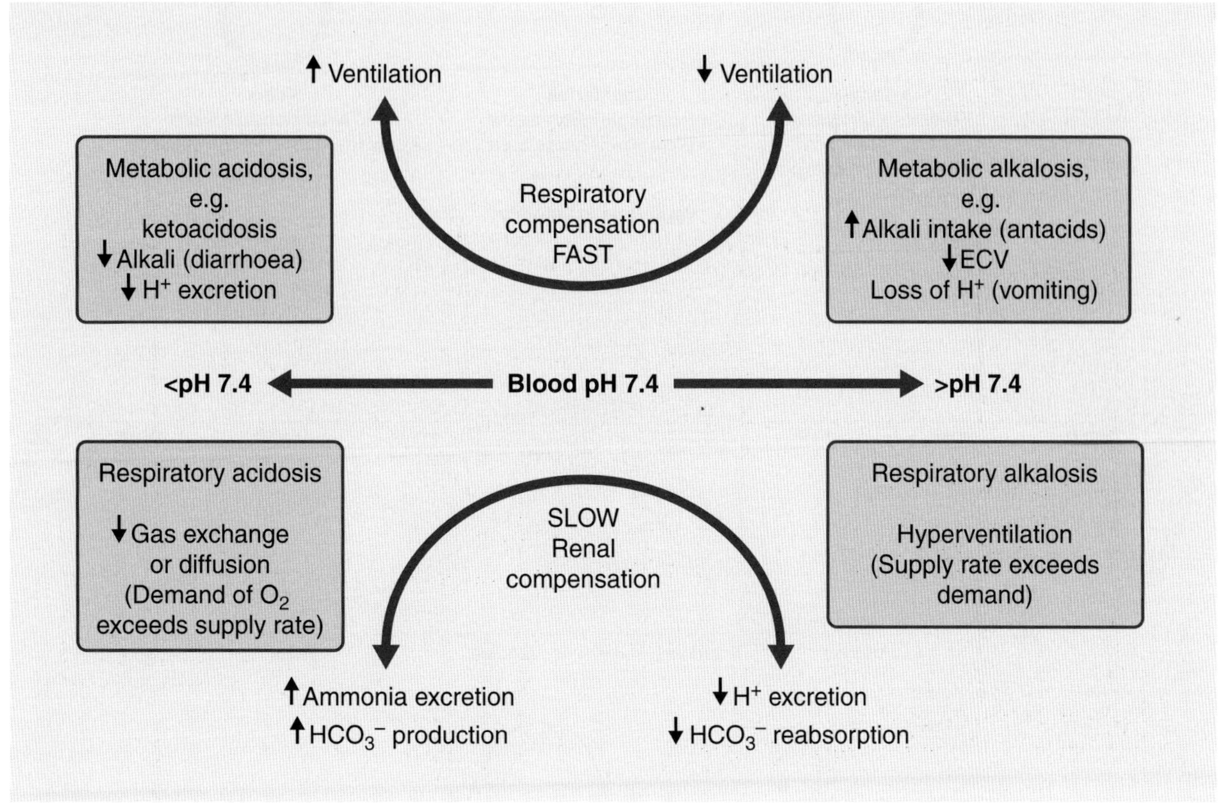


an artery and a stethoscope to hear the turbulence of blood within the blood vessels (Fig. 1.25). The amount of blood that leaves the heart per minute is described as the cardiac output. This is the volume of blood ejected from the ventricles each time the heart beats multiplied by the number of beats per minute (Fig. 1.26). The amount of oxygen that reaches the cells of the tissue depends on the proportion of the cardiac output the tissue receives.

The heart's internal pacemaker, the sinoatrial node (SAN), sets the heart rate. The SAN spontaneously depolarizes and triggers a wave of electrical activity, which stimulates the heart muscle to contract (Fig. 1.27). The SAN is innervated by both parasympathetic and sympathetic nerves. Receptors throughout the body respond to changes in blood pressure and respiratory gas level. These baroreceptors and chemoreceptors transmit information to afferent nerves in the medulla of the brain (the brain-stem) that control efferent nerves to the heart, lungs and blood vessels (Fig. 1.28).

The total capacity of blood vessels in the body exceeds the volume of the blood. To maintain homeostasis and tissue requirements the cardiovascular system is carefully regulated to ensure optimal oxygenation of the tissues. The control of blood flow is regulated by alteration of the diameter of the blood vessels, which changes peripheral resistance. The diameter of the blood vessels is altered by the activity of sympathetic nerves that innervate the smooth muscle in the vessel walls. Increased sympathetic activity, or increased adrenergic stimulation, increases vasoconstriction, reducing blood flow and increasing peripheral resistance. Decreased sympathetic activity causes vasodilation, which increases blood flow and reduces peripheral resistance. Blood vessel diameter is also controlled locally by tissue metabolites. This autoregulation increases blood flow to metabolically active tissues.

## Blood

Blood is a suspension of cells in plasma (see Table 1.2). Blood cells are all derived from stem cells in the bone marrow. The majority (> 99%) of cells are red blood cells or erythrocytes. Erythrocytes contain haemoglobin, which binds to oxygen. Iron, folic acid and vitamin

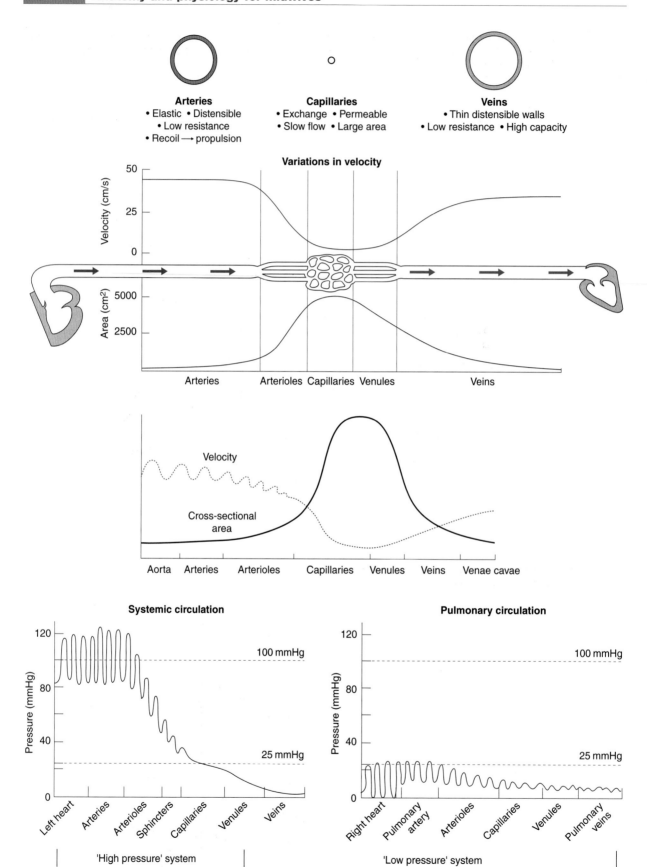

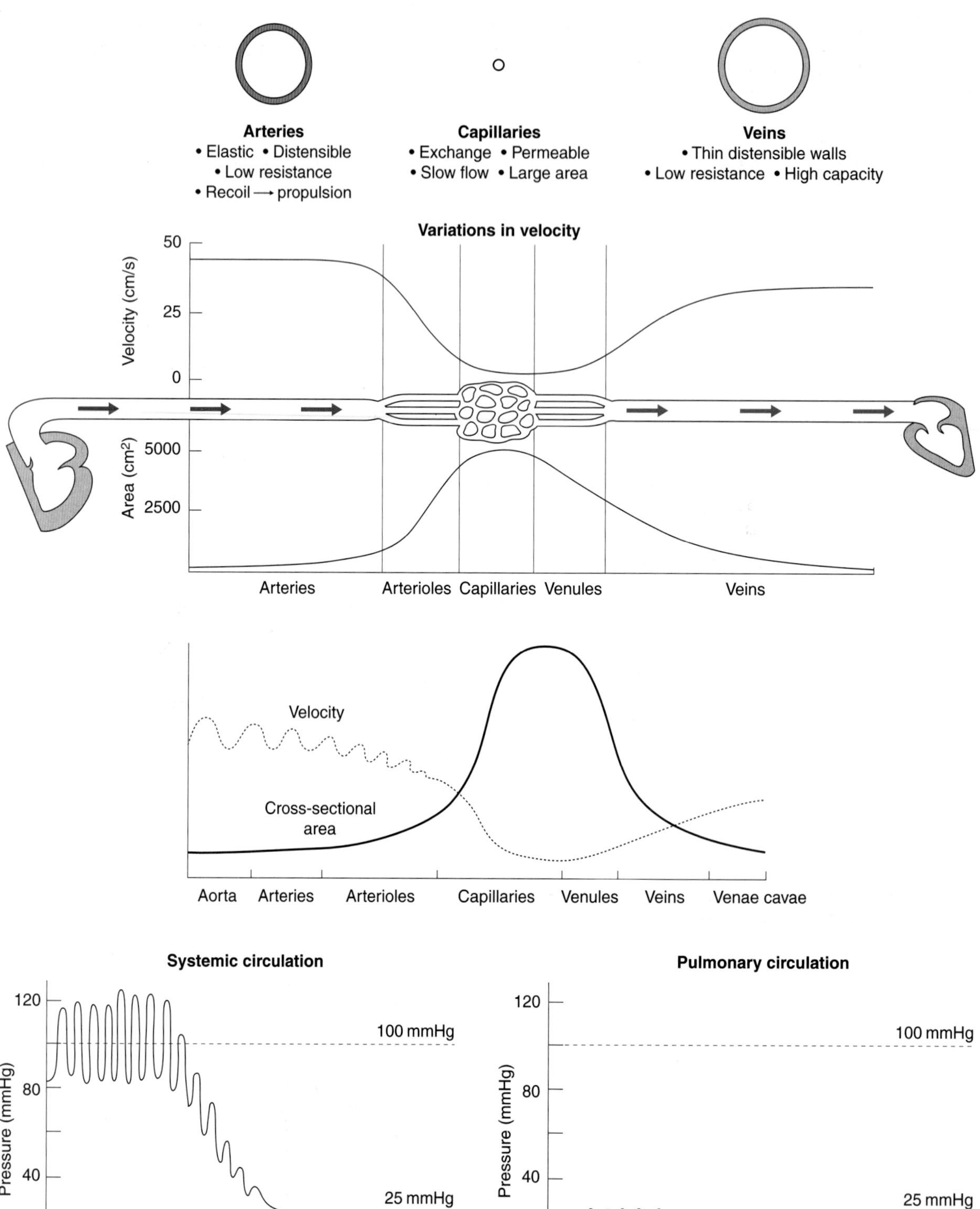
Arteries
• Elastic • Distensible
• Low resistance
• Recoil ⟶ propulsion
Capillaries
• Exchange • Permeable
• Slow flow • Large area
Veins
• Thin distensible walls
• Low resistance • High capacity
Variations in velocity
Velocity (cm/s)
50
25
0
Area (cm²)
5000
2500
Arteries
Arterioles
Capillaries
Venules
Veins
Velocity
Cross-sectional area
Aorta
Arteries
Arterioles
Capillaries
Venules
Veins
Venae cavae
Systemic circulation
Pressure (mmHg)
120
80
40
0
100 mmHg
25 mmHg
Left heart
Arteries
Arterioles
Sphincters
Capillaries
Venules
Veins
'High pressure' system
Pulmonary circulation
Right heart
Pulmonary artery
Arterioles
Capillaries
Venules
Pulmonary veins
'Low pressure' system

**Fig. 1.23** ***Blood vessels: the major role of arteries is in the generation of elastic recoil, which propels the blood around the body. The capillaries are involved in gas exchange and the veins act as capacitance vessels returning blood to the heart.***

**Fig. 1.24** ***Interior of the heart to show layers, chambers and valves. (Reproduced with permission from Brooker 1998.)***

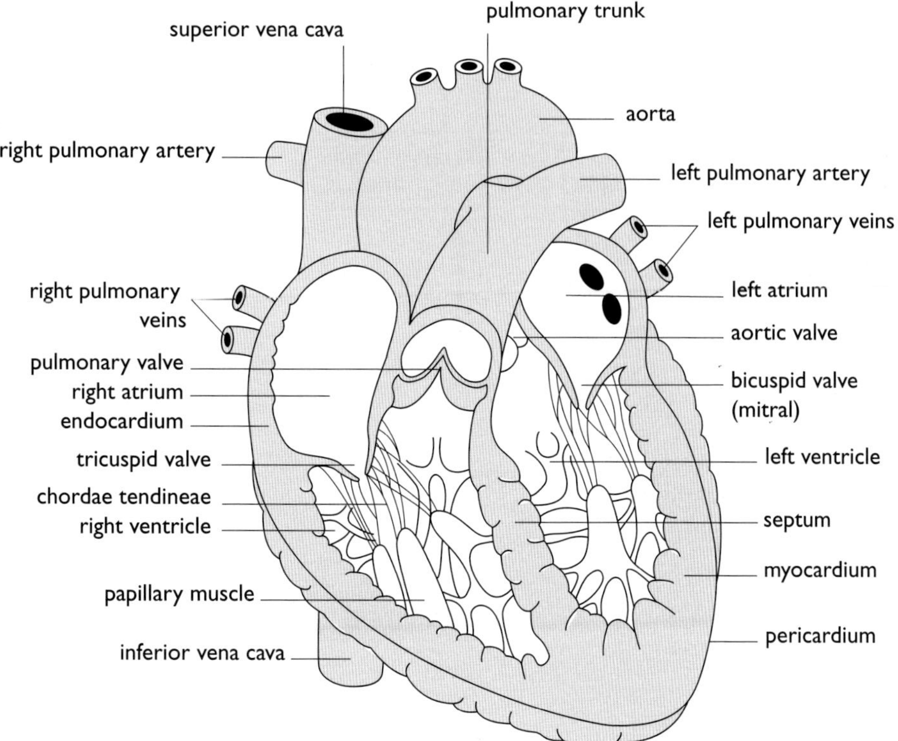


**Fig. 1.25** ***Blood pressure measurement. (Reproduced with permission from Brooker 1998.)***

| phase | blood pressure (mmHg) | | |
|---|---|---|---|
| | | 120 | systolic |
| 1 | sharp thud | | |
| | | 110 | |
| 2 | blowing or swishing | | |
| | | 100 | |
| 3 | soft thud | | |
| | | 90 | first diastolic |
| 4 | soft blowing that muffles | | |
| | | 80 | second diastolic |
| 5 | no sound | | |

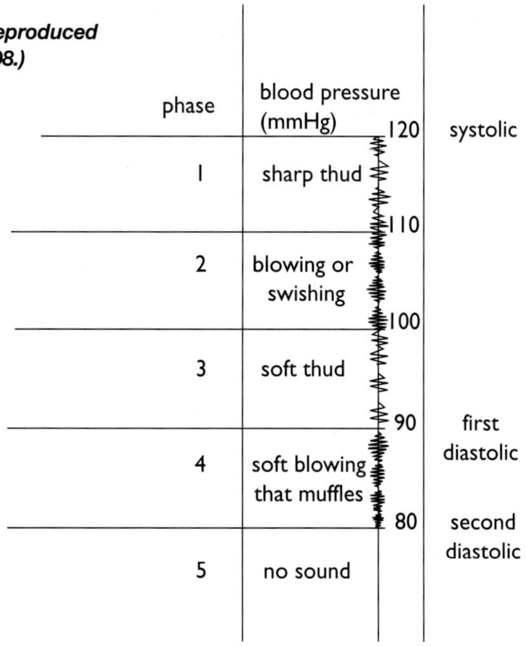

**Fig. 1.26** ***Cardiac output.***

Preload
Contractility
Afterload
⊕ ⊕ ⊖
Myocardial fibre shortening
Left ventricular size
Stroke volume × Heart rate = Cardiac output
Intrinsic rhythmicity
Extrinsic
(a) neural
(b) humoral

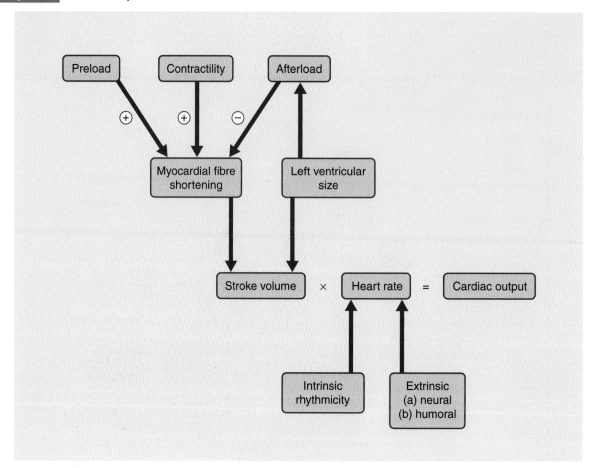

**Fig. 1.27** ***Sinoatrial node (SAN) depolarization: the conduction pathway of the heart enables the organ's coordinated and rhythmic beating.***

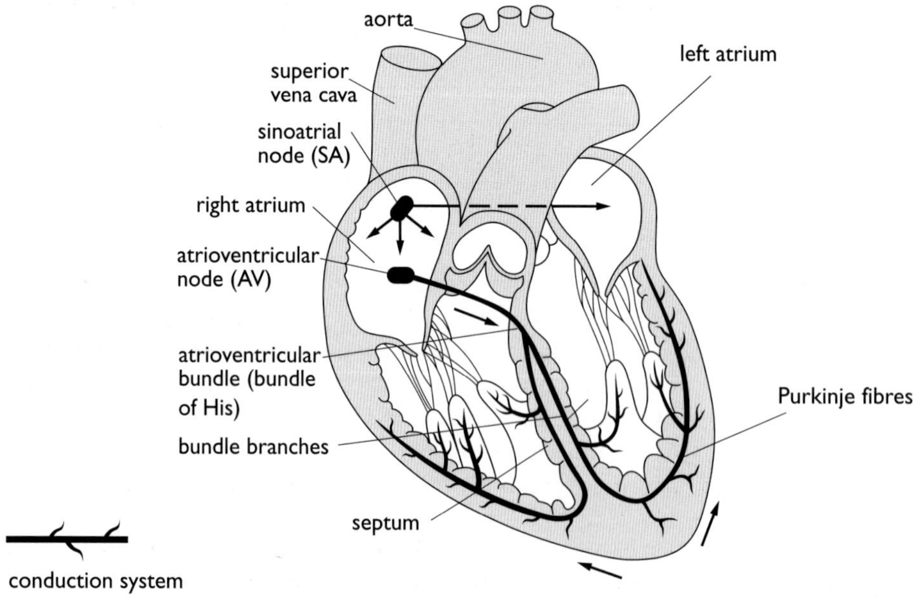

Fig. 1.28 *Regulation of blood pressure.*

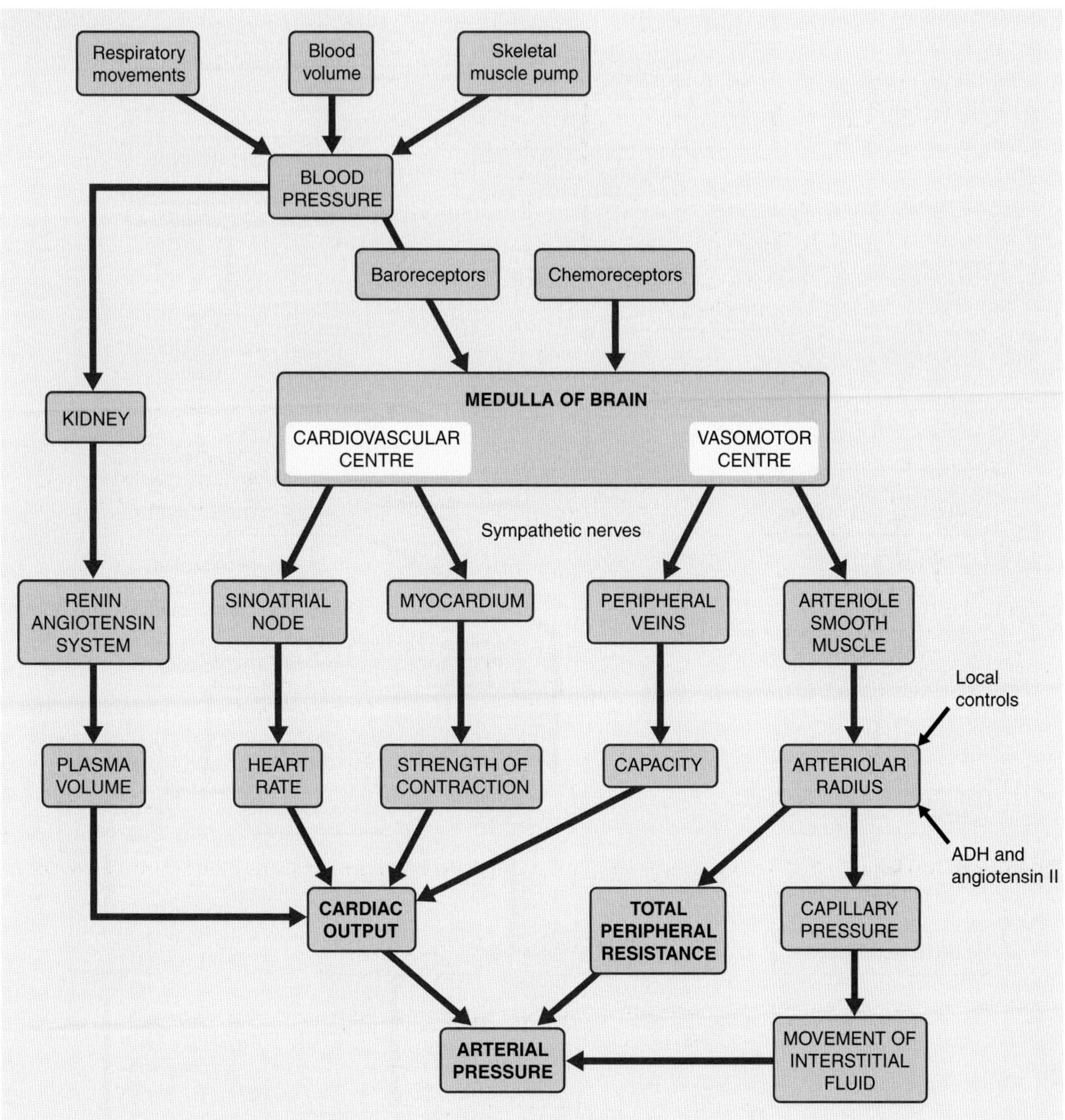


$B_{12}$ are required for the production of erythrocytes. The kidneys produce a hormone, erythropoietin, in response to low oxygen levels, which stimulates an increase in the production of red blood cells from the bone marrow. Leukocytes, or white blood cells, include polymorphonuclear granulocytes (neutrophils, eosinophils and basophils) and the agranular monocytes and lymphocytes. The role of white blood cells is the defence of the body (see Ch. 10). Platelets are cellular fragments of megakaryocytes, which are an essential component of the blood-clotting mechanism (Fig. 1.29). Plasma contains proteins (albumin, globulins and some clotting factors, such as fibrinogen), nutrients, hormones, waste products and ions.

## The lymphatic system

The lymphatic system is part of the circulatory system and consists of a network of vessels, lymph nodes and

Fig. 1.29 *Haemostasis: the blood coagulation cascade.*

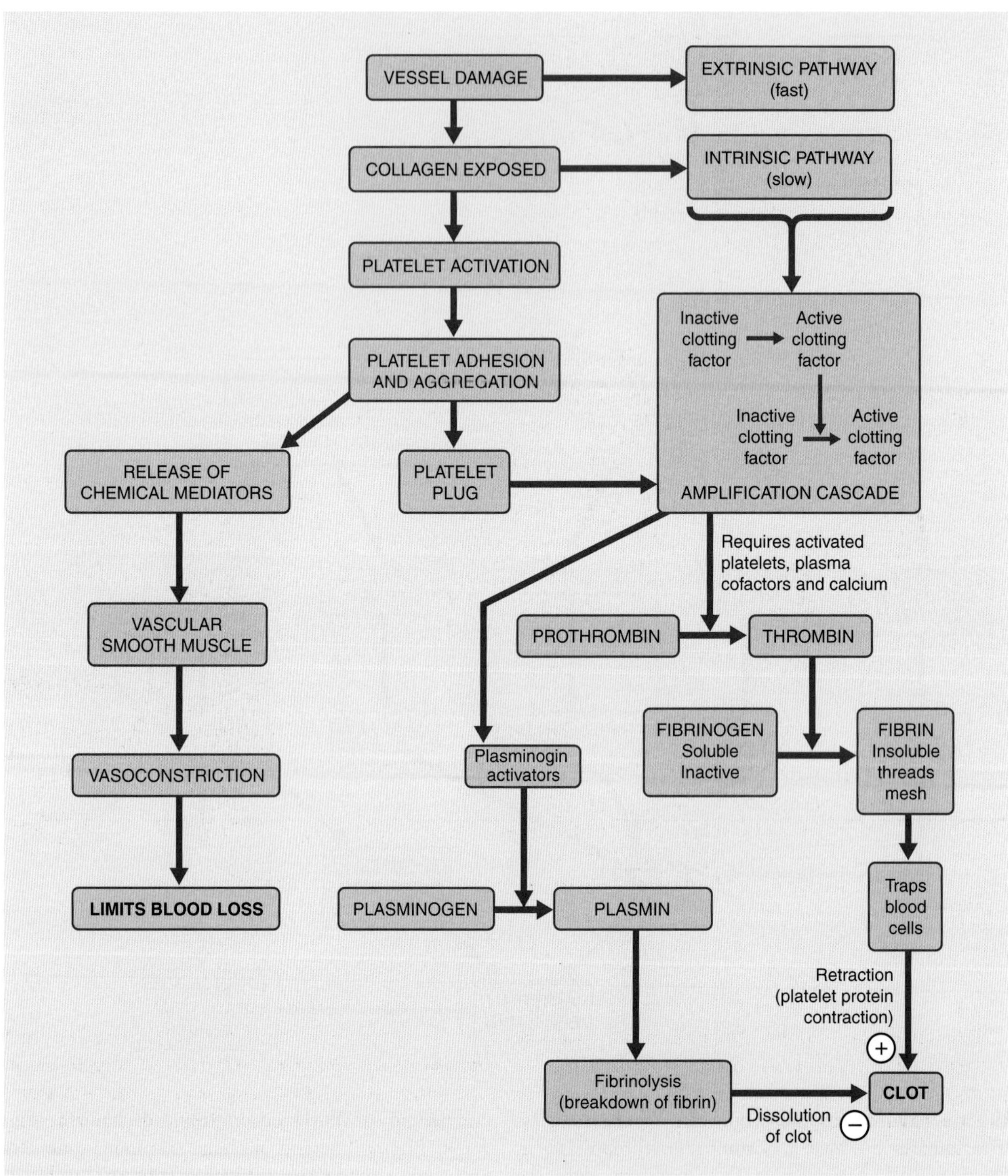


lymphatic fluid (Fig. 1.30). It collects the interstitial fluid from cells and returns it to the blood. It is important in defending the body against microorganisms (see Ch. 10). It also absorbs lipids from the digestive tract.

# Metabolism

## Energy production and storage

The cells have a continuous requirement for energy and adenosine triphosphate (ATP). The energy from

Fig. 1.30 *The lymphatic system.*

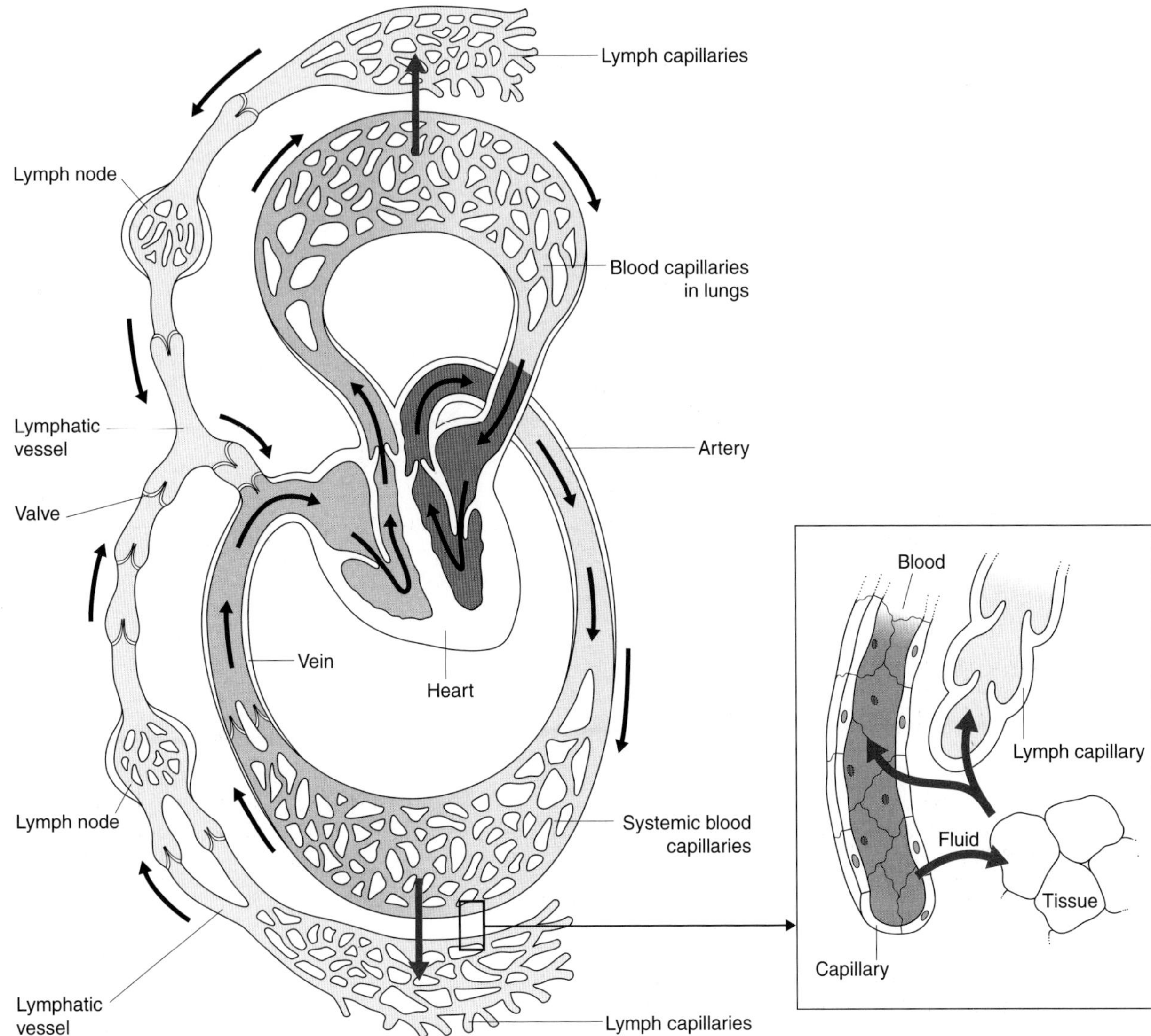


ATP drives virtually all the body processes but there is very little ATP present at any one time—just enough to provide energy requirements for only a few minutes. Every organ requires energy but some, such as muscles, have a very variable energy requirement. Meals provide fuel from food components, which are oxidized to provide ATP and heat. However, the intake of food is irregular and does not coordinate with the requirement for energy. The energy substrates from a meal are usually absorbed within 3 hours and the next meal can be hours away so animals have evolved successful methods of storing energy substrates.

The main storage forms are glycogen in liver and skeletal muscle and triacylglycerides in adipose tissue. Carbohydrates are the major fuels for the brain and nervous tissue. Oxidation of glucose occurs in several stages (Fig. 1.31). Glycolysis takes place in the cell cytosol and produces a little ATP anaerobically. If oxygen is present, there is further oxidation through the Krebs' cycle and oxidative phosphorylation (the electron transfer chain). This increased efficiency of ATP production takes place in cells that have mitochondria and adequate provision of oxygen. In tissues lacking mitochondria, such as red blood cells, or those with insufficient oxygen, such as active

Fig. 1.31 *Oxidation of glucose.*

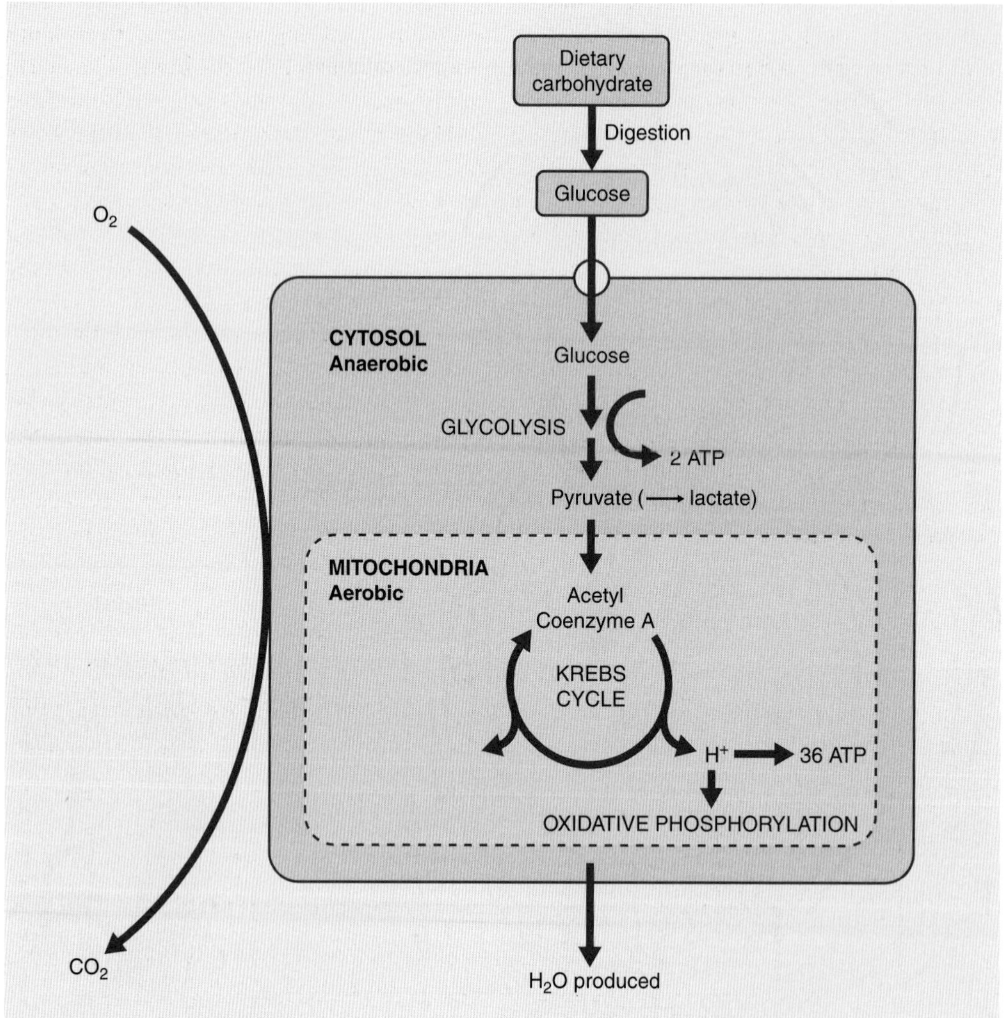


muscle, there is a build-up of the key intermediate pyruvate. Pyruvate can be converted into lactate and oxidized by the heart and kidneys or converted to glucose by the liver and kidneys.

About 500 g of the glucose polymer, glycogen, is stored: 100 g in the liver, which can release the glucose when required (by glycogenolysis) and 400 g in the skeletal muscles, which is available for use by the muscle. Triacylglycerides are stored in virtually unlimited amounts, as observed in obesity. As they do not mix with water, the storage form is very calorie dense and efficient. Triacylglycerides are composed of three fatty acids bound to a glycerol backbone. The glycerol can be converted into glucose, therefore providing a substrate for the brain to oxidize for energy. Fatty acids are released with free glycerol from the adipose tissue and can be oxidized by the liver, muscles and kidneys. Fatty acids cannot cross the blood–brain barrier and cannot be converted to glucose so they provide little substrate for the brain. Ketone bodies are water-soluble derivatives of fatty acids formed by the liver during starvation or prolonged severe exercise. When sufficient concentrations of ketone bodies accumulate, the brain and kidney use them to generate ATP. Certain amino acids are also ketogenic, and can be converted into ketone bodies. Overproduction of ketone bodies, as in uncontrolled diabetes, overwhelms the buffering capacity of the body and can cause life-threatening acidosis.

There is not a reserve storage form of protein independent of function. Protein can be metabolized to provide energy but at the expense of the breakdown of structural and functional components of the body. The use of protein as a fuel potentially damages the body so it is used only as a 'last resort' when the protein is broken down and the amino acids are converted into components of the glycolytic pathway to produce energy. However, proteins constitute a large proportion of body structure and therefore can provide a substantial source of energy when other supplies have been exhausted. Protein in excess of requirements can be irreversibly converted into glucose or triacylglycerides.

The brain consumes about a quarter of the body's daily energy production when the body is at rest. The brain's requirement for fuel drives energy metabolism. The main fuel storage form of the body is triacylglycerides but the brain cannot use fatty acids directly. Although the brain can oxidize ketone bodies, derived from fatty acids, for 80% of its energy requirements, 20% *must* come from glucose. Glucose comes from the diet or from glycogenolysis or gluconeogenesis in the liver. Other cells, therefore, utilize other substrates preferentially to glucose. The hierarchy of fuel use means the brain utilizes ketone bodies when they are available or glucose. Muscle has a major reserve of protein and glycogen. Muscle spares brain fuel by preferentially oxidizing fatty acids, thus sparing ketone bodies and glucose for the brain. The glycogen stored in the muscle is specifically available for muscle use.

The external environment is continually fluctuating and energy requirements are constantly changing. However, the body maintains homeostasis or internal stability by ensuring a constant level of amino acids and glucose in the blood, despite intermittent high loads following a meal. The level of ATP within cells is kept relatively constant although the rate of usage is variable; for instance, activity increases energy requirement of a muscle by up to 20 times. Cellular energy requirement is regulated very sensitively; different metabolic pathways predominate after a meal (called the absorptive state) to those between meals (the postabsorptive state) (Fig. 1.32). Dominance of the

**Fig. 1.32** ***Absorptive and postabsorptive states.***

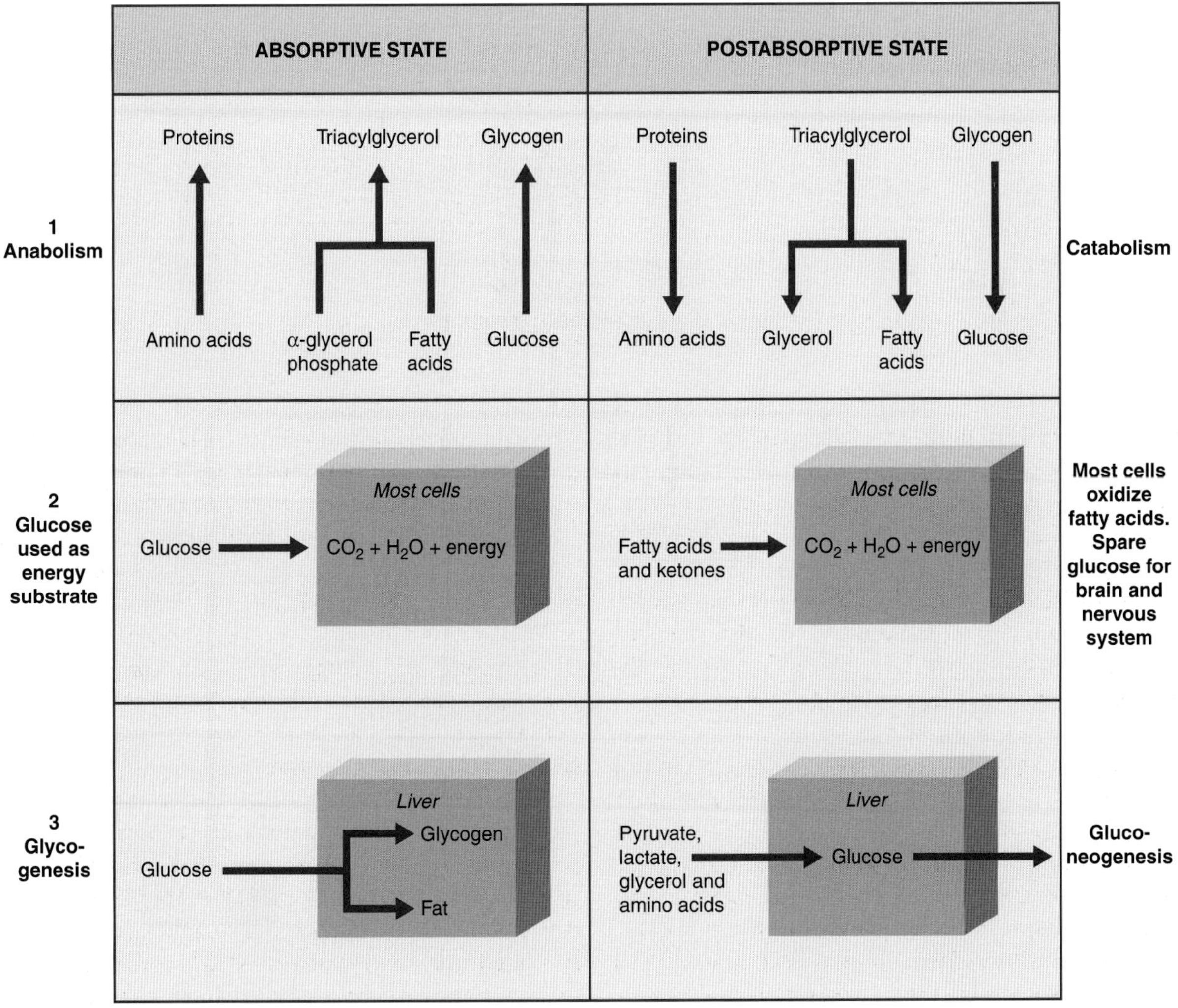

pathways is via changed enzyme activity and altered uptake of substrates, controlled by hormones. Interconversion from one metabolic step to the next is regulated by substrate activation, where the substance stimulates its own use, and product inhibition, where the product prevents the reaction from continuing. Enzymes catalysing the same reaction may exist as isoenzymes in different types of tissue, having different affinities for their substrates. This means that different concentrations of substrate are required for the biochemical pathway to progress.

## Blood sugar regulation

When plasma glucose concentration rises after a meal, secretion of insulin from pancreatic β-cells increases. Insulin stimulates the expression and insertion of glucose-transport proteins (known as 'GLUTs') into the cell membranes of tissues sensitive to insulin, such as muscle cells and adipocytes. This increases the uptake of glucose and other substrates into the cell and promotes the anabolic (storage) biochemical pathways (Fig. 1.33). Tissues that have a constant requirement for glucose, such as brain cells, do not have insulin-sensitive glucose transport. Under conditions of low glucose, pancreatic production of glucagon is increased, which acts to mobilize tissue reserves of metabolic fuels. Adrenaline, secreted from the adrenal medulla in response to sympathetic innervation, causes a rapid mobilization of fuel for 'fight or flight' (see p. 57). Adrenaline stimulates glucose production from the muscle glycogen and increases lipolysis in adipose tissue so levels of fatty acids increase to provide additional metabolic fuel.

Fig. 1.33 *The effects of insulin.*

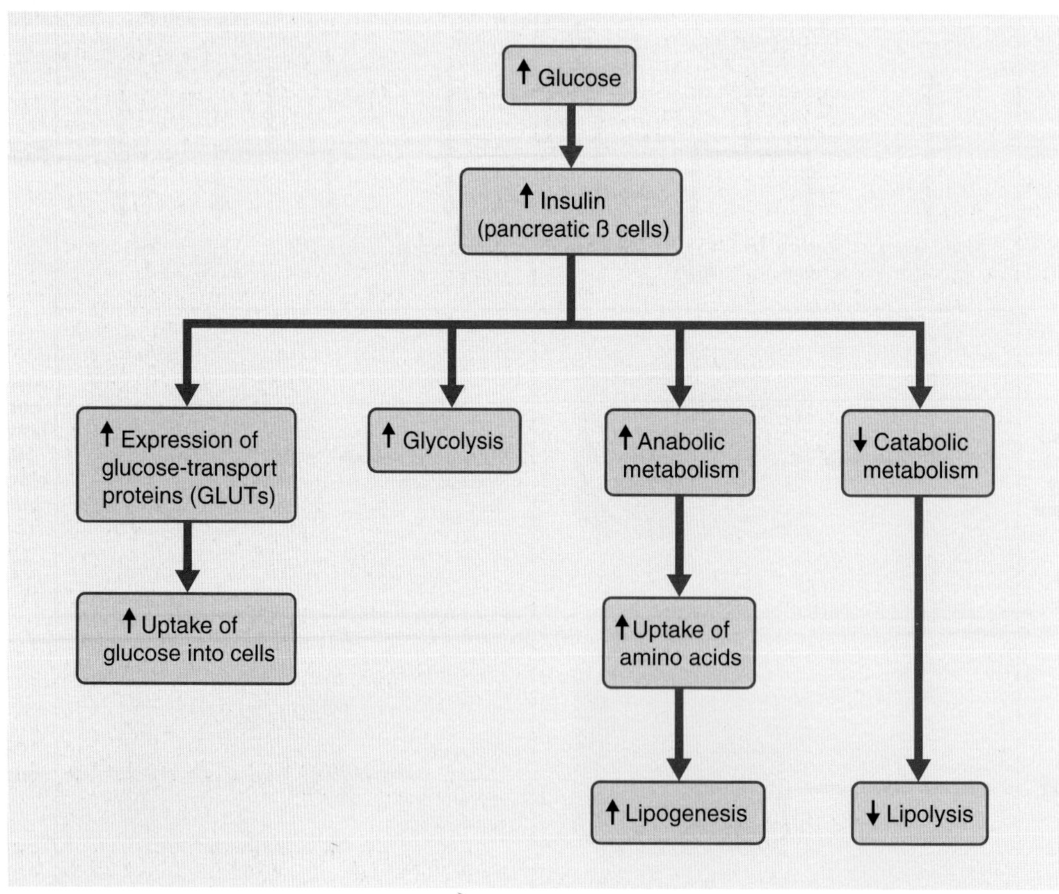

## Key points

- Cells have different anatomical structures, which are related to their physiological functions.
- Cells are organized together to form tissues which are organized into organs and the physiological systems of the body.
- The role of the physiological systems is to provide internal stability or homeostasis, which will ensure the cells' variable but essential requirements for energy are met by an adequate supply of oxygen and nutrients.
- As the enzymes that regulate cellular activity have a protein structure, they are affected by fluctuations in pH and temperature so homeostasis has to maintain optimum temperature and acid–base balance as well.

### Application to practice

The basic physiology described within this chapter relates to the non-pregnant state. During pregnancy there are many physiological changes, which are explored throughout the rest of the book.

## Annotated further reading

Alberts B, Bray D, Lewis J, Raff M, Roberts K, Watson J D 1994 Molecular biology of the cell. Garland, New York
*A beautifully written and well-illustrated text on molecular and cellular biology which is accessible, easy to read and up to date; the cell biologist's 'bible'.*

Berne R M, Levy N M 1998 Physiology, 4th edn. C V Mosby, St Louis
*A comprehensive illustrated textbook, which emphasizes physiological concepts and basic principles.*

Greenstein B, Greenstein A 1996 Medical biochemistry at a glance. Blackwell, Oxford
*A useful overview of human biochemistry which provides a synopsis using detailed flow-charts and explanatory diagrams.*

Koeppen B M, Stanton B 1996 Renal physiology, 2nd edn. University of Connecticut, Farmington
*Provides a useful reference to the area of renal physiology.*

Salway J 1994 Metabolism at a glance. Blackwell, Oxford
*A large-format book which provides a comprehensive review of basic human metabolism including inborn errors of metabolism and clinical aspects of metabolism. Metabolic pathways are summarized as segments with a clear diagrammatic pathway map on one page and an outline of the metabolism on the facing page.*

Tortora G J, Grab S R 1993 Principles of anatomy and physiology, 7th edn. Harper Collins, New York
*A clear, illustrated textbook (with CD-Rom) providing an in-depth overview of physiology and anatomy. It is targeted at students in health professions and includes clinical applications and study outlines.*

Vander A J, Sherman J H, Luciano D S 1994 Human physiology, 6th edn. McGraw-Hill, New York
*Provides a useful guide to the principles of human physiology using clear diagrams and flow-charts.*

## References

Brooker C G 1998 Human structure and function, 2nd edn. C V Mosby, St Louis, pp 15, 30, 32, 33, 88, 207, 211, 228, 277, 279, 296, 372, 383

Saffery J, Stewart M (eds) 1997 Maintaining the whole. SK220 Human biology and health, book 3. Open University Press, Milton Keynes, p 65

# 2 The reproductive and urinary systems

## Learning objectives

- To describe the structure and function of the urinary system.
- To compare the structure of the female and male reproductive systems.
- To identify differences between the male and female reproductive tracts in relation to reproduction and adaptations to facilitate childbirth.

## Introduction

This chapter reviews the basic anatomy of the reproductive and urinary systems of the human. The human urinary system differs only slightly between the male and female, mostly in relation to the structure of the external genitalia. The function of the urinary system is also essentially the same within the male and female. However, the renal system can be severely stressed by pregnancy, mostly because of its close proximity to the reproductive organs. The midwife needs to know the basics of normal renal physiology in order to understand the changes that take place in the renal system during pregnancy and how these may affect the general condition of the woman. For example, not only are the regulation and retention of fluid altered but also the excretion of glucose and other substances is affected by these changes. Drug excretion via the kidneys may be affected by pregnancy, so long-term medication may need to be changed. The effectiveness of medication may be reduced and altered drug dosage may be required. (Changes in the renal system in pregnancy are covered in Ch. 11.)

## The urinary system

The urinary system is composed of two kidneys, which produce urine, two ureters running from the kidneys to the bladder, which collects and stores the urine, and a urethra from which urine is discharged to the exterior (Fig. 2.1).

### *The kidneys*

The kidneys have a broad range of other functions (see Box 2.1) as well as producing urine. The kidneys are situated upon the posterior wall of the abdominal cavity, one on either side of the vertebral column at the level of the thoracic and lumbar vertebrae. The right kidney is slightly lower than the left owing to its relationship to the liver. Each kidney is about 10 cm long, 6.5 cm wide and about 3 cm thick. The kidneys each

**Box 2.1**
**Functions of the kidney**

- Regulation of water balance
- Regulation of pH and inorganic ion balance (sodium, potassium, calcium)
- Excretion of metabolic waste products (urea from protein, uric acid from nucleic acids, creatinine from muscle creatine and haemoglobin breakdown products)
- Removal of toxic chemicals (drugs, pesticides, food additives)
- Regulation of blood pressure (renin–angiotensin system)
- Control of formation of red blood cells (via erythropoietin)
- Vitamin D activation and calcium balance
- Gluconeogenesis (formation of glucose from amino acids and other precursors)

**Fig. 2.1** *The urinary system. (Reproduced with permission from Brooker 1998.)*

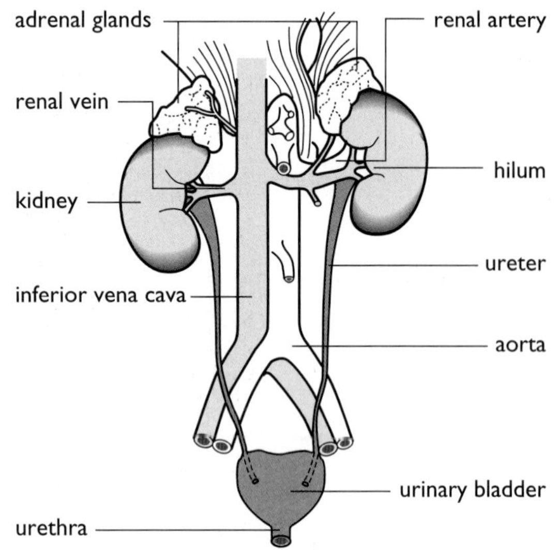


**Fig. 2.2** *The structure of the kidney (longitudinal section). (Reproduced with permission from Brooker 1998.)*

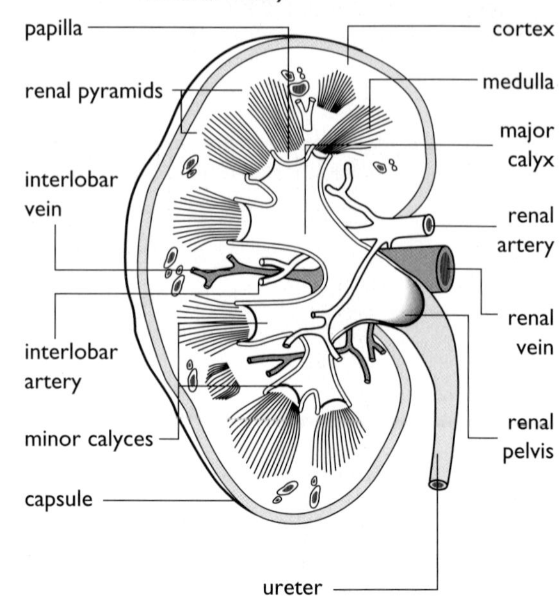


weigh about 100 grams, a small proportion of the total body mass, but they receive about 25% of the cardiac output. The renal blood supply arises from the aorta via the renal arteries and returns to the inferior vena cava via the renal veins. Each kidney is enclosed by a thick fibrous capsule and has two distinct layers: the reddish-brown cortex, which has a rich blood supply, and the inner medulla, within which the functional units of the kidney, the nephrons, can be found (Fig. 2.2).

## The nephron

Each kidney has approximately a million nephrons, which are each about 3 cm long. The nephron is a tubule that is closed at one end and opens into the collecting duct at the other. The nephron has six distinct regions, each of which is adapted to a specific function (Fig. 2.3). There are two types of nephron. Most nephrons (90%) are cortical nephrons; these have short loops of Henle and are mainly concerned with the control of plasma volume during normal conditions. The juxtamedullary nephrons, which have longer loops of Henle, facilitate increased water retention when the availability of water is short.

The renal corpuscle comprises the Bowman's capsule, a blind-ended tube, and the glomerulus, a coiled arrangement of capillaries around which the Bowman's capsule is invaginated. The glomerulus provides a large area of capillary vessels from which substances can leave, crossing the specialized flattened epithelial cells to enter the capsule of the nephron.

There is a double capillary arrangement (see Fig. 2.3) whereby afferent arterioles supply the glomerular capillaries and efferent arterioles lead from the glomerulus to a second capillary bed supplying the rest of the nephron. Differential vascoconstriction of the afferent and efferent arterioles maintains a constant blood pressure within the glomerulus, which results in a constant rate of filtration. Urine production relies on three steps: simple filtration, selective reabsorption and secretion (Fig. 2.4).

## Filtration

Filtration is a passive process that occurs through the semipermeable walls of the glomerulus and glomerular capsule. All substances with a molecular mass of less than 68 kilodaltons (kDa) are forced out of the glomerular capillaries into the Bowman's capsule. So water and small molecules enter the nephron whereas blood cells, plasma proteins and other large molecules are retained in the blood. The content of the Bowman's capsule is referred to as the 'glomerular filtrate' and the rate at which this is formed is referred to as the 'glomerular filtration rate' (GFR). The kidneys form about 180 litres of dilute filtrate each day (a GFR of about 125 ml/min). Most of it is selectively reabsorbed so the final volume of urine produced is about 1 to 1.5 litres per day.

Box 2.2 is an example of disrupted renal function in pregnancy that is detected by abnormal urine content.

**Fig. 2.3** *The nephron and double capillary arrangement. The panel on the right shows the functions of the regions of the nephron.*

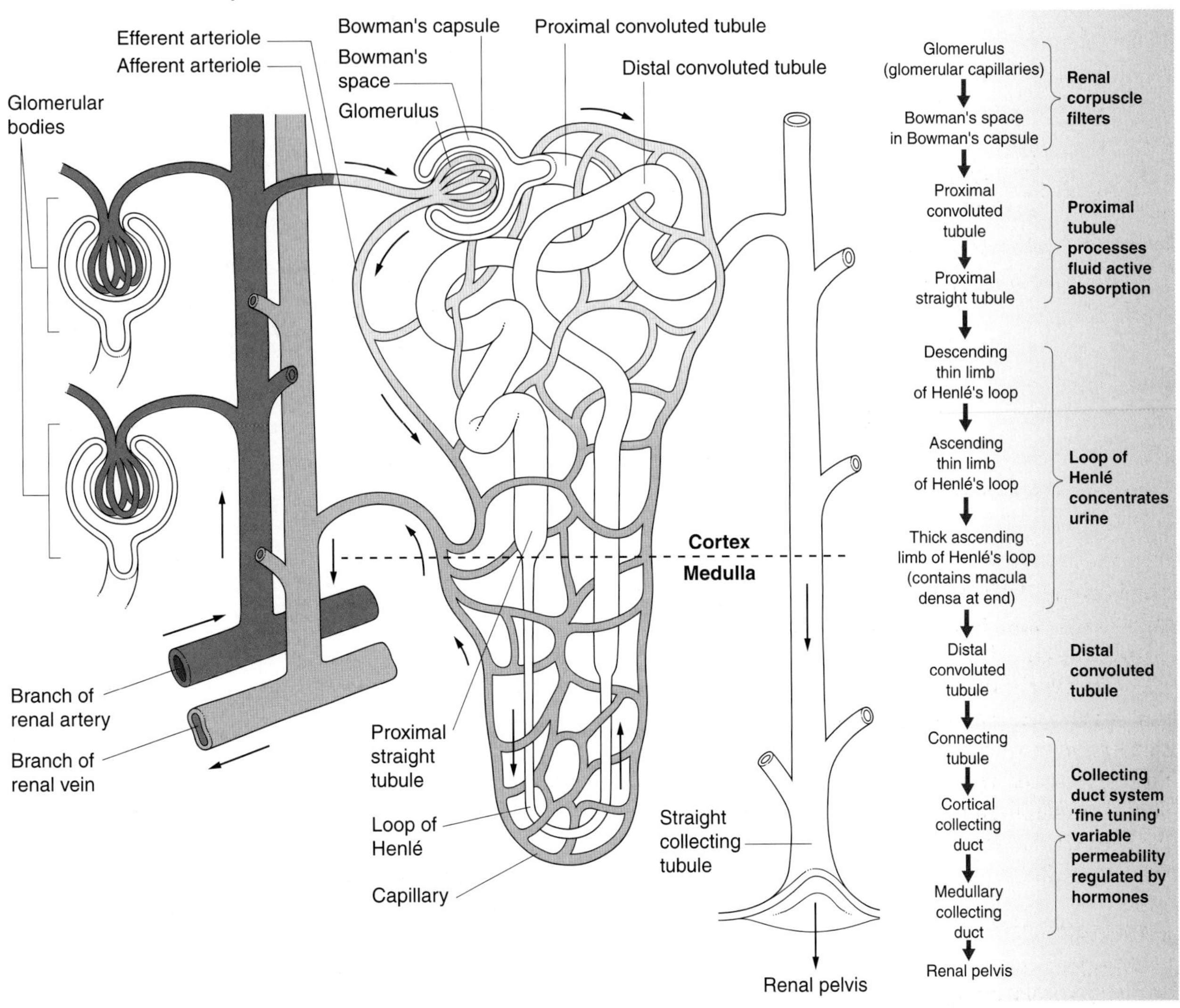


**Box 2.2**

**Hypertension in pregnancy**

Hypertensive disorders in pregnancy can disrupt renal function. The detectable presence of protein within the urine (proteinuria) may indicate that larger molecules than normal are being forced into the Bowman's capsule. This is caused by the increased blood pressure resulting in abnormal ultrafiltration.

## Selective reabsorption

The glomerular filtrate is reabsorbed from the rest of the nephron into the surrounding capillaries. The proximal convoluted tubule is the widest and longest part of the whole nephron (approximately 1.4 cm long). The cells lining it contain a large number of mitochondria to provide energy for facilitating active transport as most of the reabsorption of the glomerular filtrate takes place here. Some substances, such as glucose and amino acids, are completely reabsorbed and are not normally present in urine. Reabsorption of waste products is largely incomplete so, for instance, a large proportion of urea is excreted. The reabsorption of other substances is under the regulation of several hormones. Antidiuretic hormone (ADH) controls the insertion of proteins into the walls of the distal convoluted tubule and collecting ducts, which allows water to leave the filtrate, thus producing less urine (Fig. 2.5). The formation of concentrated urine is facilitated

Fig. 2.4 *Urine production.*

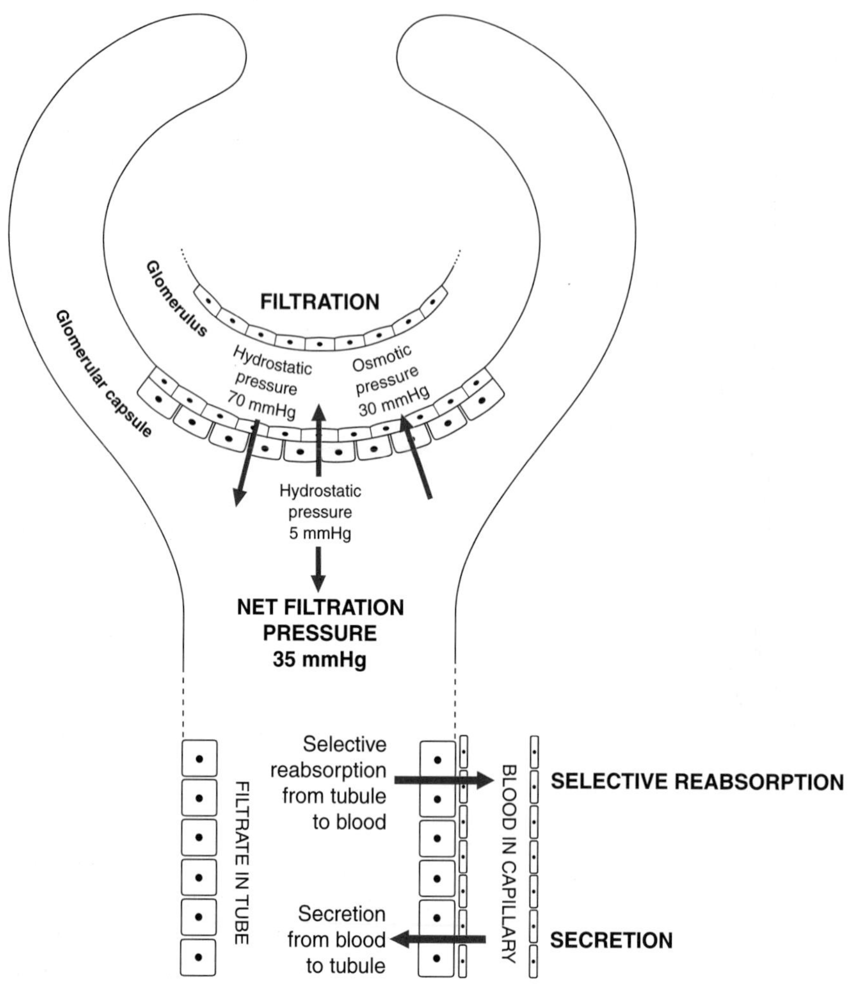


by the physical arrangement of the loop of Henle and its surrounding capillaries, which create and maintain the conditions for the reabsorption of water by osmosis (Fig. 2.6, Box 2.3). Calcitonin regulates the reabsorption of calcium and phosphate. Aldosterone affects the reabsorption of sodium (Fig. 2.7).

**Box 2.3**

**Hypertonic urine**

The evolution of the mammalian kidney has enabled mammals to become highly adapted to terrestrial living. The kidney aids water conservation by producing urine that is able to be concentrated far more than the internal body fluid environment. The scarcer water is within the environment, the longer the nephron to conserve water.

### Secretion

Some waste products may be actively transported directly into the tubules from the surrounding blood capillaries. These include hydrogen and potassium ions, creatinine, toxins and drugs. The cells of the renal tubules synthesize some substances, such as ammonia ions and peptides, which can be secreted into the filtrate.

## *The ureters*

The ureters, which are tubes about 25–30 cm long and 3 mm in diameter, transport the urine from the kidney to the bladder. From each kidney the collecting ducts open into the renal pelvis, which leads to the ureter. The walls of the renal pelvis have smooth muscle, which has intrinsic activity (i.e. not controlled

Fig. 2.5 *The action of ADH.*

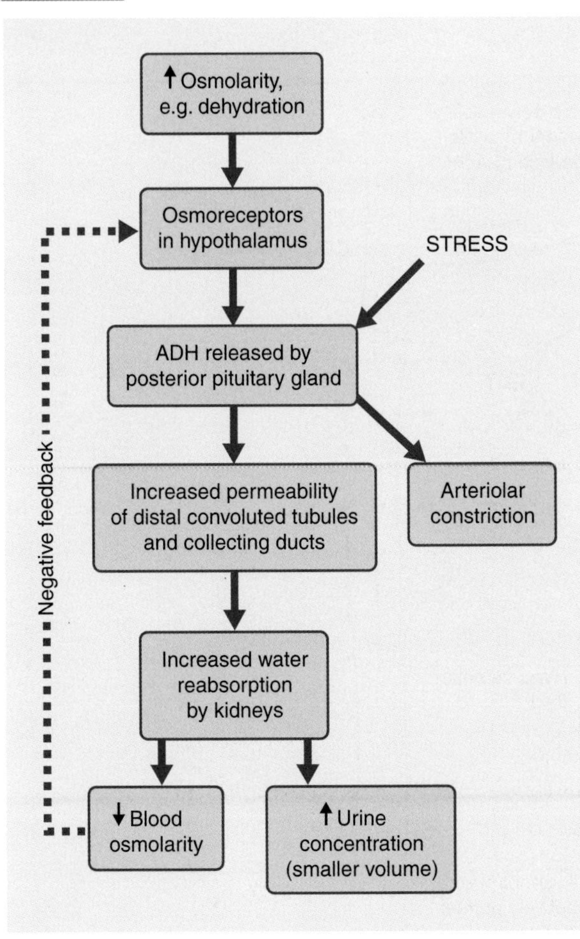


by nerves), generating peristaltic waves of contraction every 10 seconds. These waves of contraction propel urine along the ureters to the bladder. Each ureter is also lined with smooth muscle.

The ureters lie upon the posterior abdominal wall outside the peritoneal cavity, entering the bladder at an oblique angle, one at each side of the base of the specialised muscle area called the trigone which has its apex at the urethral opening. As urine accumulates in the bladder, the ureters are compressed, effectively forming a valve (the vesicoureteral valve), which prevents urinary reflux.

## The bladder

The bladder is also composed of smooth muscle and acts as a reservoir for urine. It is intermittently emptied under conscious control. Stretch receptors within the muscle and trigone provide the signals that indicate that the bladder is full. The normal capacity of the bladder is approximately 700–800 ml; however, the natural desire to void urine becomes conscious when the level of urine in the bladder reaches approximately 300 ml.

As the bladder lies below the uterus, its capacity is compromised by the growing uterus in early pregnancy. Later on, once the pregnant uterus has become an abdominal organ, the pressure on the bladder is relieved. Finally, at the end of pregnancy, bladder capacity is again compromised as the presenting part of the fetus engages, occupying space within the true pelvic cavity.

## The urethra

Urine is voided via the urethra. The female urethra is considerably shorter than the male urethra: only 4 cm in length compared with about 20 cm. This anatomical difference predisposes women towards an increased incidence of ascending urinary tract infections. Thus a colony count of more than 100 000 bacterial cells per millilitre of urine is considered to be pathologically significant. The upper internal sphincter, at the exit from the bladder, is composed of smooth muscle and is under autonomic control. The external sphincter is skeletal muscle and is under voluntary control. The urethra within the male has a dual role as the route for urine and the delivery of spermatozoa, via coitus. Structural differences related to the development of the external genitalia are covered in Chapter 5.

### Urine

Urine has a specific gravity of 1010–1030 and is usually acidic. The volume and final concentration of urea and solutes depend on fluid intake. Sleep and muscular activity also inhibit urine production. The amber colour is due to urobilin, the bile pigment. Urine has a characteristic smell, which is not unpleasant when fresh. Odour or cloudiness generally indicates an infection.

### Control of micturition

Micturition (urination) is a coordinated response that is due to the contraction of the muscular wall of the bladder, reflex relaxation of the internal sphincter of the urethra and voluntary relaxation of the external sphincter (Fig. 2.8). It is assisted by increased pressure in the pelvic cavity as the diaphragm is lowered and

Fig. 2.6 *Formation of concentrated urine.*

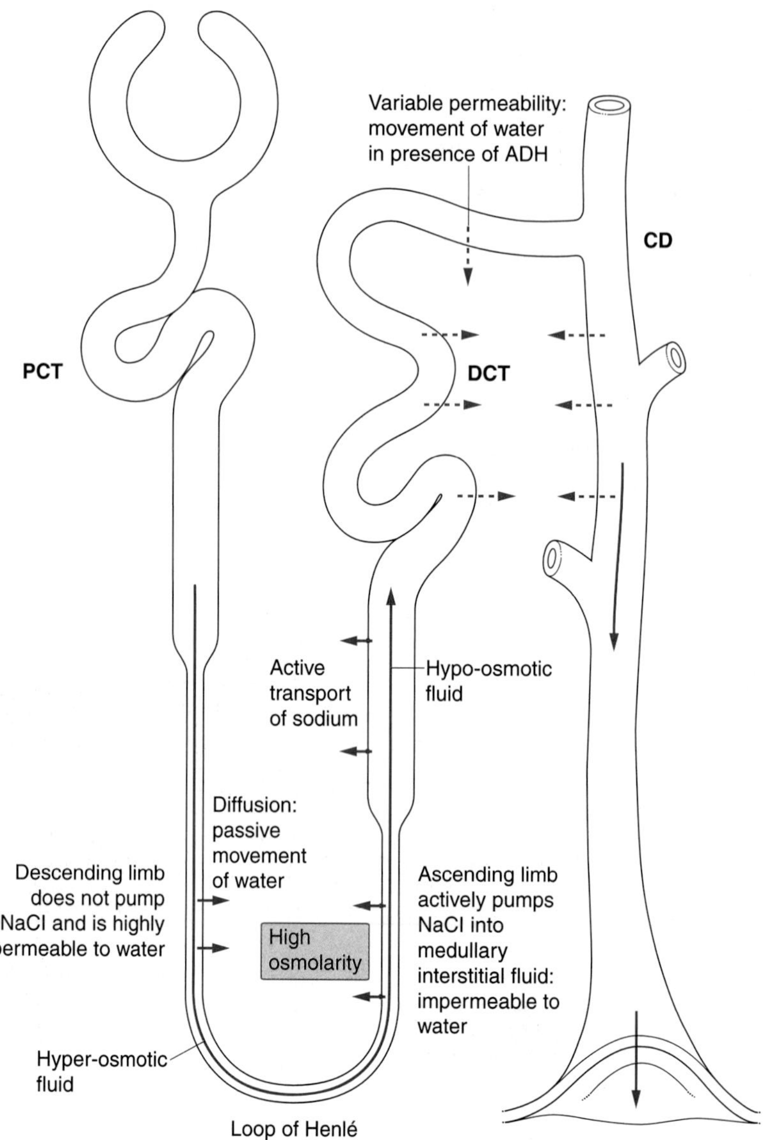


the abdominal muscles contract. Overdistension of the bladder is painful and can cause involuntary relaxation of the external sphincter resulting in incontinence and overflow. The tone of this sphincter is also affected by psychological stimuli (such as waking or getting ready to leave the house) and external stimuli (such as the sound of water or the feel of the lavatory seat). Any factor that raises the intraabdominal and intravesicular pressures (such as laughter or coughing) in excess of the urethral closing pressure can result in stress incontinence.

Accumulation of urine increases bladder wall tension, stimulating the stretch receptors of the bladder, which relay parasympathetic sensory impulses to the brain, generating awareness. However, there is conscious descending inhibition of the reflex bladder contraction and relaxation of the external sphincter. Entry of urine into the urethra irritates and stimulates stretch receptors, augmenting the sensory pathways as the bladder fills. Micturition is postponed until a socially acceptable time and place. This inhibition of the spinal reflex and contraction of the external sphincter is learned. Infants tend to develop bladder control when they are about 2 years old.

Normal physiological control of micturition requires an intact nerve supply to the urinary tract, normal muscle tone (of bladder, urethral sphincters and pelvic floor muscles), absence of any obstruction to flow,

Fig. 2.7 *Aldosterone regulation of sodium excretion.*

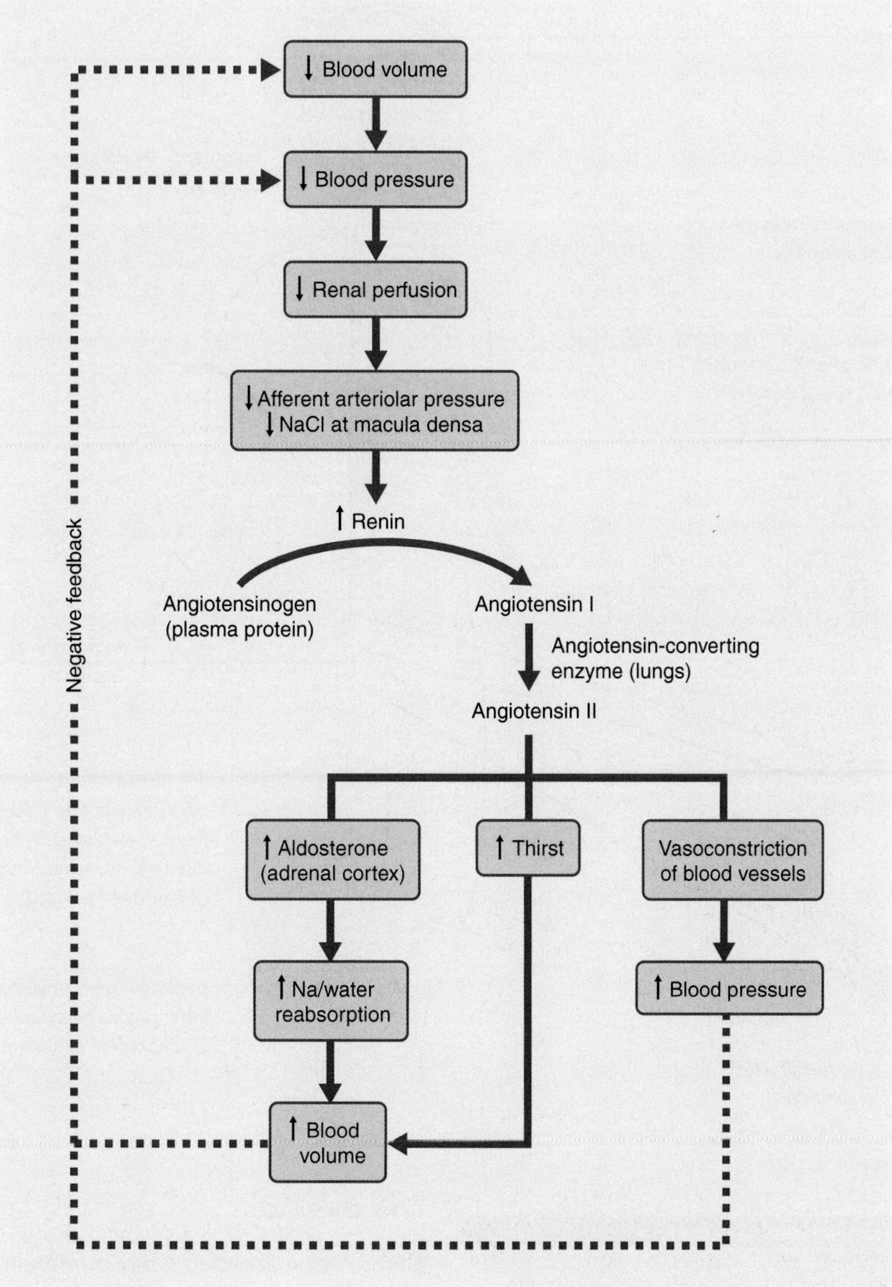


normal bladder capacity and, finally, the absence of psychological factors that may inhibit the micturition cycle (such as embarrassment and discomfort).

## The female reproductive tract

The main features of the female reproductive tract distinguishing it from the male are that the female reproductive organs are internal and in the non-pregnant state are situated within the true pelvic cavity. The female reproductive tract consists of two ovaries, two uterine (fallopian) tubes, the uterus and cervix, the vagina and external genitalia. The female reproductive system undergoes considerable changes throughout life from childhood through reproductive life (see Box 2.4) to the menopause. Superimposed on these changes are the effects of the menstrual cycle.

Fig. 2.8 *Control of micturition. (Reproduced with permission from Brooker 1998.)*

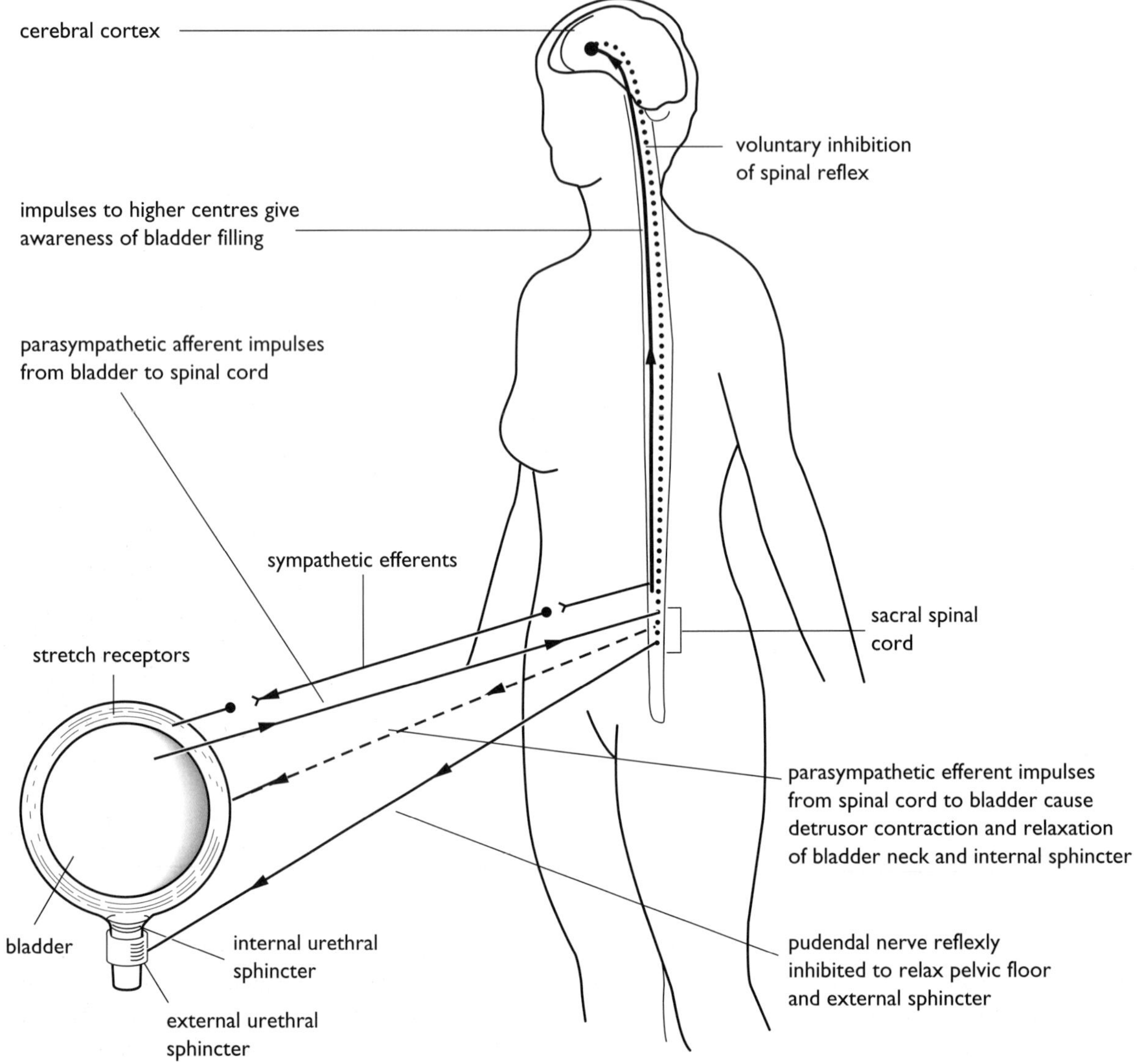


**Box 2.4**

**Changes to the genital tract at puberty**

- Hair appears on mons veneris and subcutaneous fat accumulates
- Secretory glands mature and become active
- Labia majora and minora become pigmented with melanin
- Enlargement of the clitoris occurs
- Vaginal epithelium thickens and becomes responsive to oestrogen
- Vaginal pH decreases as lactobacilli metabolize glycogen from cell secretions
- Uterus grows and cervix doubles in length

## The ovaries

The ovaries are dull-white almond-shaped bodies, approximately 4 cm long. They lie posteriorly and laterally to the body of the uterus and below the uterine tubes. They are anchored by the ovarian ligaments and attached to the posterior layer of the broad ligament, a fold within the peritoneum that extends from the uterus (Fig. 2.9). The blood supply to the ovary is via the ovarian artery, which runs alongside the ovarian ligament, and the ovarian branch of the uterine artery (see Fig. 2.12, p. 44). This dual blood supply is important in maintaining reproductive function; if the ovary becomes twisted, by a tumour or cystic growth

**Fig. 2.9** *Position of the ovary, and ovarian and broad ligaments. (Reproduced with permission from Sweet 1996.)*

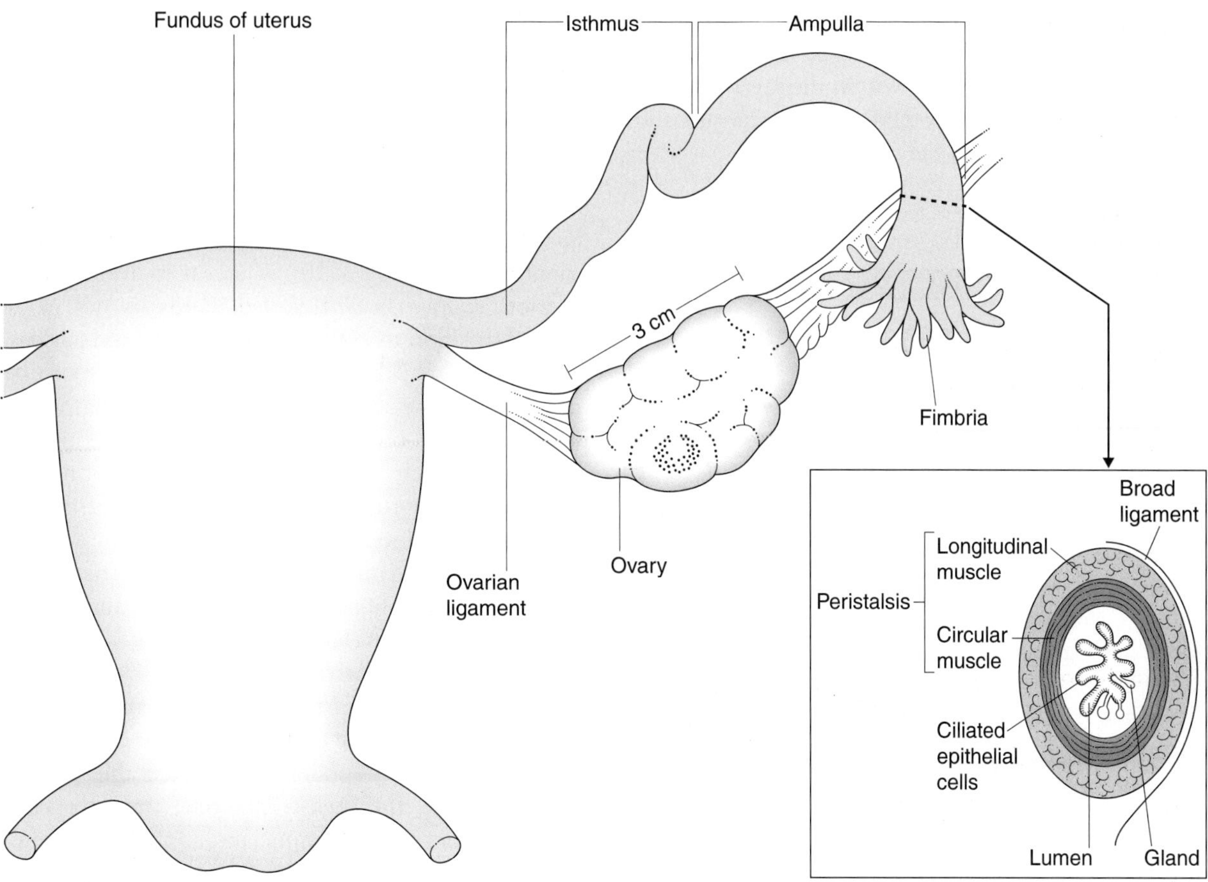


for instance, the ovarian ligament may occlude the blood supply to the ovary along the ovarian artery. This torsion of the ovary can cause ischaemia of the tissues and intense pain.

The ovaries are composed of two distinct layers: the outer layer is the cortex and the inner section is referred to as the medulla. The ovary is contained within a sheath of connective tissue, the tunica albuginea. The cortex contains the developing follicles that contain the primary oocyte and is also responsible for the production of the female steroid hormones oestrogen and progesterone (see Chs 4 and 5). The medulla is composed primarily of connective tissue and blood vessels and provides precursors to facilitate steroid production within the cortex.

## The uterine (fallopian) tubes

The uterine tubes (also known as the fallopian tubes or oviducts) are approximately 12 cm long and have walls of smooth muscle lined with ciliated epithelial and secretory cells. The distal end of the uterine tube has specialized structures called fimbriae, which surround the opening into the tube. The fimbriae lie in close proximity to the ovary and, at ovulation, assist the entry of the ovum into the uterine tube by a wafting action, which facilitates movement of the interperitoneal fluid. The lining of the uterine tubes lies in many folds (called plicae) and is composed of ciliated columnar epithelial cells interspersed with goblet cells that secret pyruvate to nourish the ovum. The cilia facilitate the movement of the ovum down the uterine tube; this is augmented by coordinated peristaltic contractions of the smooth muscle. The distal end of the uterine tube has a slightly wider area, called the ampulla, where fertilization of the ovum by the sperm usually occurs.

If both uterine tubes are completely blocked, fertilization is prevented as the sperm are unable to access the ovum. If one uterine tube is patent or only partially blocked then sperm may encounter and fertilize an ovum within the peritoneal cavity. However, if a fertilized ovum enters a partially or totally blocked uterine tube its passage to the uterus will be impeded and so the pregnancy may develop within the uterine tube or peritoneal cavity (see Box 2.5). The uterine tubes are mobile and not fixed to the ovary.

**Box 2.5**

**Tubal (ectopic) pregnancy**

An ectopic pregnancy is usually confirmed by a positive pregnancy test in conjunction with a ultrasound scan revealing an empty uterine cavity. Levels of human chorionic gonadotrophin (hCG) are also markedly lower in ectopic pregnancy. The warning sign of an ectopic pregnancy is abdominal pain at around 8 weeks' gestation. If the uterine tube ruptures then the woman may become clinically shocked owing to excessive bleeding into the peritoneal cavity. The growing fetus can be surgically removed together with the damaged uterine tube if necessary (this is referred to as a salpingectomy). Occasionally an abdominal pregnancy may ensue if implantation occurs on the peritoneum. The pregnancies rarely go to term; however, delivery of live infants via abdominal surgery have been documented. The main causes of tubal blockage are infection (pelvic inflammatory disease) and the formation of scar tissue from extensive surgery or trauma.

## The uterus

The functions of the uterus are to prepare to receive the fertilized ovum, to provide a suitable environment for growth and development of the fetus and to assist in the expulsion of the fetus, placenta and membranes at delivery. In the non-pregnant state the uterus is situated within the true pelvic cavity. It is described as being anteverted (tilted forwards) and anteflexed (curved forward), situated in a superior position to the urinary bladder (Fig. 2.10). A uterus in an abnormal position, such as a retroverted uterus, is not in an optimal position to expand in pregnancy and surgical intervention may be required to adjust its position to allow the pregnancy to proceed. The anatomical position of the uterus is maintained by the uterine ligaments, which are important in supporting the weight of the uterus, particularly during contractions (Fig. 2.11). Its blood supply is shown in Figure 2.12.

The non-pregnant uterus weighs approximately 50 g with a cavity of approximately 10 ml and is composed of three layers (Fig. 2.13). The inner layer of the uterus is the endometrium. This layer is markedly different in the body of the uterus compared with the cervix. The cells of the endometrium are ciliated and the entire cell layer undergoes considerable growth changes during the menstrual cycle; the superficial decidual layers are shed in menstruation at the end of the cycle (see Ch. 4). The vascular connective tissue, or stroma, contains many glands that secrete alkaline mucus into the uterine cavity.

**Fig. 2.10** ***The anteverted and anteflexed position of the non-pregnant uterus. (Reproduced with permission from Sweet 1996.)***

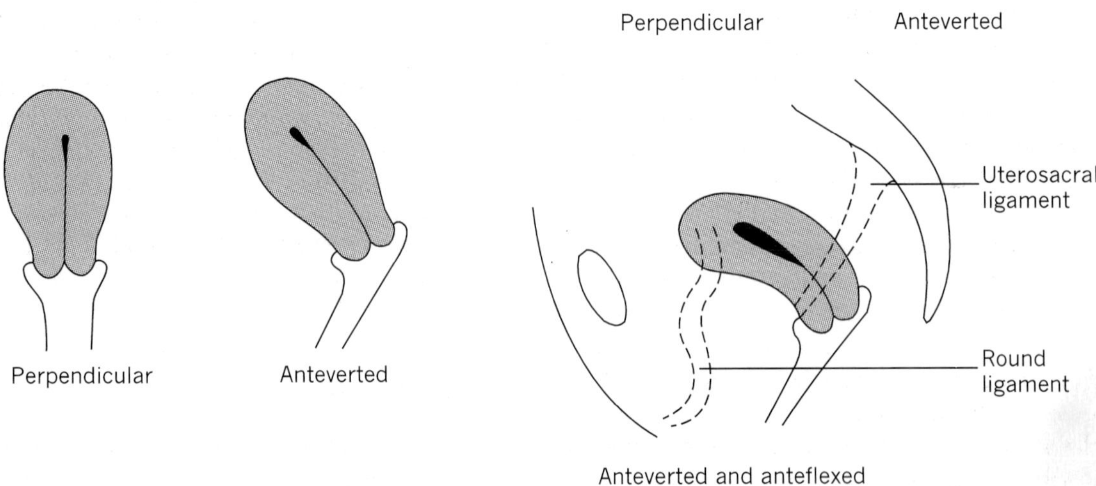

**Fig. 2.11** *The uterine ligaments (transverse and coronal sections). (Reproduced with permission from Sweet 1996.)*

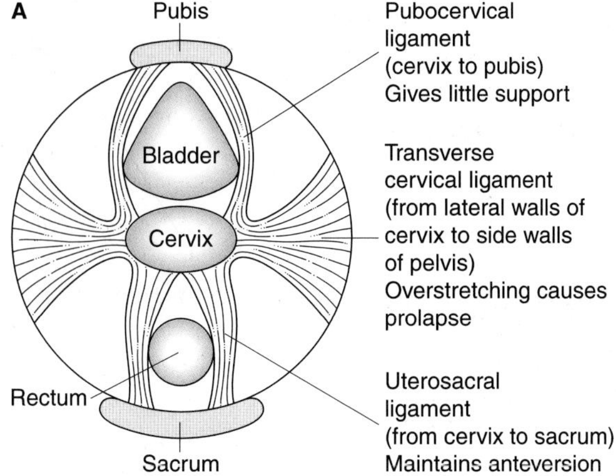


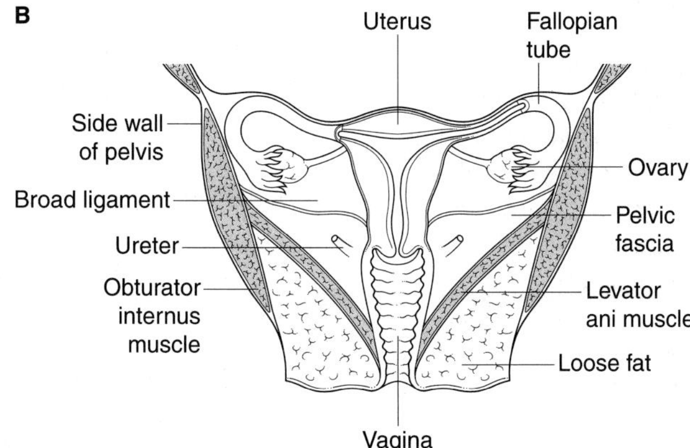


The middle layer is composed of smooth muscle, called the myometrium, which is arranged in three muscle layers (see Box 2.6). In the non-pregnant state these are not very distinctive.

The uterus has an outer layer of peritoneum that drapes over the uterus anteriorly to form a fold between the uterus and bladder, and over the uterine tubes to cover the myometrium. This is referred to as the perimetrium; it forms the broad ligament, thus maintaining the anatomical position of the uterus. The body of the uterus is about 5 cm in both length and width (excluding the dimensions of the cervix).

The uterus is innervated by both parasympathetic (arising from the second, third and fourth sacral segments) and sympathetic nerves via the presacral nerve (branching from the aortic plexus) and branches from the lumbar sympathetic chain. Both types of innervation to the uterus are via the Lee–Frankehauser plexus, which is situated in the lower region of the pouch of Douglas.

**Box 2.6**

**The uterine muscle layers**

1. *Inner layer*: fibres in the longitudinal plane that run from the anterior cervix, up over the fundus and back to the posterior edge of the cervix
2. *Middle layer*: interlaced spiral fibres concentrated in, and originating from, the fundal region of the uterus and getting less dense approaching the cervical region; the circular arrangement of the fibres is accentuated at the junctions with the uterine tubes and the cervix (internal os) thus providing closures to the expanding pregnant uterus
3. *Outer layer*: combination of longitudinal and circular fibres

## *The cervix*

The cervix is the neck of the uterus. It has an important role in protecting the uterus from infection and

Fig. 2.12 *The uterine and ovarian blood supply.*

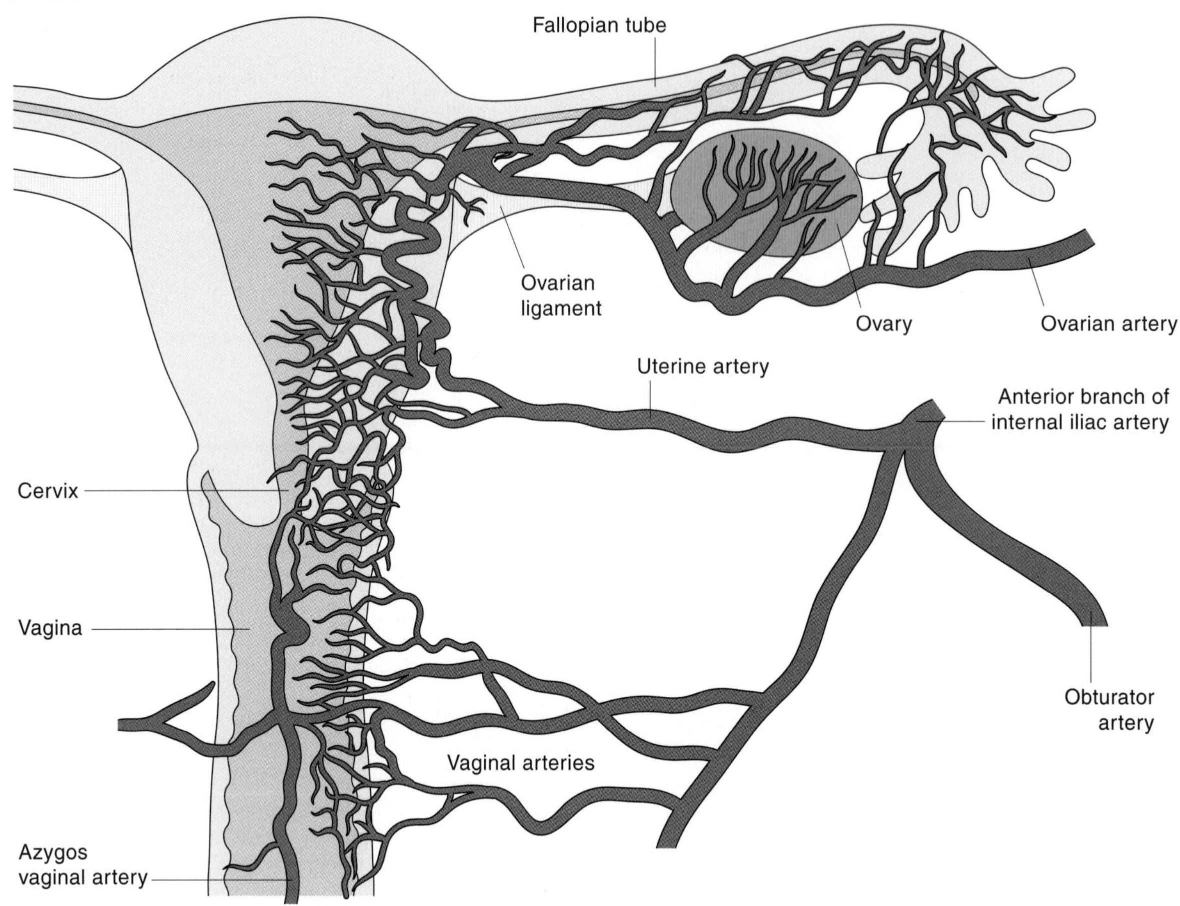


undergoes important changes preceding labour (see Ch. 13). The isthmus, an indistinct layer of tissue that forms the lower uterine segment in pregnancy (see Ch. 13), separates the body of the uterus and the cervix. The cervix is about 2.5 cm in length and is composed of dense collagenous circular fibres. The cervix is spindle shaped with an os (smooth muscle arrangement forming a constriction) at the top and bottom. The internal os forms the inner opening of the cervix at the junction with the body of the uterus. The external os is located at the bottom of the cervical canal where it projects into the vagina. Two different types of cell meet at this junction: the columnar cells of the cervical canal and the squamous epithelial cells of the outer cervix. Abnormal precancerous cells are most likely to arise at this junction. The shape of the spatula used to take cell samples during a cervical smear accommodates the curve of the external part of the cervix. The lining of the cervix does not undergo cyclical changes in growth rate although glandular activity changes. The inner tissue lies in folds that appear branched, giving it the name arbor vitae. These folds allow dilatation during delivery.

## The vagina

The vagina is a distensible muscular tube, about 8 cm long, situated within the true pelvic cavity, extending through the pelvic floor from the cervix to the vulva. The vagina is described as a potential tube because its walls are in contact but easily separated. The cervix protrudes into the vagina, normally pointing to the posterior wall of the vagina because of the anteverted and anteflexed position of the uterus. The spaces between the cervix and the upper portion of the vaginal wall are referred to as the anterior, lateral and posterior fornices (singular: fornix). The vagina has three main functions: the facilitation of coitus, as a passage for the release of the menses and as the route for the baby to be born, commonly referred to as the birth canal. It also helps to support the uterus and prevent ascending infection.

**Fig. 2.13** ***Structure of the A non-pregnant uterus and B endometrium. (B Reproduced with permission from Brooker 1998.)***

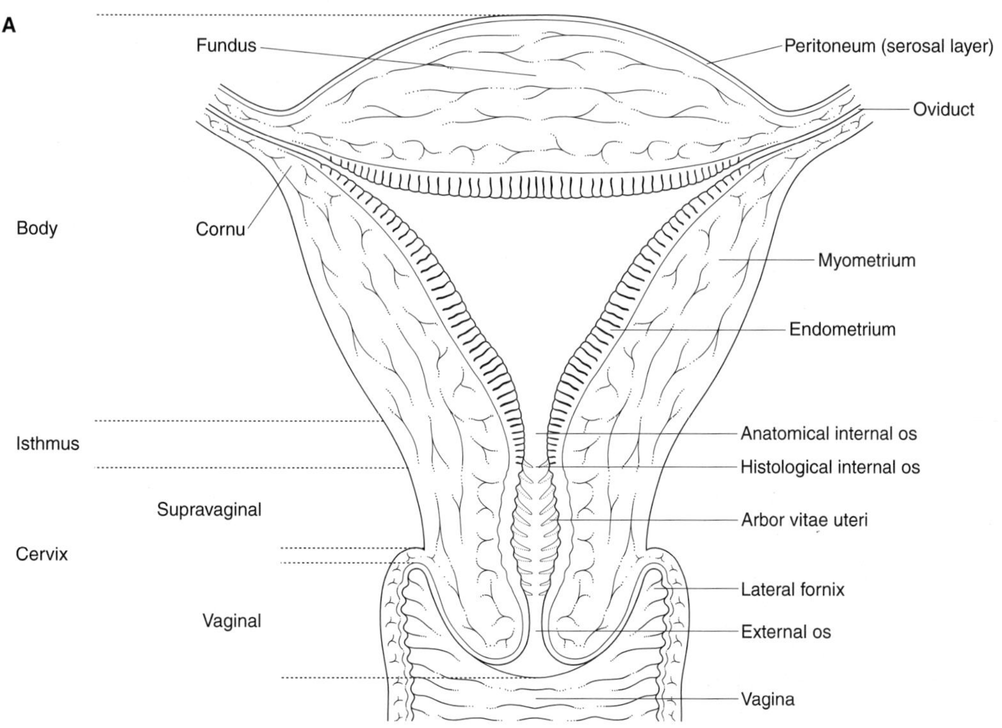


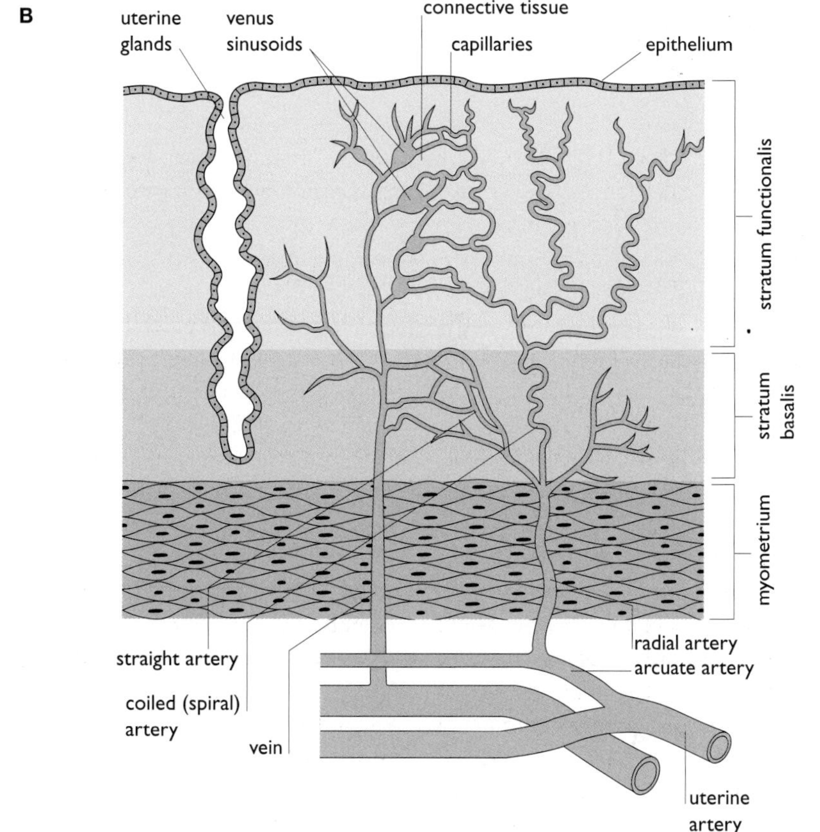

The vagina is lined by a layer of moist epithelial cells folded into ridges (called rugae) that distend during childbirth, thus facilitating the stretching of the vagina. There is also a lining of smooth muscle, which maintains the tone of the vagina. The opening of the vagina, which is a skeletal muscle sphincter, is protected by the external genitalia. It lies below the urethral opening, which is situated below the clitoris (see Fig. 2.14). The vagina does not have glands but is maintained in a moist state by secretions from the cervical glands and transudate of fluid from the blood vessels that lie below the vaginal lining.

### The external genitalia

The external genitalia are those structures that can be seen (Fig. 2.14). Most of the structures are well innervated; therefore they are very sensitive and are a source of sexual arousal responses. The external genitalia are well vascularized, which means they bleed easily if subjected to trauma but also heal rapidly.

The mons veneris is a pad of subcutaneous fat covered by skin lying over the pubic bone; it functions as a cushion during intercourse. At puberty it becomes covered with pubic hair, which is coarse and curly because of the unusually oblique hair follicles. The labia majora (singular: labium majus) are two fatty folds of tissue extending from the mons veneris in which the round ligaments terminate. The labia majora narrow where they come together between the vagina and anus. The outer surface is covered in pubic hair; the inner surface is rich in sebaceous and sweat glands. The labia majora enclose and protect the urogenital cleft. The labia minora are two smaller longitudinal fleshy folds of tissue; they are erectile and very vascular. They are pigmented, hairless and have some sweat and sebaceous glands. The labia minora enclose the clitoris anteriorly and unite posteriorly at the fourchette, which is commonly torn at the first

**Fig. 2.14** ***The female external genitalia.***

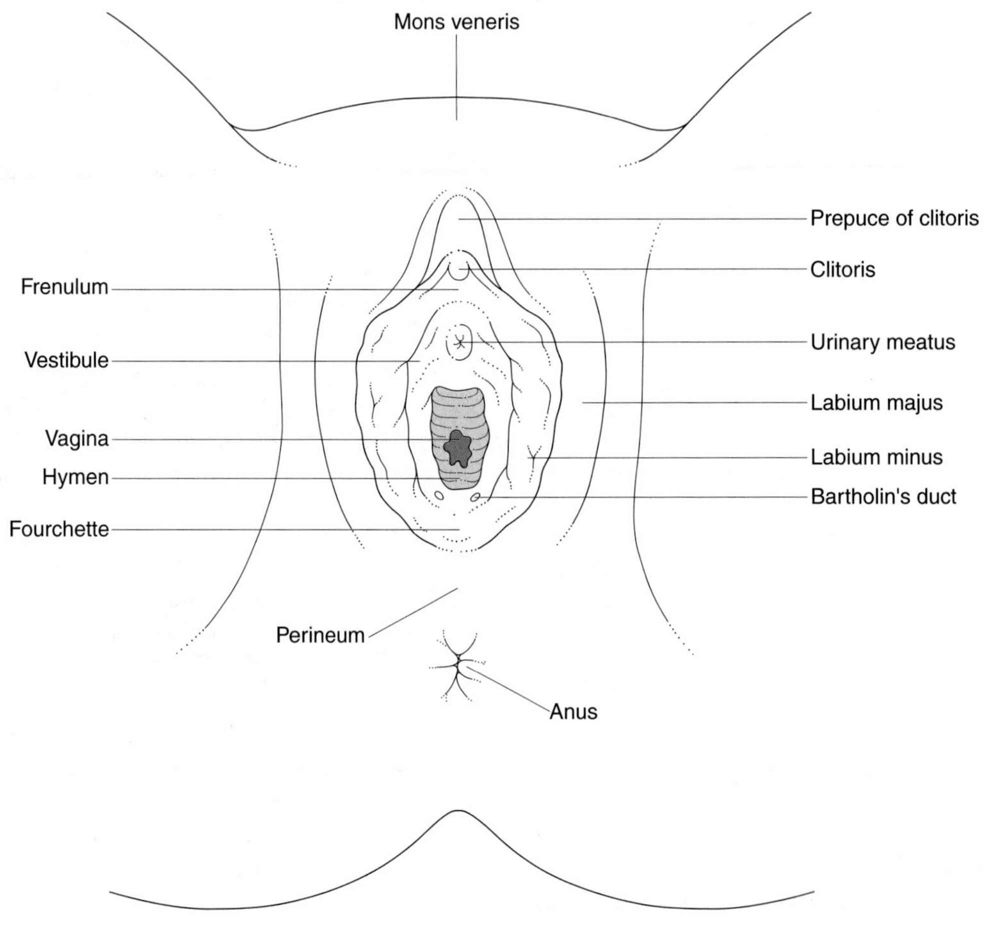

delivery. The functions of the labia minora are probably to increase the depth of the vaginal canal during intercourse and to increase retention of the ejaculate following intercourse.

The clitoris is a highly sensitive erectile body that is about 2.5 cm long exteriorly, projecting internally for up to 9 cm (O'Connell et al 1998). The erectile bodies, analogous to the spongy tissue structures of the penis, become erect and engorged on stimulation. The clitoris is an important source of sexual arousal, generating reflex lubrication responses from the surrounding tissue.

When the labia are held open, the vestibule (area from clitoris to fourchette) can be seen. It contains the external orifice of the urethra. This urinary meatus lies about 2.5 cm below the clitoris and is a characteristic vertical slit with prominent margins. It is important to identify this in women requiring catheterization. To each side, slightly behind the urinary meatus are the dimple-like exits of the Skene's ducts, which produce mucus. The vaginal orifice is partly occluded by the protective hymen, which is probably most important in preventing ascending infection before puberty when the pH of the vagina is less acidic. The Bartholin's glands lie posteriorly, each side of the vagina. These mucus-producing glands are the size and shape of haricot beans and, unless inflamed, cannot normally be seen. Their rate of secretion increases with the erection of the clitoris. The vestibular bulb posterior to the vagina is also formed of erectile spongy tissue.

Box 2.7 is an example of problems caused by mutilation of the external genitalia.

**Box 2.7**

**Female genital mutilation ('female circumcision')**

Many ethnic groups, particularly those of Muslim origin in North Africa, Indonesia and other countries, regard genital mutilation as an essential preparation for marriage. This ritual cleansing, performed in infancy, early childhood or puberty, may involve removal of the prepuce of the clitoris, removal of the labia minora and clitoris or removal of most of the labia and clitoris. The practice may include use of thorns to form stitches of the vaginal walls. Although the practice is illegal in Western Europe, it may be undertaken illicitly or girls may be mutilated in other countries. At delivery, the urogenital tissue is extremely vulnerable to trauma, which can be minimised by anterior and mediolateral episiotomy incision. Failure to deliver vaginally may result in rejection of the woman from her family.

**Box 2.8**

**Functions and characteristics of the pelvic floor**

- Its muscles are arranged in two layers: superficial and deep (see Fig. 2.15)
- It supports the internal female reproductive organs
- It provides voluntary muscle control for micturition and defaecation
- It facilitates birth by resisting descent of the descending presenting part, so forcing the fetus to rotate forward in the presence of strong regular uterine contractions

## The pelvic floor

The pelvic floor is primarily composed of soft tissues suspended within the outlet of the pelvis, forming a sling-like sheet of tissue that encloses the pelvic contents (Box 2.8). In women the main characteristic distinguishing it from that of the pelvic floor of the male is that there are three openings instead of two. As well as the anal canal and urethra, the female also has a vaginal opening.

## Pelvic shape and adaptation

The pelvis is a girdle composed of a number of bones held together by ligaments and cartilaginous and fused joints (Fig. 2.16). The dimensions of the inlet, cavity and outlet affect the passage of the fetus. This means that the fetus has to negotiate the pelvic cavity by undergoing a rotational manoeuvre. The sling-like arrangement of the gutter-shaped pelvic floor muscles means that the fetus is forced to rotate in a forward position.

Traditionally pelvic morphology has distinguished four major categories (Fig. 2.17). In practice, there is a wide variation in pelvic form combining features from all four of the categories. There are also recognized abnormalities of the pelvis including justominor pelvis (normal shape but overall dimensions smaller than normal), Nägelles pelvis (asymmetrical due to abnormal bone formation on one side), and Robert's pelvis (similar to Nägelles pelvis but the abnormal bone formation is bilateral). Pelvic shape can also be affected by disease, for example rachitic pelvis due to rickets, which is an extreme form of the platypelloid pelvis.

Fig. 2.15 *A the superficial pelvic floor muscles; B the deep pelvic floor muscles. (Reproduced with permission from Bennett & Brown 1999.)*

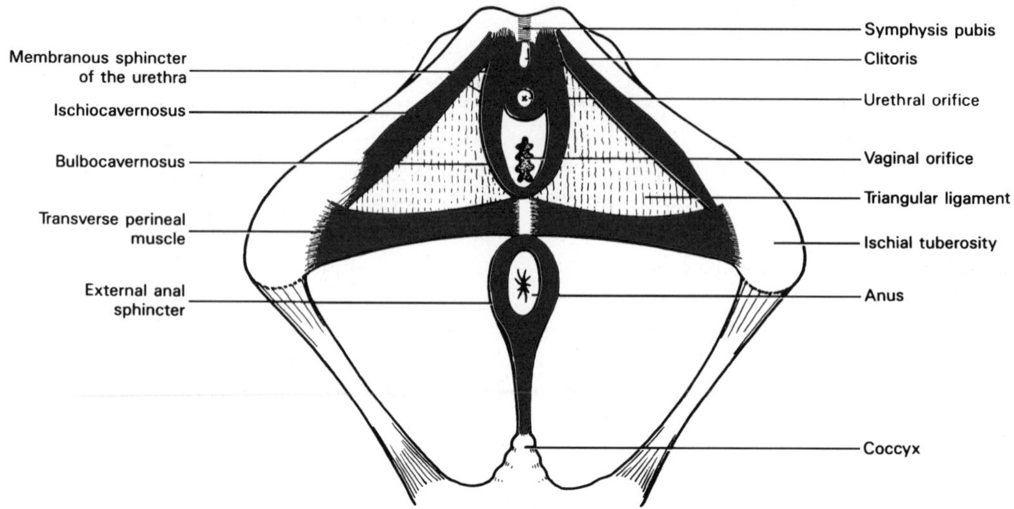


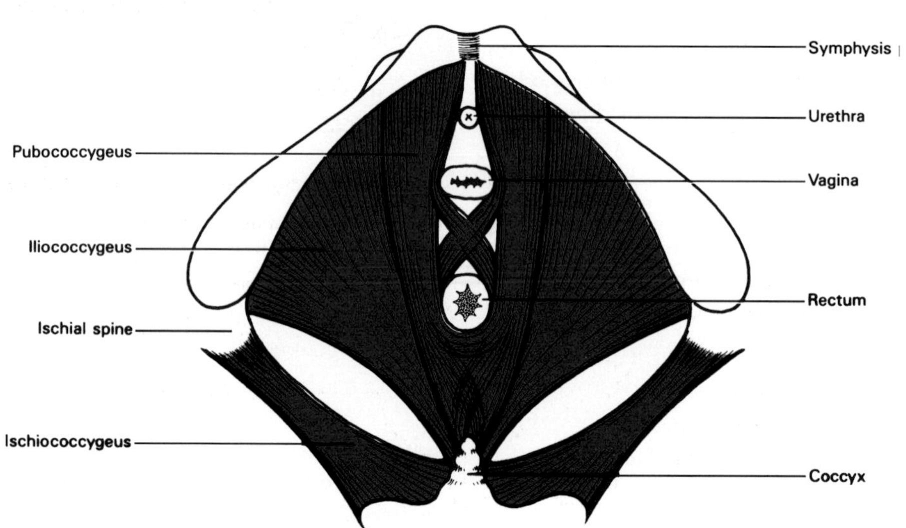


The shape of the pelvis affects the mechanism of labour (see Ch. 13); abnormal pelvic shape is associated with problems at delivery.

## The male reproductive tract

The male reproductive tract comprises a number of structures that permit gamete formation to occur below body temperature and provide conditions that allow sperm maturation and ejection (Fig. 2.18).

### The testes

The testes are suspended within the scrotal sac or scrotum. Optimal spermatogenesis in the human is achieved 2–3°C below the body's core temperature. There are a number of mechanisms to regulate the temperature of the testes. The testes are suspended outside the abdominal cavity but can be retracted upwards towards the warmth of the body by the constriction of the cremaster muscle. This muscle will also reflexly raise the testes towards the body if the inner thigh is scratched; this is used as a neurological test.

**Fig. 2.16** *The pelvic girdle: A the normal female pelvis; B innominate bone showing important landmarks; C posterior view of the pelvis to show ligaments. (Reproduced with permission from Bennett & Brown 1999.)*

A

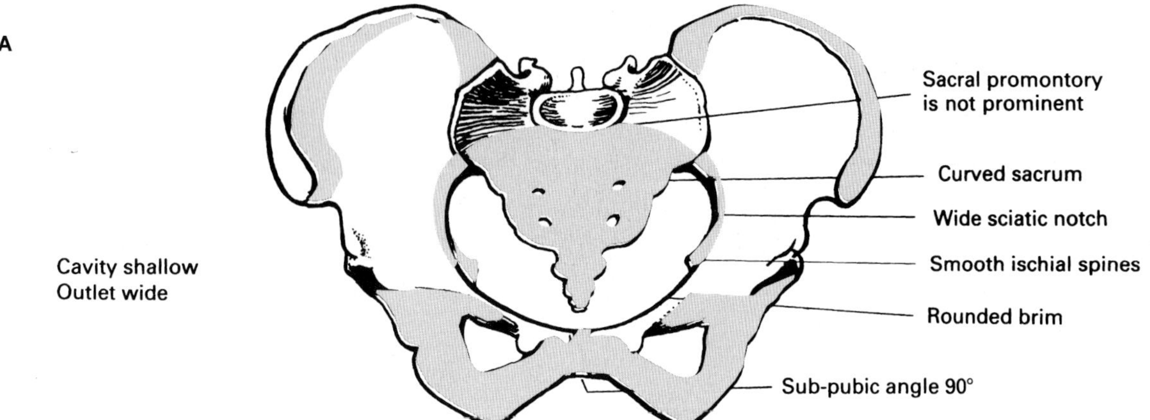


B

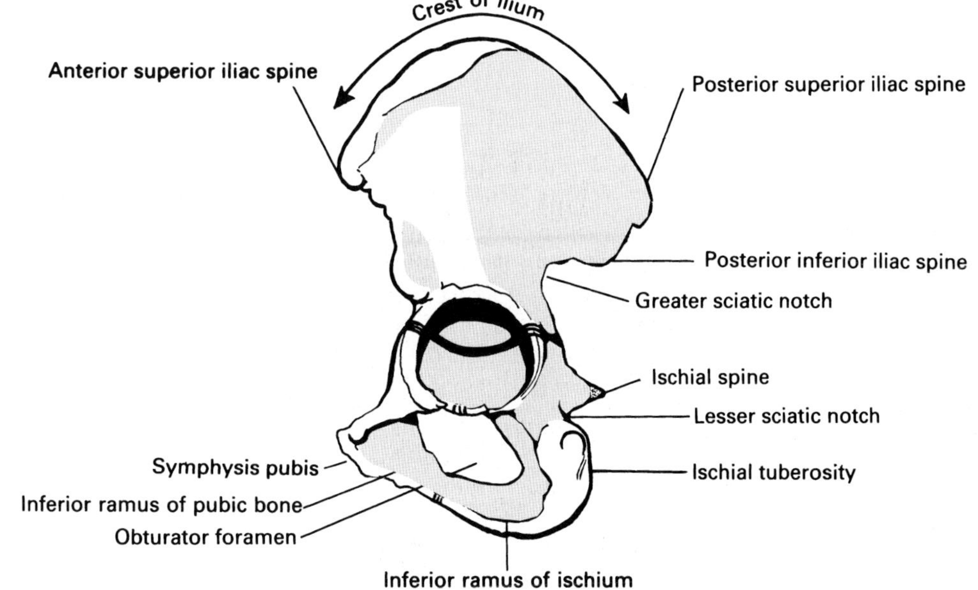


C

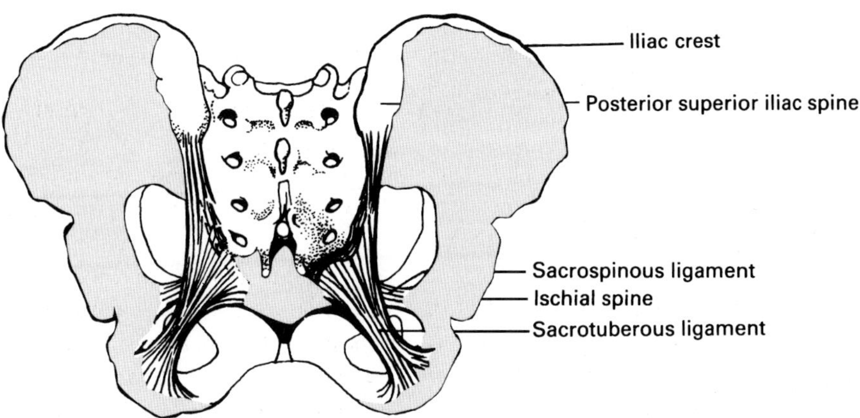

**Fig. 2.17** *Characteristics of the four categories of pelvic shape.*

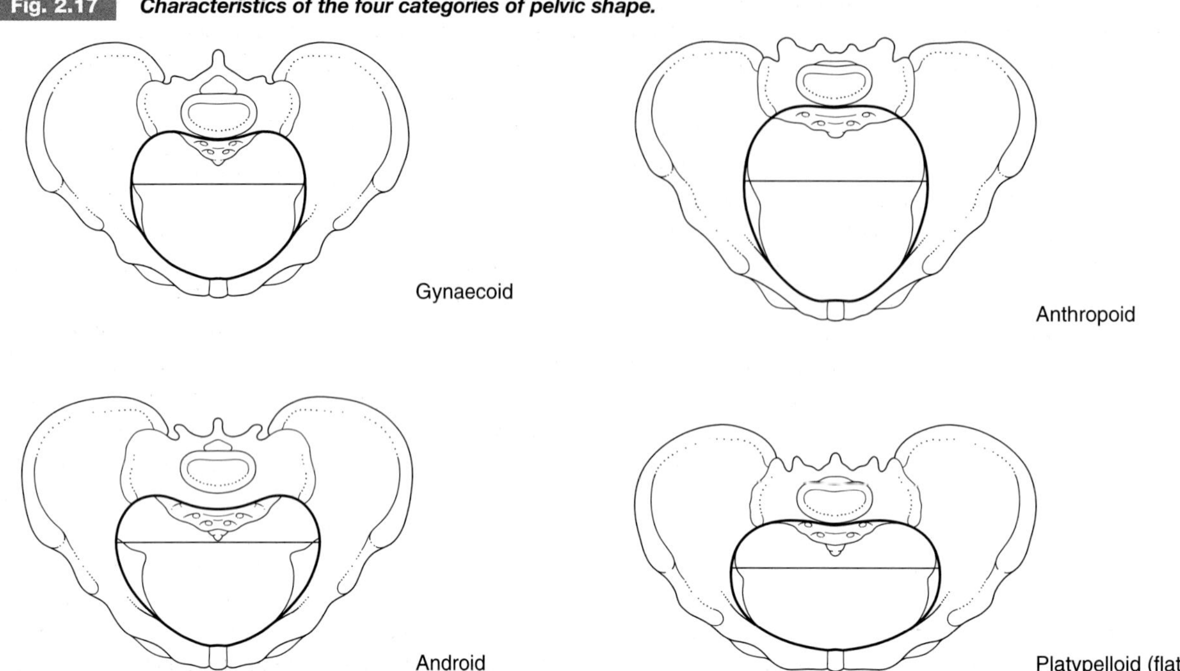


**Fig. 2.18** *The male reproductive system. (Reproduced with permission from Brooker 1998.)*

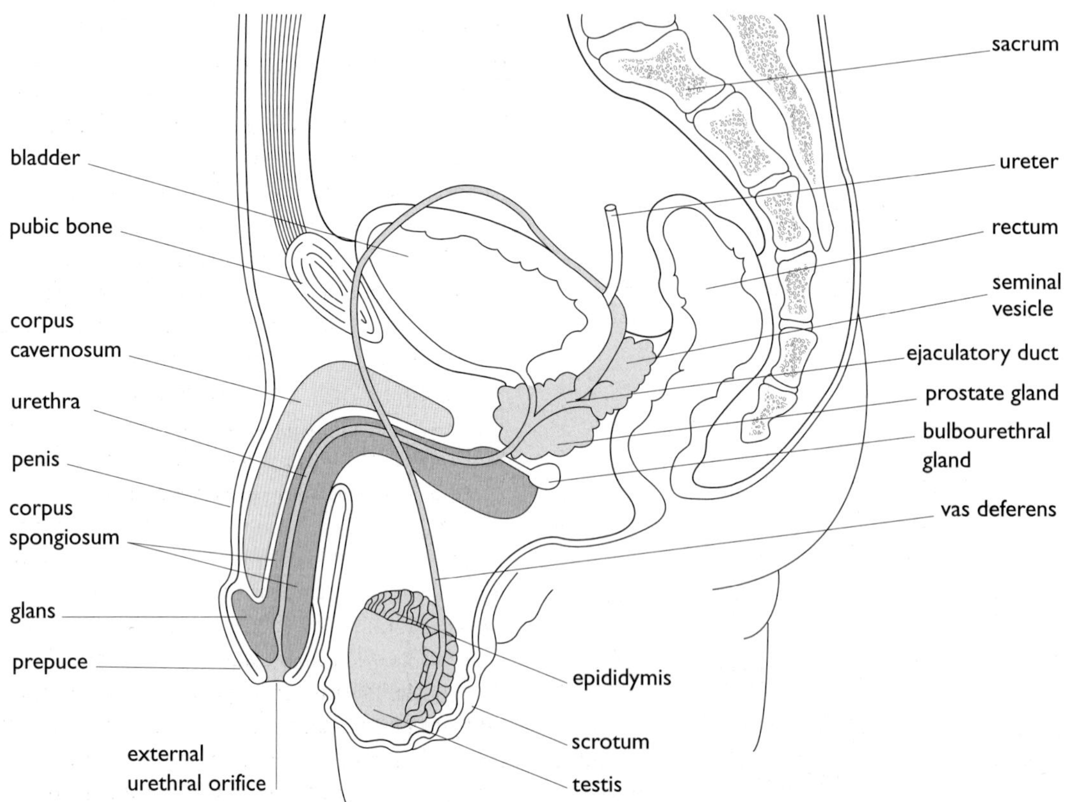

The pigmented skin of the scrotum lies in rugae (folds), which increase the surface area. The scrotum is well vascularized but has no insulating hair or subcutaneous fat. It is lined by dartos muscle, which contracts in response to cold. Blood flow to the testes allows heat to be transferred from the descending testicular arteries to the ascending pampiniform venous plexus forming a countercurrent heat exchange mechanism, which helps to maintain the lower temperature of the testes relative to the body.

The testes are a pair of glandular organs, analogous to the ovaries, that produce gametes (spermatozoa) and male sex hormones. Within the scrotum, the testes are surrounded by a thick fibrous capsule called the tunica albuginea, which penetrates internally dividing the testes into lobules. Each testis has about 200 lobules, each containing about three seminiferous tubules, about 0.2 mm in diameter and up to 70 cm long (Fig. 2.19). The seminiferous tubules are the site of spermatogenesis (sperm production). Within the tubules are spermatogenic cells and their supporting Sertoli cells. Between the tubules are the interstitial cells of Leydig, which produce testosterone.

**Fig. 2.19** ***The structure of the testis and ducts conveying sperm from the seminiferous tubules to the urethra. (Reproduced with permission from Brooker 1998.)***

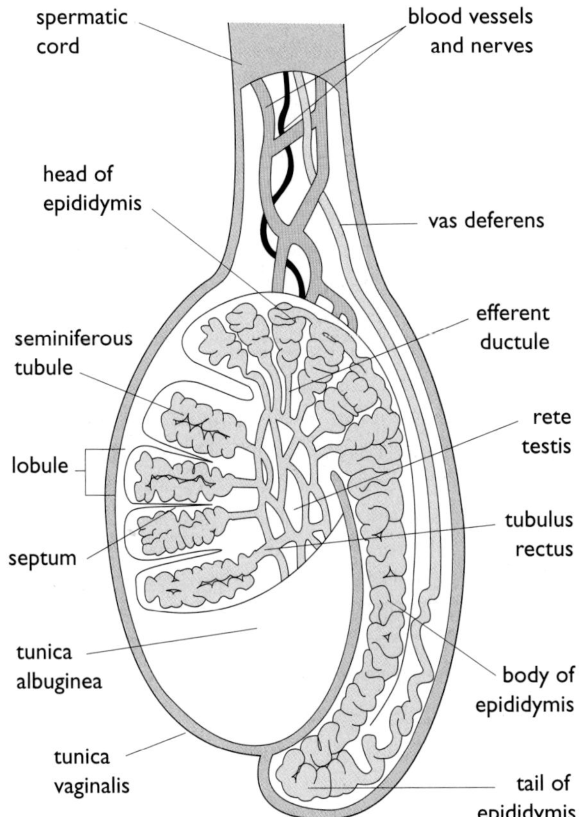


The sperm produced from the seminiferous tubules are stored in the epididymis where they are concentrated, becoming mature and motile. The epididymis is a comma-shaped convoluted tube, about 6 cm long, leading into the vas deferens. The vas deferens provides the conduit for sperm delivery during emission and ejaculation. It is a thick-walled tube leading from the tail of the epididymis to the ejaculatory duct. The vas deferens dilates into a storage reservoir, or ampulla, just before it joins with the exit of the seminal vesicle to form the ejaculatory duct. Just as infection or trauma can cause blockage of the uterine tubes, the male reproductive capacity can be also affected by blockage, of the epididymis and vas deferens for instance, impeding the passage of spermatozoa. The vas deferens, blood vessels and cremaster muscle lie closely together forming the spermatic cord.

The seminal vesicles are two pyramid-shaped membranous sacs, about 4 cm long, lying between the base of the bladder and the rectum. They produce semen, a fructose-rich viscous fluid, for sperm transport and nourishment. Secretory activity of the seminal vesicles depends on the level of testosterone. The ejaculatory ducts begin at the base of the prostate gland and terminate in the single prostatic urethra. These muscular ducts carry sperm and seminal fluid through the prostate gland. The prostate gland is a walnut-sized exocrine gland lying just below the neck of the bladder, between the rectum and pubic bone. It is a compound gland, formed of about 20–40 smaller glandular units each with its own exit into the ejaculatory duct. Prostatic fluid is a thin lubricating secretion that mixes with the sperm and seminal fluid. The prostatic gland can be palpated through the rectal wall. In elderly men, the prostate gland may undergo benign hypertrophy, which can compress the urethra and impede micturition. Prostatic carcinoma is one of the most common cancers in men in the West. The bulbo-urethral glands secrete lubricating fluid into the urethra just below the prostate gland.

The penis carries the urethra, which provides a shared passage for sperm and urine, and allows intromission: the delivery of sperm into the vagina. It has three columns of erectile tissue: two lateral corpora cavernosa and a medial corpus spongiosum (Fig. 2.20). The corpus spongiosum contains the urethra and does not engorge as much as the corpora cavernosa. This prevents trauma to the urethra and generates an appropriate angle for intromission. The tip of

Fig. 2.20 *Internal structure of the penis.*

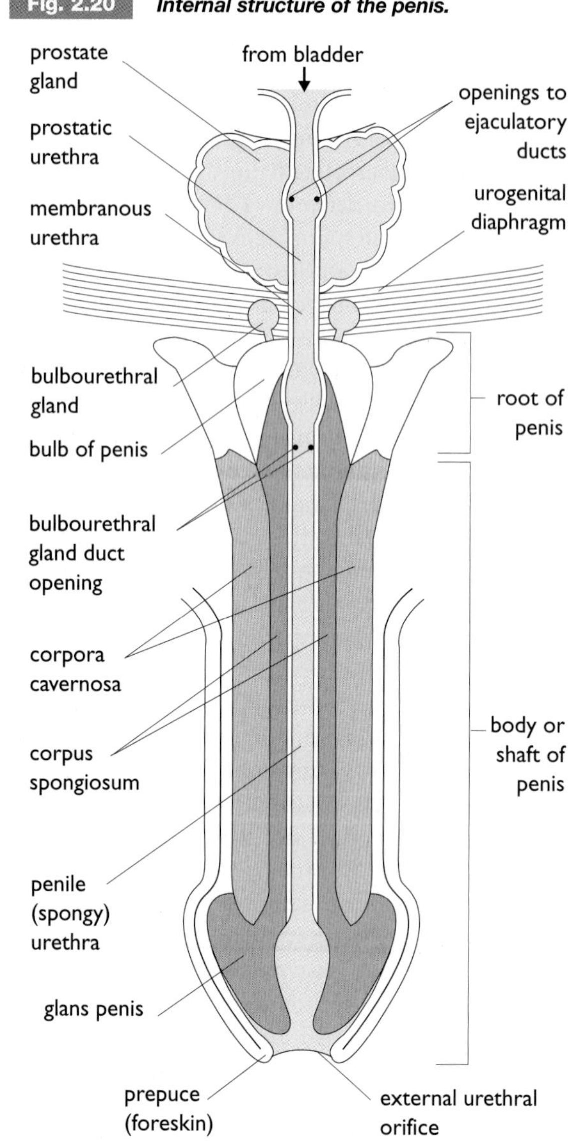


the corpus spongiosum expands to form the glans penis where the urethra opens. The penis is covered with a fold of skin or prepuce (foreskin), which can be retracted in an adult and older child. The spongy bodies of the penis become distended with blood during an erection (see Ch. 6).

# Gametogenesis

The process of gametogenesis is achieved through a specialized form of cellular division called meiosis (Fig. 2.21). The stages of meiosis are reviewed within Chapter 7. Gametogenesis is remarkably different in the male and female reproductive systems, both representing adaptation of the process of meiosis to facilitate reproduction. Gametes are specialized sex cells that contain half the genetic material of the normal cell content. Their fusion, referred to as fertilization, is described in detail in Chapter 6.

The production of spermatozoa begins at puberty within the male and results in the continual production of millions of sperm. Spermatozoa have completed all the meiotic divisions prior to ejaculation and fusion with the oocyte. In this sense, they are true gametes containing the haploid number of chromosomes. (These terms are explained in Ch. 4.)

The differences between gamete formation have evolved with the development of sexual reproduction and internal fertilization. Oocytes are relatively protected within the abdominal cavity and so it is not necessary for a large number to be produced. Movement of oocytes is passive, influenced by the structure of the uterine tube. Sperm, in contrast, must become highly motile in order to travel along the female reproductive tract. Many are lost and, of the millions contained within the ejaculate, only a few hundred will make it to the vicinity of the oocyte.

## *Spermatogenesis*

Spermatogenesis begins at puberty and continues into senescence, albeit less efficiently. The primitive germ cells, around the inner circumference of the seminiferous tubule, divide and replicate by a process called mitosis (see Ch. 4), forming many spermatogonia (Fig. 2.22). Each spermatogonium first divides into two diploid primary spermatocytes. The primary spermatocytes then undergo meiosis producing two haploid, genetically diverse secondary spermatocytes and then, after the second meiotic division, four haploid spermatids. For each cell undergoing meiosis, therefore, four gametes are produced. The spermatids undergo spermiogenesis (nuclear and cytoplasmic changes) producing the characteristic morphology (shape) of a spermatozoon. As meiosis progresses, the immature sperm are supported within Sertoli cells (see Box 2.9), which move them into the lumen of the seminiferous tubule.

The spermatozoa are stored in the epididymis where they mature for 2 weeks and may stay for up to 6 months. The shortest time between the initial meiosis and ejaculation is about 10 weeks, which is therefore the critical preconception period in men. Spermatogenesis is affected by temperature, malnutrition, alcohol, cottonseed oil (a potential source of contraception), some drugs and heavy metals.

**Fig. 2.21** *Gametogenesis. (Reproduced with permission from Brooker 1998.)*

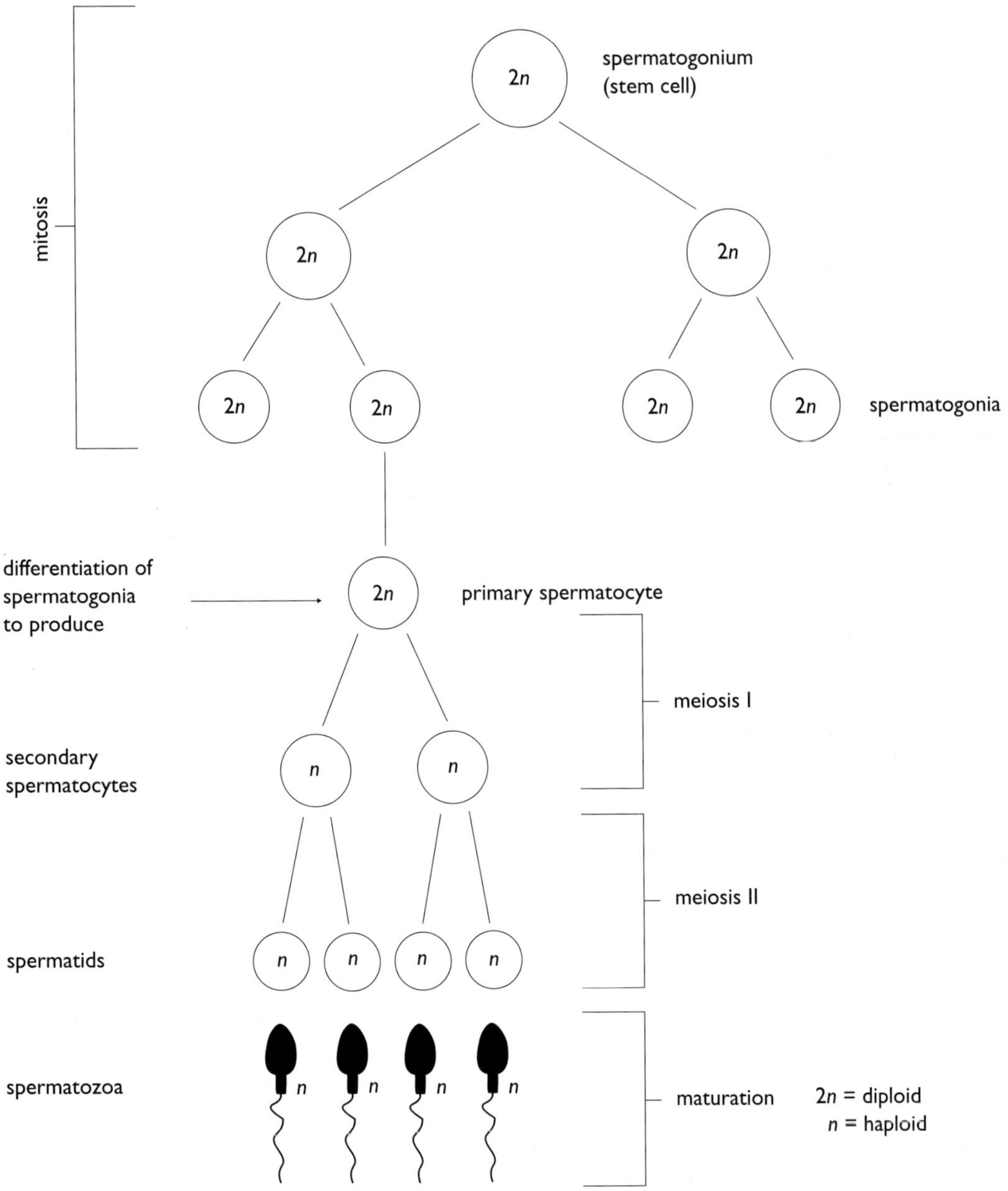

## *Steroidogenesis*

The interstitial cells of Leydig interspersed between the seminiferous tubules produce 90% of the circulating testosterone (the remainder has an adrenal origin). Testosterone is responsible for male secondary sex characteristics (see Ch. 3) and, together with FSH, controls production of sperm. Testosterone production is stimulated by luteinizing hormone (LH) from the pituitary gland (Fig. 2.23). Testosterone binds to androgen-binding protein (ABP) in the seminiferous tubules, which means that testosterone levels within the tubule can be very high while maintaining a concentration gradient that drives diffusion from outside to inside. Testosterone exerts a negative feedback mechanism on the hypothalamic–pituitary axis in a manner analogous to the feedback control by oestrogen in the female cycle (see Ch. 4). FSH stimulates the production of ABP by the Sertoli cells. Inhibin produced from the Sertoli cells inhibits FSH production. Illness and stress affect male reproductive capacity probably via the hypothalamic–pituitary axis.

**Fig. 2.22** *Spermatogenesis, showing cell stages and chromosome numbers.*

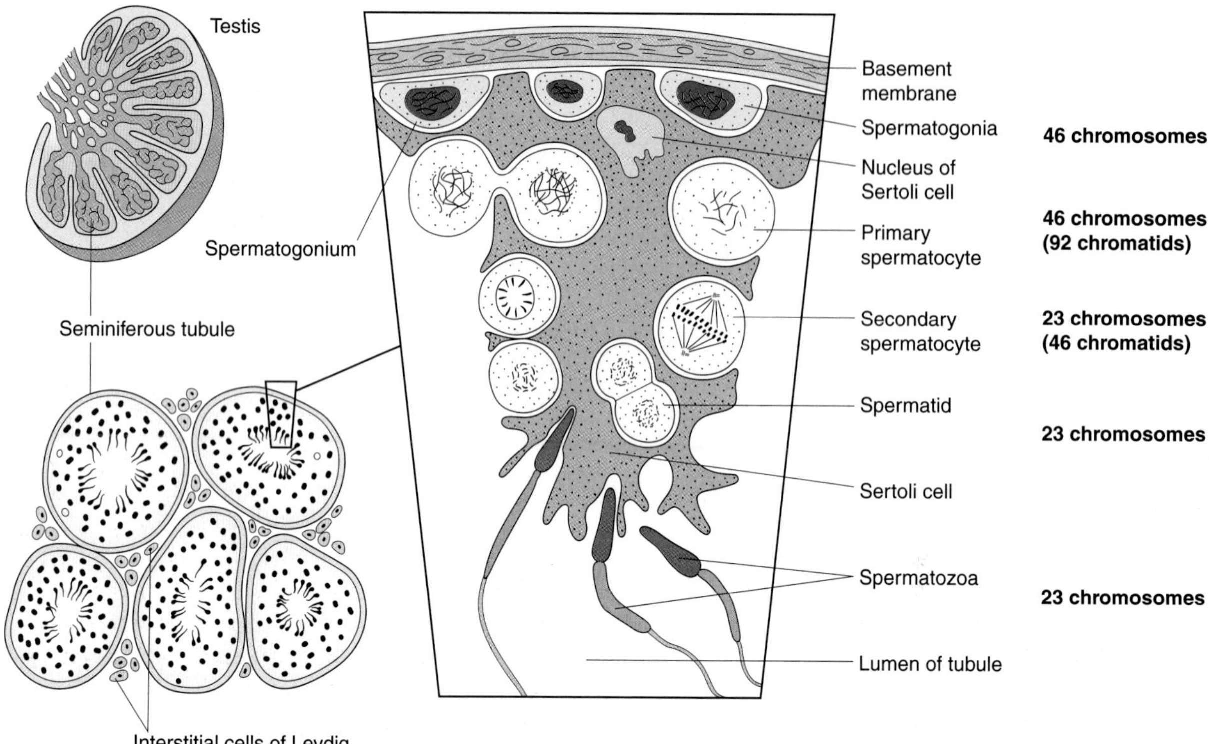


**Fig. 2.23** *Production of testosterone.*

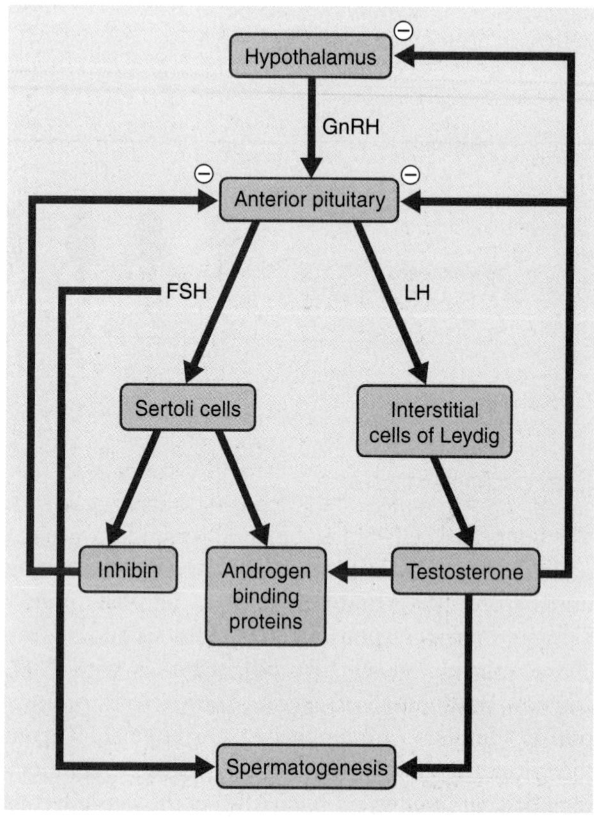


**Box 2.9**

**The role of Sertoli cells**

- Support spermatogenic cells and move them inwards
- Provide nutrients to spermatocytes and spermatids (hence their former name of 'nurse cells')
- Secrete fluid to aid release of sperm into lumen
- Act as a barrier between sperm-producing areas and lumen
- Engulf and digest cellular debris left from spermiogenesis
- Produce inhibin, which inhibits follicle-stimulating hormone (FSH) secretion
- Produce androgen-binding protein (ABP), which increases seminiferous tubule testosterone concentration
- Produce Müllerian-inhibiting hormone (MIH), which affects sexual differentiation (see Ch. 5)

## *Control of gametogenesis*

The control of gametogenesis and steroidogenesis in the male and female have some similarities. The hypothalamus regulates reproduction by secreting gonadotrophin-releasing hormone (GnRH) (see Fig. 2.23). This stimulates both FSH and LH production from the anterior pituitary gland. FSH stimulates gametogenesis: spermatogenesis in males and follicular development in females. Luteinizing hormone plays a pivotal role in steroidogenesis: increasing testosterone production from the Leydig cells in males and stimulating the increases in progesterone and oestrogen secretion in the second half of the menstrual cycle in females (see Ch. 4).

### Key points

- The renal system regulates water and electrolyte balance and is important in the maintenance of pH and the regulation of blood pressure. Waste products and foreign chemicals are excreted by the kidneys. The kidneys also have a endocrine role.
- Glomerular filtrate is formed from continuous processing of plasma and contains water and substances such as amino acids and glucose that are small enough to be filtered.
- The filtrate is modified in the nephron by reabsorption of substances into the blood and secretion of waste products into the filtrate. Reabsorption and secretion are regulated by hormones and many systems have transport maxima that can be exceeded in pregnacy, leading to urinary excretion of substances not usually present in the urine.
- Micturition (urination) is stimulated by bladder stretch receptors and controlled by learned inhibitory pathways.
- The female reproductive system produces female gametes, receives male gametes, and provides the optimum environment for fertilization, implantation and nurture of the fetus. It remains quiescent in pregnancy and generates the forces required for delivery at the end of gestation. The system is quickly restored to a fertile state at the end of pregnancy.
- Gametogenesis begins with mitosis of the primordial germ cells followed by meiosis, which reduces the chromosome number and creates infinite variation in the genetic complement of the gametes.
- The male gonads produce gametes from the seminiferous tubules and testosterone from the Leydig cells. Gametogenesis has a relatively short time-span in the male.
- The hypothalamus regulates reproduction by secreting gonadotrophin-releasing hormone (GnRH), which stimulates production of FSH and LH from the anterior pituitary, which in turn have effects on the gonads. The sex steroids produced by the gonads exert negative feedback inhibition at the hypothalamic–pituitary axis.

### Application to practice

Why is an in-depth knowledge of the female genitalia required by the midwife and how will this knowledge affect the decisions by the midwife within practice?

You might consider what the midwife needs to know in order to suture the peritoneum, to catheterize a woman during labour or to recognize the size of a baby at birth (see Ch. 5). There are many signs and 'symptoms' in pregnancy that are indicative of changes occurring within the renal system; knowledge of this will help the midwife to explain these fully to the woman.

During routine antenatal check-ups the midwife routinely performs urinalysis; are you able to explain the significance of the findings as a whole or do you think it is appropriate that midwives just observe for evidence of proteinuria?

## Annotated further reading


Burnett C W F 1979 The anatomy and physiology of obstetrics: a short textbook for students and midwives, 6th edn. Faber, London

*Although this is a rather old text, it still provides a useful introduction to reproductive anatomy and physiology, especially for students who have very little experience of reproductive science. Clear black-and-white line drawings of anatomical structures*

Johnson M H, Everitt B J 2000 Essential reproduction, 5th edn, Chapter 3 Testicular function. Blackwell Science, Oxford

*An integrated, up-to-date and well-organized research-based textbook that explores comparative reproductive physiology of mammals including anatomy, physiology, endocrinology, genetics and behavioural studies*

Mirouri N, Patel P 1998 Mosby's crash course: renal and urinary systems. C V Mosby, St Louis

*This well-illustrated book provides a useful reference text for students requiring specific knowledge of the renal and urinary systems*

Verralls S 1993 Anatomy and physiology applied to obstetrics, 3rd edn. Churchill Livingstone, New York
*This book was the first modern text that focused specifically on reproductive anatomy and physiology for midwives. It provides a useful introduction and is well illustrated and easy to read.*

Readers also are recommended to read chapters on the renal and reproductive systems in a physiology textbook, such as those listed at the end of the previous chapter.

## References

Bennett V R, Brown L K 1999 Myles' textbook for midwives, 13th edn. Churchill Livingstone, Edinburgh, pp 940, 941, 942, 949

Brooker C G 1998 Human structure and function, 2nd edn. C V Mosby, St Louis, pp 344, 345, 363, 470, 471, 473, 476, 483

O'Connell H E, Hutson J M, Anderson C R, Plenter R J 1998 Anatomical relationship between urethra and clitoris. Journal of Urology 159:1892–97

Sweet B, 1996 Mayes' midwifery, 12th edn. Baillière Tindall, London, p 29

# 3 Endocrinology

## Learning objectives

- To introduce the terminology used within endocrinology.
- To define the different types of hormones, their functions, main sites of production and mechanism of effects.
- To describe the role of the sex steroids.
- To relate endocrinology to the physiological process of reproduction.

## Introduction

This chapter presents an overview of endocrinology and examines the role of hormones in the regulation of human physiology. Throughout the chapter, links to reproductive physiology will be highlighted and referenced to other chapters in the book where the relevant interactions will be described more specifically.

The endocrine system, in conjunction with the nervous system, coordinates, regulates and adjusts the internal physiology in response to changes in the external environment. The nervous system tends to react in situations where an immediate response is required whilst the endocrine system is involved in sustaining body functions over a longer period (Table 3.1). For example, shivering is induced by neuromuscular activity to counteract a drop in the environmental temperature whereas many body cycles, such as the menstrual cycle, are almost entirely orchestrated through hormonal systems. However, the two systems do interact with one another and so some rapid responses have a hormonal component. For instance, the release of adrenaline and the fear-fight-flight reflex and hormonal release are often regulated by a neuronal pathway via the hypothalamus. The advantage of the endocrine system over the nervous system is that it can instigate a much more diffuse response in all body tissues at about the same time.

**Table 3.1** *Comparison of the nervous and endocrine systems*

| | Nervous system | Endocrine system |
|---|---|---|
| Source of signal | Brain | Endocrine gland |
| Signal | Neurotransmitter and action potential | Hormone |
| Usual route | Efferent nerve | Blood |
| Response rate | Fast | Slow |
| Specificity | Specific | Diffuse |
| Target | Single | Multiple |
| Type of effect | Immediate effect | Long-term control and integration |

## What is endocrinology?

The endocrine system originally appeared to be a relatively simple system of discrete glands (Fig. 3.1) that secreted chemical messengers, or hormones, into the blood where they would be carried to specific target cells at a distant site, inducing a reaction. However, it is now clear that hormone production is rather more complex. Some organs that have other functions also produce hormones. For instance, the heart produces atrial natriuretic peptide (ANP), which affects renal sodium reabsorption and hence blood pressure. Some hormones are produced by several different glands—such as somatostatin, which is produced by the hypothalamus, pancreas and gut. Although the trophoblast is the prime site of hCG production it can also be produced by other tissues, albeit in very low concentrations (Iles & Chard 1991). The placenta appears to be capable of synthesizing a very broad range of hormones and releasing factors that interact with both maternal and fetal physiology. Some substances such as noradrenaline can act as both hormones and neurotransmitters depending on their mode of delivery and whether they are released from a gland or from a nerve. The hypothalamus produces neurohormones that are important in the interaction between the endocrine and nervous systems.

Overall, the endocrine system (in partnership with the neural system):

- coordinates the homeostatic balance
- regulates various physiological systems such as the digestive system and reproductive system
- facilitates differentiation of the sexes in the embryonic stage and the manifestation of the secondary sexual characteristics at puberty
- modifies and induces behavioural changes within the individual.

**Fig. 3.1** *The endocrine glands. (Reproduced with permission from Brooker 1998.)*

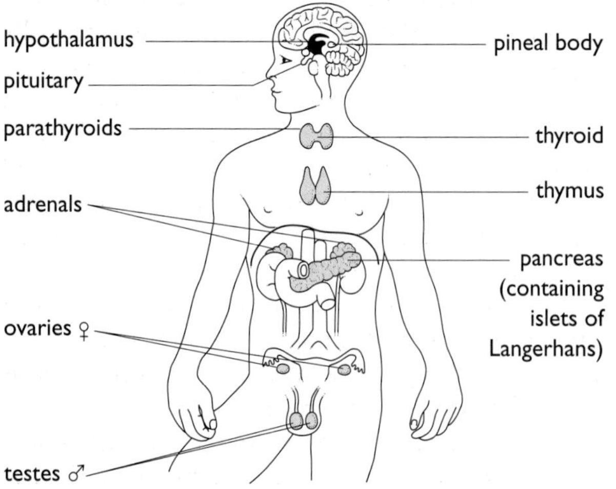


## The evolution of endocrinology

The evolution of the endocrine system has its rudiments within the activity of single-cell organisms. The unicellular organisms developed the ability to be attracted to chemicals, described as a chemotactic response, or to chemicals that were vital for the functioning of the organism, described as a chemotrophic response. Equally these organisms developed the ability to recognize noxious chemicals (toxins) and were thus able to avoid them. As the cell reacted to chemical signals interacting with receptor sites upon the cell membrane and within the cytoplasm, this led to the development of active mobility.

As multicellular organisms developed, the group of unicellular organisms that were the prototypes of multicellular organisms evolved chemical communication as an extension of the chemotrophic response. As multicellular evolution progressed further, the cells began to get more differentiated and specialized. Regulation therefore became the function of more specialized types of cells. This is reflected in the developmental sequence of a fetus, beginning with the division of a single cell (see Ch. 7). With each successive division, the resulting cells are slightly different from the original zygote cell (although differentiation during the initial divisions may be induced by the presence of maternally derived factors within the cytoplasm of the zygote). Although this differentiation is primarily under genetic control, it is achieved through a process of induction from chemical signals produced by one cell type that influence the division of other neighbouring cells. The altered gene expression of the dividing cells results in a changed morphology and developmental pathway.

As organisms became larger and more complex, cell-to-cell communication became more complicated. It evolved in two ways: the endocrine system (of chemical transmission via the circulating blood system) and the neural system (via transmission of an action potential—see Ch. 1). Under the traditional approach to biological science, the endocrine and neuronal systems were always considered in isolation; however, they are now considered to be extensions of the same system that are highly interactive. Many endocrine responses are initiated by a neuronal influence. Many neurotransmitters and neuromodulators have also been found to be endocrine hormones.

## Classification of hormones

The classical concept of a hormone being secreted into the blood and having an effect at a distant site is also no longer applicable as hormones can have a local effect (see below). Endocrine means 'secreted inwards' and is applied to hormones that fit the classical description of being secreted into the bloodstream and having an effect at a distant target. There are also exocrine hormones, which are 'secreted outwards' into ducts. These include hormones that are secreted into the vas deferens and uterine tubes.

A number of hormones have a local or paracrine effect, diffusing short distances to act on neighbouring cells or cells separated only by an intracellular space. Examples of a paracrine response are the effects of testosterone and Müllerian-inhibiting hormone (MIH) on sexual differentiation (see Ch. 5). If the hormone produced acts upon the same cell that originally produced it, it is described as autocrine. For example, an autocrine hormone may induce cellular division or signal the programmed death of the cell (apoptosis). If it affects adjacent cells, it is described as a juxtacrine hormone.

Neuroendocrine hormones are synthesized in specialized neurons, and their effects can also be paracrine in nature (these are usually described as neurotransmitters and neuromodulators). Oxytocin is an example of a neuroendocrine hormone. It is released from the posterior lobe of the pituitary gland and influences the contractility of the myometrium (see Ch. 13) and myoepithelial cells in the breast (see Ch. 16). In these respects oxytocin has an endocrine effect, but in many mammals it also modifies female behaviour by inducing parental behaviour in the presence of the sex steroids (Insel 1992).

A pheromone is a hormone produced by one organism that induces a response within another. Releaser pheromones stimulate rapid behavioural responses. Primer pheromones act via the neuroendocrine system to produce delayed responses. Receptors for pheromones are found on the vomeronasal organ close to the nasal cavity of mammals, which use pheromones to indicate identity of kin or family territory. The human vomeronasal organ was formerly thought to be atrophied in adults but recent evidence suggests a functional pathway. Pheromones have been implicated in sexual attraction and the synchrony of menstrual cycles within a cohort of women (McClintock 1971).

### *Hormone structures*

Hormones can be classified according to their structure (see Table 3.2). Steroid hormones and eicosanoids (the prostaglandin family of hormones) are lipids. The other classes are protein and peptide hormones and monoamines.

#### Steroid hormones

The steroid group of hormones consists of the sex steroids, the glucocorticoids, mineralocorticoids, thyroid hormones and 1,25 dihydrovitamin D3. Steroid hormones are derived from cholesterol and acetate (Fig. 3.2). As well as being the precursor for the steroid hormones, cholesterol is also an important structural component of cell membranes.

The first and common step in the biosynthesis of sex steroids is the formation of pregnenolone, which is rate-limiting, and therefore important in controlling production of sex steroids. Pregnenolone is produced on the inner mitochondrial membrane whereas the next stages take place in the smooth ER.

The three classes of sex steroids are structurally related, which offers the opportunity for interconversion. This means that a genetic defect in one of the steps can result not only in a deficiency of the normal amount of the product but also in an excess of another sex steroid. For instance, a genetic deficiency of the enzyme that converts 17α-hydroxyprogesterone to the precursor of cortisol results in increased levels of 17α-hydroxyprogesterone, which is converted into androstenedione and then into androgens. The unusually high level of androgens can cause masculinization of the female fetus. These structural similarities mean that the steroid hormones can affect the activity of other steroid hormones by exerting agonistic and antagonistic properties (see below). However, the effects of the hormones vary depending on their structure (see Table 3.3).

The main role of androgens is in the development and maintenance of masculine characteristics and fertility. Similarly, the dominant role of oestrogens is in development and maintenance of feminine characteristics and fertility. The key role for progesterone is the preparation for pregnancy and its maintenance.

**Table 3.2** *Classification of hormones and examples*

| | | |
|---|---|---|
| Lipid hormones | Steroid hormones | Sex steroids e.g. androgens, oestrogens and progestogens<br>Glucocorticoids e.g. cortisol<br>Mineralocorticoids e.g. aldosterone<br>Thyroid hormones<br>1,25 dihydrovitamin D3 |
| | Eicosanoids | Prostaglandins<br>Leukotrienes |
| Protein hormones | Gonadotrophic glycoproteins | Follicle-stimulating hormone (FSH)<br>Luteinizing hormone (LH)<br>Human chorionic gonadotrophin (hCG)<br>Thyroid-stimulating hormone (TSH) |
| | Somatotrophic polypeptides | Prolactin (PRL)<br>Human placental lactogen (hPL)<br>Growth hormone (GH) |
| | Cytokines | Insulin<br>Activins and inhibins<br>Müllerian-inhibiting hormone (MIH)<br>Interferons<br>Growth factors |
| Small peptides | | Gonadotrophin-releasing hormone (GnRH)<br>Oxytocin (OXY)<br>Antidiuretic hormone (ADH or vasopressin)<br>β-endorphin<br>Vasoactive intestinal peptide (VIP) |
| Monoamines | Catecholamines | Adrenaline, noradrenaline and dopamine<br>Melatonin<br>Dopamine |

Adapted from Johnson & Everitt 1995.

As steroid hormones are lipid soluble, they are able to freely diffuse across the cell membrane. The receptor sites for thyroid hormone and the sex steroids are found within the nucleus. Receptors for the other steroid hormones are within the cytoplasm, from where the hormone–receptor complex is transported into the nucleus. Steroid hormones have their effect by altering ribonucleic acid (RNA) synthesis and subsequent protein synthesis (Box 3.1). The activated receptor binds to specific segments of DNA in promoter regions of the gene in that section of DNA, affecting the rate of transcription and gene expression. Protein synthesis can be increased (or decreased) within 30 minutes so the effects of steroid hormones are, therefore, relatively slow in action compared with those of protein hormones. The term 'anabolic steroids' describes the effect of steroid hormones in influencing new tissue growth.

The other class of lipid hormones are eicosanoids, which have an important role in reproduction. They are formed from an arachidonic acid precursor, generated by the activity of either phospholipase C or phospholipase $A_2$ (Fig. 3.3). Arachidonic acid production appears to be the rate-limiting step. Phospholipase $A_2$ is present in an inactive form in lysosomes in cells that are released if the cell membranes become unstable. Prostaglandins are synthesized by most tissues of the

**Box 3.1**
**Action of steroid hormones**

- Transported in plasma bound to binding protein
- Hormone released and diffuses into target cell
- Hormone diffuses into nucleus
- Binds to specific receptor
- Affects DNA transcription
- Affects mRNA synthesis
- Affects protein synthesis
- Altered functional response of cell

**Fig. 3.2** *Steroid hormone production.*

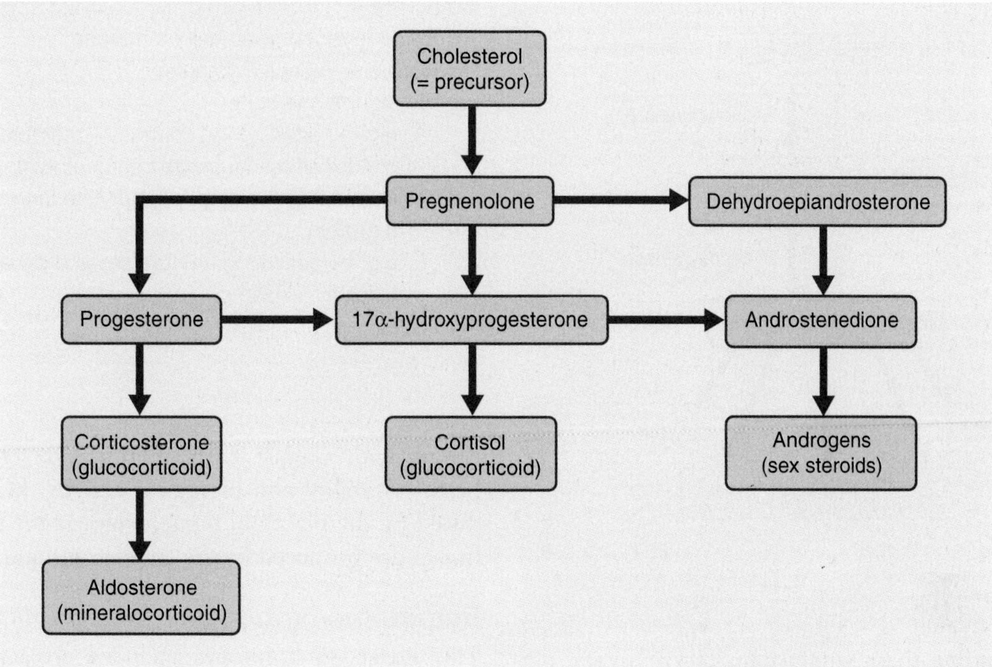


**Table 3.3** *Biological activity and effects of the sex steroids*

| Sex steroid | Family members (and approximate biological activity) | Main effects |
|---|---|---|
| Androgens | 5α-dihydrotestosterone (100%)<br>Testosterone (50%)<br>Androstenedione (8%)<br>Dehydroepiandrosterone (4%) | Differentiation of male embryo<br>Secondary sex characteristics<br>Spermatogenesis<br>Sexual and aggressive behaviour<br>Growth promoting, protein anabolism, ossification and erythropoiesis |
| Oestrogens | Oestradiol-17β ($E_2$) (100%)<br>Oestriol ($E_3$) (10%)<br>Oestrone ($E_1$) (1%) | Female secondary sex characteristics<br>Prepares uterus for ovulation and fertilization<br>Vascular effects—increased blood flow, neovascularization<br>Growth-promoting effects on endometrium and breasts<br>Primes endometrium for progesterone action<br>Mildly anabolic<br>Increases calcification of bones<br>May be associated with sexual behaviour |
| Progestogens | Progesterone (100%)<br>17α-hydroxyprogesterone (17α-OHP) (40–70%)<br>20α-hydroxyprogesterone (5%) | Prepares uterus for pregnancy<br>Maintains pregnancy<br>Stimulates glandular growth of breasts<br>Affects sodium and water excretion<br>Mildly catabolic<br>Relaxes smooth muscle tone<br>Affects appetite and thirst, metabolic rate, sensitivity to carbon dioxide |

Adapted from Johnson & Everitt 1995.

Fig. 3.3 *Formation of eicosanoids.*

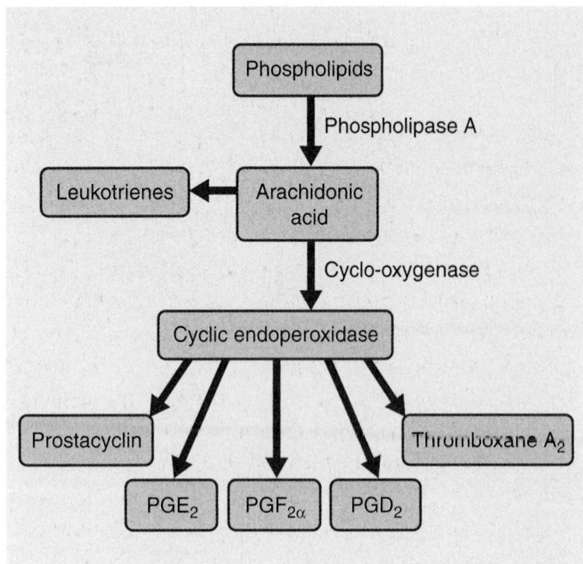


body including the myometrium, cervix, ovary, placenta and fetal membranes. They have a short half-life and are metabolized quickly so they are difficult to measure. They have an important role in amplifying signals at the onset of labour (see Ch. 13). Leukotrienes are another group of cellular signalling molecules that seem to be important in pregnancy.

## Protein, peptide and monoamine hormones

These hormones bind to receptors located on or within the cell membrane. They initiate plasma membrane depolarization and a cascade of second-messenger systems and chemical changes within the cytoplasm, generating a faster response than steroid hormones. They primarily affect the functioning of the cell by stimulation or inhibition. Their action is initiated through the activation of G-proteins located within the cell cytoplasm, which initiate various chemical reactions (Box 3.2). G-proteins may open ion channels or stimulate phosphorylation of internal proteins, thus generating the signalling cascade. Many peptide hormones function as neurotransmitters in the brain.

### *Gonadotrophic glycoproteins*

This group includes FSH, LH and hCG, all of which are structurally similar to thyroid-stimulating hormone (TSH). Their structure is a globular protein composed of two common chains and two unique chains with unique carbohydrate side chains that bestow stability and biological activity. hCG is produced by the placental tissue, whereas the other hormones are produced by the anterior pituitary gland.

**Box 3.2**
**Action of peptide hormones**

- Binds to receptor on cell membrane
- Hormone–receptor complex
- Altered internal state
  - — e.g. by opening ion channel in membrane
  - — e.g. by affecting enzyme such as tyrosine kinase which may phosphorylate (and activate) a protein
  - — e.g. by activating a G-protein and causing calcium release
- Altered cell response

### *Somatomammotrophic polypeptides*

This group of hormones includes prolactin (PRL), human placental lactogen (hPL) and growth hormone (GH), which have marked effects on tissue growth including the breasts. Their structure is a single polypeptide chain. PRL and hPL are involved with lactation. GH has a role in puberty including breast development. Although PRL and GH are pituitary hormones, the placenta also produces them in addition to hPL. The activity of the placental hormones is different from that of the pituitary hormones, however. For instance, placental GH has a higher affinity for the PRL receptor than does pituitary GH.

### *Cytokines*

Cytokines are small polypeptide chains. There is a large number of cytokines including inhibin, activin, epidermal growth factors and MIH (see Chs 5 and 13). Cytokines have a broad range of activity. They are usually made in a variety of cell types rather than in a specific gland. Cytokines act on many different cell types, often interacting with and modulating each other's responses. Several cytokines have similar and overlapping functions. They usually have paracrine activity and often modulate or mediate the actions of other types of hormone.

### *Small peptide hormones*

This group of hormones includes GnRH, a decapeptide (i.e. a chain of 10 amino acids) from the hypothalamus, and other releasing hormones, oxytocin,

ADH, β-endorphin (described in Ch. 13) and vasoactive intestinal peptide (VIP). Most of these small peptide hormones are initially produced in the form of large inactive polypeptide precursors, or prohormones. The prohormone is converted by enzymes to its smaller active form, often locally close to the target cell, before it can exert an endocrine influence. Some of the 'pro'-fragments also exert a biological effect.

### *Monoamine hormones*

This group includes catecholamines (dopamine, adrenaline and noradrenaline) and melatonin, all of which are derived from tyrosine (an amino acid) and may have a role in the neuroendocrine control mechanisms. The medulla of the adrenal gland is a modified sympathetic ganglion; its cell bodies release adrenaline and noradrenaline (in the ratio 4:1) into the blood. Its effects, therefore, augment sympathetic nervous system activity. Dopamine released from the hypothalamus affects prolactin secretion (see Ch. 16). Melatonin, from the pineal gland, may have a role in seasonal and environmental influences on reproductive capability, which are particularly important in species other than humans.

## Hormone transport

Peptide and protein hormones are water soluble and are carried dissolved in the blood, whereas steroid hormones circulate bound to plasma proteins. When hormones are secreted into the blood supply, a large proportion become protein bound, leaving only a small proportion free (unbound and able to access the target cell) and physiologically active. There are many types of hormone-binding proteins, all of which are colloidal in nature. Some hormones bind with great affinity to specific proteins. Other proteins may bind to numerous different hormones with different affinity rates that may be affected by the concentration of the hormone. Therefore, the amount of hormone present may affect its activity. For instance, oxytocin at high concentrations binds to ADH (or vasopressin) receptors within the renal tubule. During labour, levels of oxytocin do not normally rise until the end of the first stage. However, exogenous oxytocin can be administered to augment uterine contractions. If the administration of oxytocin is high and prolonged, however, water retention can occur because oxytocin also stimulates the ADH receptors. This overlap in the biological activity of hormones is described as promiscuity.

## Hormonal regulation

One of the most important functions of the endocrine system is maintenance of the internal environment. This 'steady' state is described as homeostasis (see Ch. 1). Homeostatic mechanisms buffer changes within the external environmental conditions. For example, mammals have evolved to be homeothermic (warm blooded) so that the chemical processes essential for physiological function proceed under optimal conditions of temperature. Fluctuations in temperature are monitored and the homeostatic mechanisms ensure that body temperature is held within narrowly defined limits. Homeostasis is achieved through the integration of the neural system with the endocrine system, commonly referred to as feedback systems.

As mentioned above, hormonal release is often instigated by neurological stimulation. Hormone release may also be stimulated by another hormone. Factors that facilitate the release of hormones are referred to as positive influences and factors that inhibit the release of hormones are termed negative influences.

### *Positive feedback*

Positive feedback describes a specialized chain of events involving one or more hormones in which there is a cycle of positive effects, amplifying the original signal (Fig. 3.4). An example of positive feedback is the maintained production of prolactin secretion from the

**Fig. 3.4** *Negative and positive feedback.*

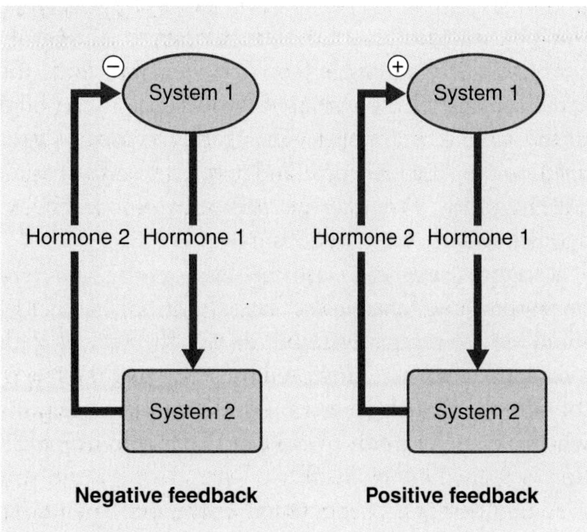

anterior pituitary gland during lactation. Suckling of the infant stimulates prolactin secretion, which maintains lactation. If suckling decreases or stops then the amount of stimulation decreases and prolactin production is reduced. Other examples of positive feedback include coagulation of blood and parturition.

### Negative feedback

Negative feedback describes a similar specialized chain of events involving one or more hormones, except here there is a cycle of negative influence (Fig. 3.4). An example of negative feedback is that the anterior lobe of the pituitary gland produces TSH, which stimulates the thyroid gland to produce thyroid hormone. TSH production is, however, inhibited by the presence of thyroid hormone.

### Activation and deactivation

Hormones may be released by the presence of a certain stimulus. For example, insulin release depends on plasma glucose levels. Many specific metabolic pathways are activated by the build-up of specific metabolites within the internal environment. Similarly, some hormones may be inhibited by the presence of a signal. This may be another hormone, such as adrenaline, neurological, such as light stimulation inhibiting melatonin release from the pineal gland, or chemical, such as insulin inhibiting the release of glucagon.

### Agonist and antagonist effects

The physiological overlap of oxytocin and ADH is an example of an agonist effect. Oxytocin can elicit the same biological response as ADH because it can bind to the same receptor sites. Therefore, oxytocin is agonistic to the ADH receptor and may be described as an ADH agonist. Progesterone acts as a glucocorticoid agonist and affects metabolism (see Ch. 11).

Receptor sites can also be blocked by different hormones and chemicals. These hormones occupy (bind to) the receptor site but do not themselves elicit a receptor response. However, by occupying the receptor site, they block the action of the specific hormone which normally binds to the site. This type of inhibition is termed antagonistic.

A number of environmental chemicals can mimic the effects of hormones. These are detailed in Box 3.3.

**Box 3.3**

**Environmental influences upon hormonal expression**

A number of environmental chemicals, such as phthalates (plasticizers) and PCBs (polychlorinated biphenyls), exert hormone-like effects. The chemicals may mimic or antagonize endogenous hormones, disrupt synthesis and metabolism of endogenous hormones and/or affect receptor expression. These oestrogenic contaminants were initially linked to abnormal sexual development in wild animals and fish but effects on humans are also under investigation. The pesticide DDT has been associated with reduced sperm counts and decreased libido. Chemicals used in plastics have been demonstrated to have oestrogenic properties. Degradation of alkylphenols used in detergents releases oestrogenic compounds. These environmental chemicals have been implicated in the increased incidence of testicular cancer, hypospadias (incomplete fusion of the urogenital folds of the penis), cryptorchidism (undescended testicles), breast cancer and endometriosis. It has also been suggested that fetal development, particularly of reproductive organs, may be affected by exposure to these compounds. The protective effect of phytooestrogens (see Ch. 4) may be related to interaction with environmental contaminants.

## Hormone action

The effects of hormones depend on a number of factors including affinity of the hormone for the receptor, agonist–antagonist effects, receptor number and hormone levels. Receptor number is important in the selection of the dominant follicle (see Ch. 4) and the increased sensitivity of the uterus to oxytocin in early labour (see Ch. 13). A lack of receptor expression can cause abnormal development, such as testicular feminization in the absence of androgen receptors (see Ch. 5). Hormone levels are affected by local circulation, stability, metabolism and excretion. Many hormones are inactivated within the blood, liver and their specific target cells. The breakdown of hormones is achieved by the action of various enzymes.

Hormone secretion may fluctuate with time. For instance, secretion of testosterone and prolactin exhibit circadian rhythms (characteristic pattern of changes during a 24-hour period), whereas GnRH, FSH, LH and PRL are released in a pulsatile fashion. A continuous infusion of these hormones would diminish their response as the constant occupancy of the receptors uncouples them from the second-messenger system, effectively exhausting the cell. A high blood flow increases dissipation of hormones and is likely to increase a systemic endocrine response but to decrease a paracrine response.

Levels and metabolism of binding proteins will also affect the activity of hormones. The protein-bound hormone complex renders the bound hormone inactive but also protects the hormone from enzymatic degradation. Hormone turnover may be affected by multiple sites of production. Different tissues may have different feedback mechanisms controlling hormone production. Replicating hormone production occurs physiologically from the placental cells, but also pathologically from tumours. Hormones and their metabolities may be excreted via the kidney during the formation of urine. As the rate of excretion of many hormones is proportional to the rate of secretion, excretion rate indicates secretion rate. Generally, peptide hormones are readily metabolized by blood enzymes and are easily excreted so their half-life in the blood is short compared with that of protein-bound steroid hormones.

Levels of hormones may change within the tissues themselves as hormones can be converted to a form with a higher biological activity. For instance, the enzyme 5α-reductase in many of the target tissues for testosterone converts testosterone to 5α-dihydrotestosterone, which has twice the biological activity. A deficiency of this enzyme can cause poor development of the male external genitalia (see Box 3.4). A hormone may be metabolized by its target cell. Peptide hormones are endocytosed and catabolized and the receptors are recycled.

**Box 3.4**

**5α-reductase deficiency**

In the Dominican Republic, there is an increased incidence of an autosomal recessive condition resulting in 5α-reductase deficiency (Imperato-McGinley et al 1986). 5α-reductase is the enzyme that converts testosterone to the more biologically active 5α-dihydrotestosterone within the target cell. The lack of enzyme means that there is a diminished response to testosterone during fetal sexual development (see Ch. 5) so an affected baby may have small and ambiguous genitalia, appearing female at birth (testicular feminization). However, at puberty the surge in testosterone production is adequate to stimulate the cells, therefore the child then develops male external genitalia. This condition is known as 'Guevodoces' (penis-at-twelve).

## Endocrine glands, hormones and reproduction

Hormones can influence the ability of the target cell to respond by regulating the number of hormone receptors. Prolonged exposure to a low concentration of hormone may increase the number of receptors expressed by the cell (described as 'upregulation'). Conversely, prolonged exposure to a high concentration of hormone might decrease the number of receptors for that hormone (described as 'downregulation'). For instance, the expression of oxytocin receptors is downregulated on prolonged exposure to oxytocin; this may explain the lack of response to exogenous oxytocin in induction of labour (see Ch. 13). Hormones can also affect receptors for other hormones, increasing or decreasing their effectiveness. When one hormone has to be present for another to have its full effect, it is described as permissive.

The endocrine glands and their main functions are summarized in Table 3.4.

### *The pituitary gland*

The pituitary gland has two main lobes, the anterior lobe (or adenophysis) and the posterior lobe (or neurohypophysis) (Fig. 3.5). The anterior lobe originates from the primitive oral cavity, whereas the posterior lobe is a continuation of the hypothalamus. The anterior lobe produces hormones such as LH and FSH that regulate gametogenesis and steroidogenesis by the gonads (see Ch. 4). The maintenance of lactation is achieved through the production of prolactin (see Ch. 16). The anterior lobe also produces TSH, growth hormone, adrenocorticotrophic hormone (ACTH) and melanocyte-stimulating hormone (MSH). The poster-ior lobe of the pituitary gland secretes oxytocin and ADH, which is also known as vasopressin.

### *The thyroid gland*

The thyroid gland lies in front of the trachea, posterior to the larynx, and produces thyroid hormones. Thyroxine ($T_4$) is circulated and converted to an active form tri-iodothyronine ($T_3$) within the target tissues. Thyroid hormones affect all tissues in the body and regulate metabolic rate, growth, brain development and function. During pregnancy, the fetus initially utilizes maternally derived thyroxine so the maternal thyroid gland hypertrophies (increases in size) to

**Table 3.4** *The endocrine system*

| Endocrine gland | Main function(s) |
|---|---|
| Hypothalamus | ■ Regulates homeostasis<br>■ Controls pituitary function<br>■ Integrates nervous and endocrine systems |
| Pituitary | 'Master gland'<br>■ Stimulates other endocrine glands |
| Pineal body | ■ Produces melatonin during nocturnal period<br>■ Involved in biological rhythms and body 'clock' |
| Thyroid | ■ Affects metabolism and growth |
| Parathyroid glands | ■ Maintenance of calcium homeostasis |
| Thymus | ■ Development of immune system |
| Adrenal glands | Medulla:<br>■ Secretion of catecholamines (adrenaline and noradrenaline)<br>Cortex:<br>■ Secretion of corticosteroids<br>— glucocorticoids affect metabolism and responses to stress<br>— mineralocorticoids affect electrolyte and fluid homeostasis<br>■ Sex steroids |
| Pancreas | ■ Insulin and glucagon control cellular uptake of glucose and regulate cellular metabolism affecting blood glucose<br>■ Somatostatin = growth hormone-inhibiting hormone |
| Gonads (testes or ovaries) | ■ Produce sex steroids that affect reproductive cycles and gamete formation |
| Kidney | ■ Erythrocyte production stimulated by erythropoietin |
| Heart | ■ Atrial natriuretic peptide lowers blood pressure |
| Adipose tissue | ■ Appetite suppressed by leptin<br>■ Affects steroid hormone metabolism |

compensate for this. This is achieved by the thyrotrophic effect of hCG and a placentally derived hormone called human chorionic thyrotrophin. The increase in thyroid activity increases the basal metabolic rate of the pregnant woman, resulting in an increase of maternal and fetal oxygen consumption.

### *The parathyroid glands*

Calcium balance is maintained by the action of the parathyroid glands (Fig. 3.6) and so in pregnancy the fetal demands for calcium mean there is an increase in calcium uptake by the maternal system to counteract this.

### *The adrenal glands*

The adrenal glands produce mineralocorticoids such as aldosterone, which are principally involved in the regulation of the electrolyte balance of the body (see Ch. 2). The adrenal glands also produce glucocorticoids such as corticosterone and cortisol, which are involved in the regulation of carbohydrate metabolism, the body's responses to stress and the regulation of the immune system. Carbohydrate metabolism is altered during pregnancy but it would appear that the fetal maternal interaction concerning carbohydrate metabolism is mediated through the action of other hormones (see Ch. 11).

### *The gonads*

The gonads are responsible for the production of the sex steroids. In the male, the testes predominantly produce testosterone. In the females, the ovary produces oestrogens and progesterone. The endocrine cells of the gonads lack the enzymes to produce mineralocorticoids and glucocorticoids. The gonadal function of the regulation of reproduction is discussed in Chapter 4.

## Fetal endocrinology

The fetal placental unit produces hormones that not only regulate fetal physiology but also interact with the maternal physiology to maintain and direct the pregnancy towards a successful outcome. Production of oestradiol involves cooperation between the maternal and fetoplacental systems (see Ch. 11). The fetal endocrine system is also involved in the differentiation and development of the sexes (see Ch. 5).

Fig. 3.5 *The pituitary gland and its secretions.*

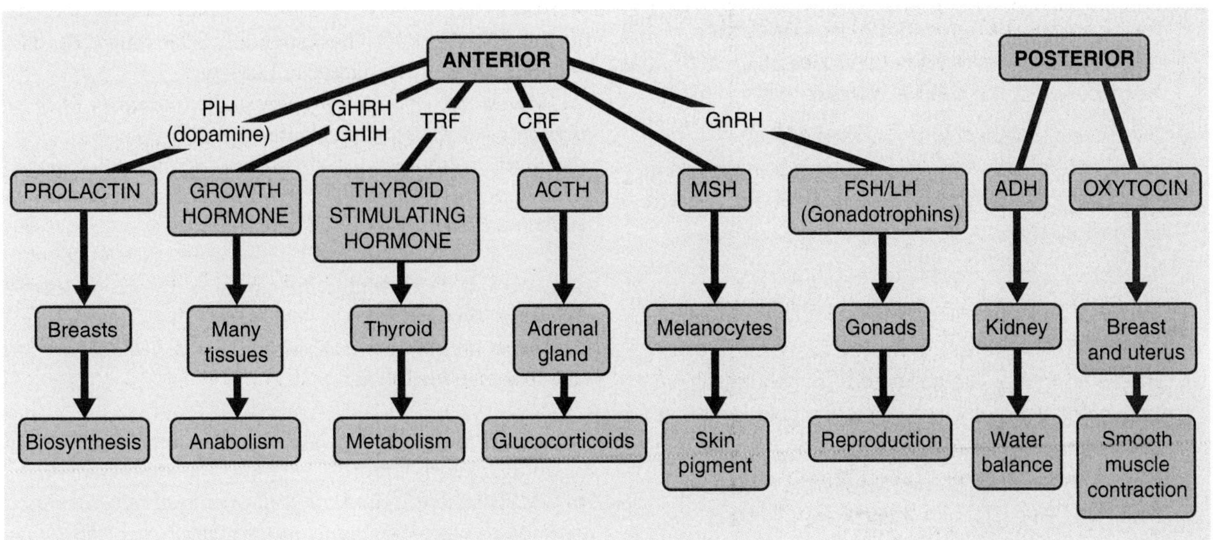


Fig. 3.6 *The parathyroid glands.*

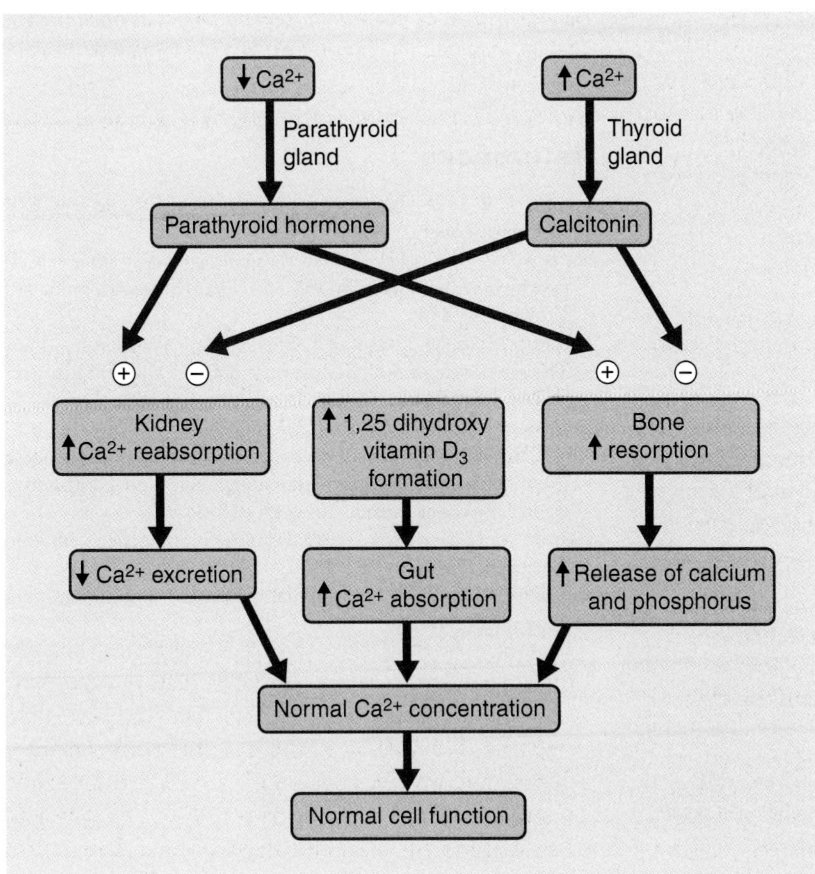

## Key points

- The endocrine system and the nervous system interact and are involved in communication and maintenance of the internal environment.
- The classic description of a hormone as a substance released from a gland and transported in the blood to its target organ(s) cannot be applied to all hormones.
- Hormones can be classified structurally as monoamine, protein, peptide or lipid (steroid) hormones.
- Steroid hormones are produced from cholesterol precursors and include mineralocorticoids (such as aldosterone), glucocorticoids (such as cortisol) and sex steroids (oestrogen, progesterone and testosterone).
- Steroid hormones circulate bound to plasma proteins and exert their effect by altering protein synthesis in their target cells.
- Peptide hormones and catecholamines circulate in the plasma and affect signal transduction in their target cells.
- Hormonal effects are modulated by binding proteins, receptor expression, hormone metabolism and agonist/antagonist effects.
- Testosterone and oestrogen are responsible for the development and maintenance of sexual characteristics and fertility. Progesterone is involved in preparation for and maintenance of pregnancy.

### Application to practice

During pregnancy, apart from the growth of the fetus, there is much tissue growth and development within the mother that is controlled by the action of hormonal changes within the maternal system and interactions with hormones produced by the fetal–placental complex.

Throughout the entire antenatal, perinatal and postnatal periods the midwife should be able to observe these physiological changes and use them to form an assessment of the progression and well-being of the pregnant woman and fetus.

It is important to remember that all the changes occur through the action of hormones at all levels.

## Annotated further reading

Carlson N R 2000 Physiology of behaviour, 7th edn. Longman Higher Education, Harlow

*An interesting and comprehensive exploration of how physiological processes regulate and influence the behaviour and psychology of organisms. It describes sexual behaviour in depth, relating it to endocrine and neurological interactions.*

Greenstein B 1994 Endocrinology at a glance, Blackwell Science, Oxford

*Introduces the study of endocrinology in a clear, precise but easy-to-understand way.*

Johnson M H, Everitt B J 2000 Essential reproduction, 5th edn. Blackwell, Oxford

*An integrated, up-to-date and well-organized research-based textbook that explores comparative reproductive physiology of mammals including anatomy, physiology, endocrinology, genetics and behavioural studies.*

Sonnenschein C 1998 An updated review of environmental estrogen and androgen mimics and antagonists. Journal of Steroid Biochemistry and Molecular Biology 65:143–150

*An exploration of potential problems and hazards to reproduction in relation to environmental contamination.*

## References


Brooker C G 1998 Human structure and function, 2nd edn. C V Mosby, St Louis

Iles R K, Chard T 1991 Human chorionic gonadotrophin expression by bladder cancers: biology and clinical potential. Journal of Urology 145:453

Imperato-McGinley J, Gautier T, Peterson R E, Shackleton C 1986 The prevalence of 5 alpha-reductase deficiency in children with ambiguous genitalia in the Dominican Republic. Journal of Urology 136:867–873

Insel T R 1992 Oxytocin—a neuropeptide for affiliation: evidence from behavioral, receptor autoradiographic and comparative studies. Psychoneuroendocrinology 17:3–35

Johnson M H, Everitt B J 1995 Essential reproduction, 4th edn. Blackwell, Oxford, p 29

McClintock M K 1971 Menstrual synchrony and suppression. Nature 229:244–245

# 4 Reproductive cycles

## Learning objectives

- To describe follicular development, ovulation and subsequent events in the ovary.
- To describe the hormonal changes in the non-fertile menstrual cycle.
- To outline the principles of hormonal regulation of reproduction and to identify factors that affect this regulation.
- To describe the effects of the hormonal changes on the female reproductive system.
- To relate the cyclical fluctuation in hormone levels to other changes in female physiology.

## Introduction

The function of the ovary is both to release oocytes and to produce the steroid hormones oestrogen and progesterone. Relatively few oocytes are produced during a woman's reproductive life, compared with the number of male gametes. The cyclical pattern of hormone release has cyclical effects on the whole body, and behaviour, of the woman. The effects are particularly pronounced on the genital tract facilitating its functions in gamete transport and the implantation and development of the conceptus. The first part of the cycle, the follicular phase, is dominated by the release of oestrogen produced by the developing follicles (Fig. 4.1). This oestrogen-dominant phase prepares the woman for ovulation, receipt of the sperm and fertilization of the oocyte. In the second half of the cycle, the luteal phase, the effects of progesterone are dominant. The physiological changes in this phase of the cycle prepare the woman's body for pregnancy and promote implantation and nurture of the conceptus should fertilization be successful. Progesterone is secreted from the corpus luteum; thus this phase of the cycle is known as the luteal phase.

Ovulatory cycles are usually of a duration of 24 to 32 days; the follicular phase is 10 to 14 days and the luteal phase between 12 and 15 days. Longer cycles usually have a prolonged follicular phase and delayed ovulation.

## The follicular phase

### Developmental stages

The stages of cell division leading to the production of the female gamete begin early in fetal life. The process is halted until ovulation, then halted again until fertilization. Although dramatic progress in the development of an oocyte takes place during the follicular phase, the development of the follicle begins about 3 months prior to the menstrual cycle in which it is released at ovulation (Fig. 4.2). At the beginning of the cycle, a number of follicles are recruited to undergo initial development, stimulated by LH. One follicle is selected to continue development as the dominant follicle. It is this follicle that releases the ovum at ovulation. The remnants of the follicle then become the corpus luteum.

In the female fetus, the primitive germ cells migrate to the ovary at 21 days postfertilization and proliferate by mitotic division producing about 10 million primary oocytes per ovary by 20 weeks of gestation (see Ch. 5). On arrival in the primitive ovary, the primitive germ cells are called oogonia. Initially, the

**Fig. 4.1** ***Phases of the menstrual cycle.***

| | Day 0 (Menstruation →) | 5 | 14 (Ovulation ↓) | 28 |
|---|---|---|---|---|
| Ovary | Follicular phase | | Luteal phase | |
| | Follicular development | | | |
| Dominant hormone | Oestrogen<br>*Preparation for ovulation* | | Progesterone (+ oestrogen)<br>*Preparation for pregnancy* | |
| Uterus | Proliferative phase | | Secretory phase | |
| | Menstruation | Endometrial growth | Glandular secretion | Ischaemia |

oogonia proliferate by mitotic division until they enter meiosis. When the oogonia enter meiotic division, they become known as oocytes. These degenerate throughout fetal life so the female neonate is born with a finite number of 250 000–500 000 oocytes; this is all the oocytes she will ever have. Degeneration of the oocytes continues throughout postnatal life; there are less than 200 000 oocytes left at puberty and numbers continue to fall. However, if one assumes a reproductive life of about 35 to 40 years, the maximum number of ova released from the ovaries will be no more than a few hundred.

## *Arrested meiosis*

Meiosis is a specialized cell division involved in the production of gametes (see Ch. 7, p. 136 for a detailed description). In it, the number of chromosomes is reduced from 46 (known as the diploid number) to 23 (the haploid number). In the first part of meiosis, the chromosomes pair up and exchange genetic material. In humans, two or three exchanges of DNA occur per chromosome pair ensuring that the combination of genes will be unique (Box 4.1). The chromosomes then separate into the two daughter cells, each containing 23 chromosomes as pairs of chromatids. In the second meiotic division, these sister chromatids finally segregate into the daughter cells or gametes.

**Fig. 4.2** ***Ovarian follicles. (Reproduced with permission from Brooker 1998.)***

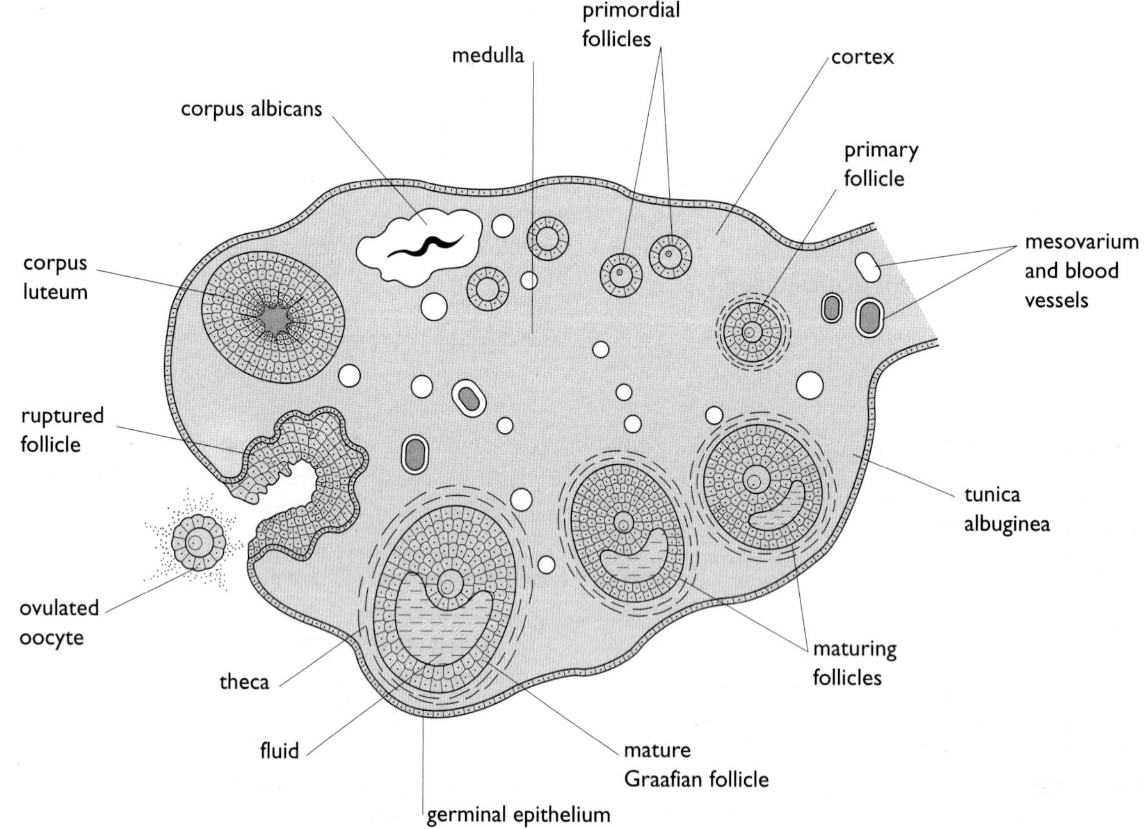

**Box 4.1**

**Gamete formation**

- Cell proliferation (mitosis)
- Genetic reshuffling and reduction (meiosis)
- Packaging of chromosomes
- Gamete maturation

In the female mitosis stops in the fetal period whereas in the male the mitotic division begins at puberty and continues until senescence (see Box 4.2). The termination of mitosis in the female, and entry into meiosis, is under the control of meiosis initiation factors produced by the granulosa cells (Eppig, Ward-Bailey & Coleman 1985). The primary oocytes, which are diploid, begin meiosis during fetal development but are arrested during the first meiotic division (Fig. 4.3). This happens at a stage of the first meiotic division that is called the 'diplotene stage' of prophase I (see Fig. 7.11, p. 138). During this stage nuclear material is exchanged between chromosomes within the germinal vessel in the nucleus. This is achieved by areas of fusion (called chiasmata) forming between adjacent chromosomes (see Ch. 7). The arrested diplotene state is known as the dictyate stage (Eppig 1996).

The meiotic cycle resumes when ovulation occurs following puberty in response to FSH and LH and secretions from the granulosa cells. However, the arrested stage may last for over 50 years; as meiotic structures called spindles (see Fig. 7.11, p. 138) become increasingly fragile with increasing maternal age. This leads to an increased number of abnormalities such as Down's syndrome and failed implantation.

**Box 4.2**

**Oogenesis compared with spermatogenesis**

- Mitosis—fetal in female, after puberty in male
- Meiosis—halted in female, can last many years
- Relatively few oocytes released
- Release is episodic at ovulation not a continuous stream
- Organization is comparable to testis—stromal tissue containing primordial follicles (tubules) and glandular tissue—interstitial glands (Leydig cells)
- Mitotic proliferation is less
- Time-course of gamete production is much longer

**Fig. 4.3** ***Arrest of oocyte meiosis. (Reproduced with permission from Brooker 1998.)***

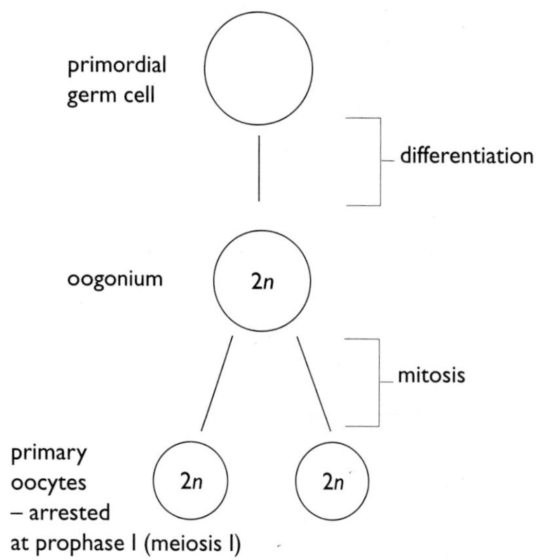


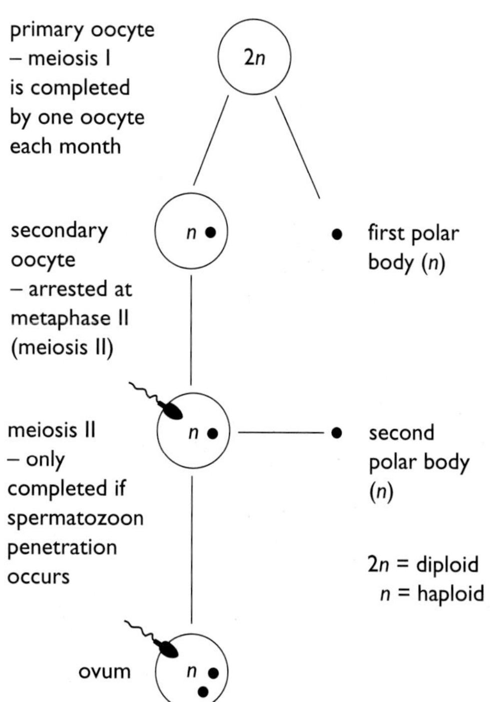


*NB* Polar bodies eventually degenerate within the ovum

## Primordial follicles

Development of a mature female gamete depends on complex interactions between the developing gamete and the surrounding cells forming the outer layers of the follicle. During first meiotic prophase, the oocyte stimulates organization of the surrounding cells to form the granulosa cells (flattened cuboidal epithelial cells) of the primordial follicles. These follicular cells secrete a basement membrane around the outside forming a cellular unit (Fig. 4.4). The primitive oocyte is about 18 μm in diameter. A few follicles may resume development spontaneously and incompletely throughout fetal and neonatal life. However, regular recruitment of the primordial follicles into the pool of growing follicles begins at puberty when levels of FSH increase.

## Preantral (primary) follicles

From puberty, a few primordial follicles restart their development each day forming a continuous stream of growing preantral or primary follicles. Most of these early follicles fail to develop fully and undergo atresia. As the majority of the follicles regress rather than progress through development, the ovary has a dense population of atretic follicles resulting in an irregular corrugated outer surface of the ovary. The development of primordial follicles into preantral follicles takes about 85 days. Initiation and progress through this early follicular development is independent of pituitary hormones but there may be paracrine regulation by cytokines, such as epidermal growth factor (EGF) (Box 4.3). These developing follicles do not secrete significant amounts of steroid hormones. Further follicular development requires pituitary support (secretion of FSH and LH).

Early in the cycle, the concentration of FSH is sufficient to support the further development of some preantral follicles. The preantral follicles that are optimal for further development are of the appropriate size and maturity to respond and have adequate FSH receptors. Recruitment of the follicles is related to the interaction between the FSH concentration and the number of FSH receptors on the developing follicles. Therefore, the number of follicles surviving is related to the amount of FSH present. The antral development phase, ovulation and luteal phase comprise one cycle in the human. In other mammalian species, antral expansion occurs in the luteal phase of the previous cycle thus shortening non-fertile cycles.

**Fig. 4.4** *Follicular development. (Reproduced with permission from Brooker 1998.)*

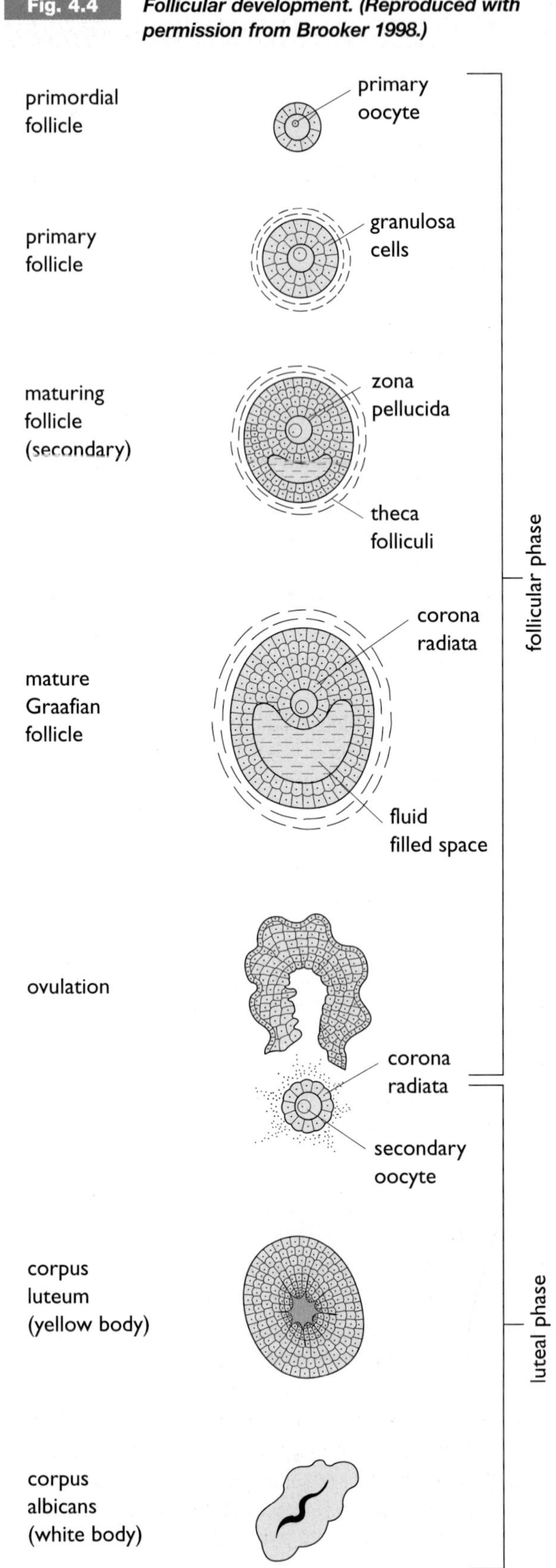

**Box 4.3**

**Cytokines and growth factors**

### Inhibin and activin

The gonadotrophins (FSH and LH) stimulate the production of the cytokines, activin and inhibin. The cytokines modulate actions of steroid hormones and gonadotrophins. Inhibin appears to affect only reproduction (see Fig. 4.7, p. 80) whereas the closely related activin affects cell growth and differentiation in other tissues. Inhibin is produced by the granulosa cells of small antral follicles in response to FSH (Roberts et al 1993) and suppresses FSH secretion. Levels peak mid cycle but remain high in the luteal phase, because the corpus luteum produces inhibin in response to LH. Inhibin production in the pituitary has a local inhibitory effect on FSH release (Hillier 1991). Inhibin stimulates androgen output by the thecal cells and moderates aromatizing activity of the granulosa cells (Hillier 1991). Activin is produced by granulosa cells, which also secrete follistatin, which may modulate the effects of activin. The thecal cells of the dominant follicle also produce activin (Roberts et al 1993). The anterior pituitary gland also produces activin, which is co-secreted with the gonadotrophins and enhances FSH production. It inhibits pituitary production of growth hormone, ACTH and prolactin. It may also have a role in embryogenesis (Hamilton-Fairley & Johnson 1998). Activin is present in follicular fluid but is inhibited by follistatin. Activin suppresses the androgen output by thecal cells but stimulates aromatizing capacity of granulosa cells. It therefore inhibits progesterone production. Activin is present early in the cycle, and inhibin later in the cycle, thus producing a balance between androgen output and conversion.

### Follistatin

Follistatin was identified in 1987 as an inhibitor of FSH secretion (Roberts et al 1993). It is synthesized in the ovary and inhibits activin activity by acting as an activin-binding protein.

### Interleukins

Interleukin 1 (IL-1) is a polypeptide cytokine, usually produced by activated macrophages. However, it is also produced by granulosa cells in a hormone-dependent manner with a peak production mid-cycle. IL-1 affects follicular maturation and a number of aspects of ovulation including increasing production of prostaglandins, collagenase, nitric acid and hyaluronic acid (Hurwitz et al 1992) and steroidogenesis. It is not known whether other members of the interleukin family are involved in follicular development.

### Epidermal growth factor (EGF)

EGF is produced by many tissues including granulosa cells. It appears to inhibit FSH-stimulated oestrogen and inhibin production and proliferation and differentiation of granulosa cells. EGF may be involved in the selection of the dominant follicle (Hamilton-Fairley & Johnson 1998).

### Transforming growth factors (TGF)

Transforming growth factors, TGF-$\alpha$ and TGF-$\beta$, have been identified in thecal cells (Adashi et al 1989). TGF$\alpha$ has similar properties to EGF and suppresses granulosa cell differentiation. It also regulates differentiation of other cell types including fetal ovaries and ovarian carcinoma cells. Members of the TGF-$\beta$ family are structurally similar to inhibin and increase FSH receptor expression, positively modulating granulosa cell proliferation and differentiation.

### Insulin-like growth factors (IGFs)

Insulin-like growth factors stimulate mitotic division and cell differentiation. Their effects are mediated by insulin-like growth factor binding proteins (IGF-BP). In follicular development, they appear to coordinate the production of steroid hormones from the granulosa and thecal layers of the follicle (Giudice 1994). IGF-I enhances follicular development and hormone production. IGF-II enhances the response to insulin. IGF-BP bind to the IGFs decreasing the concentration of free growth factor. Decreased levels of binding proteins are associated with follicular growth and increased concentrations of binding proteins are found in atretic follicles (Mason et al 1993). The large follicles from women with polycystic ovaries have lower concentrations of growth factors and higher concentrations of binding proteins (Mason et al 1994). IGFs seem therefore to have an important role in follicular growth, maturation and ovulation. In pregnancy, IGFs and their binding proteins play essential roles in modulating fetal growth and development (see Ch. 9).

### Tumour necrosis factor (TNF)

Tumour necrosis factor was initially identified as having a role in inflammation and in inhibiting tumour growth. It is produced by follicular cells and stimulates steroidogenesis, and may have a role in ovulation.

## *Antral follicles*

Usually about 15 to 20 preantral follicles are rescued from atresia and undergo initial stages of development and marked enlargement in response to the increasing FSH concentration at the beginning of each cycle. Several components contribute to the growth of the follicle: the oocyte enlarges, the follicular cells divide and further stromal cells are recruited to form the expanded outer layers of the follicle. The oocyte itself increases in size to 60–120 μm. It synthesizes large amounts of ribosomal RNA (rRNA) and messenger RNA (mRNA) to increase its protein stores ready for the maturation of the oocyte and fertilization, but does not resume meiosis. The follicular cells divide into several layers of granulosa cells, which secrete an amorphous transparent jelly, the zona pellucida. The zona pellucida is formed from condensation of glycoprotein and accumulates between the granulosa cells and the oocyte, acting as an extracellular coat of the oocyte. It has an important role in sperm binding and penetration during fertilization (see Ch. 6). Although the zona pellucida acts to separate the oocyte from the avascular granulosa cells, cytoplasmic processes penetrate the zona pellucida forming gap junctions at the oocyte surface. These allow delivery of low molecular weight substrates, such as nucleotides and amino acids, and cellular signalling molecules into the oocyte. Gap junctions also exist between granulosa cells.

The third component of follicular growth is condensation of ovarian stromal cells on the basement membrane (membrana propria) of the follicle. These recruited cells form a loose matrix of spindle-shaped cells around the follicle, known as the thecal layer. The cells differentiate into two layers: the theca interna, an inner layer of highly vascular glandular cells, and the theca externa, a poorly vascularized fibrous capsule.

The granulosa cells acquire receptors for FSH and oestrogen and the theca interna cells acquire receptors for LH. Synthesis of steroid hormones by the follicle requires cell cooperation (Fig. 4.5) (Hillier, Whitelaw & Smyth 1994). Interstitial glands lie within the stroma and between the developing follicles. They are formed of steroidogenic cells and produce androgens for secretion and aromatization in follicles. LH stimulates the theca interna cells to synthesize androgens (testosterone and androstenedione) from acetate and cholesterol but these cells initially have limited capacity to synthesize oestrogens. Androgens from the theca interna cells diffuse to the avascular granulosa cells. The granulosa cells are unable to synthesize androgens but can aromatize androgens to oestrogens (oestradiol-17β and oestrone). The enzyme aromatase is involved in the steroid biosynthesis pathway leading to increased oestrogen production. FSH stimulates production of insulin-like growth factor I (IGF-I), which stimulates aromatase activity and hence oestrogen production. Small amounts of LH are required to amplify follicular oestrogen production. The steroids are secreted into the bloodstream, where they have a systemic effect, and into the follicular fluid, where they may have a paracrine role. Androgens also stimulate aromatase. Oestrogens stimulate granulosa cells to proliferate and express further oestrogen receptors. Therefore, oestrogen further stimulates oestrogen output—an example of positive feedback. This increases the amount of circulating oestrogen from the most advanced or ‘dominant’ follicle (therefore monitoring oestrogen output is a guide to the maturity of the most mature follicles). The dominant follicle, which undergoes the most growth, will enlarge from 20 to 200–400 μm diameter. The dominant follicle produces oestradiol, which inhibits FSH secretion. However, the dominant follicle develops exquisite sensitivity to FSH and can continue to respond to the decreasing concentration of FSH. The smaller follicles, destined to become atretic, lose their responsiveness to FSH and do not develop LH receptors (Scheele & Schoemaker 1996).

### The dominant antral follicle

The single follicle emerging as dominant undergoes preovulatory growth. This dominant follicle produces more oestrogen, which inhibits production of FSH from the pituitary gland. This is an example of negative feedback where a product limits its own production. The effect of oestrogen inhibiting production of FSH is that further development of the other follicles is limited. These follicles with fewer FSH receptors exposed to a diminishing supply of FSH are least able to respond to FSH and therefore undergo a downward spiral and become atretic.

Angiotensin-II (A-II), the product of the renin-angiotensin system (RAS, see Ch. 2), may be involved in oocyte maturation and ovulation. There is a RAS that is specific to the ovary (Lightman et al 1987) and A-II occurs in high concentrations in preovulatory follicles. Symptoms of ovarian hyperstimulation syndrome include serious metabolic and fluid disturbances which are associated with abnormal control of the RAS. It has also been suggested that A-II may have

Fig. 4.5 *'Two-cell model' of steroid synthesis.*

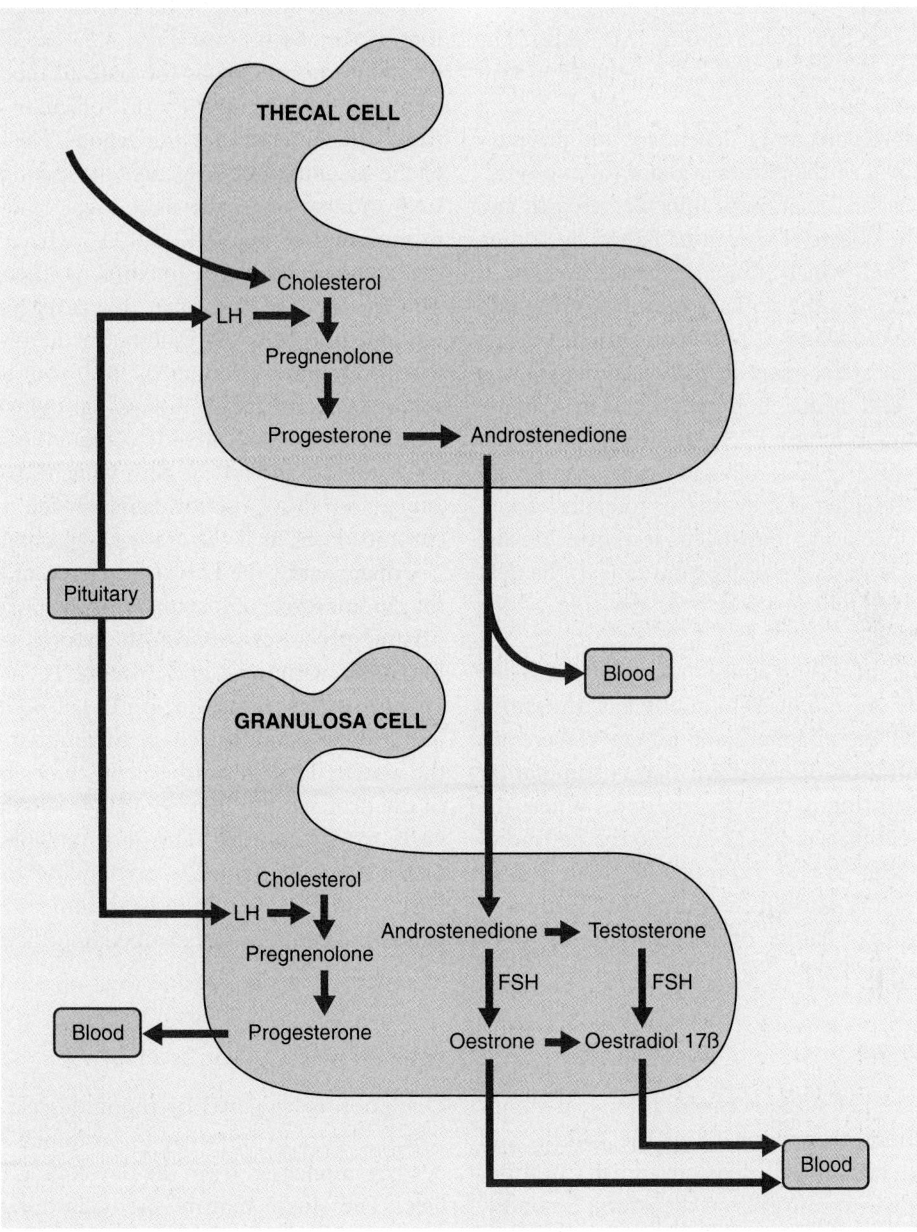


a role in the formation and maintenance of the corpus luteum, regulation of progesterone production and angiogenesis (Hamilton-Fairley & Johnson 1998). The biggest or dominant follicle, which is best able to respond to FSH, further develops on the pathway to expansion and ovulation. Oestrogen and FSH stimulate the mid-cycle expression of LH receptors on the outer layers of granulosa cells of the dominant follicle, which means that it will be able to respond to the mid-cycle surge of LH secretion. Entry into the preovulatory phase depends on both the expression of these receptors and a surge of LH from the anterior pituitary gland.

The granulosa cells continue to divide and increase in size. However, most of the increase in follicular size is due to accumulation of follicular fluid formed from mucopolysaccharides, secreted from granulosa cells, and serum transudate. The fluid coalesces forming an antrum (or cleft) filled with follicular fluid. The antrum separates the granulosa cells into two regions: the corona radiata (a rim of granulosa cells) around the oocyte and the outer membrana granulosa. The oocyte becomes isolated and suspended in the fluid connected to the rest of the granulosa cells by a thin strand of cells, the cumulus oophorus (egg stalk). The oocyte does not increase in size but continues to synthesize RNA and protein.

Follicular development is dependent on pituitary support. Removal of the pituitary gland (hypophysectomy) results in the cessation of follicular growth and the death of the oocyte. This can be halted by adding back LH and FSH, which stimulate further growth. It takes 8 to 12 days for the primary follicle to grow into the antral follicle. Failure of follicular growth for any reason results in a restarting of the cycle of follicular development, and hence both a longer first phase of the cycle and a longer cycle. It seems likely that women who regularly have a longer than normal menstrual cycle have either a slow rate of follicular development and increasing oestrogen secretion or the dominant follicle starts developing but fails so the next most appropriate follicle takes over the role as the dominant follicle.

Although the increasing concentration of oestrogen (predominantly oestradiol, $E_2$) initially has a negative feedback on the hypothalamus and pituitary, there is a critical concentration of oestrogen that is stimulatory provided it lasts for a critical duration. When the diameter of the follicle is 18–22 μm and the oestradiol concentration reaches 600–1200 pmol/l, there is positive feedback on the anterior pituitary gland leading to a sudden increase or 'surge' of LH release (Hamilton-Fairley & Johnson 1998) (Fig. 4.6).

## The LH surge

The effect of the LH surge is twofold. First, it stimulates the terminal growth phase of the follicle and oocyte, halting further cell division and maturation, culminating in its expulsion from the ovary. Secondly, it causes endocrine changes within the follicular cells that result in a different hormone secretory profile in the second half of the cycle.

Within a few hours of the LH surge, there are dramatic changes in the oocyte, which resumes meiotic division. There may also be a positive signal from the granulosa cells or a reduction of gap junction communication, which decreases the flow of meiosis-arresting substances to the oocyte. Progression though the remainder of the first meiotic division results in half the chromosomes (as paired chromatids) and almost all the cytoplasm being enclosed in the secondary oocyte, which is destined to become the ovum. The remaining chromosomes and very little cytoplasm are enclosed in a membrane forming a very small cell, known as the first polar body (see Fig. 4.3, p. 71). Thus the secondary oocyte keeps the bulk of the materials that were synthesized earlier in follicular development; these are conserved for the zygote. The chromosomes of the secondary oocyte enter the second meiotic division and go on to the next stage of division, called metaphase (see Fig. 7.4, p. 131), where they align on the spindle. However, meiosis is then immediately arrested for a second time; this is regulated by cytostatic factors. Meiosis resulting in the production of a mature female pronucleus will not resume until successful fertilization following ovulation. By this time, the oocyte will already contain the sperm nucleus. Thus, there is actually no time when the oocyte is a true gamete in the sense of being a cell with only 23 chromosomes, as is the case of a spermatozoon.

Concurrently, the LH surge promotes maturation of the cytoplasmic compartment of the oocyte. The cytoplasmic processes between the oocyte and the granulosa cells withdraw and contact is lost. The Golgi apparatus (see Table 1.1, p. 3) synthesizes lysosome-like cortical granules, which align under the surface of the oocyte. Protein synthesis continues but the profile of the proteins synthesized changes as the oocyte prepares for fertilization. The gonadotrophin surge stimulates the cumulus cells surrounding the oocyte (see Fig. 4.4, p. 72) to secrete hyaluronic acid, which disperses the cumulus cells embedding them in a mucus-like matrix (Eppig 1980).

## Ovulation

Ovulation is triggered by the mid-cycle surge of LH, which occurs in response to sustained high levels of oestrogen released from the developing dominant follicle. The single mature preovulatory follicle has a diameter of 2–2.5 cm in an ovary that is approximately 3 cm long. It was this structure that de Graaff identified and named in 1672. The increased size and changed position of the follicle means that it protrudes from the surface of the ovary (see Fig. 4.2, p. 70) This results in the thinning of the layer of epithelial cells between the wall of the follicle and the peritoneal cavity. As expansion continues, the wall becomes thinner and avascular and the cells appear to dissociate.

About 36 hours after the LH surge ovulation occurs and the oocyte is expelled from the ovary (see Fig. 4.2, p. 70). The LH surge stimulates the production of a

Fig. 4.6 ***The reproductive cycle and hormone levels.***

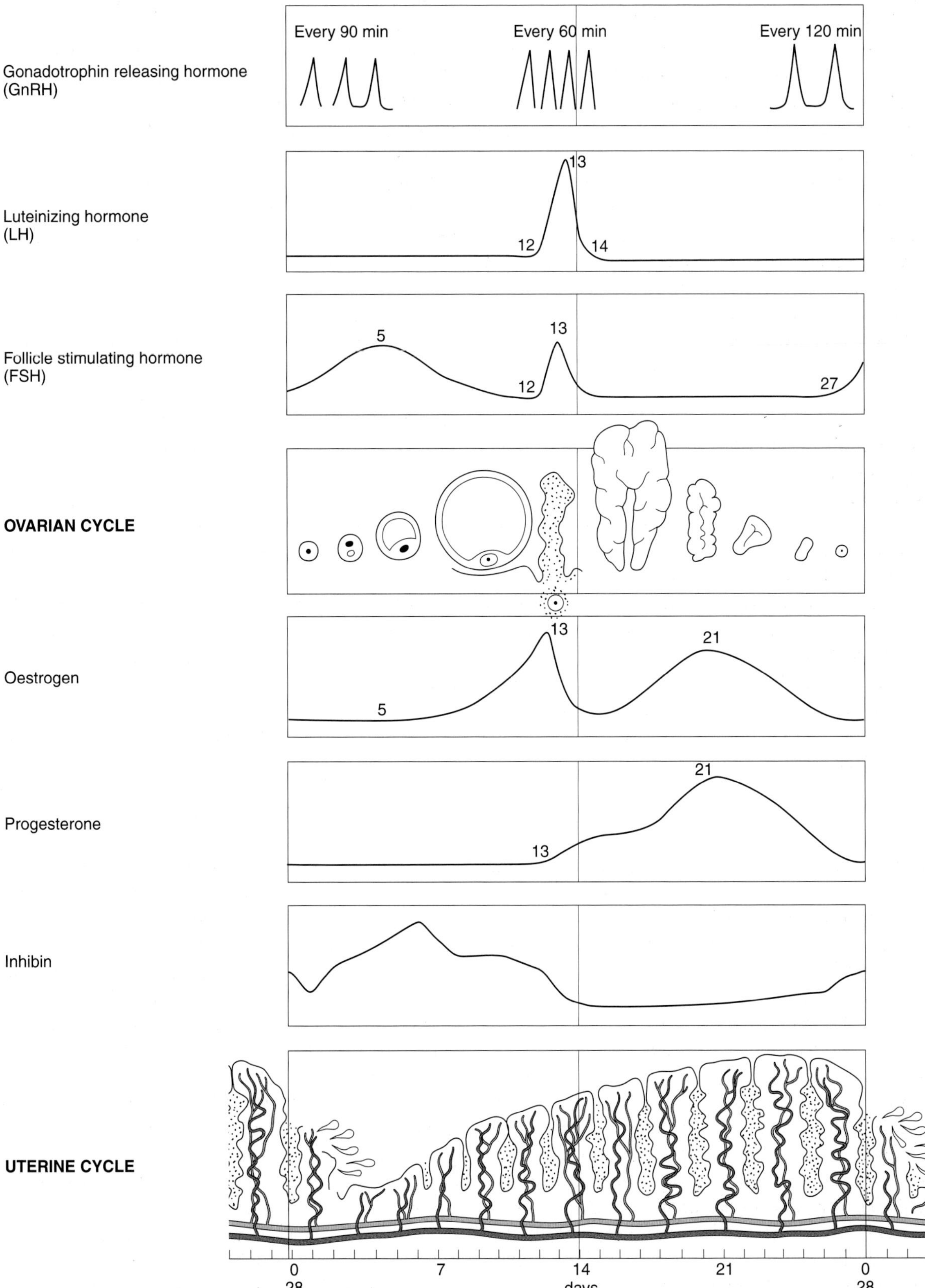

cascade of proteolytic enzymes, including renin and other trypsin-like enzymes from thecal cells, which digest the follicle wall. The biochemical changes, including generation of oxygen free radicals, that precede ovulation are similar to those seen in inflammation (Espey 1980). Plasminogen activator, which converts procollagenase to collagenase, is produced by granulosa cells resulting in the breakdown of the connective tissue. Progesterone production rises immediately after the LH surge and the preovulatory increase in progesterone may be important in follicular rupture as it decreases formation of collagen. Prostaglandins increase vascular permeability, which maintains the intrafollicular pressure as fluid begins to leak through the eroded follicular wall. Small contractile waves also ripple through the ovary increasing the intrafollicular pressure. The force is cushioned by the follicular fluid so the pressure generated is targeted at the weakened ovarian surface, causing it to rupture. As the follicle ruptures and the ovarian surface is breached, the fluid washes the oocyte, which is surrounded by the granulosa (cumulus) cells, from the ovary to the exterior. The oocyte is swept into the uterine tube by the fimbria. It is then propelled towards the uterus by peristaltic muscular activity and cilia movements of the epithelial cells lining the tube. After taking years to complete maturation, the oocyte is then viable and fertilizable for only about a day.

## The luteal phase

Within 2 hours of the LH surge, there is a transient rise in oestrogen and androgens secreted by the follicle as the thecal layers become stimulated and hyperaemic. The outer granulosa cells with their newly expressed receptors for LH no longer convert androgens to oestrogen but synthesize progesterone instead. The cells no longer bind oestrogen or FSH. The result is a marked increase in progesterone secretion, which begins several hours before ovulation.

### The corpus luteum

After ovulation, the residual parts of the follicle remaining in the ovary collapse into the space and form the corpus luteum ('yellow body'–see Fig. 4.4, p. 72). There is some bleeding and fibrotic activity in the cavity, which allows formation of a fibrin core around which the remaining granulosa cells congregate. The structure is enclosed by a capsule of fibrous thecal cells. The basement membrane between the granulosa cells and thecal cells breaks down allowing vascularization of the interior. This allows increased transport of cholesterol precursor to the lutenizing granulosa cells to maintain a high rate of progesterone secretion. A few of the thecal cells disperse to the stroma tissue. The granulosa cells first luteinize, then stop dividing and hypertrophy into large luteal cells. The luteal cells are rich in mitochondria, endoplasmic reticulum and Golgi bodies and have numerous lipid droplets and lutein, a yellow carotenoid pigment.

### Hormonal changes

Luteinization is associated with a progressive increment in progesterone secretion from the corpus luteum. The outer thecal cells form a stem cell population of smaller luteal cells which have numerous LH receptors and produce progesterone and androgens. Levels of progesterone rise until the middle of the luteal phase (see Fig. 4.6, p. 77). The corpus luteum produces oestrogen and inhibin as well as progesterone. All three hormones inhibit secretion of FSH from the anterior pituitary gland and therefore prevent further development of follicles.

It has been suggested that a cause of fertility problems may be inadequate production of progesterone at the time of ovulation and during the subsequent luteal phase. However, exogenous administration of progesterone or hCG has had limited success in clinical practice. It appears that most women have a proportion of their cycles with a low progesterone output without it affecting their fertility (Hamilton-Fairley & Johnson 1998). A shortened luteal phase can lead to intermenstrual bleeding, premenstrual spotting and short cycles.

The corpus luteum also synthesizes relaxin, secretion of which peaks in the middle of the luteal cycle (Johnson et al 1993), probably regulated by LH. Relaxin may be involved in promoting the growth of the myometrium and cervix and growth and secretory activity of the endometrium (Huang, Stromer & Anderson 1991).

Effectively, the corpus luteum is an endocrine gland producing oestrogen and progesterone. The LH surge stimulates its growth and activity. Unless fertilization occurs the life of the corpus luteum is very short, and it undergoes luteolysis (degeneration and regression) after about 6 days. The corpus luteum appears to have an age-related decrease in responsiveness to LH (Zeleznik & Hillier 1997) and so requires progressively more LH for survival. Following the LH surge, LH concentration in the luteal phase is low so luteolysis will occur. Blood flow to the corpus luteum falls and the follicular tissue becomes ischaemic. The concentrations of oestrogen and progesterone begin to fall as the degenerating corpus luteum stops hormone production. Thus luteolysis terminates a non-fertile cycle. As the level of oestrogen falls, the inhibition on the hypothalamus will be abrogated and FSH secretion will resume ready for the next cycle. The atrophying corpus luteum loses its yellow pigment, so it becomes known as a corpus albicans. It gradually contracts over a period of months, leaving a white scar.

### *Changes on fertilization*

If fertilisation occurs then hCG, which has structural similarities to LH, rescues the corpus luteum, stimulating its further growth and production of steroid hormone production up to the 10th week when placental endocrine function becomes established. Human chorionic gonadotrophin has a longer half-life than LH so it provides a sustained and more intense stimulus.

If fertilization occurs then the concentration of relaxin also continues to rise until the end of the first trimester.

## Regulation of gonadotrophin secretion

The brain controls and regulates the ovarian cycle. The gonadotrophs in the anterior pituitary secrete the glycoprotein hormones, LH and FSH (which together are known as gonadotrophins). There appear to be two distinct populations of cells in the anterior pituitary, each producing one particular type of hormone; however, fluorescent labelling shows that some cells contain both hormones. Synthesis and secretion of LH and FSH are dependent on GnRH from the hypothalamus, which acts as the common mediator of influences via the CNS. (GnRH is also known as luteinizing hormone releasing hormone, or LHRH.) The hypothalamus releases GnRH into the hypophysial portal circulation that runs to the pituitary gland.

This pathway means that control of the reproduction can be modulated and affected by other inputs from the higher brain centres. The GnRH neurons convert neural signals into endocrine signals. Stress, nutritional status and environmental influences, for instance, affect the timing and success of the reproduction. Ovulation appears to be seasonally regulated in populations experiencing seasonal variation in food availability (Bronson 1995).

There are two levels of regulation. First, the GnRH neurons of the hypothalamus have an inherent pulsatile activity. The steroid hormones, the gonadotrophins (LH and FSH) and GnRH feedback on the hypothalamic–pituitary axis (HPA) exert a second level of endocrine control. Prolactin also has an effect on the control of reproduction.

GnRH and gonadotrophins are released in a pulsatile manner (see Box 4.4). The cells releasing GnRH appear to be widely and diffusely distributed (Rance, Young & McMullen 1991) but are remarkably synchronized to produce pulses of GnRH. During the follicular phase, the pulses are of low amplitude and high frequency, occurring every 60 minutes (Clarke 1996). In the luteal phase, they are more irregular and have high amplitude and occur with a low frequency of about every 2 hours. The output of the gonadotrophins, LH and FSH, is changed by increasing or decreasing the amplitude or frequency of the pulses or by modulating the response of the gonadotrophs to the pulses. Prior to the LH surge, gonadotroph GnRH receptor density increases and the cells become more sensitive to GnRH. Inhibin and activin affect secretion of FSH without affecting secretion of GnRH. Two phenomena are observed: first, a depressant effect on output of gonadotrophins by increased oestrogen, progesterone and inhibin, and secondly, an increased surge of LH and FSH secretion induced primarily by oestradiol (Fig. 4.7). The pattern of pulsatile secretion of GnRH is regulated by a complex mechanism that allows multiple signals, such as neurotransmitters and sex steroids, to determine ovulation.

In the early part of the follicular phase, rising levels of FSH stimulate oestrogen production from the developing follicles. Rising concentrations of oestradiol have a negative feedback effect on gonadotrophin production from the anterior pituitary so FSH secretion falls. Activin and inhibin also affect FSH secretion. Inhibin is involved in the negative feedback of FSH secretion. However, the dominant follicle is exquisitely sensitive to even a diminishing concentration of FSH and continues to produce oestrogen, which markedly increases by two- to fourfold. These concentrations are maintained for 48 hours, which produces a positive feedback effect resulting in the dramatic surge of LH and FSH release seen in mid cycle prior to

**Box 4.4**

**Biological rhythms**

The study of biological rhythms is termed 'chronobiology'. All living cells, organs, organisms and groups of individuals demonstrate rhythmical changes within their internal (endogenous) physiology that can also result in external changes in behaviour. The rhythms can be categorized according to the length of the cycle or period of oscillation.

- ultradian—the rhythm is less than 1 day; for example, rapid eye movement in sleep
- circahordal—the period of oscillation is around 1 hour
- circadian—the period of oscillation is about 1 day; levels of many hormones such as cortisol fluctuate on a daily basis
- infradian—the rhythm is repeated in a cycle greater than 1 day, for example, menstrual and oestrus cycles
- circaseptram—the period of oscillation is about 1 week
- circatidal—the rhythm relates to tidal movement of water
- circalunar (synodic)—the rhythm relates to the cycle of the moon
- circannual—the rhythm has a cycle of about 1 year

These fluctuations are often affected by the external environment and appear to enable the individual to respond to forthcoming changes within the environment. Factors that influence or reset the cycle are described as entraining the cycle. In the human brain, the suprachiasmatic nuclei of the hypothalamus may influence daily fluctuations. The pineal gland, which produces the hormone melatonin at night, appears to affect the suprachiasmatic nuclei, acting as an entrainer. The circadian pattern of melatonin secretion is achieved through inhibition via a neural pathway (outside the optic nerve) that is activated by light stimulation upon the retina. Therefore, within temperate zones, light not only acts as an entrainer on a daily basis but, due to the fluctuation of the photoperiod (length of daylight exposure), entrainment of annual cycles can also be achieved.

ovulation. The effect of oestradiol is very sensitive: a low concentration has a marked and rapid effect that is evident within 1 hour and maximal within 4 to 6 hours. During the luteal phase, increased progesterone concentrations reinforce the negative feedback effects of oestradiol. The production of both LH and FSH secretion is very low, therefore the positive effect of oestradiol is blocked.

**Fig. 4.7** ***Hormonal regulation of the menstrual cycle. (Reproduced with permission from Johnson & Everitt 1995.)***

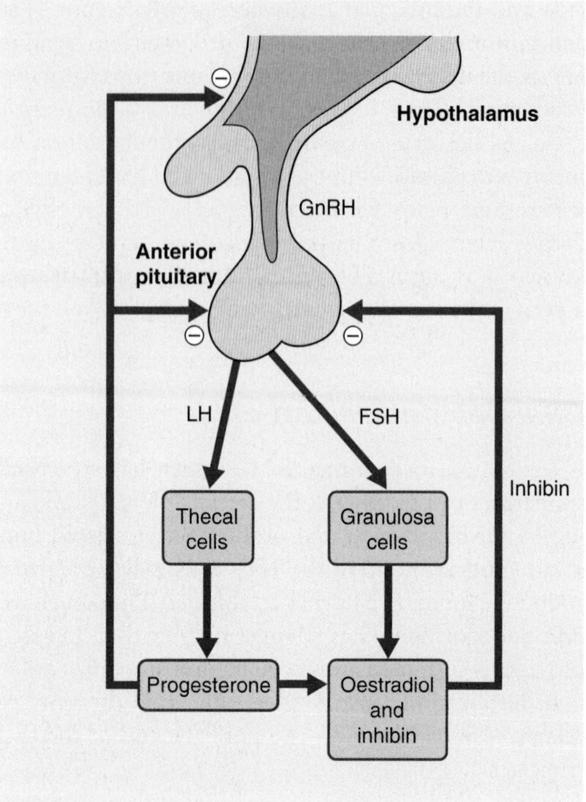


## Cyclical effects of oestrogens and progesterone

### *Effects on the uterus*

Organs that respond to hormonal changes have receptors for the hormones. Responses can change because hormone levels fluctuate or because receptor density on the target organs alters. The principal actions of oestrogen and progesterone during the monthly cycle are on the endometrium. The endometrium undergoes cyclical changes: the growth of the uterine wall in expectation of an embryo, and its degeneration if fertilization does not take place. In the first half of the cycle, the uterus goes through a proliferative phase. Oestrogen stimulates the epithelial cells of the basal layer of the endometrium to divide and proliferate, forming a thick mucosal wall with numerous endometrial glands (Fig. 4.8). Oestrogen also stimulates angiogenesis (growth of new blood vessels): extensive vascular tissue, spiral arteries and veins develop within

**Fig. 4.8** ***Cyclical effects on the endometrium.***

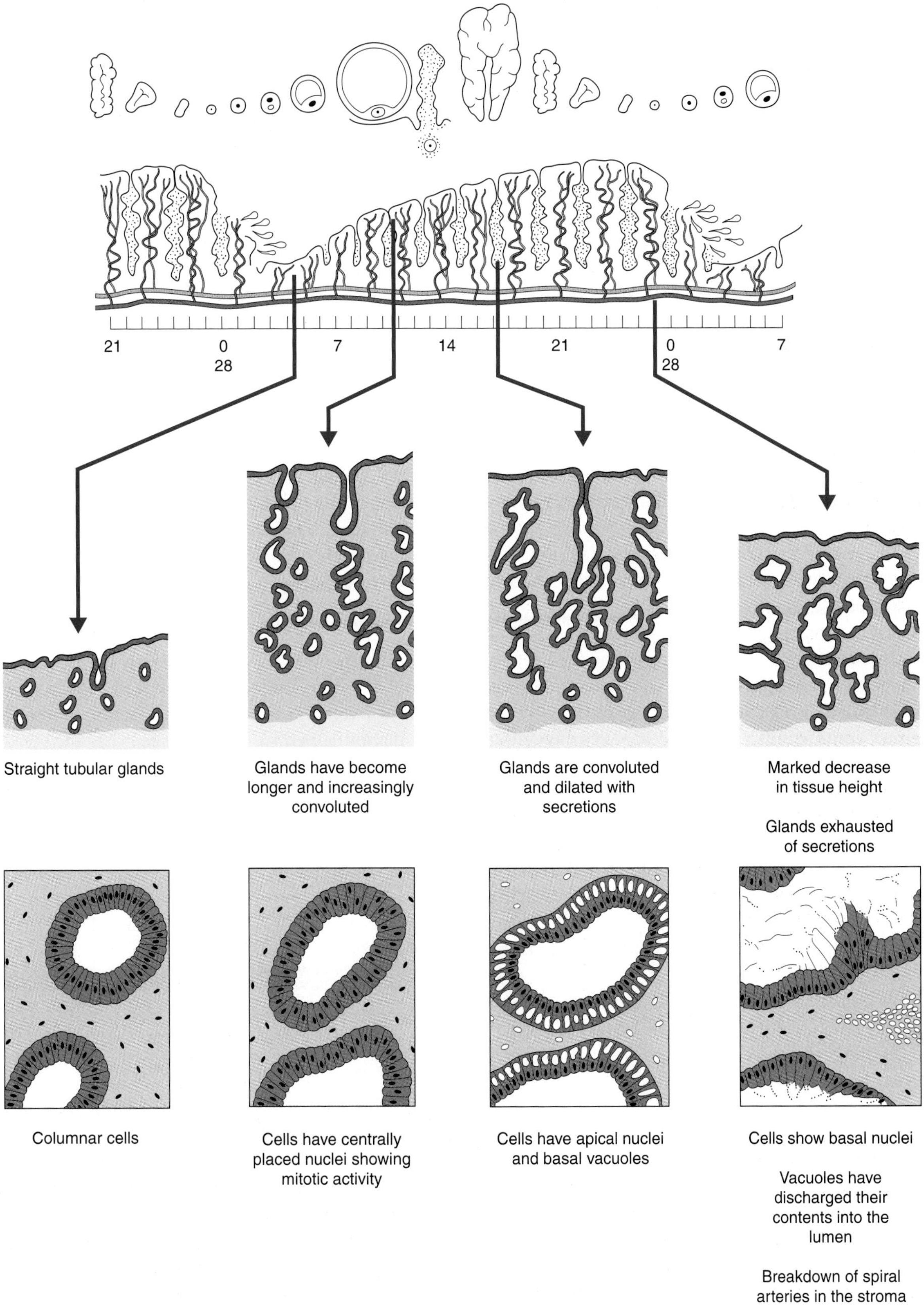

21 0 28 7 14 21 0 28 7

Straight tubular glands

Glands have become longer and increasingly convoluted

Glands are convoluted and dilated with secretions

Marked decrease in tissue height

Glands exhausted of secretions

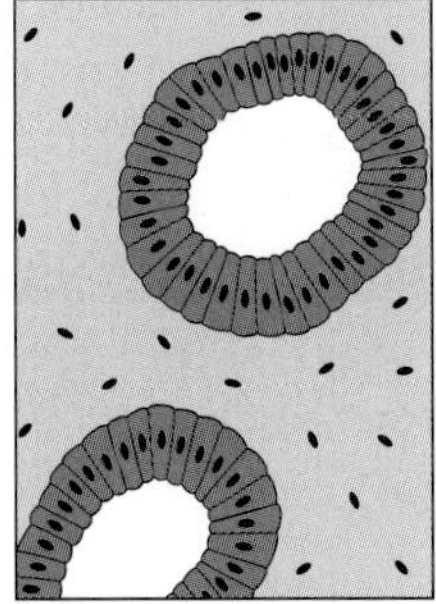

Columnar cells

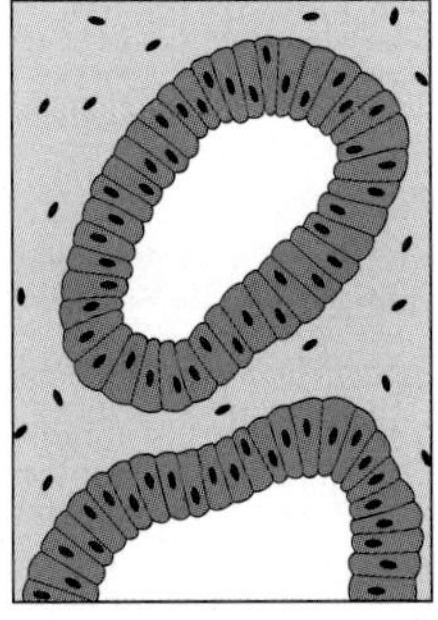

Cells have centrally placed nuclei showing mitotic activity

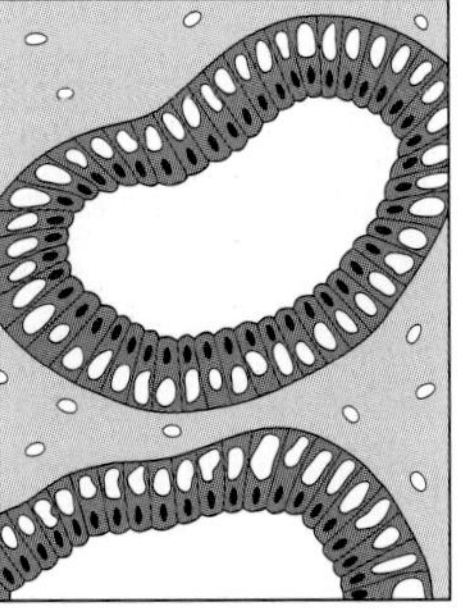

Cells have apical nuclei and basal vacuoles

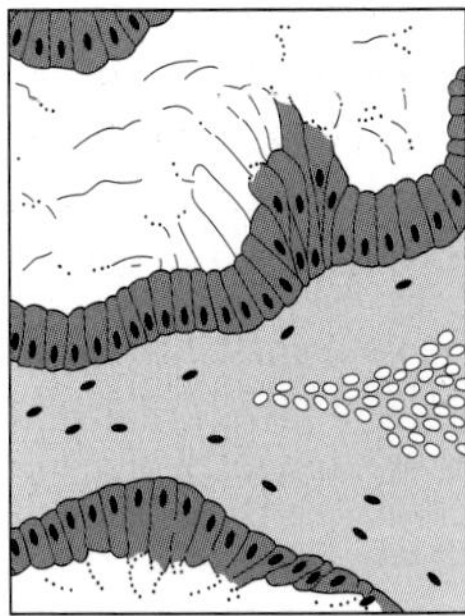

Cells show basal nuclei

Vacuoles have discharged their contents into the lumen

Breakdown of spiral arteries in the stroma

the endometrium. Within the space of a few days, the effect of oestrogen is to increase the height of the wall from 0.5 to 5 mm, a remarkable 10-fold increase. The myometrium does not grow so extensively. During the proliferative phase, oestrogen primes the endometrial cells by inducing the synthesis of progesterone receptors.

After ovulation, the cells of the enlarging corpus luteum begin to secrete progesterone, which has a dramatic effect on the secretory activity of the endometrial glands. In this secretory phase, the effects of progesterone are dominant, although oestrogen is still secreted from the corpus luteum. The spiral arteries continue growing and thus become more prominent and coiled as the height of the endometrium remains unchanged. The endometrial glands become dilated and convoluted with secretions rich in proteins, glycogen, sugars, amino acids, mucus and enzymes. The secretory products are important for the survival and nutrition of the zygote and blastocyst prior to implantation. Failure of conception results in diminishment of the corpus luteum and decreased steroid hormone production. By the 7th postovulatory day, the secretory process ceases and the glands become exhausted and regress.

Cyclical effects are particularly evident within the female reproductive tract. Activity of the myometrium is inversely related to progesterone secretion. During menstruation, when progesterone levels are low, the uterine contractions, mediated by prostaglandins, have a higher frequency and strength than in labour (Lyons et al 1991). These uterine contractions are responsible for dysmenorrhoea (period pains). Non-steroidal anti-inflammatory drugs (NSAIDs) such as aspirin inhibit prostaglandin synthesis, and are therefore effective in reducing pain. After menstruation there is a slow decline in myometrial activity during the follicular phase; it reaches negligible activity mid cycle. Thus the uterus is at its most quiescent at the time of implantation. Uterine quiescence is maintained until the late luteal phase when levels of progesterone fall. If pregnancy intervenes, levels of progesterone remain high and the myometrium remains inactive. Uterine blood flow, on the other hand, correlates positively with the pattern of oestrogen secretion. Due to low levels of oestrogen, blood supply to the endometrium during menses and early follicular phase is reduced. A marked increase occurs just prior to ovulation followed by a slight nadir. A secondary peak occurs in the luteal phase which mirrors the rise in oestrogen production. This means that endometrial blood flow is relatively high at the time of implantation but lower at menstruation, which helps to limit the blood loss at the latter time.

## *Effects on the uterine tubes, cervix and vagina*

### Uterine tubes

Oestrogen stimulates the epithelial cell activity, increasing cilia movement and secretion. This facilitates the movement of the ovum along the uterine tubes following ovulation. These effects are reversed by progesterone, which inhibits the peristaltic activity of the uterine tube smooth muscle.

### Cervix

Oestrogen relaxes the myometrial fibres supplying the cervix and increases stromal vascularization and oedema. Collagenase is activated, which causes some dispersal of the tightly bound collagen bundles into a looser matrix. The result is that the cervix becomes softer to touch. The external os everts prior to ovulation. Progesterone causes the cervical muscle to retract and the stroma to become more compact as the collagen matrix reforms. The external os becomes tighter. The change in texture of the cervix is used as part of natural family planning (see Box 4.5). The cervix is softer at ovulation and a few days before, coinciding with the fertile period. At this stage it has the consistency of lips compared with the harder 'nose-like' cartilaginous consistency of the cervix later in the cycle when the effects of progesterone are dominant.

The cyclical changes in blood flow are reflected by the composition of cervical mucus, which is copious and receptive to sperm penetration in mid

**Box 4.5**

**Concepts of natural family planning**

- Based on periodic abstinence
- Also known as 'rhythm method' or 'safe period'
- Assumes interval between ovulation and menstruation is constant
- Based on recognition of signs of ovulation and fertile phases of menstrual cycle
  - — temperature rise after ovulation
  - — increased cervical mucus and watery vaginal secretions
  - — softer consistency of cervix
- Probably most effective for birth spacing

**Table 4.1** *Changes in cervical mucus*

| Proliferative phase (follicular) | Secretory phase (luteal) |
|---|---|
| 'E' mucus | 'G' mucus |
| Oestrogen | Progesterone |
| Network of long parallel polypeptide chains | Meshwork of polypeptide strands |
| Carbohydrate side chains | Increased carbohydrate side chains |
| Forms channels 5 μm wide | Smaller space between molecules |
| High water content (98%) | Lower water content |
| Copious volume | Scanty volume |
| Clear | Cloudy |
| Acellular | Cells present |
| Spinnbarkeit = 10–20 cm (stretching between glass plates) | Spinnbarkeit ~ 3 cm |
| Dehydration: ferning | No ferning |
| Assists transport of sperm | Forms mucus plug to protect against infection |

cycle (Table 4.1). When progesterone levels are high, small volumes of thick cervical mucus are secreted that are hostile and impenetrable to sperm. The increased viscosity of the mucus in the latter half of the menstrual cycle reduces the risk of ascending infection at the time of implantation.

Both oestrogen and progesterone are secreted from the corpus luteum in the second half of the cycle. The concentrations of oestrogen and progesterone will continue to rise if successful fertilization results in secretion of hCG and consequent survival of the corpus luteum. Therefore, the effects of the hormones in the second half of the cycle on the female body portend the changes that would take place in pregnancy.

## Vagina

Oestrogen increases mitotic activity and secretion in the vaginal epithelial cells. Stimulation by progesterone results in an increased size of nucleus of vaginal epithelial cells. It is important when examining cervical cells, obtained from a smear, to relate the morphological differences to the stage of a woman's menstrual cycle. Earlier in the cycle, cells appear flatter whereas under the influence of progesterone they tend to become clumped and folded. There are also cyclical changes in the pH of the vagina as oestrogen stimulates the growth of lactobacilli (Doderlein's bacilli). These lactobacilli metabolize glycogen from the cervical secretions producing lactic acid as a metabolic by-product, which decreases pH to a level that protects the reproductive tract from opportunistic pathogenic microorganisms.

The resident flora of the vagina also produces volatile aliphatic acids, which have distinctive odours. The profile of acids changes throughout the cycle under the influence of the changing hormones, and may result in changed sexual behaviour. It is suggested that male responses to their partners are affected by the cyclical fluctuations in olfactory stimuli stimulating sexual responsiveness and interaction. These olfactory signals do not seem to be consciously perceived in humans. Another example is women who live together are often observed to demonstrate menstrual synchrony: they ovulate and menstruate at the same time. Recently, it has been demonstrated that humans have the potential to communicate by pheromones. Odourless body secretions from women in different phases of the menstrual cycle can advance or delay the phases of other women (Stem & McClintock 1998).

## Other effects

There are additional effects and benefits of oestrogen on women's health. Oestrogens appear to protect the cardiovascular system; thus women of reproductive age and normal endocrine function have a lower incidence of hypertension and a reduced risk of cardiovascular disease owing to higher levels of high-density lipoproteins (HDLs), which lower circulating levels of cholesterol. Oestrogens stimulate osteoblasts, the cells involved in bone formation, thus maintaining bone mass. Oestrogens may depress appetite and are mildly anabolic.

Postovulatory levels of progesterone are high causing a slight increase in the basal metabolic rate. The basal body temperature rises owing to the influence of progesterone on the thermoregulatory centre of the hypothalamus. A temperature rise of 0.2–0.6 °C confirms ovulation has taken place but does not predict it. In the second half of the cycle the skin may appear more pigmented and acne may worsen as progesterone increases constriction of sebaceous glands. Progesterone also increases appetite during the luteal phase (Buffenstein et al 1995). Women with premenstrual syndrome (PMS) may report cravings for carbohydrate, which are often associated with feelings of depression (Dye & Blundell 1997). These patterns of fluctuations in energy intake, appetite and depression appear to be associated with low serotonin activity. Metabolism of drugs and alcohol may cyclically alter during the menstrual cycle.

Oestrogen and progesterone affect connective tissue oedema and hyperaemia and can cause increased breast size and tenderness. Progesterone binds to renal aldosterone receptors, causing natriuresis (sodium excretion) and blocking aldosterone occupation. Aldosterone increases to restore sodium retention, so there is a net effect of sodium retention. Oestrogen stimulates angiotensinogen production, which also tends to enhance sodium retention. Thus, in the luteal phase of the cycle, salt and water retention may be increased causing generalized weight gain and premenstrual feelings of bloatedness.

## Menstruation

Menstruation is the loss of the decidual (superficial) layers of the endometrium accompanied by some blood loss. In the human, menstrual loss usually lasts 5–7 days. Humans and other primates, together with elephant-shrews and some types of bats, are the only animals that menstruate. In these species there is marked progesterone-related proliferation of the endometrium and implantation is invasive. It was suggested that menstruation evolved as a protective mechanism against sperm-borne pathogens. However, an alternative hypothesis is that cyclical regression and proliferation of the endometrium is energetically more economical in term of reproductive costs than constantly maintaining a receptive endometrium (Strassmann 1996).

The degeneration of the corpus luteum and resulting fall in oestrogen and progesterone levels cause a modest but significant decrease in endometrial tissue height so the spiral arteries are coiled tighter and compressed. This results in a reduced blood flow, ischaemia and denudement of the endometrial tissue and interstitial haemorrhage. Prostaglandins released by the spiral arteries stimulate vasoconstriction and vasodilatation resulting in rhythmic waves of contraction and relaxation in the latter. (The effect is like breaking a wire by rhythmically bending it backwards and forwards.) The waves become longer and more profound causing the decidual endometrium to break away along the natural plane of cleavage. The straight arteries in the basal layer maintain the blood supply. It is from these that new spiral arteries will regenerate. At the end of the secretory phase, there is an ischaemic phase followed by the menstrual phase leading to the next proliferative phase. Within 12 hours, the height of the endometrium falls from 4 mm to 1 mm.

Menstrual flow is usually between 35 and 95 ml and consists of endometrial debris and blood. Blood loss is limited by vasoconstriction of the spiral arteries and formation of thrombin–platelet plugs in the terminal portions of the straight arteries. When oestrogen secretion resumes at the beginning of the next cycle, it stimulates healing and new tissue growth. Menstrual blood does not coagulate in the pattern seen normally. The damaged endometrial cells secrete proteolytic and fibrinolytic enzymes, which inhibit the formation of fibrin and therefore clot formation. The average volume of blood lost is 50 ml, which accounts for 0.7 mg iron, a loss which is just matched by dietary iron absorption.

Case study 4.1 looks at the problem of calculating the length of gestation from the date of the last menstrual period.

**Case study 4.1**

Njuka is in England with her husband who is a diplomatic representative of a central African country. When they first meet, the midwife asks Njuka when her baby is due and is informed that four full moons are left to pass before the baby will come. The midwife, intrigued by this answer, asks Njuka how she knows this. Njuka explains that six full moons have passed since her last period and that is how she knows.

- How accurate is Njuka's calculation of her gestation?
- Why is it important for a midwife to be able to estimate the length of gestation?
- What other information can help in this estimation?

## Hormonal causes of infertility

Hormonal causes of infertility account for about a third of the known causes (Box 4.6).

**Box 4.6**
**Hormonal causes of infertility**

- Hypogonadotrophic hypogonadism
- Anorexic states
- Weight fluctuations
- Obesity
- Hyperprolactinaemia
- Polycystic ovary syndrome

### *Hypogonadotrophic hypogonadism*

Hypogonadotrophic hypogonadism is due to malfunction of the hypothalamic–pituitary axis and is characterized by low levels of oestrogen. Women with normal pituitary functions can be successfully treated with pulsatile exogenous GnRH from a small infusion pump. The hypothalamus is frequently entrained by the pump so normal rhythms of pulsatile secretion continue after the pump is removed. Alternatively, women can be treated with exogenous gonadotrophins. Human menopausal gonadotrophin (hMG) extracted from the urine of postmenopausal women (the effects of ovariectomy or the menopause are to decrease oestradiol concentration, which results in raised circulating levels of FSH and LH) is used because it contains both FSH and enough LH to stimulate synthesis of androgenic precursors for oestrogen production. Ultrasound monitoring of follicular development is important to assess development of excess follicles and the risk of multiple pregnancy. Ovarian stimulation can cause ovarian hyperstimulation syndrome which has serious implications because vascular permeability can suddenly increase, resulting in a movement of fluid out of the vascular system (McClure et al 1994).

### *Anorexic states and weight fluctuations*

Weight loss can also disrupt the hypothalamic–pituitary axis. Anorexic patients often have disrupted menstrual cycles, but acute weight loss (such as that associated with 'crash' dieting) even within a normal body weight range may disrupt hormone secretion. A body mass index (BMI) index greater than 19 $kg/m^2$ and at least 22% fat as a proportion of body weight seem to be necessary for the maintenance of normal ovulatory cycles. It has been suggested that the critical fat mass for fertility is equivalent to the energy requirements of pregnancy (Frisch 1990). Low body fat delays puberty and the menarche. Weight loss particularly affects LH secretion and can result in an abbreviated luteal phase.

Appetite is stimulated by the orexigenic neuropeptide Y (NPY) from the hypothalamus. NPY is involved in the regulation of food intake and energy balance. It has both stimulatory and inhibitory effects at the pituitary gland. In the well-nourished state, NPY release is acute and intermittent, a mode of secretion that potentiates GnRH-induced LH release. However, fasting decreases plasma glucose concentrations and extremes of exercise result in chronic secretion of NPY and continuous NPY receptor activation, which is inhibitory to LH release and thus fertility.

Eating causes storage of triacylglycerides in adipose cells, which stimulates the cells to release leptin. Leptin seems to be the satiety signal, which modulates the release of NPY. In starvation, leptin levels are low and NPY levels are high, which inhibits GnRH. The nutritional control of reproduction probably had an important evolutionary role in suppressing fertility at times of poor food supply. Suspending reproductive function at times of food shortage is protective.

Case study 4.2 looks at the problem of underweight in the calculation of gestation.

### *Obesity*

Paradoxically, obesity also affects fertility; obese women are overrepresented in fertility clinics and have increased incidence of menstrual abnormality and a higher risk of miscarriage. The effects of obesity may persist even after weight loss has occurred. One of the reasons is that the adipose tissue is metabolically active, producing altered ratios of oestrogens and androgens. Obesity also affects insulin secretion (obese people are more likely to demonstrate insulin resistance) and affects production of leptin.

### *Hyperprolactinaemia*

Hyperprolactinaemia can result from prolactin-secreting tumours, which are usually benign. However,

**Case study 4.2**

Lisa, a 17-year-old primipara, presents herself at the midwives' clinic, giving a vague history and saying that she thinks she might be pregnant. On palpation and abdominal examination, Lisa seems to be 26 weeks' pregnant and this is supported by a fundal height of 26 cm. The presence of fetal heart sounds confirms that Lisa is indeed pregnant. On questioning Lisa, the midwife discovers that Lisa has had only two scanty periods in the last 2 years and does not know the date of her last menstrual period. Lisa smokes 60 cigarettes a day, and has the appearance of being very underweight.

- Can you identify any possible reasons why Lisa might have irregular periods?
- Why must the midwife not assume that Lisa is 26 weeks' pregnant?
- Are there any clues that the midwife may investigate in order to estimate more precisely the actual gestation of Lisa's pregnancy?

other factors including stress, breast stimulation or examination, hypothyroidism, polycystic ovarian syndrome and dopaminergic antagonists can also raise circulating prolactin levels. Hyperprolactinaemia can cause oestrogen deficiency, amenorrhoea and galactorrhoea (milk production). The management of hyperprolactinaemia is usually by administration of bromocriptine, a dopamine agonist, although tumours may be surgically removed.

### Polycystic ovary syndrome

Polycystic ovarian syndrome (PCOS) is suspected from clinical signs and symptoms, and confirmed by ultrasound examination that shows enlarged ovaries containing more than 10 large cysts. Some women exhibit symptoms of disrupted cycles, obesity and hyperandrogenism, which causes acne, alopecia and hirsutism. The endocrine causes are hypersecretion of LH and increased levels of testosterone, insulin and prolactin. Oestrogen levels are high but not cyclical and ovulation frequently does not occur. The follicles retain the oocyte, forming ovarian cysts. Weight loss often improves the hormonal profile and alleviates the symptoms. Clomiphene citrate is an antioestrogenic drug that can be used to re-establish a normal pattern of ovulation.

## Artificial control of fertility

### Oral contraceptives

The first oral contraceptives were extracts from yam. Although yams are rich in progesterone-like compounds, the active ingredient was actually mestranol, an oestrogenic agent. The combination of progestogen and mestranol was essential for good cycle control. Natural progesterone and most other steroid hormones are digested in the gastrointestinal tract and are usually effective only if injected. Chemically modified hormones are resistant to proteolytic digestion in the gut but retain their biological activity. Many synthetic steroid hormones have been developed that have similar biological activity to the naturally occurring hormones and are metabolized very slowly by the liver, increasing their half-life. The term 'progestogens' is used to describe the family of natural and synthetic progesterone-like compounds.

The first contraceptive pills, used in Britain since 1961, were combined oral contraceptive pills (COC), combinations of an oestrogen and a progesterone. Currently the most common progestogen and oestrogen combinations used are norethisterone and ethinyloestradiol respectively (Fig. 4.9). A course of COC pills is taken for 21 days followed by 7 pill-free (or placebo) days when hormone levels fall, mimicking natural hormonal cycles and allowing a withdrawal bleed. Monophasic pills have a constant concentration of the active agents whereas biphasic and triphasic preparations attempt to mimic the characteristic fluctuations in oestrogen and progesterone throughout the cycle. Alternatively, progesterone-only preparations, known as 'minipills', containing small doses of progesterone only are taken on a continuous basis. Progesterone can also be administered as a depot injection or as slow-releasing preparation from a subcutaneous or uterine source.

### Effects on reproductive cycle

Synthetic oestrogens feed back on the hypothalamus during the antral phase of the menstrual cycle, reducing levels and the rate of the pulsatile secretion of GnRH. Therefore the release of FSH is inhibited so follicular maturation and expression of LH receptors do not occur. The oestrogens also prevent the LH surge and subsequent ovulation. Production of endogenous oestrogen is reduced.

**Fig. 4.9** ***Chemical structures of synthetic contraceptive hormones.***

Cholesterol

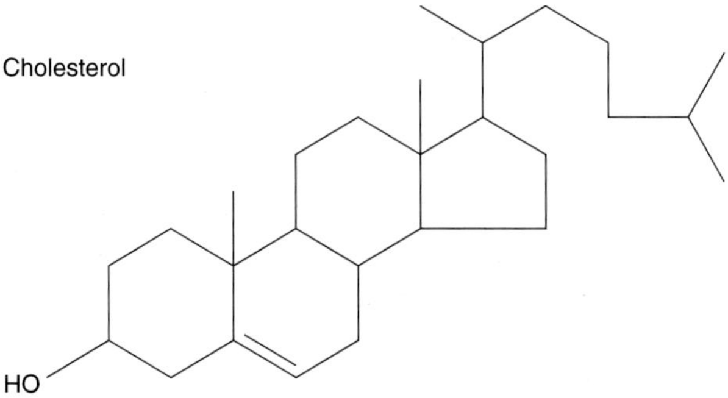

HO

Progesterone

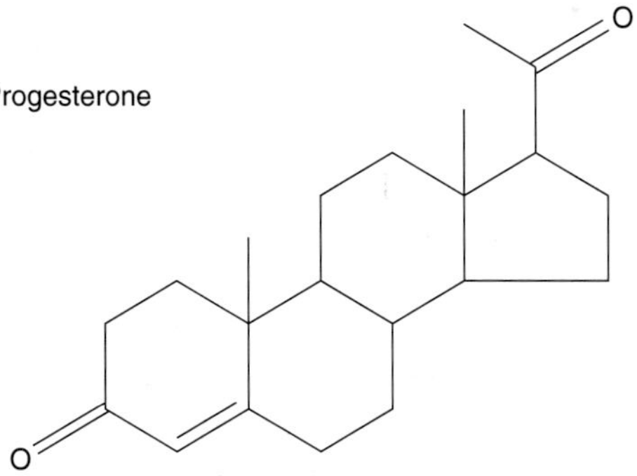

O

O

Norethisterone

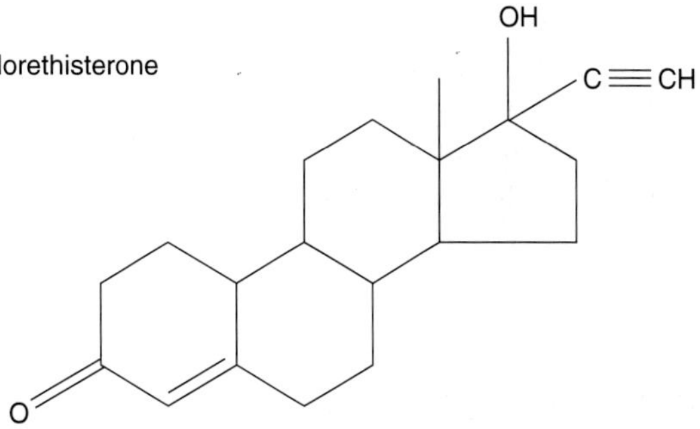

OH

C≡CH

O

Oestradiol-17ß

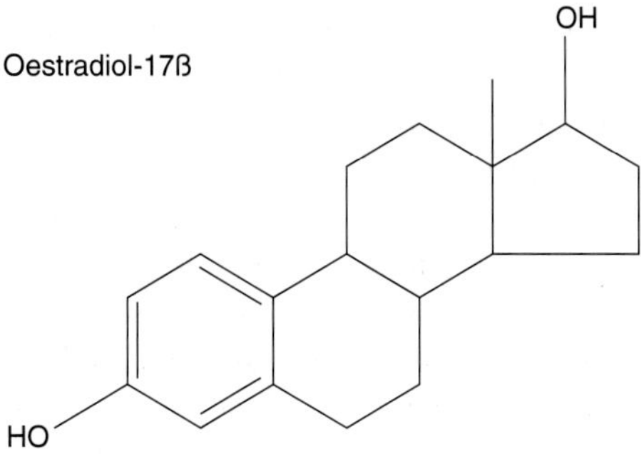

OH

HO

Gestodene

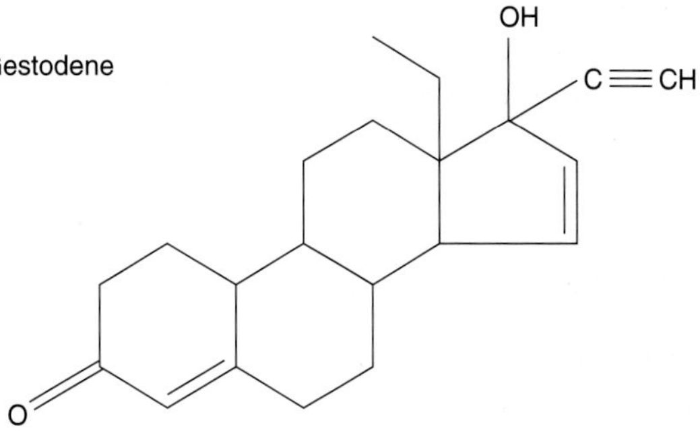

OH

C≡CH

O

Testosterone

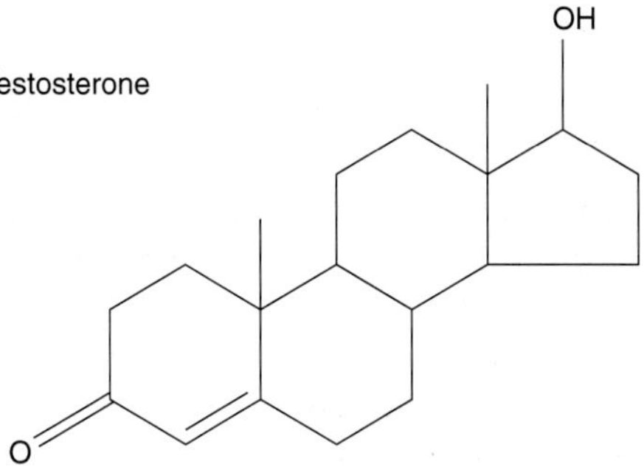

OH

O

Ethinyloestradiol

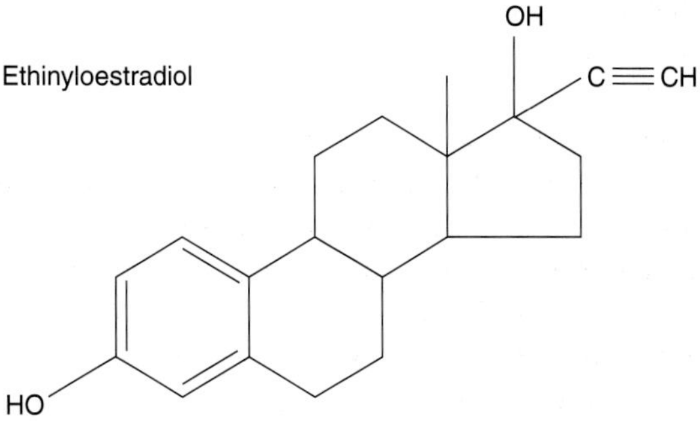

OH

C≡CH

HO

Synthetic progestogens interfere with the pulsatile secretion of GnRH and decrease the production of LH. Small doses of progesterone may not suppress ovulation but large doses do inhibit maturation of follicles and ovulation. Norethisterone also slows down the breakdown of natural progesterone by the liver. It can be used in low doses because it specifically binds to the progesterone receptors, rather than to androgen receptors as well. Progestogens also reduce secretory activity of the endometrium so it is not favourable to implantation. Under the influence of progestogens, the cervical mucus is thick and tenacious so is unreceptive to sperm. The peristaltic muscle activity and cilia movement of the uterine tube become uncoordinated so transport of the ovum and sperm are affected; this may directly affect successful fertilization. This effect on tubal motility is the reason why there is a slight increase in risk of ectopic pregnancy (implantation in the uterine tube) associated with progesterone preparations.

### *Side-effects*

Oestrogens affect coagulation factors and promote intravascular coagulation. They also tend to increase plasma lipid levels. Therefore, they can be used safely in young, healthy, motivated women who have no history of circulatory disease. However, smoking and obesity significantly increase the risk of side-effects, particularly thromboembolic complications. Although chemical contraceptive agents have been linked to an increased risk of breast cancer, the doses of synthetic hormone used in current contraceptive preparations are now extremely low so it is difficult to assess their risk. Although hormonal treatment has known thromboembolic health concerns, the morbidity complications from pregnancy and labour far outweigh the risks of using oral contraceptives.

## Puberty

Puberty describes the morphological, physiological and behavioural changes that occur as the gonads change from infantile to adult condition. Menarche is the term used for first menstrual cycle, which indicates that the levels of oestrogen and progesterone are adequate to induce development of the uterus. The equivalent step in males is the first ejaculation, which is often nocturnal. However, menarche or the first ejaculation does not necessarily mean that the adolescent body is able to reproduce. The sequence of pubertal changes is fairly constant but the starting age and the time for the changes to take place vary.

### *Physical changes*

Physical changes include the development of secondary sex characteristics, the adolescent growth spurt and marked changes in height, psychological states and fertility. All muscle and skeletal dimensions change and the body composition also alters. The earliest changes are measurable in young girls from the age of 6 years. Secondary sex characteristics become evident as secretion of oestrogen (from ovaries), and androgens (from ovaries and adrenal glands) increases. Changes are seen in the breasts, genitalia, pubic hair and voice.

### *Hormonal changes*

The hypothalamic–pituitary–gonadal axis, which has been developing since fetal life, is activated in early infancy but inhibited in childhood before being reactivated at puberty. Immediately after birth, levels of hCG and placental steroid hormones fall. LH and FSH levels increase; they are released in a pulsatile pattern, with nocturnal dominance, throughout infancy and childhood. FSH levels are higher in females and LH levels are higher in males. In the prepubertal period, FSH levels are relatively high compared with LH levels.

At puberty, the pulse amplitude of GnRH increases, resulting in the LH secretion exhibiting a pulsatile pattern. The 'on' switch is unknown but may be related to body mass or energy metabolism. Adrenal function matures independently before gonadal function. Adrenal secretion of sex steroids increases. Adrenal androgens stimulate pubic and axillary hair growth and have a small effect on growth and bone development. The timing of gonadal maturity and the onset of puberty correlate more closely with bone development than with chronological age. The central nervous system can restrain the onset by affecting the hypothalamic GnRH pattern. The age at menarche is affected by body mass, exercise, stress, nutrition and altitude (Frisch 1990).

### *Age of menarche*

Over half of early menstrual cycles are anovulatory and do not result in the release of an ovum. Ovulation usually occurs about 10 months after menarche. After a period of 5 years, the incidence of anovulatory cycles has decreased to about 20%. There are secular trends in the age of menarche. The average age of menarche in Europe is currently 12–13 years compared with a century ago when it was 14–15 years. Although there is a wide variation, the age of menarche appears to continue to fall at a rate of about 3 months per decade. Various influences on the age of menarche have been investigated, such as photoperiod and body mass. One suggestion was that the earlier age of menarche has coincided with the introduction of electricity, increasing the photoperiod and the individual's exposure to light (Bullough 1981). However, a more plausible theory is that it is related to better nutrition. Women seem to have a critical body mass for successful reproduction; if their body mass falls much below, the menstrual cycle becomes erratic and stops. Body fat levels seem to play a role. Anorexic women have lower levels of FSH and LH (see above). Moderate obesity is associated with earlier menarche but severe obesity delays it. The combination of heavy exercise and undernutrition is synergistic, as can be observed in ballet dancers and athletes (see Ch. 12). Chronic illness can also delay menarche; the exact mechanisms are unknown.

### Sequence of changes at puberty

The normal sequence in females is breast budding (at 8–13 years), growth of pubic hair, peak growth velocity (9.5–14.5 years) and then menarche (10–16.5 years). The pattern in boys is testicular growth, pubic hair growth, penile growth and growth spurt. From about 6 months of age, childhood growth depends on adequate growth hormone secretion. Growth declines progressively and reaches its slowest velocity just before the onset of the pubertal growth spurt. In boys, the growth spurt is slightly later, and is faster (9.4 cm/year compared with 8.3 cm/year in girls) with delayed fusion of the epiphyseal plates so men attain a higher adult height. The pubertal growth spurt depends on sex hormones secreted from the gonads. Optimal growth depends on both sex steroids and growth hormone; growth hormone levels are highest in the pubertal period.

## The menopause

The term 'menopause' is literally the cessation of menstrual cycles. However, the term is frequently applied to the climacteric, which is the decline of reproductive activity over a period of 2 to 3 years, usually between the ages of 45 and 55 years (median 51 years). The climacteric begins when fertility is already rapidly declining and continues until the ovaries cease secreting oestrogen.

### Effects on the reproductive system

Morphologically, the ovaries appear smaller and relatively devoid of follicles. When oestrogen secretion diminishes, the production of androgens increases. The finite number of ova become exhausted. There are advantages to the species in preventing late childbearing and ensuring the dependent human offspring are more likely to have the care and protection of their mother.

At the menopause, levels of FSH and LH are high and levels of oestrogen and inhibin are decreased. FSH increases because of the lack of a negative feedback from oestrogen influencing the anterior pituitary gland. The postmenopausal ovary continues to produce considerable amounts of androgens, thus natural menopause is not equivalent to the effects of a surgically induced menopause following oophorectomy (removal of ovaries).

### Hormone replacement therapy (HRT)

Hormone replacement therapy aims to reduce the diverse symptoms and adverse effects of the menopause (Box 4.7). In addition to the reproduction tract itself, there are many other target organs bearing oestrogen receptors, which respond to the fall in

**Box 4.7**
**Hormone replacement therapy**

- Exogenous oestrogen replaces ovarian oestrogen
- Prevents long-term consequences
- Oral route or directly to genital tract or systemically (transdermal patch or subcutaneous implant)
- Abrogates flushing and sweating
- Stimulates replication of, and secretion from, vaginal epithelial cells
- Progesterone given to induce menstruation (and prevent endometrial hyperplasia)
- Progesterone-withdrawal bleeding is major reason for non-compliance
- Protects against coronary heart disease and osteoporosis

circulating oestrogen levels. The resulting vasomotor instability produces symptoms of hot flushes, sweats and palpitations. The thermoregulatory centre in the hypothalamus falsely signals that body temperature is too high. This results in physiological processes such as increased peripheral vasodilation that attempt to reduce core body temperature. Emotional and psychological problems such as anxiety, depression, loss of libido and mood swings may occur. Insomnia is also a frequently cited problem.

All the tissues of the female reproductive tract have a high density of oestrogen receptors and are profoundly affected by oestrogen withdrawal. The uterus shrinks. The vaginal epithelium diminishes and the cells decrease production of glycogen, affecting lactobacillus colonization, so pH increases resulting in increased susceptibility to vaginal infections. Vaginal atrophy causes vaginal secretions to diminish, which may result in painful intercourse. Menopausal women have an increased frequency of urinary problems, which is probably related to oestrogen withdrawal as there are many oestrogen receptors in the urinary tract (which shares the same embryonic origin as the lower reproductive tract).

## Other effects of the menopause

Oestrogen protects the cardiovascular system. The incidence of coronary heart disease in premenopausal women and postmenopausal women treated with hormone replacement therapy is much lower than in men. Oestrogen inhibits the uptake and degradation of low-density lipoprotein (LDL) by the coronary blood vessel endothelium. It may also inhibit coronary vasospasm. Oestrogen has been shown to decrease vascular resistance (and therefore blood pressure), increase cardiac output and increase synthesis of nitric oxide (NO, a potent locally acting vasodilator). Postmenopausal women have significantly higher levels of serum cholesterol and triacylglycerides. Oestrogen withdrawal is associated with raised levels of certain blood-clotting factors and an increased tendency for thrombosis, and thus with increased risk of myocardial infarction and cerebrovascular accident (stroke).

## Key points

- The ovary produces the female gametes (ova) and steroid hormones, oestrogen and progesterone.
- Relatively few female gametes are produced during a woman's reproductive life, between puberty and the menopause.
- The meiotic division of the ovum begins in the female fetus and is suspended until ovulation, halts again, and is completed at fertilization.
- Follicular development begins about 3 months prior to ovulation but key stages in development of the follicles are stimulated by FSH in the first half of the menstrual cycle in which the ovum is released. The developing follicles produce oestrogen; usually a single dominant follicle matures and ovulates.
- The first half of the menstrual cycle (follicular phase) is dominated by oestrogen and prepares the reproductive system for ovulation, for instance by stimulating growth of the endometrial lining.
- Ovulation is triggered by the surge of LH. The ovum surrounded by a rim of cumulus cells is released and swept into the uterine tube.
- Follicular cells remaining in the ovary become the corpus luteum, which produces progesterone and oestrogen.
- The second half of the cycle (luteal phase) is dominated by the effects of progesterone, which prepare the body for pregnancy.
- LH promotes secretion from the corpus luteum. However, the effect is short lived so the corpus luteum regresses, unless rescued by hCG from the dividing cells of the embryo, and menstruation ensues.
- Pituitary secretion of FSH and LH is under the control of pulsatile GnRH release from the hypothalamus. Oestrogen and progesterone exert negative feedback effects on the hypothalamic–pituitary axis except at mid-cycle, when oestrogen exerts positive feedback leading to the LH surge and ovulation.
- The hypothalamus integrates other signals regulating reproductive function. Fertility can be disrupted by abnormal endocrine activity such as abnormal production of GnRH and hyperprolactinaemia, abnormal follicular development and extremes of weight loss or gain.
- Understanding the hormonal regulation of reproduction has allowed manipulation of fertility using chemical analogues of the steroid hormones in contraceptives.

Skeletal changes occur as the decrease in oestrogen results in increased bone resorption increasing the tendency to stoop and the likelihood of fractures. Osteoblasts (bone-producing cells) have oestrogen receptors. Oestrogen deficiency uncouples bone formation and bone resorption. This effect is increased by changes in hormones controlling calcium balance. Levels of calcitonin fall in parallel with oestrogen levels. Calcitonin inhibits the activity of oesteoclasts (bone-absorbing cells). The progressive loss of calcium from the bones and the long postmenopausal lifetime means that a woman can lose about half of her trabecular bone and about a third of her cortical bone and is therefore predisposed to osteoporosis. Collagen is lost from the skin, tendons and bones.

**Application to practice**

There are many environmental influences, both internal and external, that may affect the regulation of reproductive cycles.

It is important to realize that the menstrual cycle prepares women for pregnancy. The physiological changes, in preparation for and support of pregnancy, are initiated prior to ovulation and conception.

An understanding of the variance in the menstrual cycle is important when considering the estimated due date. Knowledge of the reproductive cycles is essential in understanding the various methods of birth control.

## Annotated further reading


Balen A H, Jacobs H S 1997 Infertility in practice. Churchill Livingstone, New York

*A description of the aetiology of infertility and the clinical applications, tests and treatments currently in use and potential future developments in fertility treatment.*

Elliot G (ed) 1991 Biological clocks. Unit 15. In: Animal physiology S324. Open University, Milton Keynes

*This chapter introduces the study of chronobiology and contains a useful overview of the physiology that generates biological rhythms within organisms.*

Eppig J J 1996 The ovary: oogenesis. In: Hillier S G, Kitchener H C, Neilson J P (eds) Scientific essentials of reproductive medicine. W B Saunders, Philadelphia, pp 147–159

*Explores ovarian function in relation to ovum development.*

Foster R G 1988 Shedding light on the biological clock. Neuron 20:829–832

*Provides an introduction to neurological aspects of chronobiology.*

Hillier S G (ed) 1991 Ovarian endocrinology. Blackwell, Oxford

*Explores the endocrine activity of the ovary in the regulation of female physiology.*

Johnson M H, Everitt B J 2000 Essential reproduction, 5th edn. Blackwell, Oxford

*An integrated, up-to-date and well-organized research-based textbook that explores comparative reproductive physiology of mammals including anatomy, physiology, endocrinology, genetics and behavioural studies.*

Loudon N (ed) 1991 Handbook of family planning, 2nd edn. Churchill Livingstone, New York

*Explains the common methods of family planning, their application and management.*

McMillen I C, Houghton D C, Young I R 1995 Melatonin and the development of circadian and seasonal rhythmicity. Journal of Reproduction and Fertility 49:137–146

*Explores the role of the hormone melatonin in the regulation of endogenous biological rhythms.*

Ridley M 1993 The red queen: sex and the evolution of human nature. Penguin, London

*A new and exciting approach to understanding reproductive behaviour and physiology from an evolutionary perspective.*

Shuttle P, Redgrove P 1978 The wise wound: menstruation and every woman. Victor Gollancz, London

*This text provides an exploration of the sociological and anthropological perspectives of human reproduction.*

Turek F W 1998 Circadian rhythms. Hormone Research 49:109–113

*Provides a useful description of circadian rhythms and their function.*

Wise P M, Krajnak K M, Kashon M L 1996 Menopause: the ageing of multiple pacemakers. Science 273:67–70

*This article explores the factors that interact and govern the ageing process within the female reproductive system.*


## References


Adashi E Y, Resnick C E, Hernandez E R, May J V, Purchio A F, Twardzik D R 1989 Ovarian transforming growth factor-beta (TGF beta): cellular site(s), and mechanism(s) of action. Molecular and Cellular Endocrinology 61(2):247–256

Bronson F H 1995 Seasonal variation in human reproduction: environmental factors. Quarterly Review of Biology 70:141–164

Brooker C G 1998 Human structure and function, 2nd edn. C V Mosby, St Louis, pp 480, 488, 489

Buffenstein R, Poppitt S D, McDevitt R M, Prentice A M 1995 Food intake and the menstrual cycle: a retrospective analysis with implications for appetite research. Physiology and Behaviour 58:1067–1077

Bullough V L 1981 Age at menarche: a misunderstanding. Science 213:365–366

Clarke I J 1996 The hypothalamic-pituitary axis. In: Hillier S G Kitchener H C, Neilson J P (eds) Scientific essentials of reproductive medicine. WB Saunders, Philadelphia, pp 120–132

Dye L, Blundell J E 1997 Menstrual cycle and appetite control: implications for weight regulation. Human Reproduction 12:1142–1151

Eppig J J 1980 Regulation of cumulus oophorus expansion by gonadotrophins in vivo and in vitro. Biology of Reproduction 23:545–552

Eppig J J 1996 The ovary: oogenesis. In: Hillier S G, Kitchener H C, Neilson J P (eds) Scientific essentials of reproductive medicine. W B Saunders, Philadelphia, pp 147–159

Eppig J J, Ward-Bailey P F, Coleman D L 1985 Hypoxanthine and adenosine in murine ovarian follicular fluid: concentrations and activity in maintaining oocyte meiotic arrest. Biology of Reproduction 33:1041–1049

Espey L L 1980 Ovulation as an inflammatory process: a hypothesis. Biology of Reproduction 22:73–106

Frisch R E 1990 The right weight, body fat, menarche and ovulation. Baillière's Clinics in Obstetrics and Gynaecology 4:419–439

Giudice L C 1994 Growth factors and growth modulators in human uterine endometrium: their potential relevance to reproductive medicine. Fertility and Sterility 61:1–17

Hamilton-Fairley D, Johnson M R 1998 The ovary. In: Chamberlain G, Broughton Pipkin F (eds) Clinical physiology in obstetrics, 3rd edn. Blackwell, Oxford, pp 396–417

Hillier S G 1991 Regulatory functions for inhibin and activin in human ovaries. Journal of Endocrinology 131:171–175

Hillier S G, Whitelaw P F, Smyth C D 1994 Follicular oestrogen synthesis: the 'two-cell, two-gonadotrophin' model revisited. Molecular and Cellular Endocrinology 100:51–54

Huang C J, Stromer, M H, Anderson L L 1991 Abrupt shifts in relaxin and progesterone secretion by aging luteal cells: luteotrophic response in hysterectomized and pregnant rats. Endocrinology 128:165–173

Hurwitz A, Loukides J, Ricciarelli E et al 1992 Human intraovarian interleukin-1 (IL-1) system: highly compartmentalized and hormonally dependent regulation of the genes encoding IL-1, its receptor, and its receptor antagonist. Journal of Clinical Investigation 89(6):1746–1754

Johnson M H, Everitt B J 1995 Essential reproduction, 4th edn. Blackwell Science, Oxford, pp 64, 65, 108, 109

Johnson M R, Carter G, Grint C, Lightman S L 1993 Relationship between ovarian steroids, gonadotrophins and relaxin during the menstrual cycle. Acta Endocrinologia 129:121–125

Lightman A, Tarlatzis B C, Rzasa P J et al 1987 The ovarian renin angiotensin system: renin-like activity and angiotensin II/III immunoreactivity in gonadotropin-stimulated and unstimulated human follicular fluid. American Journal of Obstetrics and Gynecology 156(4):808–816

Lyons E A, Taylor P J, Zheng X H, Ballard G, Levi C S, Kredentser J V 1991 Characterization of subendometrial contractions throughout the menstrual cycle in normal fertile women. Fertility and Sterility 55:771–774

McClure N, Healy D L, Rogers P A W et al 1994 Vascular endothelial growth factor as capillary permeability agent in ovarian hyperstimulation syndrome. Lancet 34:235–236

Mason H D, Margara R, Winston R M L, Seppala M, Koistinen R, Franks S 1993 Insulin-like growth factor-I (IGF-I) inhibits production of IGF-binding protein-I while stimulating estradiol secretion in granulosa cells from normal and polycystic human ovaries. Journal of Clinical Endocrinology and Metabolism 76:1275–1279

Mason H D, Willis D S, Holly J M P, Franks S 1994 Insulin preincubation enhances insulin-like growth factor-II (IGF-II) action on steroidogenesis in human granulosa cells. Journal of Clinical Endocrinology and Metabolism 78:1265–1267

Rance N E, Young W S, McMullen N T 1991 Topography of neurons expressing luteinizing hormone releasing hormone gene transcripts in the human hypothalamus and basal forebrain. Journal of Comparative Neurology 339:573–586

Roberts V J, Barth S, El-Roeiy A, Yen S S 1993 Expression of inhibin/activin subunits and follistatin messenger ribonucleic acids and proteins in ovarian follicles and the corpus luteum during the human menstrual cycle. Journal of Clinical Endocrinology and Metabolism 77(5):1402–1410

Scheele F, Schoemaker J 1996 The role of follicle stimulating hormones in the selection of follicles in human ovaries: a survey of the literature and a proposed model. Gynecological Endocrinology 10:55–66

Stem K, McClintock M K 1998 Regulation of ovulation by human pheromones. Nature 392:177–179

Strassmann B I 1996 The evolution of endometrial cycles and menstruation. Quarterly Review of Biology 71:181–220

Zeleznik A J, Hillier S G 1996 The ovary: endocrine function. In: Hillier S G, Kitchener H C, Neilson J P (eds) Scientific essentials of reproductive medicine. WB Saunders, Philadelphia, pp 133–146

# 5 Sexual differentiation and behaviour

## Learning objectives

- To discuss the advantages of sexual dimorphism.
- To describe how sexual differentiation is achieved during embryological development.
- To describe possible causes of indeterminate sex.
- To understand the phases of gonadal development.
- To explain the main differences in gonadal function between the male and female.
- To discuss factors affecting sexual behaviour.

## Introduction

Evolutionary biologists have long questioned why evolution has led to sexual dimorphism: the differentiation of the sexes into male and female. Hermaphrodism remains limited to lower life-forms, such as the annelids (worms), slugs and snails, although it is widespread throughout the plant kingdom. It is widely accepted that the development of sexual reproduction increased the speed of evolution resulting in the wide diversity of life-forms upon the planet. The essential characteristic of sexual reproduction is that the new individual is generated from two distinct packages of genes: half from the male gamete and half from the female gamete. The meiotic division that produces the gametes not only halves the normal (diploid) number of chromosomes but also randomly modifies the genes within each chromosome (see Ch. 7). Sexual reproduction results in a wide diversity of genetic material within a species enabling the species to adapt to environmental changes within two generations. The advantage of this diversity is that the population is likely to be more resilient to environmental challenges. Asexual reproduction, on the other hand, allows genetic adaptation only by mutation. The question as to why higher life-forms evolved a reproductive strategy involving dimorphism remains unanswered. However, mammalian gametes are morphologically different, which lessens the potential for same-sex fertilization, which is not far removed from self-sex fertilization, thus ensuring optimal mixing of genes.

Sexual dimorphism within many animals is genetically controlled. However, some species, such as crocodiles and tortoises, regulate sexual dimorphism by behavioural methods. They lay their eggs in environments with different ambient temperatures, which promotes the development of either male or female offspring. Intermediate temperatures of egg incubation result in the ratios of the sexes altering in relation to the differing temperature gradients. In birds, the female carries the XY chromosome, whereas some species of fish are able to change sex during a single lifetime. Differentiation of the sexes in mammals also involves sexual dimorphism of the urinary system because the two systems are closely linked in their development.

## Differentiation into male and female

In humans, differentiation into either a male or female fetus is almost always under genetic control, depending on whether the ovum is fertilized by a sperm carrying an X chromosome (female) or Y chromosome (male). However, events such as maternal pyrexia in the first trimester of pregnancy can result in abnormal cell division and development, in some cases contributing to indeterminate (ambiguous) sexual characteristics as well as other physical malformations. As in all mammals, the human female usually carries the XX chromosome arrangement whereas the male form carries the XY arrangement for reproductive function to be successful. Therefore, it is the sperm that determines the sex of the fetus (Fig. 5.1).

### The indifferent embryo

The development of the fetus, both male and female, is initially the same. Until approximately the 4th week of gestation, the fetus is in a sexually undifferentiated state. After this phase, the differentiation process is initiated by the activation of a gene, usually found only upon the Y chromosome (Sinclair et al 1990). This gene is known as the *SRY* (sex-determining region of the Y) gene. If the gene is not activated (even though the genotype is XY), the female morphological form will develop. Occasionally the *SRY* gene may be translocated on to an X gene so if it is activated then a male morphological state may develop from a XX genotype.

Abnormal numbers of sex chromosomes are often compatible with fetal development and, therefore, occur with a relative high birth frequency (Table 5.1). If there is an additional one or more X chromosomes, as in Klinefelter's syndrome (47 chromosomes, XXY), the fetus will differentiate along the male pathway, as the Y chromosome is present. The absence of a Y chromosome, as in normal female development (XX) or Turner's syndrome (45 chromosomes, X0, when 0 = an absent sex chromosome), will result in the fetus developing as a female.

The factors that activate the *SRY* gene remain unknown; however, its effects are orchestrated through its influence upon the production of androgens. The effects of these hormones upon tissue differentiation and development result in sexual dimorphism of the male during the embryonic phase. During the embryonic phase, female form develops in the absence of endocrine activity. Therefore, a genetic male may develop female characteristics if the *SRY* gene is not activated or absent (Fig. 5.2).

**Fig. 5.1** ***Paternal genetic determination of sex in humans: sex determination is genetically influenced by the SRY gene normally located on the Y chromosome, therefore it is fertilization by either a gynosperm or an androsperm that influences sexual dimorphism.***

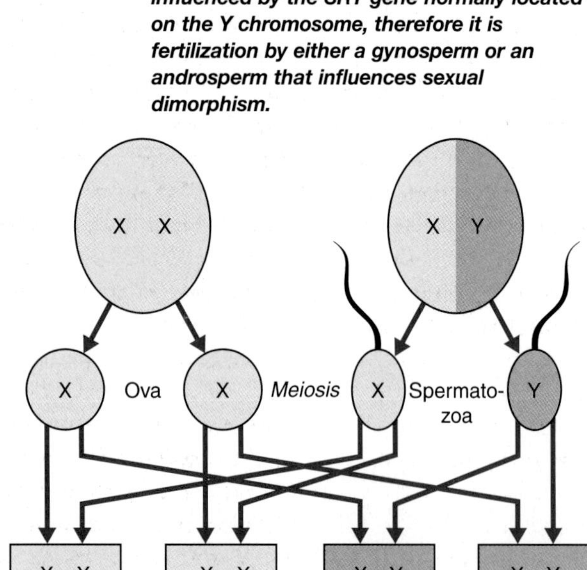


### The undifferentiated gonad

The gonads are derived from three embryonic tissue sources: the coelomic epithelium, the underlying mesenchyme and the primordial germ cells (Fig. 5.3). The primitive germ cells, which are ultimately responsible for the production of the gametes (spermatozoa and ova), originate from the yolk sac. Here, they undergo rapid mitosis before migrating from the yolk sac wall towards the developing kidneys, about 4 weeks after fertilization. The coelomic epithelium develops into the genital ridge, which is found on the medial side of the mesonephros (which develops from the mesenchyme). The genital ridges appear to produce chemotactic substances that attract the primitive germ cells, stimulating them to develop pseudopodia and undergo amoeboid movement. Colonization of the primitive gonad by the germ cells is completed during the 6th week of embryonic development. The primary sex cords develop from the gonadal ridges into the underlying mesenchyme forming the medulla and cortex of the gonad. In the testes, the medulla develops and the

**Table 5.1** *Normal and abnormal sex chromosome complements*

| State | Karyotype | Phenotype (expressed sex) | Incidence per live births | Notes and effects |
|---|---|---|---|---|
| Normal female | 46, XX | Female | | |
| Turner's syndrome | 45, X0 | Female | 0.1 per 1000 females | Females are usually short in stature, possibly with a broad chest, webbed neck, cubitus valgus (extreme outward displacement of the extended forearm) and autism. They are infertile (primary amenorrhoea) and sexually immature. Associated with younger mothers |
| 'Super female' | 47, XXX | Female | 1.0 per 1000 females | Normal in appearance and fertility, may be mentally retarded |
| Normal male | 46, XY | Male | | |
| Klinefelter's syndrome | 47, XXY (up to four X chromosomes have been found) | Male | 1.3 per 1000 males | Affected males are tall and thin with long limbs and small testes. May be infertile (azoospermia) and have gynaecomastia (breast development). May be mentally retarded. More common in sons of older mothers |
| 'Super male' | 47, XYY | Male | 1.0 per 1000 males | Affected males tend to be tall, have reduced IQ and show 'antisocial' behaviour. Some studies show increased incidence (2–3%) in institutes for the criminally insane |
| Sex reversed | 46, $XX^{sxr}$ | Male | 1.0 per 20 000 | Small piece of Y chromosome containing SRY gene is translocated on to an X chromosome |

cortex regresses; this is reversed in the development of the ovary. Two sets of primitive internal genitalia begin development. Further development will follow either the male or female route depending on the hormonal influences.

## The development of the male morphology

### *Embryological development*

The *SRY* gene is essential to the production of the male morphology. It stimulates the medulla of the undifferentiated gonad to develop into the testes and produce two hormones: testosterone and Müllerian inhibiting hormone (MIH). MIH, from Sertoli cells, inhibits the development of the paramesonephric ducts (Müllerian ducts) into female internal genitalia. Testosterone, from Leydig cells, stimulates development of the Wolffian ducts into the male internal genitalia, the epididymis, seminal vesicles and the vas differens. Sexual differentiation along the male pathway requires active diversion, whereas differentiation into a female embryo follows an inherent pattern.

The Wolffian ducts, or mesonephric ducts, initially develop as part of the embryological renal system. The adaptation of the mesonephric ducts to form the male morphology is a significant development in sexual dimorphism, in evolutionary terms. Individuals rarely have testicular and ovarian tissues. These true hermaphrodites appear to be chimeras, having a mixture (mosaic) of XY and XX (or X0) cells.

The external genitalia also have the potential to become male or female (are 'bipotential'). Steroid hormones directly influence the development of male external genitalia (unlike the female). Testosterone from the testes is converted into 5α-dihydrotestos-

**Fig. 5.2** *Sex determination factors: activation and influence of the SRY gene. Activation of this gene instigates a number of endocrine influences that determine the male morphology. In the absence of SRY gene activation, female morphology develops under a genetic influence.*

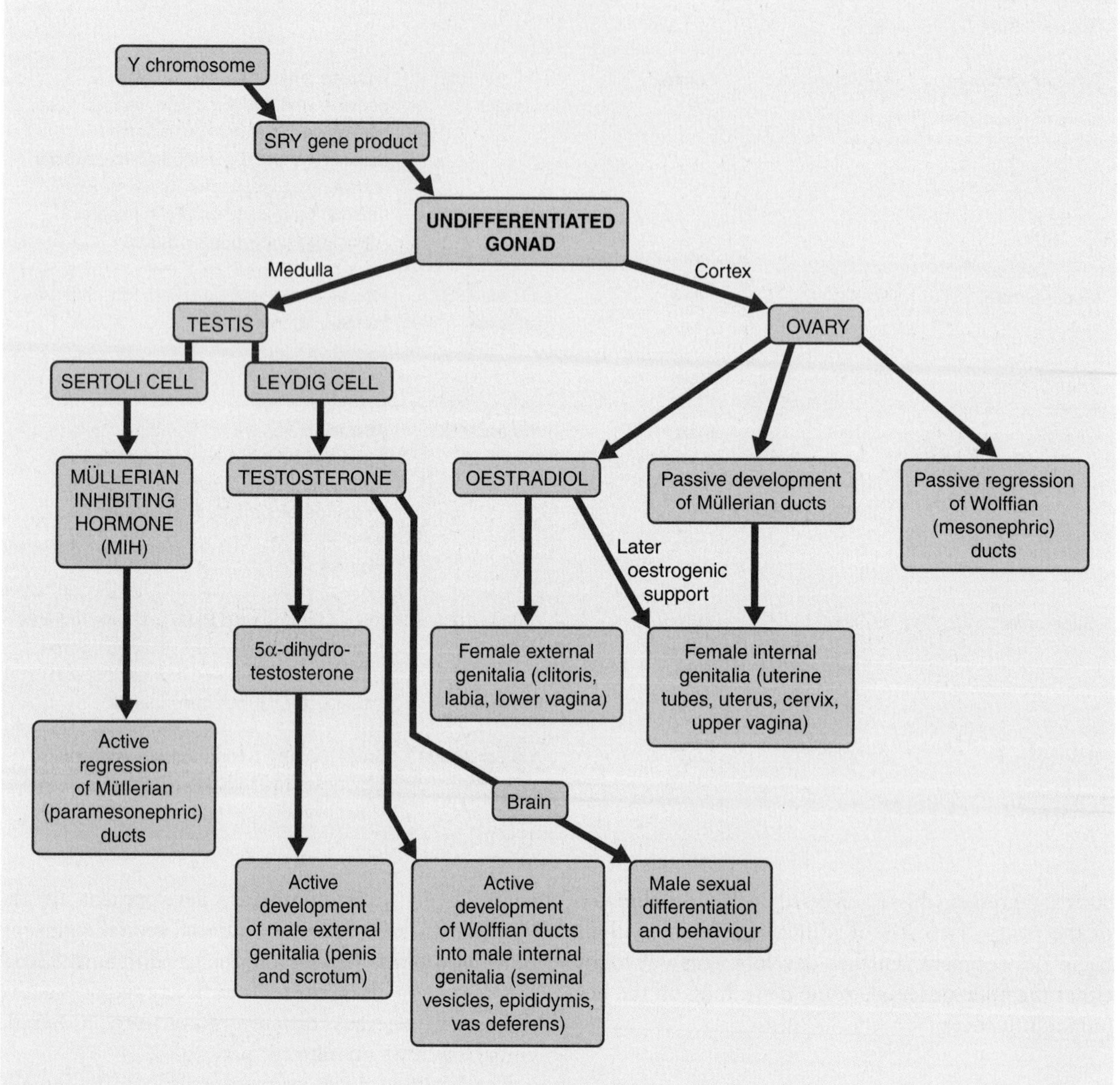


**Fig. 5.3** *Development of the internal genitalia. Once differentiation of the gonads has occurred, the resulting endocrine production coordinates the development of the internal genitalia. In the male, the reproductive tract is an evolutionary adaptation of a vestigial urological system.*

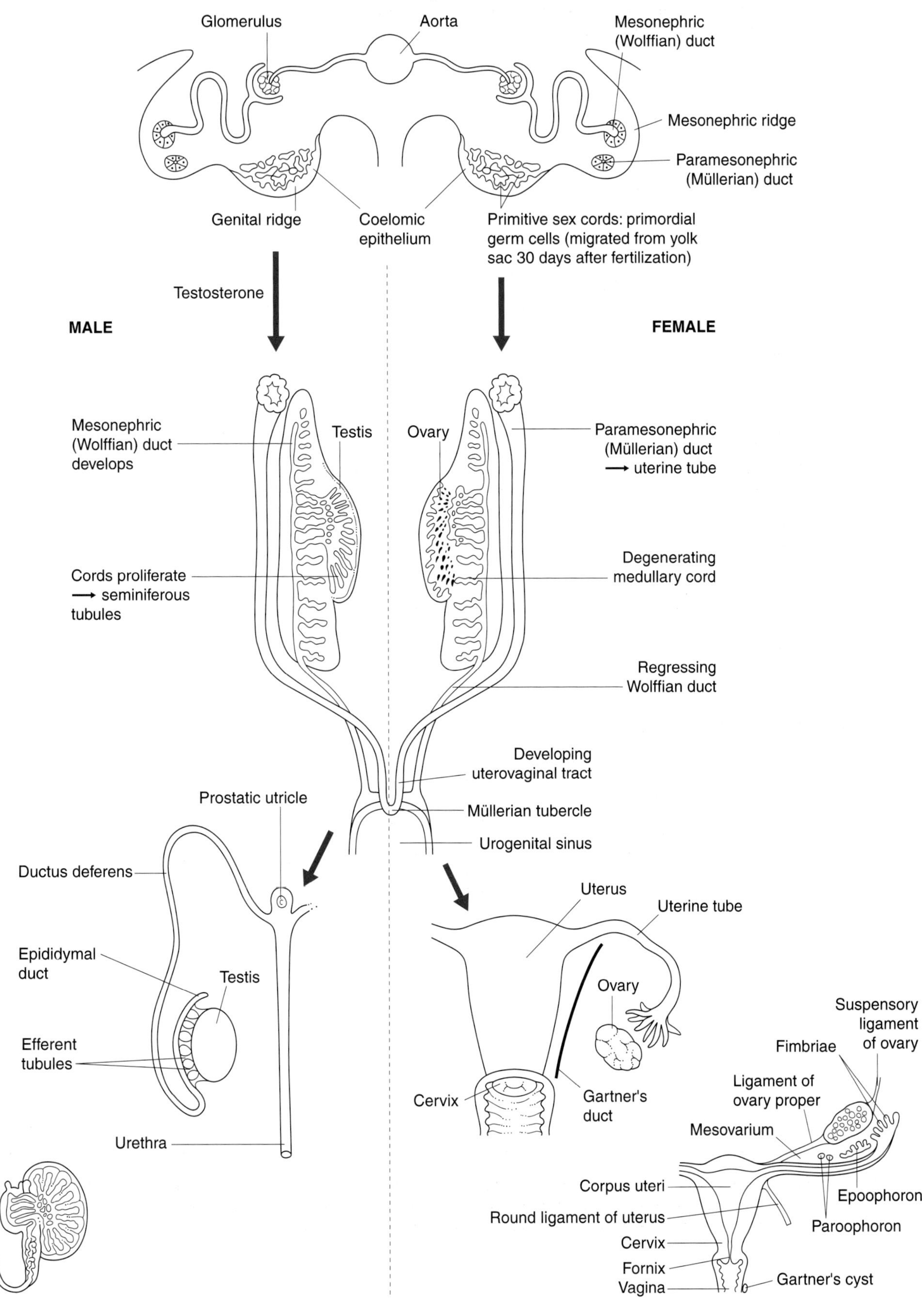
Undifferentiated gonad
Glomerulus
Aorta
Mesonephric (Wolffian) duct
Mesonephric ridge
Paramesonephric (Müllerian) duct
Genital ridge
Coelomic epithelium
Primitive sex cords: primordial germ cells (migrated from yolk sac 30 days after fertilization)
Testosterone
MALE
FEMALE
Mesonephric (Wolffian) duct develops
Testis
Ovary
Paramesonephric (Müllerian) duct ⟶ uterine tube
Cords proliferate ⟶ seminiferous tubules
Degenerating medullary cord
Regressing Wolffian duct
Developing uterovaginal tract
Prostatic utricle
Müllerian tubercle
Urogenital sinus
Ductus deferens
Epididymal duct
Testis
Efferent tubules
Urethra
Uterus
Uterine tube
Ovary
Cervix
Gartner's duct
Suspensory ligament of ovary
Fimbriae
Ligament of ovary proper
Mesovarium
Corpus uteri
Round ligament of uterus
Cervix
Fornix
Vagina
Epoophoron
Paroophoron
Gartner's cyst

terone (5α-DHT) within the target cells. Under the influence of this biologically more potent androgen, the tissues of the external genitalia form the penis and scrotum (Fig. 5.4). The urethral folds and genital swelling form the penis and scrotum. The genital tubercle expands to form the glans penis. The testes, like the ovaries, initially develop within the abdominal cavity but do not remain there. They descend to their normal position within the scrotal sac, suspended outside the abdominal cavity, just before or soon after birth. However, it is quite common (in approximately 1 in 50 liveborn males) for either one or both testes to fail to descend at this time (the condition is described as cryptorchidism). Spontaneous descent usually occurs within the first year of life. Testicular damage, potentially resulting in later failure of spermatogenesis, occurs if the testes remain within the abdominal cavity, so the testes are surgically lowered if spontaneous resolution has not occurred.

Testosterone is also converted into oestrogens within the brain. The presence of oestrogen is believed to be responsibile for differentiation of certain brain

**Fig. 5.4** ***Development of the external genitalia: formation of the external genitalia is hormonally influenced; absence of testosterone or functioning testosterone receptors will result in the female morphology developing regardless of genotype. (Adapted with permission from Johnson & Everitt 1995.)***

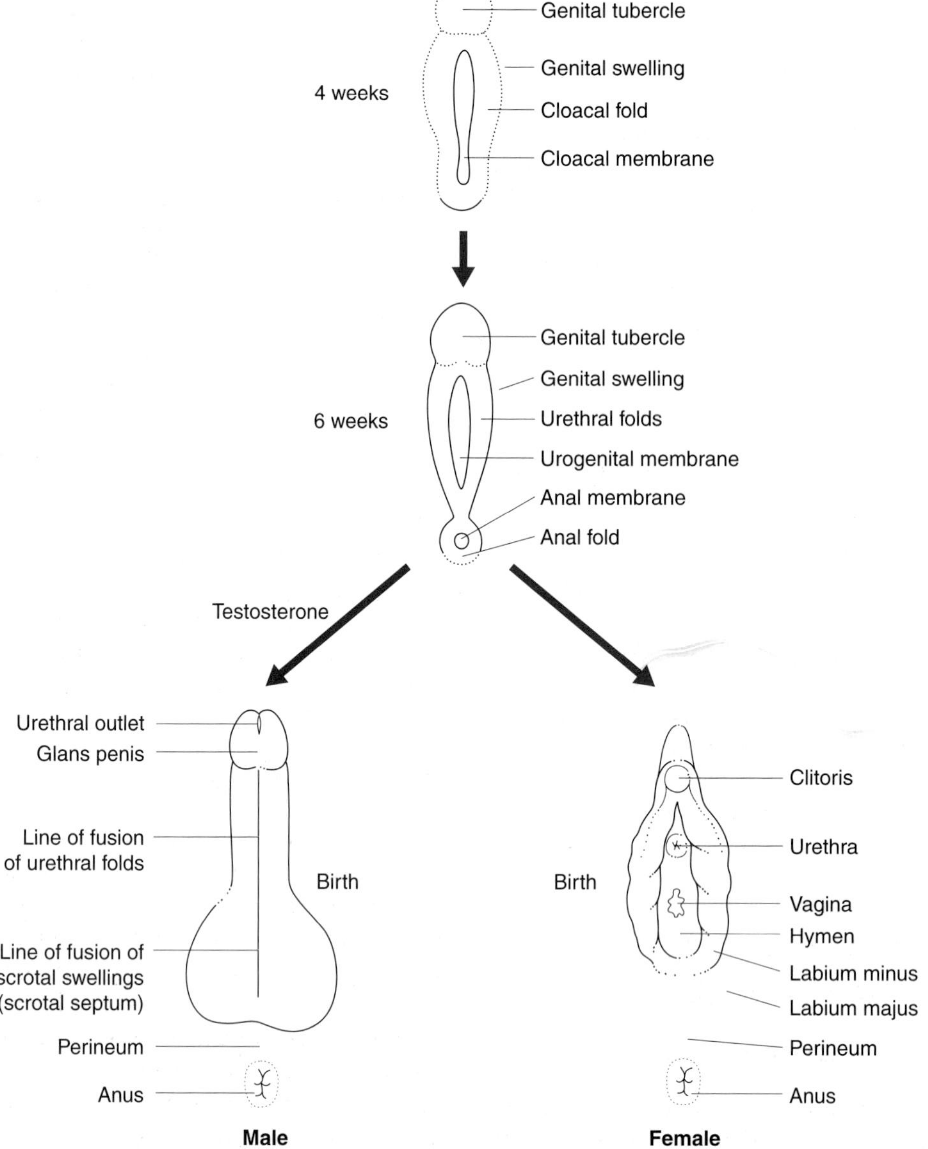

structures along a male or female pathway. This resulting difference in morphology underpins the biological explanations for behavioural patterns differing between the sexes. Male sexual activity appears to depend on the presence of testosterone above a critical threshold. Female sexual activity in the human may be cyclical in response to changes in male behaviour. There are cyclical changes in the organic acid content of vaginal secretions (derived from normal bacterial flora), which may be a mechanism of olfactory communication to the woman's sexual partner (see Ch. 4).

### *Puberty*

Following birth, the testes are endocrinologically inactive. As in the female, puberty commences when the secretory pattern of FSH and LH, under the influence of GnRH, becomes mature. FSH and LH orchestrate spermatogenesis within the male (see Ch. 2). Unlike the ovarian cycle, this is a continuous process resulting in the production of many gametes. The testes produce testosterone from the Leydig cells, which influences the development of the male secondary sex characteristics (Box 5.1). Unlike the female, the male retains the capability of spermatogenesis indefinitely but failure to achieve copulation becomes more common with the progression of age.

**Box 5.1**

**Male secondary sex characteristics**

- Enlargement of the penis
- Pubic and axillary hair growth
- Deepening of voice (due to growth of larynx)
- Masculine pattern of fat distribution
- Development of the skeletal muscle (protein anabolism)
- Secretion of skin oil glands (predisposes to acne)
- Bone growth and adolescent growth spurt (via growth hormone secretion)
- Male sexual behaviour and aggression

## The development of the female morphology

### *Embryological development*

As the X chromosome does not contain the *SRY* gene, the Müllerian ducts differentiate into the female internal genitalia, the uterine tubes and fimbriae, the uterus, cervix and upper two-thirds of the vagina. The undifferentiated gonad develops into the ovary; the cortex develops and the medulla regresses. This is the route of differentiation in the absence of testosterone and MIH. Female external genitalia form independently of any hormonal influences, therefore the ovary has little endocrine activity until puberty. The genital tubercle becomes the clitoris and the urethral folds and genital swellings remain separate, forming the labia.

#### Common abnormalities

During development, the body of the uterus, cervix and upper vagina are formed by the fusion of the two Müllerian ducts. Abnormalities may range from a simple uterine septum to the complete duplication of the reproductive system (Fig. 5.5). The failure of one of the paramesonephric ducts to develop will result in a unilateral rudimentary horn.

### *Puberty: the initiation of fertility cycles*

Puberty commences with the activation of the hypothalamus to produce GnRH in a mature pattern of secretion. It is suggested that the menarche is initiated when a critical mass of body fat, which may be genetically defined, is accumulated (Frisch 1990). GnRH stimulates the anterior pituitary to produce FSH and LH which orchestrate the reproductive cycles in the female (see Ch. 4). The ovaries begin to produce oestrogens, which influence the development of the female secondary sex characteristics. The breasts develop, the deposition of adipose tissue is responsible for the distinct female body curvature, and the growth of hair in the axilla and genital region commences.

### *The menopause*

The menopause (see Ch. 4) marks the end of the ability of the female to reproduce. The menstrual cycle ceases and the ovarian cycle is lost resulting in atrophy of the ovaries. Therefore there is a marked decrease in the amount of systemic oestrogen present in the postmenopausal woman. Modern fertility treatments can reverse the menopause to restore the menstrual cycle but not ovarian function. Hence, postmenopausal fertility treatment requires the donation of an ovum from a fertile, premenopausal woman.

Fig. 5.5 *Abnormalities of the female reproductive tract.*

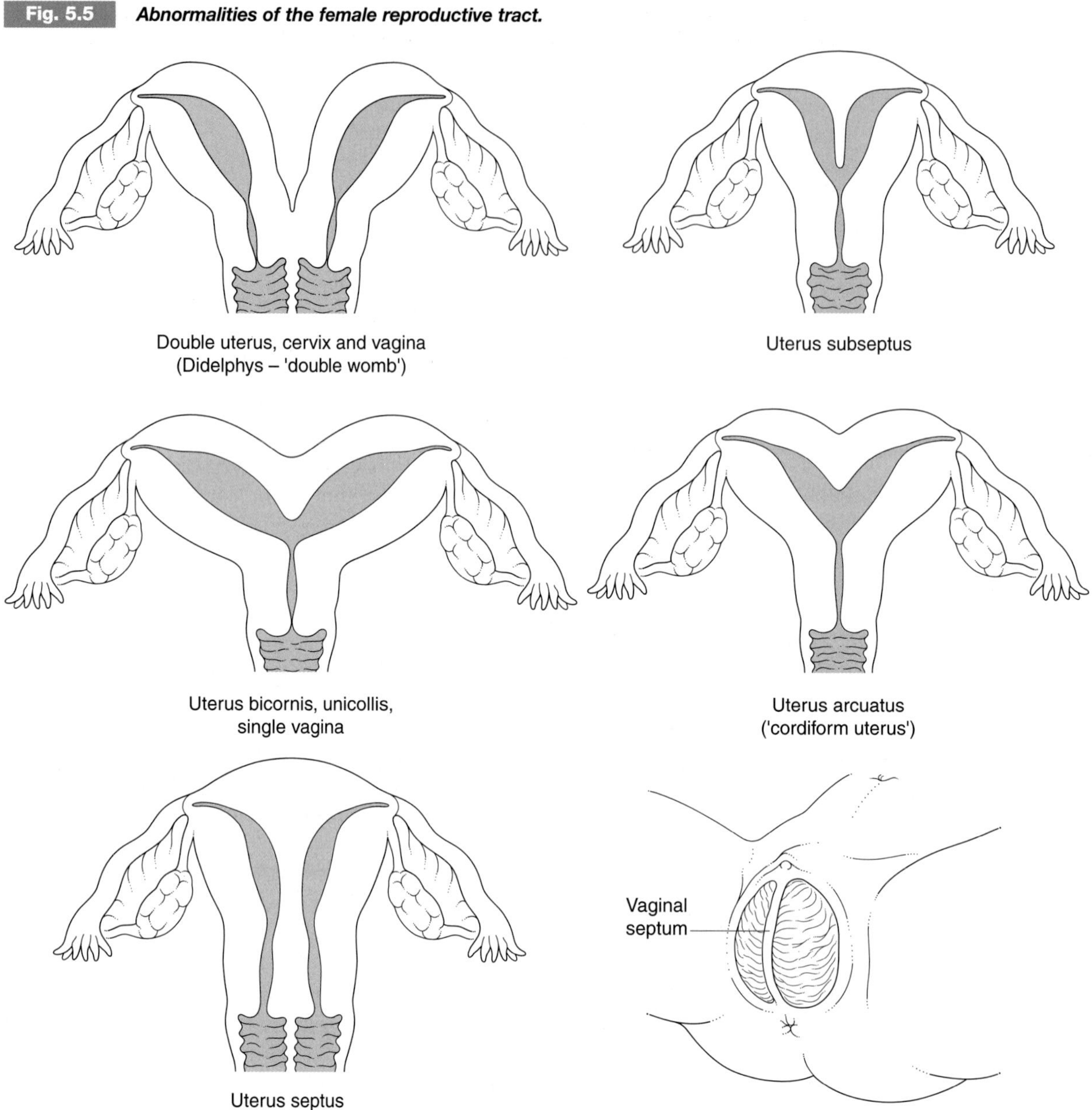


# Indeterminate sex

Indeterminate, or ambiguous, sexual features at birth are usually attributable to genetic abnormality, endocrine dysfunction (see Fig. 5.6) or developmental failure. In cases of ambiguous genitalia, the karyotype of the individual is assessed to determine the chromosomal sex (i.e. the presence of a Y chromosome for a male or the absence of a Y chromosome for a female regardless of the number of X chromosomes present within the karyotype).

## *Genetic abnormalities*

The aetiology of genetic disease is discussed within Chapter 7. There are genetic conditions that result in a range of variable sexual development, such as Klinefelter's syndrome and Turner's syndrome. These disorders have been useful in understanding the control of normal sexual development. In Klinefelter's syndrome (47, XXY) the testes form normally but the germ cells die before completing meiosis. The Y chromosome initiates development of the male gonads but

**Fig. 5.6** ***Aetiology of indeterminate sex at birth: A testicular feminization—insensitivity to androgens; B androgenital syndrome—excess androgens; C Müllerian duct syndrome—insensitivity to MIH.***

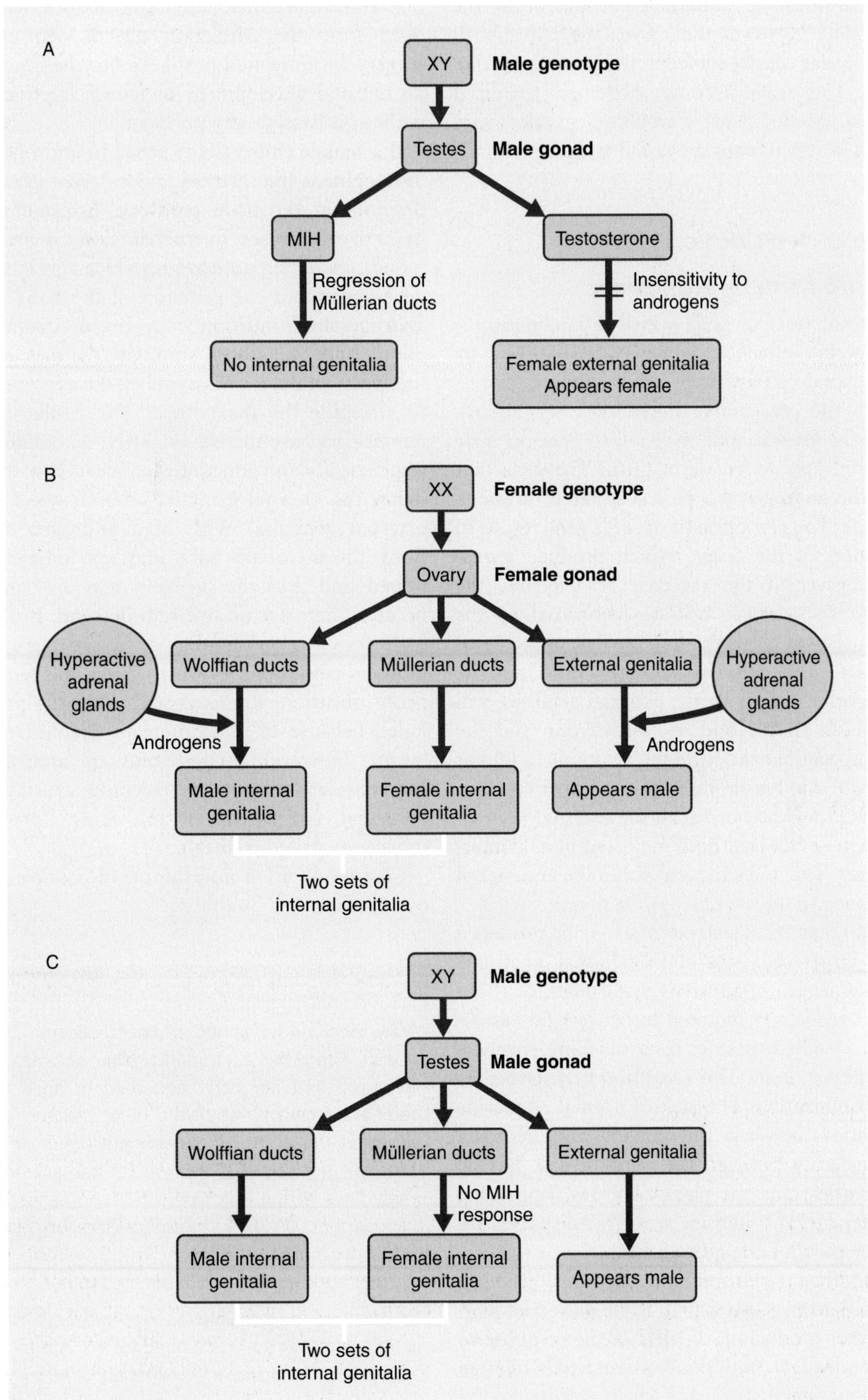

the presence of two XX chromosomes limits the completion of development. In Turner's syndrome, the single X chromosome initiates development of the ovary normally. However, the oocytes die before birth and the follicular cells become atretic, causing ovarian dysgenesis. The ovary becomes extremely regressed during fetal development, forming a streak ovary similar to a postmenopausal ovarian structure.

## *Endocrine dysfunction*

### Fetal endocrine dysfunction

The embryonic stage of male sexual differentiation is under endocrine influence. This may be disrupted by the failure, total or partial, of production of, or response to, the necessary hormones (Fig. 5.6). Therefore, the genetic male may fail to develop male genitalia, and appear female at birth. The gene that codes for the androgen receptor is situated on the Y chromosome. The activation of the *SRY* gene results in the formation of the testes, which produce testosterone. However, if the receptor is defective, the response to testosterone will be ineffectual so the Wolffian ducts will fail to develop into the male reproductive tract. The defective receptor may also be present on other tissues so the external genitalia will also be unable to respond to testosterone and the infant will appear female. MIH will continue to inhibit the growth of the female internal reproductive tract. Thus the child will be born with the external appearance of a female but lack both male and female internal structures. The testes remain within the abdominal cavity and as a result become dysfunctional.

Sufficient amounts of testosterone may be produced but if the target cells lack the functional androgen receptors (androgen insensitivity syndrome), or if the enzyme (5α-reductase) required to convert the testosterone into 5α-dihydrotestosterone is lacking, then virilization will not occur. This condition is described as testicular feminization. The lack of normal endocrine communication between the gonads and genitalia causes a disparity between the gonadal sex (having testes or ovaries) and the phenotypic sex (appearing male and female). Conditions with this disparity are described as pseudohermaphroditism.

Müllerian duct syndrome can occur if the MIH receptor is defective (persistent Müllerian duct syndrome). Either production of MIH or the response to it may be inadequate. Both the Wolffian and Müllerian ducts develop simultaneously, which results in the development of both of the male and female internal genitalia. The baby is genetically and gonadally male but retains the female internal structures, which developed from the Müllerian ducts. Men undergoing surgery for unrelated problems may be found to have an unusual development of female internal genitalia without it causing any problem.

If a female embryo is exposed to androgens during development the internal and external genitalia may develop on the male pathway. Congenital adrenal hyperplasia causes overproduction of steroid hormones, including androgens, which can influence the development of the genitalia. If the fetus is female, androgenital syndrome may occur, causing virilization. Androgens both stimulate the development of the Wolffian ducts and stimulate the external genitalia to resemble the male form. The Müllerian system remains because there is no MIH. Although the baby is genetically and gonadally female (XX with ovaries), it has the internal genitalia of both sexes and male external genitalia. With high androgen concentrations, the sex of the baby may not initially be questioned and thus the problem may be evident only because there are no testes to descend. In the 1950s, high levels of progestogenic drugs were given to mothers who had previously had a mid-term spontaneous abortion. It was thought that the pregnancies failed because of inadequate production of progesterone. However, progestogens are androgenic and can stimulate testosterone receptors causing pharmacological virilization of the fetus ('progestogen-induced hermaphrodites').

Case study 5.1 is an example of possible endocrine dysfunction.

**Case study 5.1**

Milly, who is 43, has had an uncomplicated third pregnancy. Following a chorionic villus sample, she was informed that her baby appeared to have a normal female karyotype. As Milly's other children are boys, she was thrilled to be expecting a daughter because she had decided that this will be her last pregnancy, regardless of the outcome. Milly spontaneously went into labour at 39 weeks' gestation and, following a rapid and uncomplicated delivery, a 4.2 kg male infant, of normal appearance, was presented to her.

- What are the possible reasons to explain this?
- Do you think there is a need for any further investigations and, if so, what should they be?

## *Developmental failure*

The physiological processes resulting in the development of the reproductive tracts are complex, arising from the induction and differentiation of embryonic tissue. If the tissues, such as the pronephros upon which the gonads develop, are missing then the gonads fail to develop because essential induction factors produced by the pronephros are lacking.

Induction, differentiation and growth of tissues are also affected by several other factors. Optimal development occurs at body core temperature. Maternal pyrexia at critical stages of embryonic development may severely disrupt the process. Many pathogens produce chemicals or toxins that can also severely affect embryological development (Box 5.2). There is growing concern among environmentalists over the increasing amounts of manmade chemical pollutants within the environment (see Box 3.3, p. 64). Many of these chemicals may disrupt endocrine function in a variety of ways not only by inhibition but also by mimicking the effects of endogenous hormones

Case study 5.2 is an example of ambiguous genitalia.

# Sexual behaviour

Hormonal control of sexual dimorphism results in not only physical differences between the male and female, but also behavioural differences. The differentiation of certain brain structures underpins the biological explanations for differences in sexual behaviour between the sexes. However, it is important to acknowledge that social construction also influences the development of sexual behaviour in humans (Carlson 1998).

**Box 5.2**

**Teratogens and endocrine disrupters**

- Teratogens are chemical substances that are known to interfere with embryological development and so result in the manifestation of fetal abnormalities
- Teratogens may be produced by pathogens, ingested by the mother either intentionally or unintentionally, or may be present within the external environment
- Many drugs such as Thalidomide (used in the late 1950s as an antiemetic agent within early pregnancy) are now known to produce physical deformities

**Case study 5.2**

The midwife examines a newborn baby and is concerned over the appearance of the genitalia. Initially the parents had been congratulated upon the birth of a daughter but on closer examination the labia appears fused and the clitoris seems unusually large. A paediatrician who explains his concern to the parents examines the baby.

- What are the possible causes for this ambiguity?
- What investigations will be performed to establish the true sex of the baby?
- Why is it important to confirm the sex of the baby before registering the birth?
- What are the implications of assigning the wrong sex at birth?

The correct assignment of sex at birth is thought to be important in gender development, sexual orientation and attitudes later in life. Young children appear to demonstrate gender-related patterns of energy expenditure, parental rehearsal, explicit sexual behaviour and attentiveness to personal appearance. It is suggested that children recognize their own gender identity by the time they are about $2\frac{1}{2}$ years old and ambiguity may have long-term developmental consequences. It is not clear whether there is any link between transexualism and biological or social gender ambiguity.

Human sexuality is complex; sex appears to serve a social, as well as a reproductive, function. There is a wide diversity of sexual behaviour patterns within humans ranging from complete homosexuality, to bisexuality, to complete heterosexual behaviour. Traditionally, in Western cultures, heterosexual behaviour has always been regarded as normal and any other variation as being abnormal. This assumption was based upon many animal observations where copulation appeared to be involved only in reproduction. Justification of such behavioural patterns has been strongly argued from a sociological perspective. Recently, however, there has been an increasing amount of evidence arising from biological perspectives that attempts to explain the existence of diverse sexual behaviour (Crew 1994).

Anatomical studies have shown that there may be biological differences within certain brain structures associated with the expression of homosexual behaviour in both males and females (LeVay & Hamer 1993). These studies can be criticized for many reasons; for instance, they are small, and the differences have been demonstrated only upon postmortem inspection. It has been questioned whether these changes might be caused by death and whether the samples studied were representative of the entire population. Many of the males studied died from AIDS-related conditions; the possibility of physical changes in the brain being affected by these conditions needs to be excluded.

The emergence of genetic fingerprinting has enabled the identification of parents. Many biologists formerly accepted that many animals pair-bonded, reproduced and then cooperated to bring up their young, sometimes on a seasonal basis or for life. However, recent genetic studies have revealed that the offspring of many animals were conceived outside the pair-bonding arrangement. Promiscuity appears to be widespread throughout the animal kingdom. Society often portrays the human male as sexually promiscuous but studies have shown that females are six times more likely to commit adultery at the time of ovulation than during any other time of the menstrual cycle (Ridley 1993). Animal studies have also revealed that some animals use sex as a means of providing social stability. Studies of the Bonobo (pygmy chimpanzee) show that sex is used as a form of greeting, bonding and submission and that a full range of sexual behaviour from homosexuality to heterosexuality is present (de Waal 1995).

The programming of sexual behaviour may occur by endocrine organizational influences within the embryological period. However, reproductive behaviour may also be influenced by the endocrine system on a cyclical basis as well. Human females copulate throughout the menstrual cycle but sexual motivation appears to increase during the ovulatory period and to decrease during the luteal phase.

Some animal studies have shown that the presence of sex steroids is required for positive sexual behaviour to be initiated. An example of this is the female rat who is receptive to the male only at certain times. During the fertile period, the female will adopt a specific position for mating called lordosis, which is induced by the presence of oestrogens and progesterone. The sex steroids also appear to make the female chemically attractive to the male by the production of pheromonal substances. Therefore sexual behaviour in the female rat can be described in three ways:

1. receptive—develops an ability to copulate
2. proceptive—increase in sexual motivation
3. attractive—physiological changes that arouse sexual interest in the male.

Some animals have a visual signal to the attractiveness component—such as the female baboon who advertises her sexual receptiveness by developing swollen genitalia. These components of female sexual behaviour are most clearly evident in animals who have an oestrus cycle, where ovulation is stimulated by copulation to maximize the chance of fertilization. In the human female, it appears that all three components are present throughout the cycle, which suggests that sexual activity in humans has evolved to have a social role. In many animals, it appears that various forms of stimuli produced by the female thus influence male reproductive behaviour that promotes successful reproduction. Human male sexual behaviour, however, may have developed to be more responsive to the social aspects of sex.

## Key points

- Females have two X chromosomes whereas the presence of the *SRY* region on the Y chromosome causes maleness. If there is an abnormal number of sex chromosomes, the presence of a Y chromosome leads to the phenotypic expression of maleness.
- If the embryo has a Y chromosome, the indifferent gonads differentiate into testes, which produce testosterone and Müllerian-inhibiting hormone. Testosterone promotes male differentiation of the internal and external genitalia. Müllerian-inhibiting hormone causes the structures that would have formed the female internal genitalia to regress.
- The endocrine changes at puberty cause development of secondary sex characteristics and the start of reproductive maturity.
- Indeterminate or ambiguous sex at birth can be due to genetic, endocrine or development problems.
- An abnormality of sex chromosome number is frequently associated with effects on fertility and mental ability.
- Sexual behaviour has been associated with endocrinology, brain development and cultural factors.

**Application to practice**

Knowledge of sexual differentiation is essential in the examination of the newborn.

Abnormalities of the sex organs and genitalia have their aetiology in the failure or dysfunctioning of the endocrine system. This may have a genetic origin or may be influenced by external factors such as pollutants.

## Annotated further reading

Goodfellow P N, Lovell-Badge R 1993 SRY and sex determination in mammals. Annual Review of Genetics 27:71–92

*Describes the possible mechanisms by which the SRY gene determines sexual differentiation.*

Hawkins J R 1993 The SRY gene. Trends in Endocrinology and Metabolism 4:328–332

*Comprehensive review of the literature about how the SRY gene influences the development of the male morphology.*

Johnson M H, Everitt B J 2000 Essential reproduction, 5th edn. Blackwell, Oxford

*An integrated, up-to-date and well-organized research-based textbook that explores comparative reproductive physiology of mammals including anatomy, physiology, endocrinology, genetics and behavioural studies.*

Parker L A 1998 Ambiguous genitalia: etiology, treatment, and nursing implications. Journal of Gynecology and Neonatal Nursing 27:15–22

*Provides a useful reference and overview of abnormal genitalia development within human development including implications for care of a baby born with ambiguous genitalia.*

Werner M H, Huth J R, Gronenborn A M, Clore G M 1996 Molecular determinants of sex. Trends in Biochemical Sciences 21:302–308

*This article explores the complex interactions of genes and proteins that promote development of the male gonads and regression of the female reproductive structures.*

## References

Carlson N R 1998 The physiology of behaviour, ch 10. Allyn & Bacon, Boston, pp 290–323

Crew D 1994 Animal sexuality. Scientific American 271(1): 96–102

Frisch R E 1990 The right weight, body fat, menarche and ovulation. Baillière's Clinics in Obstetrics and Gynaecology 4:419–439

Johnson M H, Everitt B J 1995 Essential reproduction, 4th edn. Blackwell Science, Oxford, p 10

LeVay S, Hamer D H 1993 Evidence for a biological influence in male homosexuality. Scientific American 270(5):44–49

Ridley M 1993 The red queen: sex and the evolution of human nature. Penguin, London

Sinclair A H, Berta P, Palmer M S et al 1990 A gene from the human sex-determining region encodes a protein with homology to a conserved DNA-binding motif. Nature 346: 240–244

Waal F B M 1995 Bonobo sex and society. Scientific American 272(3): 82–88

# 6 Fertilization

## Learning objectives

- To describe the physiological processes involved in coitus.
- To describe the morphology and characteristics of the male and female gametes and how they are adapted to their specific function.
- To discuss factors thought to be involved in the conception of either a male or female baby.
- To describe capacitance, the acrosome reaction and the cortical reaction in the stages of fertilization.
- To describe events in the first week after fertilization: the first mitotic divisions, cell cleavage, compaction, hatching, implantation and maternal recognition of pregnancy.
- To outline the relevance and implications of parental imprinting.
- To discuss the approaches used in assisted reproduction technologies.

## Introduction

Fertilization is a series of processes that culminate with the union of the male gamete, the sperm, and the female gamete, the oocyte, to form a diploid zygote. Following fertilization, one cell progressively divides into six billion cells ($6 \times 10^{12}$), forming a unique individual, in about 38 weeks. Understanding fertilization is important for following events during pregnancy and understanding some of the causes of infertility and failed pregnancy. From this understanding, conditions can be mimicked allowing Both in vitro fertilization to be achieved and, conversely, strategies for preventing fertilization to be developed (the basis for contraception).

Mammalian fertilization occurs within the female reproductive tract. Less than one in a million sperm, or spermatozoa, reach the oocyte. The sperm are deposited in the vagina during intercourse (coitus) and then make the long journey through the female reproductive tract (equal to about 100 000 times their own length). The hazards and challenges imposed on the successful fertilization are thought to help ensure that the individual sperm that actually fertilizes the oocyte is strong and healthy. Following fertilization the zygote undergoes cleavage divisions whilst travelling through the uterine tube to the uterus where it implants in the uterine wall.

## Coitus

Coitus in the human lasts on average for 4 minutes. Masters and Johnson (described in Levin 1998) described a four-phase model for sexual responses in human. This is known as the EPOR model:

- E—excitment phase, when stimuli increase sexual arousal or tension
- P—plateau phase, when arousal becomes intense; if the level of stimulation is inadequate, arousal subsides and there is no further progression to the next phase
- O—orgasmic phase, which is a few seconds of involuntary climax during which sexual tension is relieved, usually accompanied by a wave of profound pleasure

- R—resolution phase, when sexual arousal is dispersed; in males, it is believed that there is an absolute refractory period in which further sexual arousal and orgasm are impossible.

### In the male

Initial stimulation of the penis can be both psychogenic (from thoughts and visual stimuli) and tactile (via touch receptors in the penis and perineum). Penile erection is a vascular phenomenon in humans. There are three components: increased arterial flow, relaxation of the sinusoidal spaces and venous constriction. In the excitement phase, increased inflow of blood converts the low-volume, low-pressure vasculature to a large-volume, high-pressure system (Andersson & Wagner 1995). The arterioles and arteriovenous shunts dilate so there is an increase in blood flow to the erectile vascular tissues (cavernous and spongiosum bodies, see Ch. 2). The corpus spongiosum does not increase in turgor as much as the two corpora cavernosa so the urethra is not compressed. Blood outflow is limited by compression and constriction of the veins so the sinusoids (blood-filled spaces) enlarge. This results in hardening and erection of the penis as the blood volume is increased by about 50%.

The control of an erection is by stimulation of parasympathetic nerves, and probably simultaneous inhibition of sympathetic outflow, which reduces arterial smooth muscle tone causing dilatation and increase in blood flow. Various neurotransmitters appear to be involved in mediating the erectile response: acetylcholine, VIP, endothelin, NPY and NO all increase vasodilation (Argiolas & Melis 1995). Failure of erection (impotence) can be caused by damage to the spongy bodies, impaired flow in the vessels supplying the penis, drugs that interfere with neurotransmitter action or psychogenic factors. Descending pathways are both excitory (such as those initiated by the perceived attractiveness of the partner) or inhibitory (such as anxiety or guilt). The role of testosterone in erections is not clear; there is little difference in hormone levels between men with and without erectile problems.

Erectile dysfunction can be caused by abnormalities of circulation or of neural inputs affecting the nervous control of erection. Local atherosclerosis can affect blood flow as can nicotine, which has vasoconstrictive properties. Some types of erectile dysfunction (impotence) can be treated pharmacologically with intracavernous injection of prostaglandin $E_1$ (alprostadil) or papaverine, which are vasoactive drugs causing increased relaxation of the vascular smooth muscle. Sildenafil citrate (Viagra) selectively inhibits the breakdown of the signals that raise intracellular calcium. The effect therefore is to increase calcium, which regulates smooth muscle activity and erectile function. Neurogenic erectile dysfunction arises from lesions in the nervous system, such as peripheral nerve damage in diabetes mellitus.

As the penis becomes erect, the testes increase their blood volume and are drawn up towards the perineum. The dartos muscle contracts so the scrotal skin thickens and contracts. As stimulation proceeds, the plateau phase of emission occurs, where the muscles of the prostate, vas deferens and seminal vesicle undergo coordinated responses that propel spermatozoa and seminal fluid into the urethra. Ejaculation, the orgasmic phase, is where the sperm are expelled from the urethra following contraction of the urethra smooth muscle. This is accompanied by contraction of the pelvic floor muscles and the accessory muscles including the vesicular urethral sphincter, which prevents retrograde ejaculation into the bladder. The composition of ejaculate changes because the contractions are sequential and there is relative little mixing of the components:

| *Fraction* | *Dominant gland* | *Particularly rich in* |
|---|---|---|
| initial | prostate | acid phosphatase |
| mid | vas deferens | sperm |
| late | seminal vesicles | fructose. |

### In the female

Women have similar responses in coitus to those of men. Tactile stimulation of the perineal region and the glans clitoris as well as psychogenic stimuli elicit the response. The corpora of the clitoris and the labia undergo vascular engorgement. Increased blood flow to vagina increases transudation and vaginal lubrication. The vagina increases in width and length and the uterus is elevated upwards, which lifts the cervical os to produce a 'tenting effect'. At orgasm, vaginal and uterine contractions increase in intensity. Sexual responses in the female tend to be more prolonged. Detumescence of the female organs is similar to detumescence of the penis. Orgasm in women seems to be learned whereas in men it is a reflex action; female orgasm is not essential for pregnancy.

Systemic effects occur in both male and female: heart rate and blood pressure increase, accompanied

by peripheral vasodilation. This is followed by the resolution phase.

# The gametes

## Male gametes

The sperm (Fig. 6.1) develop in the seminiferous tubules of the testes (see Ch. 2). At about 17–20 μm long, the sperm cell is one of the smallest human cells. It retains fertilizing ability for about 2 to 5 days once deposited in the female reproductive tract. The nuclear material of the male gamete is carried in the head of the sperm. At the pointed head end of the sperm is the acrosome, a vesicle containing digestive enzymes. The sperm body, or mid piece, has a plentiful supply of mitochondria providing energy for movement. The tail has a whip-like movement and can generate the propulsion for the sperm to swim about 30 cm per hour. Abnormalities in human sperm morphology (such as having no tail, two tails or a coiled tail, or no head, two heads or a small head) are very common. Table 6.1 summarizes these and their possible causes.

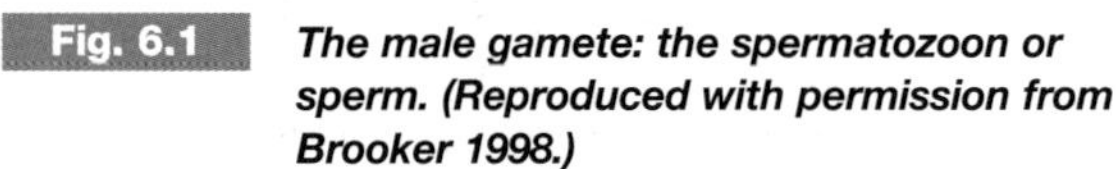

**Fig. 6.1** ***The male gamete: the spermatozoon or sperm. (Reproduced with permission from Brooker 1998.)***

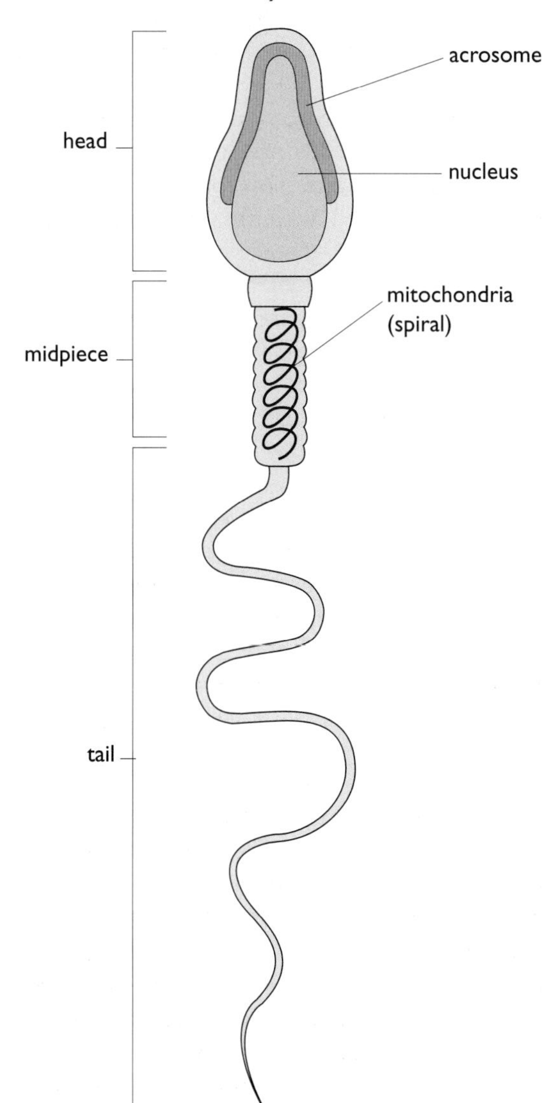


### Sperm competition

It has been proposed that morphologically abnormal sperm, rather than being due to errors in production, have a role to play in fertilization (Baker & Bellis 1988). This highly controversial theory suggests that there are two types of sperm: 'egg-getters' and 'blockers'. The morphologically abnormal sperm may be adapted to non-fertilizing roles, particularly preventing passage and successful fertilization by a competitor's sperm. However, the theory has been contested because the metabolic cost of producing non-fertilizing sperm is high and sperm competition is probably better achieved by better swimming and fertilizing ability rather than by producing sperm to compete in other ways (Harcourt 1991).

## Female gametes

The ovum (i.e. the oocyte surrounded by the corona radiata) is expelled from the mature follicle of the ovary (see Ch. 4) and picked up by the fimbria of the uterine tube. The oocyte is the largest human cell, approximately 120–150 μm in diameter, and is, therefore, just visible. In comparison, follicular cells are typical-sized human cells of about 10 μm diameter. A rim of these follicular cells known as cumulus cells or the corona radiata surrounds the released oocyte. During follicular growth, the oocyte accumulates RNA and protein and numerous large mitochondria, which provide for the needs of the dividing zygote. At birth, meiotic division has been suspended (see Ch. 7). The lifespan of the human oocyte is thought to be about 6 to 24 hours. This means that fertilization requires coitus within a fertile period of about 4–5 days before ovulation. Sperm have a viability of up to about 5 days so sperm in the reproductive tract up to 5 days before ovulation have a chance of fertilizing the zygote.

**Table 6.1** *Abnormalities of sperm*

| Type of abnormality | Description | Possible causes |
|---|---|---|
| Azoospermia (aspermia) | No sperm present within the ejaculate | Primary testicular failure; blockage to the vas deferens i.e. infection or trauma |
| Oligozoospermia (oligospermia) | Reduced numbers of sperm in the ejaculate (low sperm count) | Gonadotrophin insufficiency; drugs (social and medical, alcohol, toxins, etc.) |
| Idiopathic oligospermia | Low sperm count but physiological parameters normal | Unexplained |
| Teratozoospermia (teratospermia) | Abnormal morphology, e.g. giant heads, double tails | Genetic, toxins, viral infection |
| Asthenospermia | Reduced (or lack of) mobility | Toxins, infection |
| Sperm agglutination | Sperm clump together in groups | Infection<br>Production of antigens against sperm (autoimmune response) |

## *Sex of the zygote*

In meiotic division, the cells have their genetic complement reduced from 46 to 23 chromosomes. Each normal sperm will have 22 autosomes and either an X or a Y sex chromosome. If the oocyte is fertilized by a sperm bearing an X chromosome (a gynosperm) the zygote will be female and if it has a Y chromosome (an androsperm) the offspring will be male (see Ch. 5). Theoretically, there will be equal numbers of gynosperm and androsperm. However, the sex ratio is not constant. The number of male babies born exceeds the number of female babies all over the world. There are even more male conceptions occurring but male embryos have a higher failure rate (Bromwich 1991).

It was observed that the incidence of male babies was markedly higher in cultures where menstruating women were considered unclean and had a ritual cleansing period (niddah) before resuming sexual relations (Harlap 1979). It was therefore suggested that sperm bearing X and Y chromosomes swim at different rates. If there is a longer period between menstruation and the first intercourse, sperm deposition is less likely to occur much before ovulation so a recently ejaculated sperm will achieve fertilization. It is hypothesized that androsperm, which are slightly smaller than gynosperm and have rounder heads, can swim faster.

There are a number of methods that are proposed to alter the sex chromosome ratio in sperm and allow sex selection. The difference in mass of gynosperm and androsperm in some species is much more marked than it is in humans. Bulls' sperm, for instance, can be differentially centrifuged. The bottom fraction in the tube will be enriched with the heavier gynosperm, which can be used to impregnate cows to increase the female dairy proportion of the herd. Separation of human androsperm and gynosperm seems more difficult but is practised albeit with questionable success rates. Although a number of practices may have no scientific foundation, an increased number of female babies are born as the father ages, infants with blood group O are more likely to be male and environmental pollution seems to increase the number of female babies born. Sex selection is practised but usually not at the time of fertilization. In some parts of the world, selective abortion or infanticide is reported. In the West, sex selection is evident in that couples who have both a male and a female child are less likely to have further children.

Case study 6.1 looks at the question of sex determination.

In the days leading up to ovulation, the epithelial cells lining the uterine tubes become more ciliated and smooth muscle activity of the tubes increases. At ovulation the fimbriae of the uterine tube move closer to the ovary and rhythmically stroke its surface. These sweeping movements, together with the currents generated by the moving cilia, facilitate the capture of the ovum released at ovulation. Ovum capture is remarkably efficient. Some women have only one functional ovary and one functional uterine tube; even if the

**Case study 6.1**

Molly, who has four healthy daughters, is expecting her fifth child. She jokes with the midwife that she knows that this will be a girl as well. The midwife asks her why and Molly informs her that her husband works on an oil rig and is always home for 10 days and then away for 10 days. She laughingly states that every time she has conceived she has always started her period on the day her husband returns home.

- What factors in Molly and her husband's life may influence the sex of their children?
- How unusual is it to have five children all of the same sex?

ovary and uterine tube are from opposing sides, pregnancy can still occur. The oocyte is transported towards the uterus by movements generated by peristaltic contractions of the uterine tube aided by cilia movement. The oocyte has no inherent motility but is washed along by tubal fluid secreted by the epithelial cells and serum transudate. It takes about 3 or 4 days to reach the uterus. Initially the movement through the ampulla, where fertilization is most likely to occur, is slow, but the zygote travels faster through the isthmus into the uterus. The junction between the uterine tube and the uterus relaxes under the influence of progesterone and allows the oocyte through. If the oocyte has not been fertilized, it degenerates and is phagocytosed.

## Stages of fertilization

### Sperm deposition

Spermiogenesis (see Ch. 2) occurs in the seminiferous tubules but although the sperm are morphologically mature they are not fully motile. The sperm develop swimming ability during a maturation phase of 4–12 days in the epididymis. At intercourse, about 300 million sperm are released in about 3 ml of seminal fluid (Box 6.1), which is deposited in the vagina. Repeated ejaculation normally results in a fall in sperm concentration but numbers of motile sperm tend to rise in men who are infertile, suggesting that impaired transport through the male genital tract affects motility (Matilsky et al 1993). The sperm coagulate in the vagina, which appears to facilitate their retention and to buffer them against the normally unfavourable acidic environment (pH~4–5) of the vagina. The pH of the vagina is increased by the buffers in the seminal fluid favouring sperm motility and access to the cervix.

**Box 6.1**
**Composition of ejaculate**

- 40–250 million sperm
- Prostatic fluid (30%): citric acid, acid phosphatase, magnesium and zinc ions
- Seminal fluid (60%): fructose (energy source for sperm), alkaline
- pH 7.0–8.3
- Volume: 2–6 ml

The coagulum dissolves in about 20–60 minutes. Between days 9 and 16 of the menstrual cycle, during the fertile period of the few days preceding and including ovulation, the watery composition of cervical mucus facilitates passage of sperm (see Table 4.1, p. 83). The cervical mucus interacts with the sperm. The cervical mucus provides protection and nourishment of the sperm. It also acts as a reservoir and may filter morphologically abnormal sperm. Most sperm (99%) do not enter the uterus. A few hundred sperm reach the uterine tubes within a few hours of coitus; this first wave of rapid transport probably depends on rhythmic muscular movements of the female reproductive tract. However, muscular activity of the female genital tract does not seem to be essential for fertilization; some sperm will be stored in cervical crypts and then travel in a relatively slow second wave through the cervical mucus, reaching the uterine tube a few days after ejaculation. A chemoattractant, probably present in follicular fluid or released from the follicle, guides the sperm to the ovum.

### Capacitation

Ejaculated sperm are unable to fertilize an oocyte immediately. In vitro, there may be a delay of several hours before unprepared sperm can fertilize an oocyte. However, in vivo (and in sperm reclaimed from the uterus) the action of female enzymes and the oestrogen-stimulated high salt concentration of the uterine secretions speed up the preparation of the sperm. These biochemical and functional changes undergone by the sperm in the uterus and uterine tubes are known as capacitation. The changes include the stripping of the glycoprotein coat from the sperm plasma membrane and reorganization of the sperm surface molecules (DeLamirande, Lederc & Gagnon

1997). Biochemical changes include raised intracellular pH and calcium concentrations. The modifications alter ion channels in the membrane allowing a transmembrane flux of ions, which initiate hyperactivation of the sperm. Sperm metabolism changes from oxidative to glycolytic. The hyperactivated sperm tail movements change to become whiplash-like so the sperm thrusts vigorously forward, moving from the isthmus of the uterine tube to the ampulla (Mbizvo 1995). The accentuated lateral head movements generate a boring action, which aids access to the oocyte. The tail is also involved in sperm movement within the oocyte (Van Blerkom et al 1995).

## *Access to the oocyte*

The first barrier preventing access of the sperm to the oocyte is the outer layer of cumulus cells, the corona radiata, embedded in an intercellular matrix of carbohydrates, protein and hyaluronic acid. Hyaluronidase, released from the sperm acrosome, breaks down the hyaluronic acid matrix between the follicular cells so sperm can pass through to the zona pellucida. The hyperactive swimming movements of the sperm aid penetration of the corona radiata. The gradual release of sperm from the reservoir of cervical mucus and their activation close to the oocyte means the time-limit of fertility is extended.

## *Binding to the zona pellucida*

The oocyte is surrounded by the zona pellucida, which is about 14–15 μm thick. It is an extracellular matrix composed of sulphated glycoproteins that were produced by the growing oocyte. It is permeable to some viruses, immunoglobulins and enzymes. Before ovulation, cytoplasmic processes from the corona radiata cells penetrated the zona pellucida, allowing communication to, and nourishment of, the oocyte via gap junctions. When these are withdrawn in response to the LH surge, they may leave gaps in the zona pellucida that offer easier access for sperm penetration, thus facilitating fertilization (Familiari et al 1992). The zona pellucida acts as a barrier that allows sperm of the same species through to the oocyte.

The zona pellucida is antigenic: anti-zona pellucida antibodies may be the cause of some cases of infertility. The composition of the zona pellucida changes with the cortical reaction after fertilization so it prevents polyspermia but allows secretions of the uterine tube to reach the oocyte during the early stages of cell division. The zona pellucida also has a role in preventing the blastocyst from prematurely implanting into the wall of the uterine tube before it reaches the uterus. It is possible that an excessively thick zona pellucida could cause problems with blastocyst hatching and subsequent implantation.

Sperm attach to receptors on the surface of the zona pellucida, digesting a pathway through to the oocyte plasma membrane. Complementary molecules on the zona pellucida and the sperm plasma membrane interact, permitting interaction of the two gametes. The sperm receptor on the zona pellucida is a glycoprotein known as the ZP3 molecule (Tulsiani, Yoshida-Komiya & Araki 1997). The structure of this receptor varies between species, which may help to protect against fertilization of an oocyte by a sperm of a different species. Although there is a species-specific egg–sperm recognition, sperm of some mammalian species can interact with the ZP3 receptor of other species even though fertilization does not follow. This is the basis of the hamster egg penetration assay where the ability of human sperm to penetrate the zona pellucida is tested with hamster oocytes.

The interaction with the zona pellucida seems to occur in two stages (Wasserman 1987). At first, the capacitated sperm loosely and reversibly adhere to the surface of the zona pellucida. Then, the sperm become strongly and irreversibly bound to the zona pellucida. Many sperm bind to the oocyte zona pellucida but usually only one will penetrate and fuse with the oocyte plasma membrane.

## *The acrosome reaction*

After binding to the zona pellucida, the sperm undergo the acrosome reaction (Fig. 6.2). This is initiated by the raised intracellular calcium concentration following binding to the ZP3 receptor. However, it can also be triggered by follicular fluid and progesterone (Brucker & Lipford 1995). The outer acrosome membrane fuses with the covering plasma membrane of the sperm. Small vesicles containing acrosomal enzymes are pinched off and their contents are released. The inner acrosomal membrane then forms the covering of the head of the sperm. A tunnel is digested through the zona pellucida by acrosin, an enzyme that remains bound to the inner acrosomal membrane, and the acrosomal enzymes released from the vesicles. The

Fig. 6.2 *The acrosome reaction.*

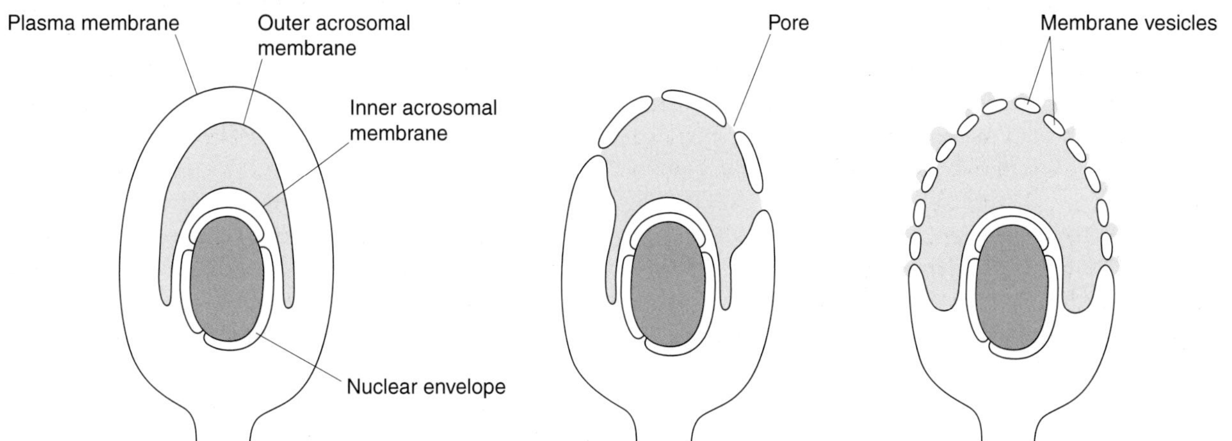


lurching movements of the sperm propel it forward through the zona pellucida and the perivitelline space so that its head is in contact with the oocyte vitelline (surface) membrane. Penetration through the zona pellucida requires both hyperactivated sperm and lysis of the zona pellucida.

## Gamete fusion

The acrosome reaction triggers changes in the sperm membrane that allow fusion to occur. Adhesion molecules present on the oocyte and sperm membranes are important in sperm–egg fusion (Blobel et al 1992). The head of the sperm is drawn into the oocyte microvilli on the surface of the oocyte envelope. The sperm plasma membrane is then incorporated into the oocyte membrane. In the mouse, it has been shown that a layer of actin filaments in the cortical region of the oocyte may also contribute to the incorporation of the sperm head. Fusion of the sperm membrane with the vitelline membrane of the oocyte takes about 10 to 20 minutes. In human fertilization, the sperm tail remains motile and is incorporated into the oocyte (Payne et al 1997). It is thought that any paternal mitochondria entering the oocyte are selectively expelled (Kaneda et al 1995). The zygote and resulting embryo have only maternal mitochondria (Gyllensten et al 1991); the oocyte seems to lose mitochondrial DNA with increasing maternal age, a factor that may be important in fertility. As well as the male nuclear component, the fertilizing sperm also contributes the centriole and microtubule-organizing centre, from which the first mitotic spindle will develop (Van Blerkom et al 1995).

## The cortical reaction

Once fusion has occurred, entry of other sperm into the oocyte (polyspermia), which would potentially produce a non-diploid zygote, is prevented. Non-diploid zygotes are usually not viable but some can develop into tumours such as hydatidiform mole or choriocarcinomas. The incidence of non-diploid zygotes increases with alcohol, drug use, anaesthesia and fertilization of 'aged' oocytes (i.e. aged in terms of hours after ovulation). When the sperm fuses with the oocyte, there is increased potassium conductivity, which depolarizes the membrane.

The changed membrane potential itself may be important in blocking further sperm fusion but it also results in calcium release from intracellular stores, which promotes fusion of the cortical granules with the oocyte membrane (Hoodbhoy & Talbot 1994). The calcium increase starts from the site of fusion and moves as a wave through the oocyte sequentially activating about 4000 cortical granules (Fig. 6.3). The trigger for this calcium-induced calcium rise may be a soluble cytosolic factor from the fertilizing sperm. The resulting calcium oscillations may last for several hours (Palermo et al 1997), and may be involved in activation of the embryo. The contents of the cortical granules (enzymes such as proteases and peroxidase and polysaccharides) are released into the perivitelline space and diffuse through the zona pellucida to digest the ZP3 sperm receptors. The zona pellucida loses its ability to bind to sperm and induce the acrosome reaction. The changed texture of the zona pellucida is described as 'zona hardening'. This reaction is known as the zona reaction. The composition of the oocyte plasma membrane is also altered.

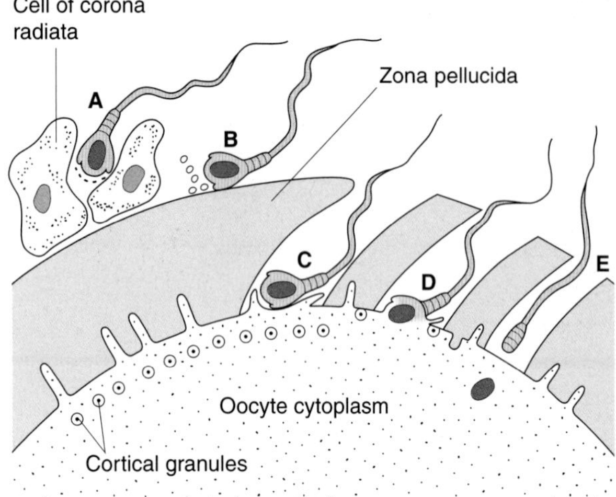


**Fig. 6.3** *Fertilization. A Acrosome reaction; B binding to zona pellucida; C penetration of zona pellucida; D fusion of oocyte and sperm, and cortisol reaction; E fertilization.*

## *Events leading to the first mitotic division*

### Possible benefits of arrested meiosis

The chromosomes of the oocyte had been arrested in metaphase of the second nuclear division (see Fig. 7.11, p. 138). It has been suggested that growth of the oocyte requires a diploid number of chromosomes. Meiotic arrest in the diplotene stage of metaphase means that both maternal and paternal alleles can be expressed during oocyte maturation. Observation of in vitro fertilization has shown that the human meiotic spindle is unstable and very sensitive to external influences.

As a species, humans have a high frequency of aneuploidy in products of fertilization. This results in zygotes and embryos with the wrong number of chromosomes, for example Down's syndrome with 47 chromosomes (see Table 7.1, p. 139). Down's syndrome is an example of a chromosome complement that is compatible with fetal survival; other examples are just as likely but may result in failed implantation or failed in utero development. Aneuploidy is mostly due to non-disjunction of bivalent chromosomes in the first meiotic division (see Fig. 7.11) and is associated with pregnancy loss or mental retardation if the fetus survives (Griffin 1996). The frequency of aneuploidy increases with increased maternal age; ageing oocytes seem more prone to errors in meiosis and normal segregation of chromosomes. Other factors have been found to disrupt meiosis such as alcohol abuse, chemotherapy and smoking (Zenzes, Weng & Casper 1995). Arrest in the second meiotic division may help to prevent aneuploidy and the inclusion of an extra or absent chromosome in the oocyte.

### Completion of the second meiotic division

The calcium rise that triggers the cortical reaction is also the stimulus for the oocyte to increase its metabolism. Calcium regulates the cell cycle (Whittaker 1995); it promotes resumption of meiosis, probably via activation of M-phase-promoting factor (MPF), and completion of second meiotic division (Fig. 6.4). The increase in oxidative metabolism is preceded by a rise in intracellular pH. The 23 paired chromatids then separate, half being expelled as the second polar body into the perivitelline space. A pronuclear membrane appears around the remaining 23 chromosomes forming the female pronucleus, thus completing the meiotic division.

### Decondensation of the sperm nucleus

The genetic material of the mature sperm is very tightly packed in the head. After the head of the sperm enters the cytoplasm of the oocyte, it is affected by cytoplasmic factors that cause the chromatin threads of the DNA to unravel and spread out. This decondensation of the sperm nucleus takes place while the sperm pronucleus is moving towards the pronucleus of the oocyte. The centrioles radiate microtubules in a formation known as a sperm aster, which aids the movement of the two pronuclei (Schatten 1994). Then oocyte histones begin to associate with the male chromosomal material (see Ch. 7). As the developing pronuclei near each other in the centre of the cell, they synthesize DNA in preparation for the first mitotic division and the chromosomes replicate into chromatids.

### First mitotic division

In the first mitotic division, the two pronuclei membranes first break down and the male and female chromosomes become organized around a mitotic spindle ready for the first cell division. The combination of the male and female chromosomes is called syngamy. Fertilization is complete about 18–24 hours after fusion, and the fertilized oocyte is known as a zygote (the steps of fertilization are summarized in Box 6.2). A cleavage furrow then appears and the zygote becomes two identical cells.

The random assortment of nuclear material in meiosis and the random exchange of nuclear material

Fig. 6.4 *Fertilization and the generation of the second polar body.*

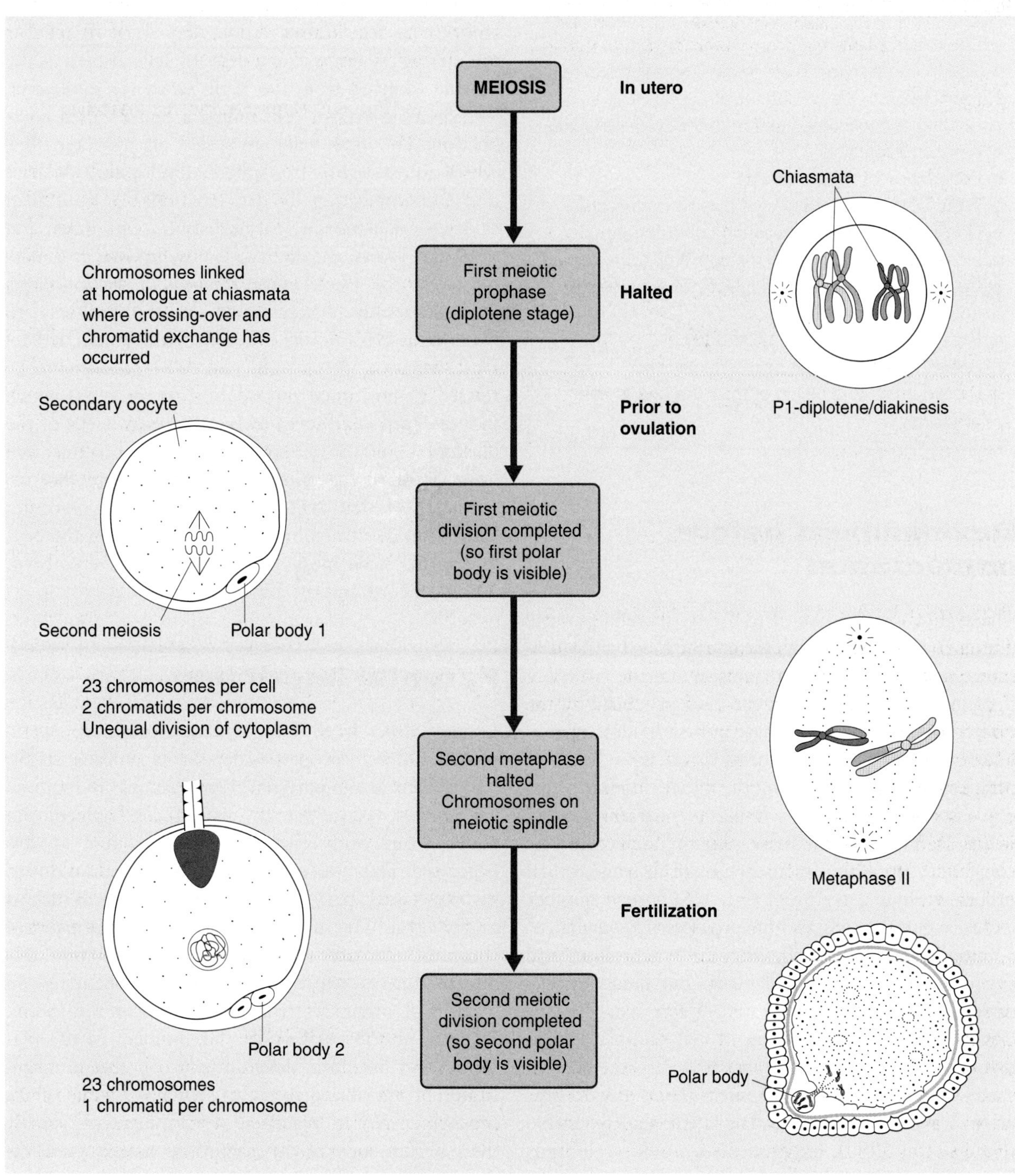


creates new combinations of genes so the gametes are both haploid and genetically unique. Fertilization of one gamete with another results in a unique combination of genetic material in the zygote, which is important in variation of the species (see Ch. 7). Whether the sperm carries a X or Y chromosome will determine the primary sex of the zygote so it will differentiate into either a female or male embryo (see Ch. 5). Fertilization restores the diploid number of chromosomes and initiates the cleavage of the zygote.

**Box 6.2**
**Sequence of steps in fertilization**

- Deposition of sperm
- Sperm capacitation in the female reproductive tract
- Penetration of the corona radiata
- Binding of capacitated sperm to the zona pellucida
- Acrosome reaction
- Penetration of zona pellucida
- Fusion of sperm with oocyte plasma membrane
- Cortical reaction and prevention of polyspermia
- Increased respiration and metabolism by the oocyte
- Completion of the second meiotic division of the oocyte
- Extrusion of the second polar body
- Decondensation of the sperm nucleus
- Development and fusion of the male and female pronuclei

## Development before implantation

The zygote spends about 4 to 6 days travelling to the uterus. It is moved through the uterine tube by the peristaltic action of the smooth muscle and the sweeping movements of the cilia and the fluid produced by the ciliated epithelium. The embryo at first divides approximately every 15 hours; the division time becomes progressively shorter. During the initial cleavage steps, the embryo is enclosed within the restraining zona pellucida and its total mass remains approximately constant. Cytoplasmic factors regulate cleavage, which occurs without net growth (Fig. 6.5) so cell number increases but the cells become progressively smaller.

Initially, the cleavage divisions are synchronous and each cell (blastomere) is identical, but then the cells divide at an independent rate. (When synchrony is lost, the pattern of doubling of cell number is also lost.) In humans and mice embryos at the eight-cell stage, each of the cells is totipotent (i.e. is able to generate all types of cell line) and its fate is not irreversible (Hardy et al 1990). Experiments on mouse embryos have demonstrated that each of the cells has the capability of independently developing into an embryo. Cells from different origins can also be combined to form a mosaic or a chimera. In human in vitro fertilization, a single blastomere can be removed from the blastocyst at this stage for genetic testing without prejudicing the outcome for the embryo if it is transferred to the uterus (see Ch. 7).

After the eight-cell stage, the cells change morphologically so some of the cells at the outer edge of the embryo become flatter. About day 4, as it reaches the uterus, the embryo is a mass of cells known as the morula (derived from the Latin word for mulberry). The dividing ball of cells enters a phase called compaction. The inner cells are sealed off by outer cells, which adhere tightly in a sphere, developing a polarity and communicating by gap junctions. A fluid-filled cavity, or blastocoele, forms between the inner and outer cell layers; the embryo is now known as a blastocyst. By the 64-cell stage, the cells of the conceptus are irreversibly differentiated on the pathway to becoming embryonic or extraembryonic tissue. Differentiation into a particular cell type seems to be related to positional information of the cells, which induces particular genes to be expressed. Cells of the blastocyst initially differentiate into two distinct cell lines. Most of the outer layer of cells form the trophoblast, which will develop into the placenta, chorion and extraembryonic tissue. Most of the cells of the inner cell mass will develop into the embryo, umbilical cord and the amnion (Fig. 6.6).

## Parental imprinting

Chromosomes from the oocyte and sperm appear to possess different properties depending on their origin; both maternal and paternal chromosomes are required for normal zygote formation and development but genes from both chromosomes are not always expressed. This is described as imprinting and is due to gamete-specific patterns of DNA modification such as methylation. This means that, although the pairs of chromosomes carry the same genetic information, this information is expressed differently depending on whether it originates from the oocyte or the sperm. Paternal imprinting favours development of the placenta and inhibits development of the embryo. Maternal imprinting seems to switch off some of the genes involved in placental development. Normally the paternal copy of the X chromosome is preferentially activated in cells derived from the trophoblast. Conversely, in the inner cell mass the paternal and maternal chromosomes are randomly inactivated (see Ch. 7). X-chromosome inactivation is irreversible except in oogonia. Parental genetic imprinting is lost (reordered) on formation of the new gametes, which have new parental imprinting on the new formation of new chromosome sets.

**Fig. 6.5** *Development before implantation.*

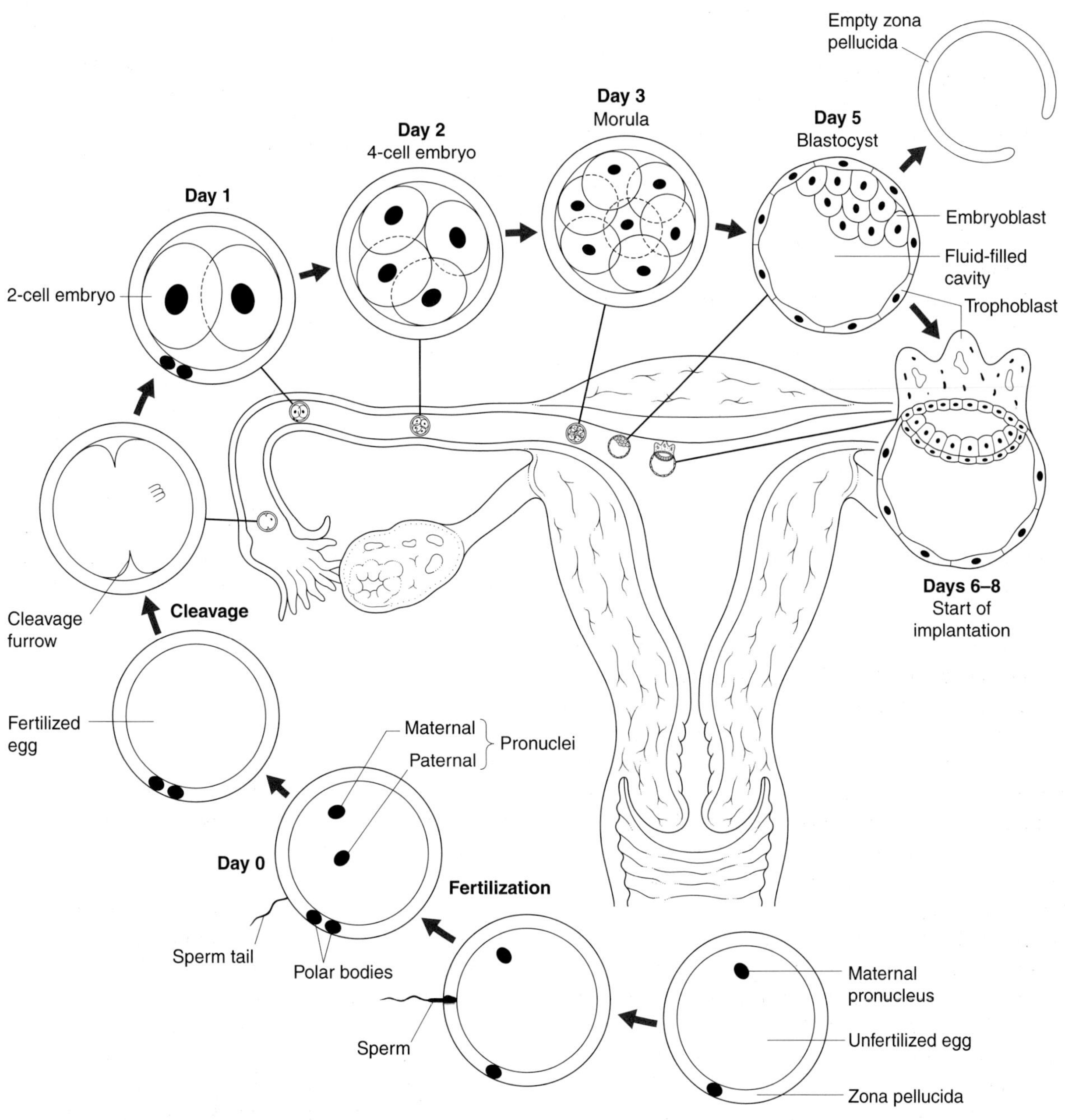


In mice embryo cells, removal and replacement of one of the pronuclei with another of opposite sex (so both pronuclei are of the same sex) results in abnormal development. If both the pronuclei are female, early embryo development appears normal but placental development is impaired. If both pronuclei are male, placental development appears normal but embryonic development is extremely stunted. Hydatidiform mole development in the human occurs as a result of diandric diploids—that is, when two sperm fertilize an oocyte and the maternal chromosome complement does not participate in development (Jacobs et al 1980). The result is extreme overdevelopment of the placental tissues and extreme underdevelopment of the embryonic tissues. This situation could also arise from the fertilization of an oocyte with a diploid sperm.

Fig. 6.6 *The pathway of cell division.*

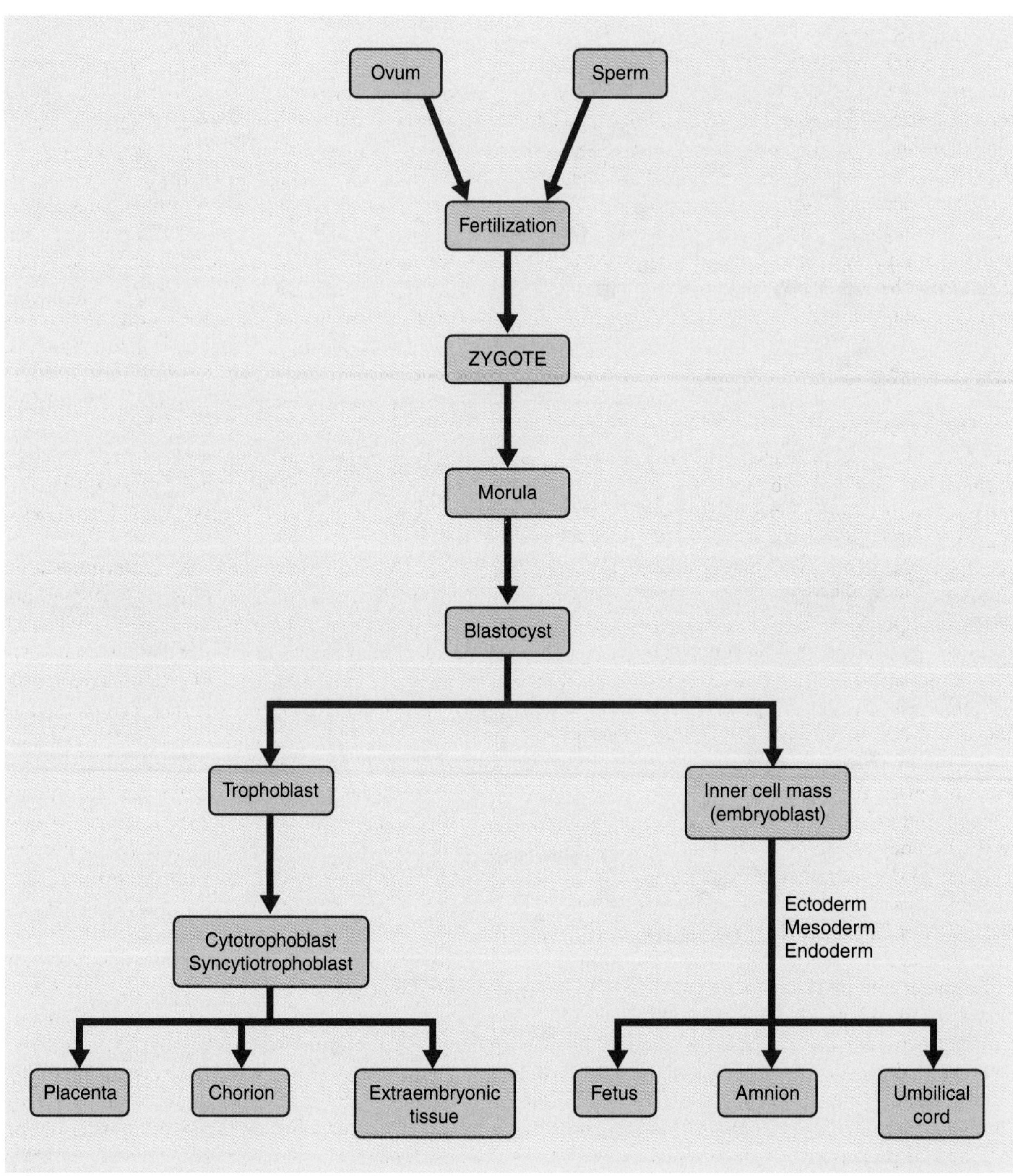


Digynic triploids (i.e. two maternal and one paternal chromosome sets) can occur if the polar body is retained.

Human oocytes can be induced to undergo spontaneous cleavage in the absence of fertilization by a sperm and develop into parthenotes. Early stages of cleavage, therefore, seem to be maternally imprinted. However, mouse parthenogenic oocytes arrest after the first cleavage divisions, at the time the embryonic genes would be expressed. Some maternal genes are expressed in the blastocyst but overall embryonic genes are required for blastocyst formation.

## Twins

The incidence of twins in the UK is 1 in 80 deliveries. Approximately two-thirds of the twins are dizygotic (fraternal or non-identical) and one-third is monozygotic (identical). Dizygotic twins arise from multiple ovulation and two fertilized oocytes implanting and developing. Monozygotic twins are derived from one fertilized oocyte; the single embryo divides and then splits. Although it is possible that a two-celled embryo could split and result in twins, most twins in practice result from the subdivision of the inner cell mass at the blastocyst stage (Fig. 6.7).

## Implantation

The blastocyst may remain free floating in the uterine cavity before it hatches and implants at day 7. The accumulated fluid in the blastocyst expands and contracts. This blastocyst expansion, together with the digestion and thinning of the zona pellucida by uterine enzymes, results in 'hatching' of the blastocyst at about 6–7 days' postfertilization. The disappearance of the zona pellucida allows the cells of the blastocyst to come into contact with the epithelium of the uterus. The blastocyst consists of at least 100 cells but some apoptosis has already occurred (Hardy, Handyside & Winston 1989). In most blastocysts there is a degree of degeneration of some trophoblasts and some of the inner cell mass. After hatching the blastocyst grows in mass as well as in cell number. Embedding or nidation of the blastocyst normally occurs in the upper part of the body of the uterus (the fundal region). The blastocyst implants at the embryonic pole, where the inner cell mass lies. The inner cell mass forms the embryonic disc (see Ch. 9).

The outer cells of the blastocyst secrete proteolytic enzymes and collagenase, which break down and destroy some of the cells of the endometrial surface, forming a depression in which the blastocyst lies. Implantation in humans is a very invasive mechanism. Uterine muscle activity is low at this time because secretion of progesterone is high. Once implantation has occurred, the lining of the uterus closes over the blastocyst and the pregnancy is established. The trophoblastic cells absorb nourishment from the decidua and secrete hCG which stimulates growth and secretory activity of the corpus luteum to produce steroid hormones, which support the growth of the decidua. Critical amounts of hCG are required for blastocyst survival.

## Maternal recognition of the pregnancy

Successful implantation requires two-way communication between mother and embryo. Many signals are involved in the crucial role of maintaining the corpus luteum, regulating uterine vascular permeability and maternal immunosuppression. Not all of the signals have been identified. hCG is involved in maintaining the corpus luteum and its essential endocrine role. hCG is luteotrophic, binding to the LH receptors and stimulating a progressive rise in progesterone and oestrogen secretion. Levels of hCG are abnormally low if implantation is inadequate, if trophoblast cell division is insufficient, if implantation is ectopic or if growth of the corpus luteum is deficient (Check, Weiss & Lurie 1992). Secretion of hCG from the trophoblast is regulated by trophoblastic GnRH. hCG also binds to the embryonic trophoblast cells and affects the differentiation of cytotrophoblast into syncytiotrophoblast (see Ch. 8).

Implantation and the three stages of apposition, adhesion and penetration require the endometrium to change and to become responsive. The endometrial stroma is modified (see Ch. 8); vascular permeability increases, and the endometrial cells become hypertrophied and produce prolactin. The processes inducing the changes are known as decidualization; the changed uterine lining is called the decidua. The initial changes begin in the luteal phase of the menstrual cycle. The uterine glands become more tortuous, the spiral arteries develop and the endometrium becomes thicker and oedematous. Uterine secretions increase and intercellular spaces develop.

Effectively, an implantation-receptive window occurs at about day 20 to 23 of the cycle (6 to 8 days after ovulation). The timing of the endometrial changes have to coincide with the time that the fertilized ovum enters the uterus (Csemiczky et al 1998). Problems with coincident timing can cause infertility or impaired fertility. During this receptive period, tiny microvilli-like protrusions, called pinopods, develop on the surface of the endometrium (Coticchio & Fishel 1998). The pinopods absorb fluid and molecules from the uterine lumen. This tends to decrease the size of the uterine cavity and to increase the chance of apposition between the embryo and the endometrium. Progesterone stimulates pinopod formation, as well as increased uterine secretions, increased blood flow and oedema.

Fig. 6.7 *The pathway of development for dizygotic and monozygotic twins. (Reproduced with permission from Larsen 1997.)*

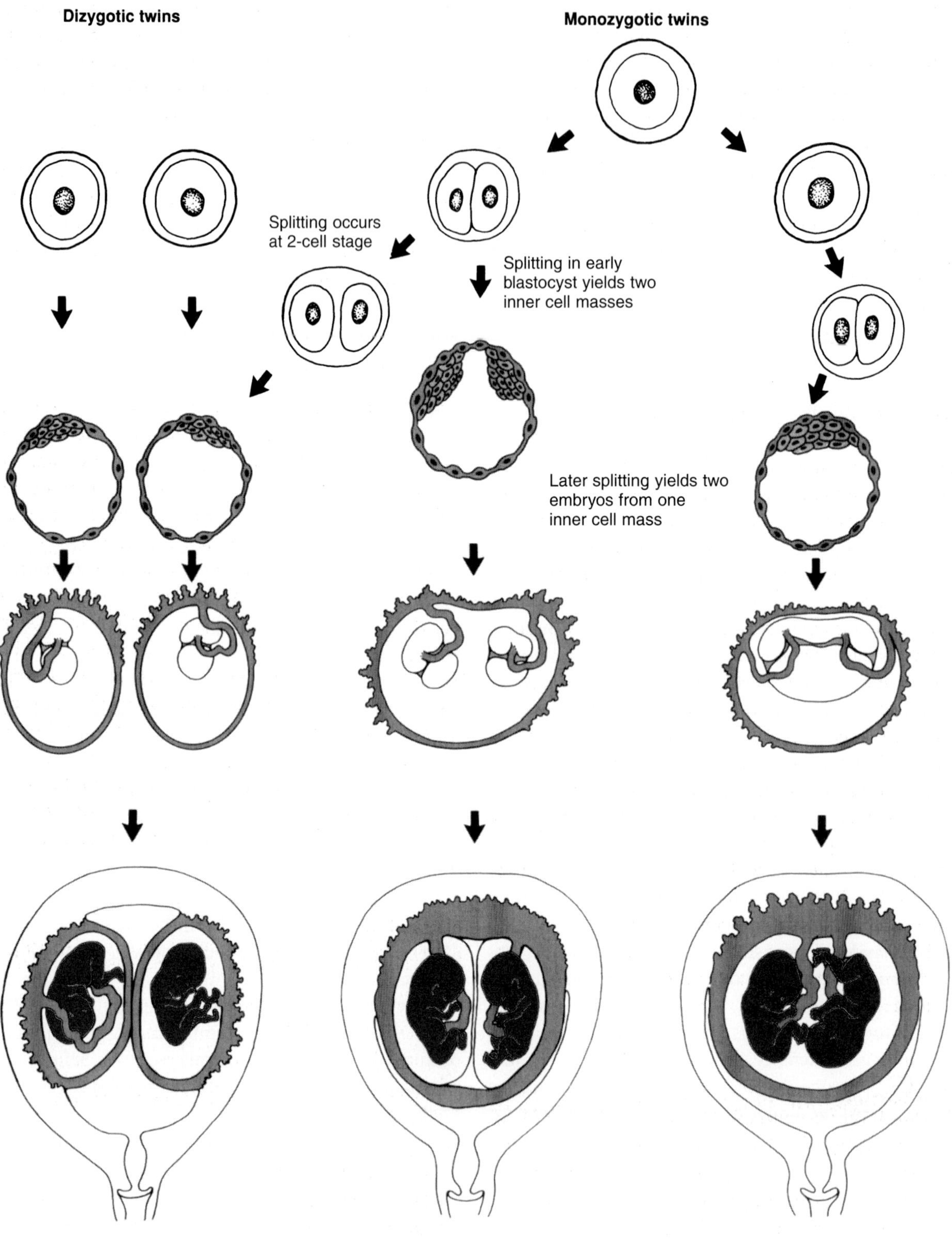

Embryo-derived platelet-activating factor (ED-PAF) influences vasodilation and oedema of the decidua. It increases vascular permeability, induces thrombocytopenia, regulates prostaglandin synthesis and activates platelets. Prostaglandins are also involved in regulating decidual factors. Other substances involved in signalling between the mother and embryo include inhibin, interferon, cytokines and other growth factors (see Box 4.3, p. 73) and adhesion molecules and a putative early pregnancy factor (EPF), which seems to have an immunosuppressive role (Coticchio & Fishel 1998). Growth factors such as endometrial leukaemia-inhibiting factor (LIF) (Hambartsoumian 1998) and EGF (Artini et al 1994) are critical to implantation.

## Artificial fertilization

Subfertility is thought to affect about 15–20% of couples. However, this figure depends on how subfertility is defined as couples may also experience delays in achieving second and subsequent pregnancies. In practice, infertility cannot be cured but may be treated; medical intervention attempts to optimize conditions that will aid conception. The study of infertility is a relatively new field, open to new research. It involves not just biological aspects of fertility but also social and psychological aspects. Many couples seeking fertility treatment will not succeed. In the UK, fertility treatment is regulated by the Human Fertilisation and Embryology Act 1990 and monitored by Human Fertilisation and Embryology Authority (HFEA).

If gametes are available, either from the couple themselves or from a donor, assisted conception techniques can be used. Laboratory techniques can be used to prepare the gametes and bring them closer together to enhance fertility (Box 6.3). Such techniques can be utilized in situations where there is damage to the uterine tubes (the site of normal fertilization), endometriosis, which may alter the uterine environment, male infertility (reduced number, motility or fertilizing ability of sperm) or coital dysfunction. They are also used to treat unexplained fertility where they will test the fertilizing ability of the sperm or where preimplantation diagnosis of genetic disorders is advisable.

IVF (in vitro fertilization) is now a routine procedure for certain types of infertility. Gamete intrafallopian transfer (GIFT) and zygote intrafallopian transfer (ZIFT) are related procedures, which require patent uterine tubes.

**Box 6.3**

**Commonly used assisted reproduction procedures**

|  |  |
|---|---|
| In vitro fertilization and embryo transfer | IVF + ET |
| Gamete intrafallopian transfer | GIFT |
| Zygote intrafallopian transfer | ZIFT |
| Intracytoplasmic sperm injection | ICSI |
| Donor insemination | DI |
| Intrauterine insemination | IUI |

### *In vitro fertilization*

There are a number of stages in a cycle of IVF treatment (Box 6.4) (Van Steirteghem, Liebaers & Devroey 1996). The couple may have more than one cause of infertility. IVF can also be used with oocyte donation, for instance, where the woman has ovarian dysfunction (such as premature menopause or Turner's syndrome) or has a high risk of transmitting a serious chromosomal abnormality. Ovarian stimulation is used to increase the number of mature oocytes that will be harvested as some are likely to fail to be fertilized. The method is based on suppressing the natural menstrual cycle by inhibiting the LH surge with a GnRH agonist and then stimulating follicular development with hMG (which contains FSH and LH). Ultrasound techniques can be used for both follicular assessment and the retrieval of oocytes. When several follicles have grown to a particular size

**Box 6.4**

**Stages in an IVF cycle**

- Patient selection
- Ovarian stimulation
- Oocyte retrieval
- Semen preparation
- Possible cryopreservation of gametes (variable success rates)
- Insemination
- Assessment of fertilization
- Embryo cleavage
- Embryo replacement
- Cryopreservation of excess embryos
- Detection of pregnancy

(17–18 mm), ovulation is induced with human gonadotrophin. The oocytes are collected at a pre-ovulatory stage so they are not truly mature. Progesterone or hCG is necessary to support the luteal phase. The collected oocytes are then cultured. The semen is prepared by separating the motile sperm from the seminal fluid and allowing them to capacitate. The capacitated sperm are introduced to the oocyte within a few hours of oocyte retrieval. The oocyte is enclosed by the corona radiata. The presence of the first polar body shows that the oocyte is at the metaphase II (see Fig. 7.11, p. 138) stage and ready to be fertilized.

After about 18 hours after insemination, the oocytes are denuded by mechanical removal of the cumulus cells. If fertilization has occurred, two distinct pronuclei, and usually two polar bodies, will be observable under a microscope. Twenty-four hours later, embryonic cleavage is evident and the quality of the embryo can be assessed morphologically for its potential to continue developing by the number of anucleate fragments and the evenness of the cells. Embryos with fragmented or uneven cells rarely continue developing. At the four-cell stage, a blastomere could be removed for preimplantation diagnosis (Handyside et al 1992). Two or three embryos are then selected for transfer to the uterus about 48 hours after the two-cell stage. The zona pellucida tends to harden in culture and has to be eroded mechanically or by acid digestion to aid hatching prior to the transfer. Multiple births are common with IVF, particularly in younger women, as two to three embryos may be replaced.

## Other procedures

In GIFT, the gametes are collected and prepared as for IVF but they are immediately transferred to the uterine tubes so fertilization occurs in vivo. In ZIFT, the fertilized oocyte is transferred into the uterine tube before cleavage. Excess embryos can be cryopreserved (carefully frozen using protectant fluid and specific rates of freezing and thawing). Increased hCG levels 10 to 12 days after fertilization confirm a successful pregnancy; levels of hCG usually double every 1.3 days.

Where there is severe male infertility the sperm are unable to fertilize the oocyte. Several techniques have been developed to micromanipulate the gametes to allow the sperm direct access to the oocyte. In PDZ (partial zona dissection) a small hole is made in the zona pellucida to allow the sperm to enter the perivitelline space. In SUZI (subzonal sperm injection) several sperm are injected into the perivitelline space. Both of these techniques have now been superseded by ICSI where a single sperm is injected directly into the oocyte (Palermo et al 1997). The advantage of this method is that it is successful even with very severe sperm dysfunction. Sperm do not need to be motile and can even be harvested from the epididymis by microepididymal sperm aspiration (MESA) or percutaneous epididymal sperm aspiration (PESA). The success rates of ICSI are usually high because the oocyte and endometrium are healthy and apparently not damaged by the procedures (although the egg is pierced and the cytoplasm disrupted). It will be important to monitor the health of children born following assisted conception procedures. For instance, the fertility of male offspring resulting from a fertilization with a sperm incapable of normal fertilization may be affected. Also male offspring born following ICSI from fathers with Y-chromosome deletions may inherit the same deletion (Chandley 1998).

Case study 6.2 is an example of artificial fertilization.

**Case study 6.2**

Elizabeth is a 42-year-old primipara who has been married for 20 years to Thomas. They had never used contraception. After initial investigations at a subfertility clinic, they were told that Thomas had a very low sperm count and that the sperm present were morphologically abnormal and displayed little motility. After eight attempts of IVF, Elizabeth and Thomas were offered ICSI and as a result a pregnancy occurred.

- Should the advice that the midwife gives to Elizabeth and Thomas be any different to that given to a normal fertile couple?
- What kinds of anxieties and concerns would Elizabeth and Thomas have and how might these be addressed?

## Key points

- The male gamete (sperm) is one of the smallest human cells and is motile, whereas the female gamete (oocyte) is one of the largest human cells and is immotile.
- Fertilization is the union of the sperm and the oocyte, resulting in a diploid zygote.
- Coitus requires circulatory and neuronal activity resulting in erection of the penis by increasing blood volume. Sexual arousal causes analogous physiological changes in the female.
- Although sex selection is practised in the husbandry of domesticated animals, there is little evidence to suggest it can be successfully manipulated in humans.
- In the female reproductive tract, the ejaculated sperm undergo changes, described as capacitation, which alter their tail movements and metabolism and enable them to fertilize the oocyte.
- The acrosome reaction, and release of enzymes, results in digestion of a pathway through the follicular cells and zona pellucida. Interaction between the sperm and the oocyte is mediated by species-specific receptors.
- Fusion of the gametes results in the cortical reaction (which prevents polyspermia), metabolic changes, completion of the oocyte meiotic division and initiation of the first mitotic division.
- The embryo or zygote undergoes cell cleavage as it is moved towards the uterus.
- As the number of cells increases, the embryo is described as a morula. The inner and outer cells undergo compaction and differentiate.
- The accumulation of fluid causes the embryo to 'hatch' out of the zona pellucida and it is then described as a blastocyst. The blastocyst has an outer layer of trophoblast cells (the future placenta) and an inner cell mass (the future embryo).
- The trophoblast cells secrete hCG, which promotes the survival and further growth of the corpus luteum.
- Maternal recognition of the pregnancy allows embryonic development and uterine receptiveness to be coordinated.
- Implantation occurs about 7 days after fertilization.
- Assisted fertility techniques have been developed for couples who have subfertility.

### Application to practice

Primarily, the midwife is not involved with the treatment of infertility. However, with the advance of technology there are an increasing number of conceptions and successful pregnancies as a result of fertility treatment.

An understanding of the complexities and interventions required to achieve conception is essential in order for the midwife to support women and partners. A knowledge of fertilization is also required in the understanding of contraceptive techniques.

## Annotated further reading

Balen A H, Jacobs H S 1997 Infertility in practice. Churchill Livingstone, New York

*Provides an overview of human infertility problems, aetiology and possible interventions.*

Bancroft J 1989 Human sexuality and its problems. Churchill Livingstone, New York

*A comprehensive, multidisciplinary account of the determinants of human sexuality. It covers sexual development, anatomy and physiology, biochemistry and endocrinology in addition to sociological and psychological aspects.*

Carlson B M 1994 Human embryology and developmental biology. C V Mosby, St Louis

*An illustrated account of development of the human embryo from conception to birth including the molecular and mechanistic basis of human development and recent research findings.*

Coticchio G, Fishel S 1998 Conception to implantation. In: Chamberlain G, Broughton Pipkin F (eds) Clinical physiology in obstetrics, 3rd edn. Blackwell, Oxford, pp 439–466

*A detailed account of this early period of embryo development by authors working in the field of fertility treatment.*

Furse A 1997 The infertility companion: a user's guide to tests, technology and therapies. Thorsons, London

*A useful and sensitively written reference on all aspects of human infertility including practical information on the medical help available, the procedures involved, potential side-effects of fertility drugs, complementary therapies and emotional aspects of fertility treatment.*

Gerhart J, Kirschner M 1997 Cells, embryos and evolution. Blackwell, Oxford

*This text explores how the origin of phenotypic variation in relation to evolutionary adaptation is achieved in the development of and the processes within the eukaryotic cell.*

James W H 1997 Sex ratio, coital rate, hormones and the time of fertilization within the cycle. Annals of Human Biology 24:403–409

*This article examines the relationship between coital rates, the timing of conception within the menstrual cycle and the sex ratios of the offspring produced.*

Johnson M H, Everitt B J 2000 Essential reproduction, 5th edn. Blackwell, Oxford

*An integrated, up-to-date and well-organized research-based textbook that explores comparative reproductive physiology of mammals including anatomy, physiology, endocrinology, genetics and behavioural studies.*

Larsen W J 1993 Human embryology. Churchill Livingstone, New York

*A good introduction to embryology which is clearly written and illustrated.*

## References


Andersson K E, Wagner G 1995 Physiology of penile erection. Physiological Review 75:191–236

Argiolas A, Melis M R 1995 Neuromodulation of penile erection: an overview of the role of neurotransmitters and neuropeptides. Progress in Neurobiology 47:235–255

Artini P G, Battaglia C, D'Ambrogio G et al 1994 Relationship between human oocyte maturity, fertilization and follicular growth factors. Human Reproduction 9:902–906

Baker R R, Bellis M A 1988 Kamikaze sperm in mammals. Animal Behaviour 36:936–939

Blobel C P, Wolfsberg T G, Turck C W, Myles D G, Primakoff P, White J M 1992 A potential fusion peptide and an integrin ligand domain in a protein active in sperm-egg fusion. Nature 356:248–252

Bromwich P 1991 The sex ratio, and ways of manipulating it. Progress in Obstetrics and Gynaecology 7:217–231

Brooker C G 1998 Human structure and function, 2nd edn. C V Mosby, St Louis, p477

Brucker C, Lipford G B 1995 The human sperm acrosome reaction: physiology and regulatory mechanisms. Human Reproduction Update 1:51–62

Chandley A C 1998 Chromosome anomalies and Y chromosome microdeletions as causal factors in male infertility. Human Reproduction 13 (suppl 1): 45–50

Check J H, Weiss R M, Lurie D 1992 Analysis of serum human chorionic-gonadotropin levels in normal singleton, multiple and abnormal pregnancies. Human Reproduction 7:1176–1180

Coticchio G, Fishel S 1998 Conception to implantation. In: Chamberlain G, Broughton Pipkin F (eds) Clinical physiology in obstetrics, 3rd edn. Blackwell, Oxford

Csemiczky G, Wramsby H, Johannisson E, Landgren B M 1998 Importance of endometrial quality in women with tubal infertility during a natural menstrual cycle for the outcome of IVF treatment. Journal of Assisted Reproduction and Genetics 15:55–61

DeLamirande E, Leclerc P, Gagnon C 1997 Capacitation as a regulatory event that primes spermatozoa for the acrosome reaction and fertilisation. Molecular Human Reproduction 3:175–194

Familiari G, Notola S A, Macchiarell G, Micara G, Aragona C, Motta P M 1992 Human zona pellucida during in vitro fertilization: an ultrastructural study using saponin, ruthenium red and osmium thiocarbohydazide. Molecular Reproduction and Development 32:51–61

Griffin D K 1996 The incidence, origin and etiology of aneuploidy. International Review of Cytology 167:263–296

Gyllensten U, Wharton D, Josefsson A, Wilson AC 1991 Paternal inheritance of mitochondrial DNA in mice. Nature 352:255–257

Hambartsoumian E 1998 Endometrial leukemia inhibitory factor (LIF) as a possible cause of unexplained fertility and multiple failure of ovulation. American Journal of Reproductive Immunology 39:137–143

Handyside A H, Lesko J G, Tarin J J, Winston R M L, Hughes M R 1992 Birth of a normal girl after in vitro fertilisation and preimplantation diagnostic testing for cystic fibrosis. New England Journal of Medicine 327:905–909

Harcourt A H 1991 Sperm competition and the evolution of non-fertilizing sperm in mammals. Evolution 45: 314–328

Hardy K, Handyside A H, Winston R M L 1989 The human blastocyst—cell number, death and allocation during late preimplantation development in vitro. Development 107:597

Hardy K, Martin K L, Leese H J, Winston R M L, Handyside A H 1990 Human preimplantation development in vitro is not adversely affected by biopsy at the 8-cell stage. Human Reproduction 5:708–714

Harlap S 1979 Gender of infants conceived on different days of the menstrual cycle. New England Journal of Medicine 291:1445–1448

Hoodbhoy T, Talbot R 1994 Mammalian cortical granules: contents, fate and function. Molecular Reproduction and Development 39:439–448

Jacobs P A, Wilson C M, Sprenkle J A, Rosenheim N B, Migeon B R 1980 Mechanism of origin of complete hydatidiform mole. Nature 286:714–717

Kaneda H, Hayashi J L, Takahama S, Taya C, Lindal K F, Yonekawa H 1995 Elimination of paternal mitochondrial DNA in intraspecific crosses during early mouse embryogenesis. Proceedings of the National Academy of Sciences USA 92:4542–4546

Larsen W J 1993 Human embryology, 2nd edn. Churchill Livingstone, New York, p 481

Levin R J 1998 Sex and the human female reproductive tract—what really happens during and after coitus. International Journal of Impotence Research 10(suppl 1):514–521

Matilsky M, Battino S, Ben-Ami M, Gesleivich Y, Eyali V, Shalev E 1993 The effect of ejaculatory frequency on semen characteristics of normozoospermic and oligozoospermic men from an infertile population. Human Reproduction 8:71–73

Mbizvo M T 1995 Functional motion changes during sperm transport to the site of fertilization and in vitro applications: a review. International Journal of Andrology 18:1–6

Palermo G P, Avrech O M, Colombero L T et al 1997 Human sperm cytosolic factor triggers $Ca^{2+}$ oscillations and overcomes activation failure of mammalian oocytes. Molecular Human Reproduction 3:367–374

Payne D, Flaherty S P, Barry M F, Matthews C D 1997 Preliminary observations on polar body extrusion and pronuclear formation in human oocytes using time-lapse video cinematography. Human Reproduction 12:532–541

Schatten G 1994 The centrosome and its mode of inheritance; the reduction of the centrosome during gametogenesis and its restoration during fertility. Developmental Biology 165:299–335

Tulsiani D R P, Yoshida-Komiya H, Araki Y 1997 Mammalian fertilization: a carbohydrate mediated event. Biology of Reproduction 57:487–494

Van Blerkom J, Davis P, Merriam J, Sinclair J 1995 Nuclear and cytoplasmic dynamics of sperm penetration, pronuclear formation and microtubule organization during fertilization and early preimplantation in the human. Human Reproduction Update 1:429–461

Van Steirteghem A, Liebaers I, Devroey P 1996 Assisted reproduction. In: Hillier S G, Kitchener H C, Neilson J P (eds) Scientific essentials of reproductive medicine. W B Saunders, Philadelphia, pp 230–241

Wasserman P M 1987 The biology and chemistry of fertilisation. Science 235:553–560

Whittaker M 1995 Regulation of the cell division cycle by inositol phosphate and the calcium signalling pathway. Advances in Second Messenger and Phosphoprotein Research 30:299–310

Zenzes M T, Wang P, Casper R F 1995 Cigarette smoking may affect meiotic maturation of human oocytes. Human Reproduction 10:3213–3217

# 7 Overview of human genetics and genetic disorders

**Learning objectives**

- To describe the packaging of genes in the chromosome and how they are expressed.
- To describe the characteristics of dominant, recessive and X-linked genetic traits.
- To interpret a pedigree chart and make simple genetic predictions.
- To understand the principles of genetic screening.
- To relate current genetic research to midwifery practice.
- To discuss evolutionary influences upon human reproduction.

## Introduction

The science of genetics is reductionist in nature. It focuses on cellular nuclear biochemistry and how these interactions produce the unique morphology of individual organisms through protein synthesis. Biological determinism is the belief that every aspect of human life can be explained in terms of human biology, particularly genetics. Characteristics are passed from one generation to the next in the form of genes. In sexually reproducing species, the genes are assorted and packaged into the gametes. Variations between genes affect survival so the individuals with the best-adapted characteristics to cope with environmental conditions have an advantage. This is described as Natural Selection.

The study of genetics focuses on inherited characteristics, particularly those that are considered abnormal, how these arise and their effects on the individual's physiology and behaviour. Genetics is a predictive science and its rules are based upon the application of mathematical statistics and probability. Evolutionary effects on genetics which may determine the penetration of recessive genetic disorders such as cystic fibrosis into gene pools are discussed. The impact of genetics upon antenatal screening is of particular relevance for midwives.

## A brief history of genetics

The influence of genetic interactions is associated with the work of an Austrian monk called Gregor Mendel in the 1860s. Mendel's breeding experiments on peas describe how characteristics of parents are passed on to their prodigy, for example the height, colour and petal shape of pea flowers. Mendel proposed that 'particles of inheritance' were transmitted from one generation to the next. He correctly identified the concept of genes long before the structures of DNA and chromosomes were understood.

Historically, genetics has been associated with the study of eugenics. This term was first used by Francis Galton (a cousin of Charles Darwin) who advocated that the overall population could be improved by the use of selective breeding. This was a strong influence in the philosophy of Nazi Germany, but also had supporters throughout the Western world in the first half of the twentieth century.

Recently there has been a change in the way the sciences of genetics and evolution are presented from the spontaneous model that began with Charles Darwin's theory of Survival of the Fittest.

Neo-Darwinists advocate that survival of a species is not necessarily by the fittest but by those that are most likely to reproduce successfully. This is reflected in the work of Richard Dawkins who describes genes and groups of genes as being selfish in the respect that in order to replicate and be successful they use organisms that contain them as a vehicle to ensure survival (Dawkins 1989). Obviously reproduction is vital to ensure that this occurs.

This controversial view portrays organisms solely as mechanical methods of survival to pass genes on to as many offspring as possible. However, there are a number of arguments against this view. Organisms are not perfectly adapted; for instance, humans seem to have some non-advantageous genes such as those coding for the vermiform appendix. It could be argued that these genes have not been obliterated because other, linked genes are advantageous and effectively protect them. The other important point is that species not only interact with their environment but also positively alter their environment.

The environment interacts with genes (the nature–nurture debate) and has a tremendous influence on how they are expressed, affecting susceptibility and resistance to disease. Genes may act in competition with each other, which may explain certain pathophysiological conditions and their aetiology. Some organisms may use their genes to alter the phenotype of another animal to increase their chances of survival. For example, infection with the trematode parasite causes its snail host's shell to become thicker (Dawkins 1999).

Within the modern medical world there now exist moral dilemmas surrounding the screening for, detection of and termination of abnormal fetuses. Current research on genetics is not solely medical (Box 7.1) as it can be applied to population studies, such as tracing the origins of human migration movements, and genealogy, such as tracing the real families of children of the Argentinean 'Disappeared' (Jones 1994).

**Box 7.1**

**Areas of genetic research**

- Screening for fetal abnormality
- Genetic counselling for parents with a family history of genetic disorders
- Identification of fetal sex in the early (indifferent) embryological phase
- Cloning of whole organisms
- Gene manipulation, not only to eradicate disease, but also to improve existing disease states
- Treatment by gene manipulation in animals to produce human proteins, hormones, etc.
- Genetic modification
- Identification of individuals by genetic 'fingerprinting'

## Genes and chromosomes

Genes are the units of inheritance. Each gene is a length of DNA on a chromosome that contains the coded information to direct the synthesis of a specific protein chain. The differences between organisms are related to different proteins being synthesized that have different structures and functions. Effectively the genes act as a blueprint, or instruction manual, for the total development of the organism and how it will function and change during its lifetime (Box 7.2). Chromosomes are packages of DNA in the nucleus, on which the genes are linearly arranged. Chromosomes have two arms: a shorter p arm and a longer q arm, with a centromere between them. Chromosomes are important in cell replication and the passing of the genetic message from one generation to the next. Usually the DNA, about 180 cm per nucleus, exists as an unstructured mass of threads in the nucleus. However, when the cell is undergoing division the DNA becomes organized and compacted into chromosomes, which can be visualized by microscopy (see Ch. 1). This chromosomal organization allows biologists to identify genes and localize them to a particular chromosome to follow their pattern of inheritance.

**Box 7.2**

**Genetics as a language**

Genetics can be considered as a language based on the DNA molecule. Linguistic development and evolution have a number of similarities. Studies looking at the origins of a particular word and how it has evolved to be slightly different in different languages are similar to the changes in genes (Jones 1994). Genetic mutations are analogous to new words being introduced into the language (such as 'email').

- Genetics = language
- Vocabulary = genes
- Grammar = rules about the arrangement of information
- Literature = the instructions to make a human
- Alphabet = four bases of DNA
- Word = codon (three 'letter' code for an amino acid)

Each cell has the same genetic information in its nucleus as the original zygote (fertilized ovum) and all of the cells derived from it. Different cells behave in different ways because they express different subsets of information from the DNA.

## The structure of DNA and RNA

Watson, Crick, Franklin and Wilkins elucidated the biochemical structure of DNA in 1953. Their description of the helical structure revealed how the molecule was able to replicate itself and thus explained the cellular mechanism of reproduction. DNA is composed of two strands of sugar phosphate molecules that are joined together to form long chains (Fig. 7.1). The strands of DNA are made up of repeating units called nucleotides. The DNA nucleotide has three components: a deoxyribose sugar, a phosphate group and a base. There are four types of bases: thymine and cytosine, which have single-ring structures, and adenine and guanine, which have double-ring structures. DNA exists as a double-stranded molecule wound into a helix. The strands are kept together by hydrogen bonding between the bases. The bases are different sizes and have a different potential number of hydrogen bonds so they always pair in the same ways. Adenine and thymine pair with two hydrogen bonds; cytosine and guanine pair with three. This means that the sequence of the bases is complementary; the sequence of bases on one strand can be deduced from the sequence on the other strand.

## DNA replication and cell division

The arrangement of base pairs of the two strands is like the rungs of a ladder or teeth of a zip. When DNA replicates, the strands unwind and the hydrogen bonds holding the base pairs together separate (unzip). Each strand acts as a template for the synthesis of another new strand of complementary DNA bases to form from nucleotides that enter the nucleus through the nuclear pores (Fig. 7.2). So two new DNA double helices are formed, each with one strand of 'old' DNA and a newly synthesized strand. Thus the replication is described as semiconservative. Replication occurs as part of mitosis, or cell division. Replication of DNA

**Fig. 7.1** *The structure of DNA.*

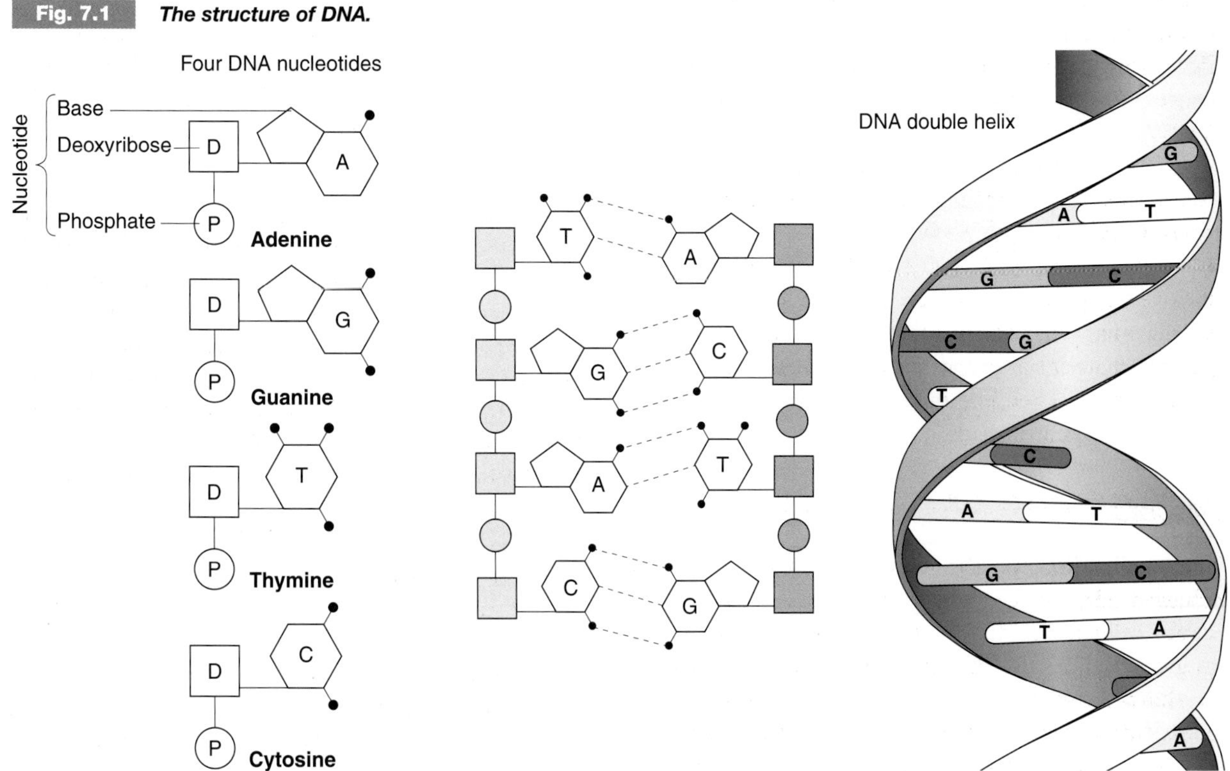

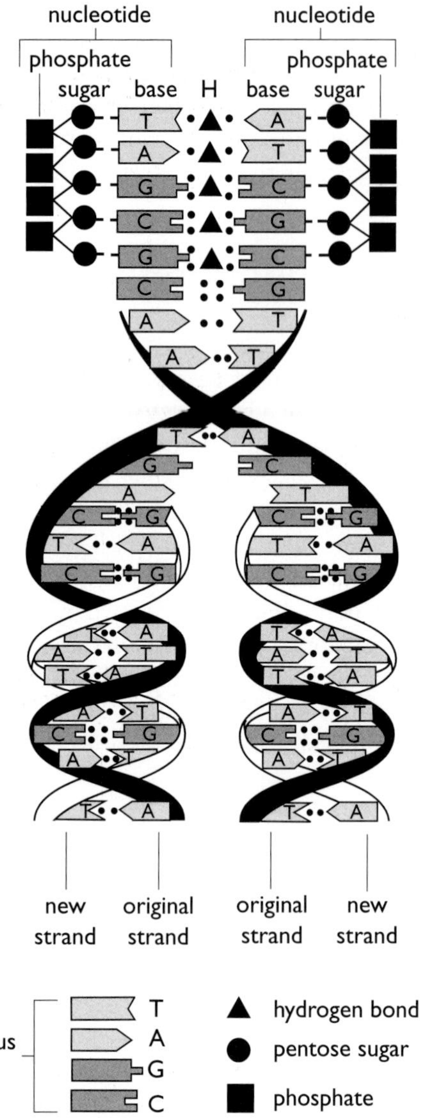


**Fig. 7.2** *DNA replication. (Reproduced with permission from Brooker 1998).*

means that the chromosomes have double their nuclear material in preparation for dividing into two separate cells. Therefore the chromosome is formed of two identical chromatids.

### *Mitosis*

The replication of the entire human genome is achieved through the process of mitosis, which is part of the cell cycle (Fig. 7.3). Cellular replication results in growth of tissues through hyperplasia (an increase in the number of cells); each cell has the identical genetic message (DNA content) to its parent cell. Mitotic rates are different for different types of cells.

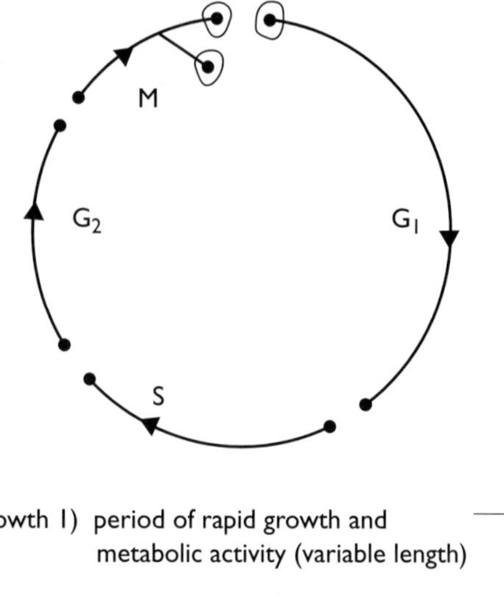


**Fig. 7.3** *The phases of the cell cycle and cell content. (Reproduced with permission from Brooker 1998.)*

Cells that divide fast (have a high mitotic index) include skin and gut epithelial cells, spermatogonia and tumour cells. With increased age the mitotic rate slows down so skin renewal, for instance, takes longer and the appearance of the skin is more aged. Drugs used to treat cancers also inhibit mitosis so their side-effects are mostly clearly manifested in normal cells with high mitotic rates, causing problems with nutrient absorption and decreasing male fertility. Many cells have an extremely slow rate of mitosis, such as brain, heart and liver cells, and do not regenerate or heal well after injury. Mitosis is a continuous process but for ease of description is traditionally described in distinct phases; prophase, metaphase, anaphase and telophase (Fig. 7.4). Interphase is the name given to the gap between mitotic divisions.

## The genetic message

The structure of DNA allows both ease of replication and duplication of the genetic message prior to cell division, and also a method of directing protein synthesis and ultimate cell function. The DNA message is interpreted as a specific protein product. Proteins are synthesized at the ribosomes of the cell whereas the

Fig. 7.4 *The stages of mitosis. (Reproduced with permission from the Open University 1987.)*

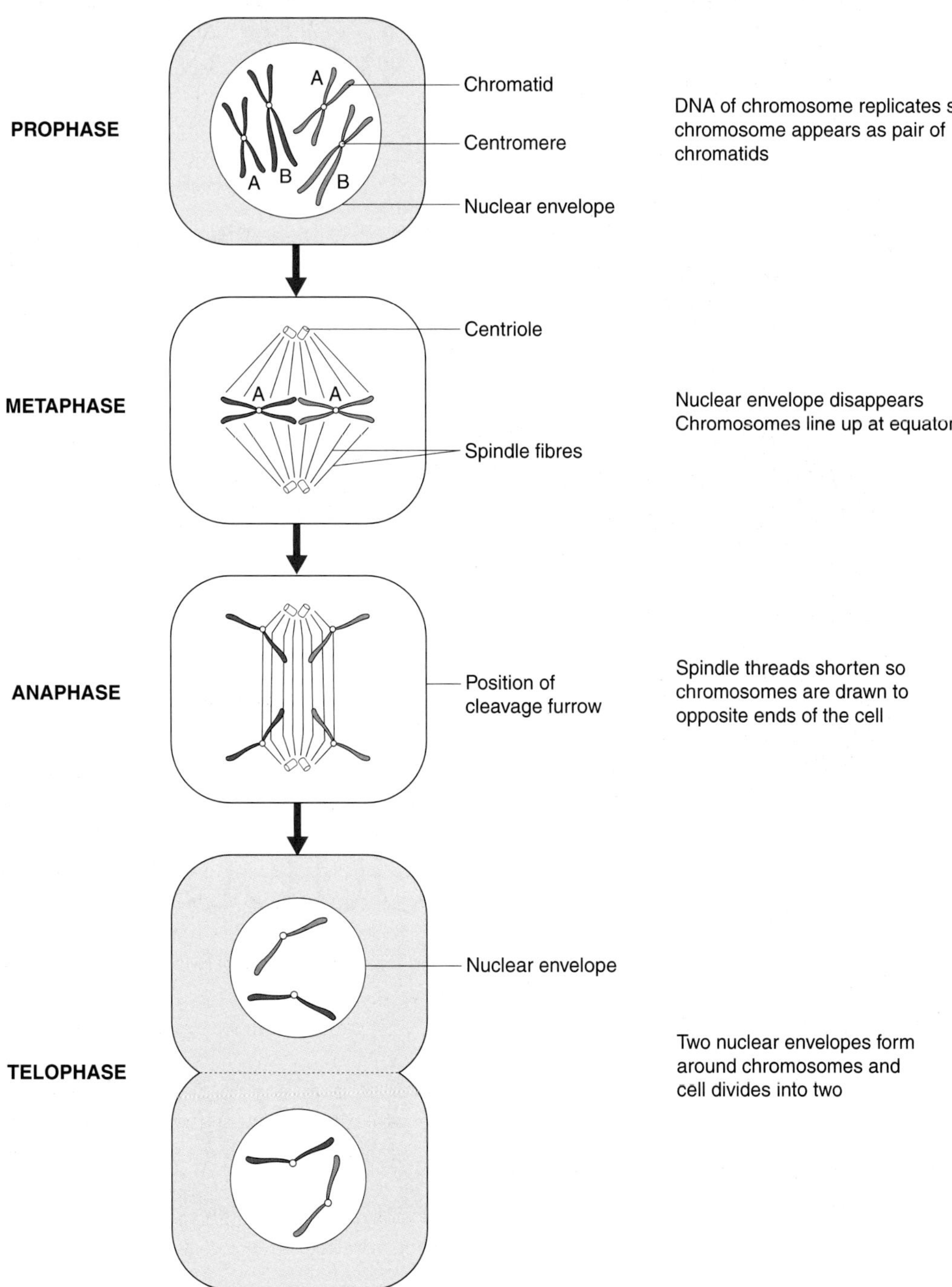


encoded information, in the form of DNA, remains within the nucleus. The information is carried from DNA to the site of protein synthesis by the second type of nucleic acid, RNA. Whereas DNA is a double strand, RNA exists as a single strand of sugar phosphate units, and has ribose sugar units (instead of deoxyribose) and similar complementary base molecules to those found in DNA, except that uracil instead of thymine pairs with adenine. RNA also exists as different forms with different functions. It is messenger RNA (mRNA) that carries the message from the nucleus to the ribosome, as a complementary strand of mRNA is formed using a stretch of unwound DNA as a template.

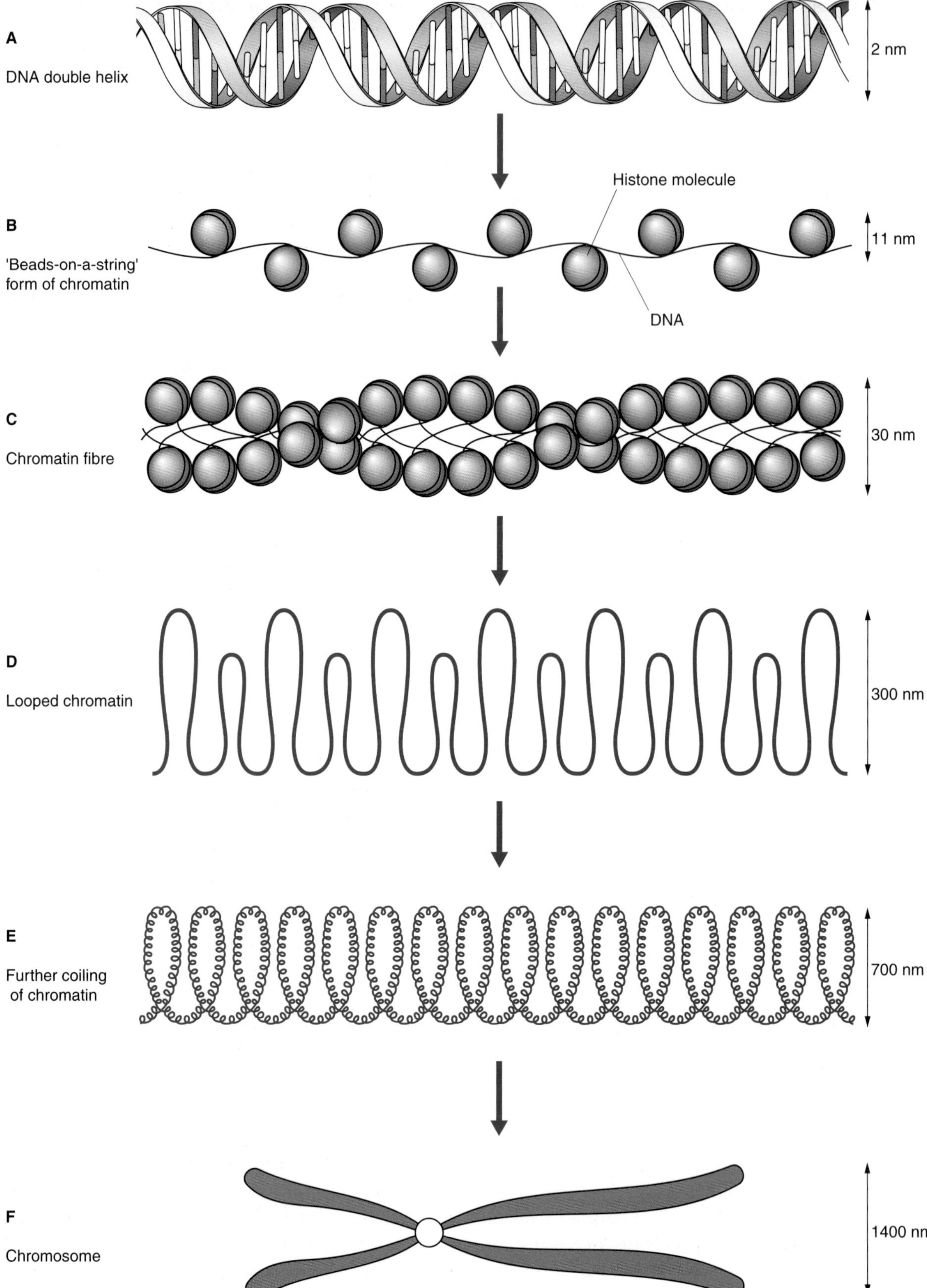
A
DNA double helix
2 nm
Histone molecule
B
'Beads-on-a-string' form of chromatin
11 nm
DNA
C
Chromatin fibre
30 nm
D
Looped chromatin
300 nm
E
Further coiling of chromatin
700 nm
F
Chromosome
1400 nm

**Fig. 7.5** ***A–F The stages of DNA packaging; in order for transcription to take place, the chromosomes must be uncoiled and 'unzipped' in the reverse process to that shown. (Adapted with permission from Goodwin 1997.)***

## *Transcription*

The process starts with the DNA strands separating like a zip pulling open in the middle. This is the reverse process to the way it coils when condensing into chromosomes (Fig. 7.5). Only one strand of DNA, the coding or 'sense' strand, is used as the template; the other is described as non-coding or 'non-sense'. The mRNA chain is built as the bases pair with the DNA template; this is called transcription (Fig. 7.6).

The whole gene is transcribed but not all of it is used so the primary transcription product mRNA is modified (cut and spliced) into functional mRNA (Fig. 7.7). The parts of the mRNA that are removed have been copied from parts of the gene called introns and those

**Fig. 7.6** ***Transcription.***

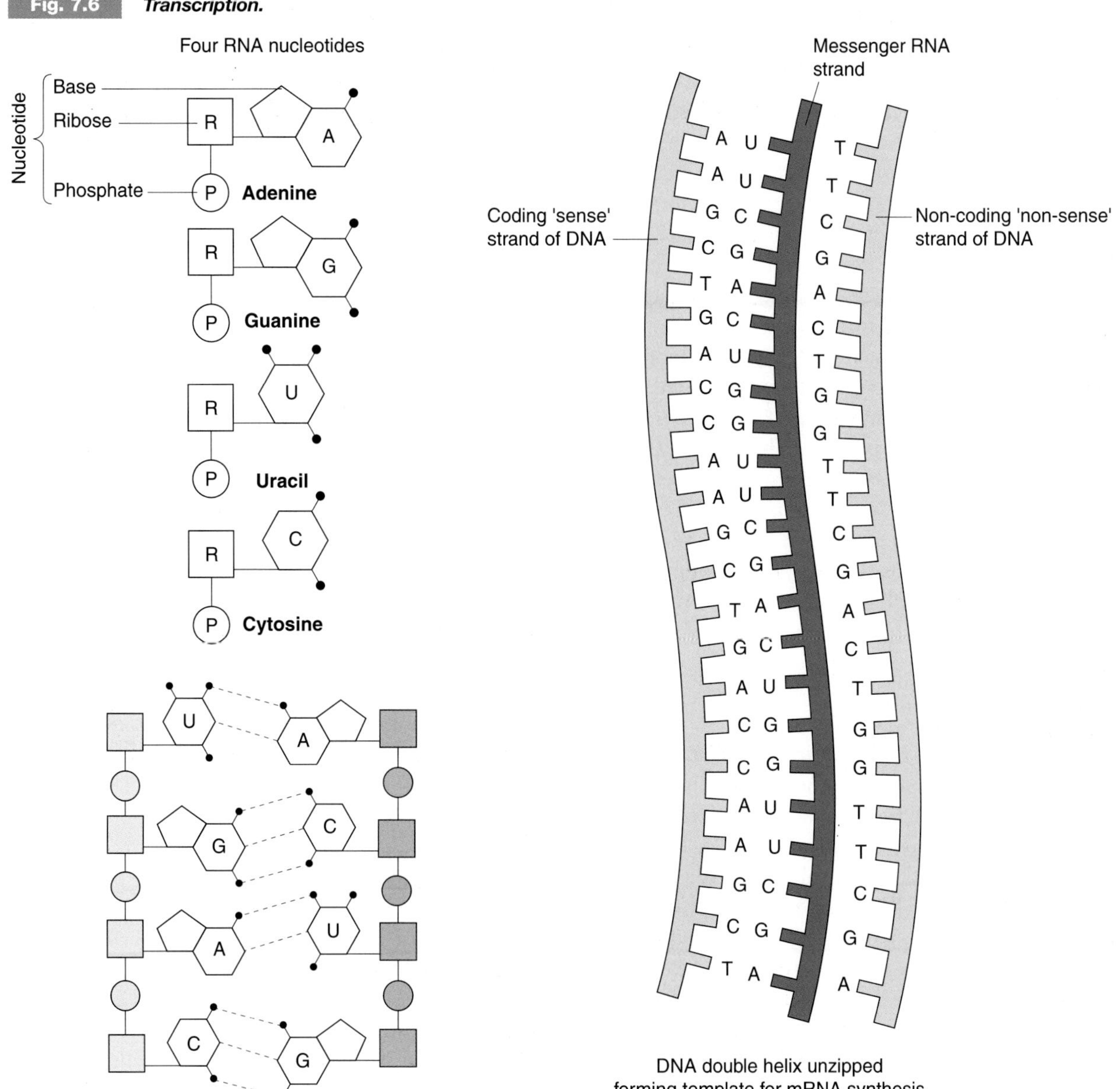

Fig. 7.7 *Splicing. (Reproduced with permission from Goodwin 1997.)*

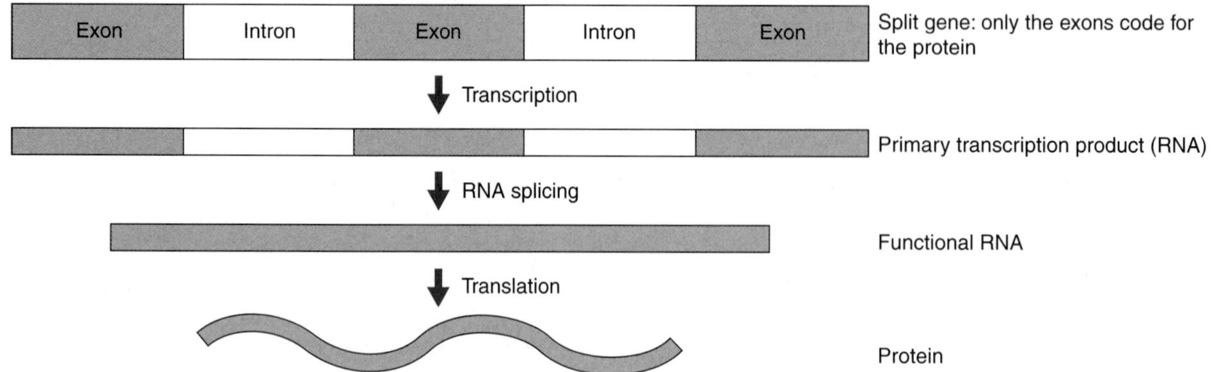


that are retained come from the parts of the DNA known as exons. It is estimated that only about 2–5% of the total genome (genetic code or DNA) is composed of exons and actually codes for protein synthesis. Some of the DNA modulates genetic expression, switching the process of protein synthesis on and off; these control genes are referred to as operator, regulator and inducer genes. Introns form the majority of the DNA sequence and do not appear to be involved in coding for protein synthesis, although they may allow different proteins to be formed from the same length of DNA. Much of the genome may be composed of redundant genes that are no longer activated. These unused stretches of DNA are used to compare tissue samples for DNA fingerprinting. The Human Genome Project aims to read and publish all the three billion DNA bases in order to 'map' human genetic composition; this may provide insights in the function of this apparently superfluous DNA. (The genome is the name given to the total number of genes found within an organism.)

### Protein synthesis

When transcription and post-transcription modification are complete, the finished functional mRNA strand detaches from the DNA and leaves the nucleus, via a nuclear pore, to go to the ribosomes. Ribosomes are structures formed of two subunits made of protein and another type of RNA, ribosomal RNA (rRNA). mRNA attaches to ribosomes and the sequence of bases of the mRNA is decoded to direct the synthesis of a protein; this step is called translation (Fig. 7.8). The mRNA sequence is 'read' three bases at a time. A particular sequence of three bases is called a codon; each codon prescribes that a specific amino acid is incorporated into the final amino acid chain of the overall protein structure. There are 20 amino acids; however, as a three-base genetic code allows the potential of $4 \times 4 \times 4 = 64$ permutations, most amino acids are coded for by more than one codon (Fig. 7.9).

Another form of RNA in the cytoplasm, called transfer RNA (tRNA), carries amino acids to the ribosome to be incorporated into the protein chain. There are different types of tRNA, each one with a specific binding site for a particular amino acid at one end and an 'anticodon', which recognizes the codon on the mRNA at the other end. The first amino acid of a new protein is methionine. The next amino acid joins to the carboxyl group of methionine with a peptide bond. Successive amino acids join, forming a chain of amino acids until a 'stop' codon on mRNA signals the end of the chain. The sequence of amino acids determines the primary structure of the protein. The further configuration of the protein is determined by the interactions between different amino acids on the chain, which change the protein shape into a 'folded' structure, the final shape determining its function. Hence the sequence of bases of the gene, or region of DNA determines the sequence of amino acids, which in turn prescribes the structure and function of the protein.

## Mutation

The copying of DNA has to be accurate. If mistakes are introduced into a region of DNA that is expressed as a protein (i.e. into an exon), the altered sequence of amino acids can change the structure of the protein. This change in base sequence of DNA is described as a mutation. It is estimated that mutations occur every

Fig. 7.8 *The stages of protein synthesis translation.*

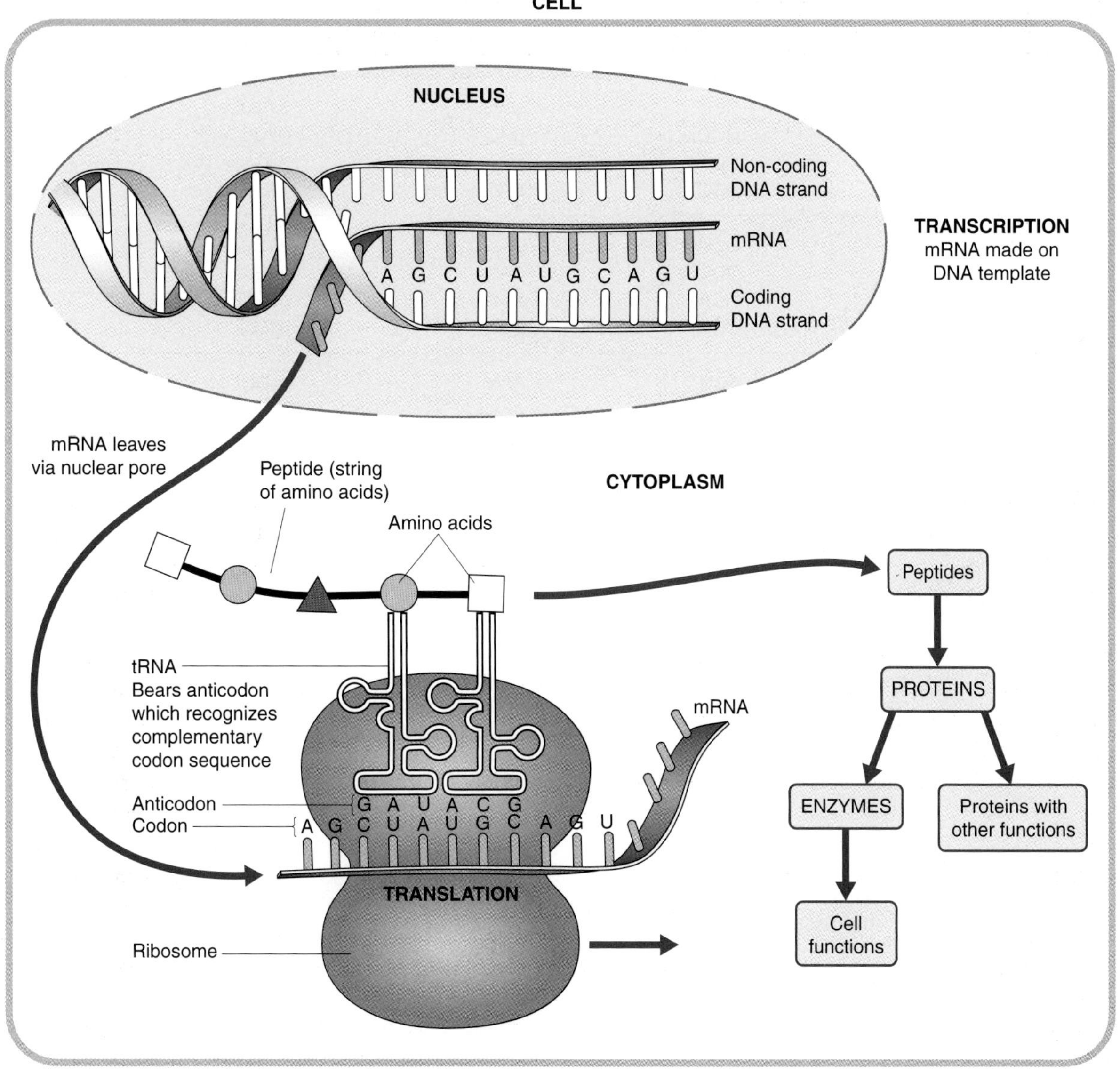


DNA makes RNA (transcription) makes protein (translation)

half hour in each person but a mutation in a functional gene only occurs once in five generations. A mutation can be described as 'descent with modification'. In mitosis, there are accumulated errors in copying the genetic message. Each chromosome has a specialized length of DNA at its end, which gets shorter with each successive division. About four bases seem to be lost with each successive cell division.

A base pair can sometimes be spontaneously replaced by a different base pair thus altering the codon and ultimately the amino acid sequence. Age, environmental pressure, radiation and chemicals increase mutation rate. One notable example is haemophilia, the sex-linked genetic condition that afflicted male members of the European Royal Family for several generations. The spontaneous mutation for changed haemoglobin structure may have occurred in one of the gametes forming the zygote that became Queen Victoria. This type of mutation is referred to as a substitution. Mutations may also occur by the complete insertion of new codons or by the deletion of a complete codon, thus altering protein structure by introducing or deleting amino acids in the protein. This can be complicated if codons are duplicated and repeated one after the other—for example in fragile X syndrome.

Fig. 7.9 *Codons and the amino acids they code for. (Reproduced with permission from the Open University 1988.)*

| First letter | Second letter: U | | C | | A | | G | | Third letter |
|---|---|---|---|---|---|---|---|---|---|
| U | UUU | Phe | UCU | Ser | UAU | Tyr | UGU | Cys | U |
| | UUC | | UCC | | UAC | | UGC | | C |
| | UUA | Leu | UCA | | UAA | stop | UGA | stop | A |
| | UUG | | UCG | | UAG | stop | UGG | Trp | G |
| C | CUU | Leu | CCU | Pro | CAU | His | CGU | Arg | U |
| | CUC | | CCC | | CAC | | CGC | | C |
| | CUA | | CCA | | CAA | Gln | CGA | | A |
| | CUG | | CCG | | CAG | | CGG | | G |
| A | AUU | Ileu | ACU | Thr | AAU | Asn | AGU | Ser | U |
| | AUC | | ACC | | AAC | | AGC | | C |
| | AUA | | ACA | | AAA | Lys | AGA | Arg | A |
| | AUG | Met | ACG | | AAG | | AGG | | G |
| G | GUU | Val | GCU | Ala | GAU | Asp | GGU | Gly | U |
| | GUC | | GCC | | GAC | | GGC | | C |
| | GUA | | GCA | | GAA | Glu | GGA | | A |
| | GUG | | GCG | | GAG | | GGG | | G |

The abbreviated names of amino acids are:

**Ala** = alanine
**Arg** = arginine
**Asn** = asparagine
**Asp** = aspartic acid
**Cys** = cysteine
**Gln** = glutamine
**Glu** = glutamic
**Gly** = glycine
**His** = histidine
**Ileu** = isoleucine
**Leu** = leucine
**Lys** = lysine
**Met** = methionine
**Phe** = phenylalanine
**Pro** = proline
**Ser** = serine
**Thr** = threonine
**Trp** = tryptophan
**Tyr** = tyrosine
**Val** = valine

Many mutations occur in the non-coding areas of DNA, so protein structure and function are not affected by the change; these mutations are described as 'silent' as they have no effect. If the mutation results in a different codon that codes for the same amino acid as the original, there will also be no effect. However, a different base, or a missing base, will cause a change in the final sequence of amino acids of the protein, which may have serious effects on protein structure and function. An example is sickle cell anaemia (Box 7.3 and Fig. 7.10).

## Meiosis

Each species has a characteristic number of chromosomes; humans have 46 chromosomes, arranged as 23 pairs. One chromosome of each pair is maternally derived (from the ovum); the other is paternally derived (from the sperm). (The members of each pair are called homologous—see below.) Human gametes contain only 23 chromosomes—that is, half the normal number of chromosomes in other human cells.

**Box 7.3**

**Sickle cell anaemia**

Most haemoglobin in adults is HbA, which has two α- and two β-peptide chains forming the haemoglobin molecule. Sickle cell anaemia is an example of a single point mutation where the substitution of one base changes the codon and results in the substitution of one amino acid (Fig. 7.10). Uracil replaces adenine so, instead of glutamic acid, valine is inserted in the protein chain at position 6. Valine has a different charge to glutamic acid so the protein folds differently. The result is that the protein structure of the β-chain of haemoglobin is changed, which affects the molecular shape and oxygen-binding properties. The red blood cells distort into a characteristic sickle shape, particularly at low oxygen tension. Sickle cell anaemia is inherited as an autosomal recessive condition; affected patients have two mutant haemoglobin S genes, one from each parent. The parents are heterozygotes (HbA/HbS) and are thus clinically normal but carry the sickle cell gene. Homozygotes (HbS/HbS) have chronic haemolytic anaemia and are prone to infarction; lifespan is shortened.

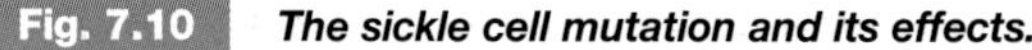

**Fig. 7.10** ***The sickle cell mutation and its effects.***

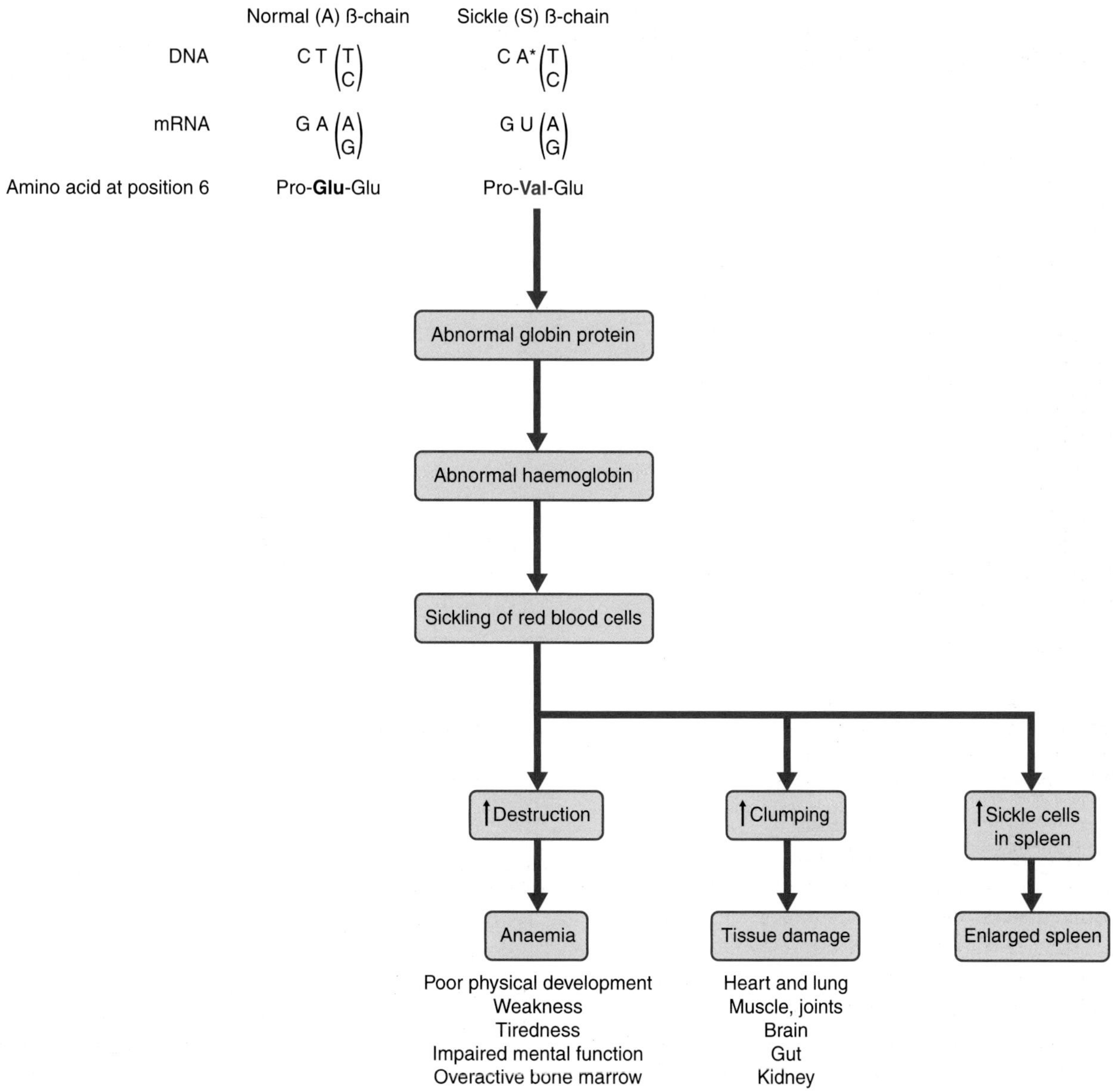

| | Normal (A) ß-chain | Sickle (S) ß-chain |
|---|---|---|
| DNA | C T (T/C) | C A* (T/C) |
| mRNA | G A (A/G) | G U (A/G) |
| Amino acid at position 6 | Pro-**Glu**-Glu | Pro-**Val**-Glu |

Abnormal globin protein

Abnormal haemoglobin

Sickling of red blood cells

↑Destruction → Anaemia: Poor physical development, Weakness, Tiredness, Impaired mental function, Overactive bone marrow

↑Clumping → Tissue damage: Heart and lung, Muscle, joints, Brain, Gut, Kidney

↑Sickle cells in spleen → Enlarged spleen

This reduction from the diploid number of chromosomes (46) to the haploid number (23) is accomplished by meiosis. Meiosis results in gametes, or sex cells, that are not identical to their parent cells. These gametes are haploid and during meiosis the genetic instructions are randomly assorted, thus generating unique combinations. Meiosis is also described as 'reduction division' because the number of chromosomes is reduced from 46 (i.e. 23 pairs) to 23. It occurs in two successive divisions, each of which can be divided into steps (Fig. 7.11).

In anaphase I, there is random segregation of each member of the chromosome pairs with a maternal and a paternal chromosome randomly going to a particular end of the cell. This would theoretically generate $2^{23}$ (i.e. 8 388 608) different possibilities of gamete combination. However, the crossing over of genetic material between the chromosomes adds far more variation. The chances of any two individuals arising from different pregnancies inheriting exactly the same genome are infinitely small.

The longer an oocyte is immobilized at prophase I the greater is the chance of failure of separation of the homologous chromosomes. Often genetic abnormalities arise as extra genetic material is incorporated into the genome. If an extra chromosome is inserted, the condition is referred to as trisomic (Table 7.1). Most combinations of trisomy are not seen, but there is no

**Fig. 7.11** *The stages of meiosis A–J. (Reproduced with permission from Goodwin 1997.)*

**Division I of meiosis**

**PROPHASE I**

Chromosomes appear, divided into chromatids Red chromosomes have been inherited from the mother, grey chromosomes from the father

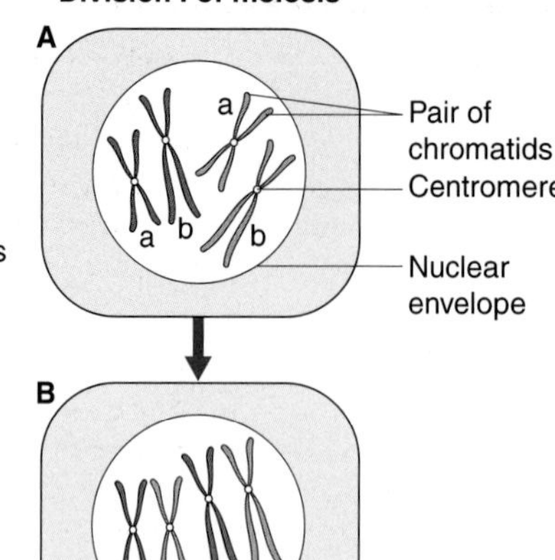


B

Chromosomes pair up: the two chromosomes (a) form one pair, the two chromosomes (b) form another

C

Chromatids cross over and exchange material

D

**METAPHASE I**

Nuclear envelope disappears and chromosomes line up at equator of cell

E

**ANAPHASE I**

Chromosomes pull away and move to opposite poles of the cell

F

**TELOPHASE I**

Nuclear envelopes develop around both sets of chromosomes and cell divides into two

**Division II of meiosis**

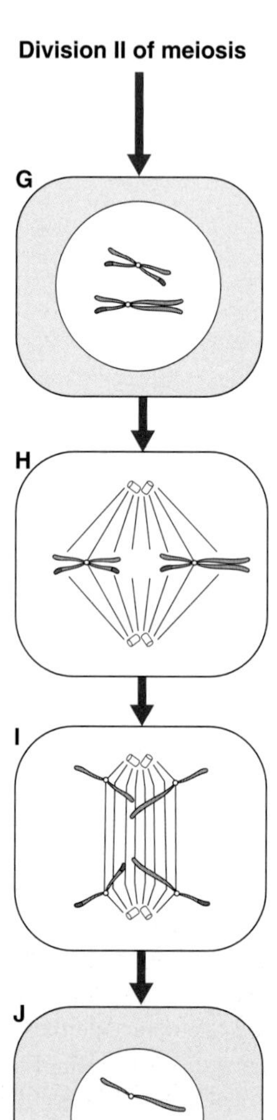


**PROPHASE II**

Beginning of division II (Only one of the two cells of stage F is shown here – the upper one)

**METAPHASE II**

Nuclear envelope breaks down and chromosomes align themselves at the equator

**ANAPHASE II**

Centromeres divide and chromatids separate and move to opposite poles

**TELOPHASE II**

New nuclear envelopes enclose the two sets of chromatids (i.e. chromosomes) and cell divides into two

**Table 7.1** *Examples of chromosome disorders*

| Disorder | Example | Incidence | Outcome | Notes |
|---|---|---|---|---|
| Polyploidy | Triploidy 69 chromosomes (69, XXX, 69, XXY, 69, XYY) | Occurs in 2% of conceptions but early spontaneous abortion is normal | Lethal | Usually arises from fertilization of oocyte by two sperm or from a diploid gamete. 69, XXY is most common Polyploid cells occur normally in the bone marrow and liver as a stage of cell division |
| Trisomy | Trisomy 13 | 1/5000 livebirths | Patau's syndrome | Usually due to non-disjunction of chromosomes or chromatids at anaphase. Trisomy increases with increased maternal age and is sometimes associated with radiation or viral infection. There may be a familial tendency |
| | Trisomy 18 | 1/3000 livebirths | Edward's syndrome | Maternal age effect. Incidence at conception much higher—most affected fetuses abort spontaneously. More female fetuses seem to survive |
| | Trisomy 21 | 1/700 livebirths | Down's syndrome | Incidence at conception is higher. Maternal age effect; the extra chromosome is maternal in 85% cases. The most serious complications are mental handicap and congenital heart problems |
| | 47, XXY | 1/1000 male births | Klinefelter's syndrome | Trisomies involving sex chromosomes usually result in a less serious outcome. Condition is usually diagnosed during investigations for infertility |
| | 47, XYY | 1/1000 male births | | Often asymptomatic, some effects on IQ. Only XX and XY offspring observed |
| Monosomy | Monosomy X | 1/5000 female births, much higher at conception | Turner's syndrome | Due to non-disjunction in either parent; 80% of affected females have maternal X so it is the paternal chromosome that is missing |
| Deletion and ring chromosome | Wolf–Hirschhorm syndrome (partial deletion of short arm of chromosome 4) Cri du chat syndrome (partial deletion of short arm of chromosome 5) | Incidence of deletions and/or duplications is 1/2000 births | Chromosome imbalance of autosomes is usually associated with mental retardation and multiple dysmorphic features | A deletion is the loss of part of chromosome. A ring chromosome is due to deletions in both arms of a chromosome and the fusion of the proximal sticky ends. Microdeletions are deletions that can just be detected by light microscopy |
| Duplication | | | | Duplication is where there are two copies of a segment of chromosome. This is more common and less harmful than deletions |

*continued*

**Table 7.1** *Examples of chromosome disorders – contd*

| Disorder | Example | Incidence | Outcome | Notes |
|---|---|---|---|---|
| Inversion | | | The carriers of balanced inversions and translocations are healthy because the cells have all the genetic material but gamete formation is affected so there is a high rate of miscarriage and malformation | A segment of the chromosome is inverted through 180° between breaks. Usually does not cause clinical problems but unbalanced gamete may result |
| Translocation | Reciprocal | | | Translocations involve transfer of chromosomal material between chromosomes. Two chromosomes are broken and repaired abnormally or there is recombination between non-homologous chromosomes at meiosis. Reciprocal translocations involve transfer of material between two chromosomes |
| | Robertsonian (centric fusion) | | | Robertsonian translocation involves transfer of material, which leaves a large chromosome, and a fragment of a chromosome, which is unable to replicate; most common centric fusion translocations are 13/14 and 14/21. Balanced carriers have 45 chromosomes and are healthy. Gametogenesis is affected |

reason to believe that certain chromosomes are more susceptible to failed disjunction. Those seen are probably those that are compatible with fetal survival, although they may cause congenital abnormalities or affect neonatal survival. Sometimes extra chromosomal material may become attached to a chromosome, making it abnormally long. Rarely a condition called triploidy occurs where the chromosomes of the zygote are in triplicate rather than the normal duplicate complement. This condition is not compatible with embryo survival but is sometimes found in products of a failed conception (early miscarriage) and is associated with a high incidence of hydatidiform mole (see Ch. 6). Imperfect disjunction also causes conditions where the genome is lacking part or a whole chromosome. For example, there is only one X chromosome present in Turner's syndrome (see Ch. 5) and Wolf–Hirschhorm syndrome is caused by loss of chromosomal tissue from chromosomes 4 and 5.

## Autosomes and sex chromosomes

Each gene has a specific location on a specific chromosome, which is referred to as a locus (plural loci). Each chromosome may have 1000–2000 different genes, each with its own location and function. The visualization of the chromosomes from a cell is described as a karyotype (Box 7.4). Of the 23 pairs of chromosomes that constitute the human genome, 22 pairs of chromosomes can be seen in both sexes; these are referred to as the autosomes and contain the autosomal genes. The 23rd pair of chromosomes comprises the sex chromosomes; these are homologous within the female (i.e. XX) but in the male the XY arrangement consists of a pair of non-homologous chromosomes. The sex chromosomes provide the mechanism for the determination of sex and the differentiation into male morphology, which is usually

**Box 7.4**
**Karyotyping**

Karotyping is the method of visualizing the chromosomes in an ordered display of the chromosomes as they appear in the nucleus of a cell during metaphase of mitosis. For a fetal karyotype, a sample of amniotic fluid is removed. The cells are centrifuged to concentrate the fetal cells. The supernatant can also be used diagnostically for biochemical tests such as investigation of enzyme deficiencies, protein defects and gene alterations. Alternatively, cells may be taken from the chorionic villus. A karyotype of adult cells is usually derived from a sample of venous blood, where the anuclear red blood cells are lysed and the washed remaining cells are, therefore, white blood cells containing nuclei.

The fetal cells or white blood cells are grown in cell culture. The time taken for this depends on the number of cells in the original sample. Contamination of the sample can interfere with the success of the method. Colchicine, a chemical poison, is added to the culture medium to prevent spindle formation. Thus mitosis in all cells is halted at the metaphase stage when the chromosomes are maximally contracted and well defined as paired chromatids (therefore they take on the typical X-shaped appearance). The cells, all halted at the same stage, can be separated from the culture medium. Exposure of the cells to hypotonic saline causes the nucleus to swell so the chromosomes are spread out. The cells are then fixed and stained. Visualization of the karyotype is done by computer-aided photographic techniques. The chromosomes are ordered according to size with the homologous autosomes being paired together. The chromosomes of pair number 1 are the longest and those of pair number 22 are the shortest. The position of the centromere is also used to sort the chromosomes into order. Stains that bind preferentially to some areas of the chromosome, producing a distinct pattern of bands, can be used to identify the chromosomes. Karyotypes can be used to identify gross abnormalities such as additional or missing chromosomes and missing or duplicated parts of chromosomes. However, a normal karyotype does not reveal the presence of abnormal genes at specific loci. In order to identify such genes, the chromosomes are stained, which produces a pattern or banding enabling an abnormal gene or a marker gene to be identified. A marker gene is a gene that is often found in close proximity to an abnormal gene; the closer the marker gene to the abnormal gene the higher is the association.

Occasionally, results from karyotyping may be complicated by mosaicism. Mosaicism, a different number of chromosomes in different populations of cells, may occur for instance where the chorionic tissue has a different number of chromosomes to the fetus.

dependent on the inheritance of a Y chromosome (see Ch. 5). As well as sex determination and identity, other genetic traits can be inherited on the sex chromosomes (see below).

### Alleles

Each pair of autosomes is homologous; this means that their gene arrangements, although not necessarily the specific gene at each locus, are identical. So although the genes at a specific locus code for a specific physiological feature these features in themselves may vary. For instance, the genes at a particular locus may code for eye colour—but this could be blue eye colour on the chromosome inherited from one parent and brown eye colour on the chromosome inherited from the other parent. Genes that code for the same physical feature but produce variations in that feature are called alleles.

If the genes are identical alleles, then the structure and coding of the pair are referred to as being homozygous. If the genes are differing alleles then the pair is referred to as being heterozygous. If one copy of a gene is required for a protein to be expressed (i.e. for the feature to be 'visible' in the resultant individual), the gene is described as being dominant. If two copies are required, the gene is described as being recessive. Autosomal traits (genetic instructions carried on the autosomes) can be expressed either as dominant or recessive traits. Simple inheritance of these traits can be predicted diagrammatically (see Figs 7.12 and 7.16).

## Prediction of genetic outcomes

Genetic predictions forecast the chance of an ovum carrying a specific combination of genes being fertilized by a sperm carrying a specific combination of genes. The convention is to show the dominant gene as a capital letter. The genetic potential is described as the genotype; how it is expressed is called the phenotype. Combination diagrams and Punnett squares give the same results, predicting the chance of a particular outcome (Figs 7.12 and 7.13).

The genetic rules that dictate eye colour follow the traditional form of dominant and recessive interaction (see Box 7.5). However, it is important to realize that, like so many other physiological states, expressed characteristics may be the outcome of multifactorial genes where more than one gene is involved. The environment may also influence the expression of genes. For instance, inheriting genes for tall stature does not necessarily mean the child will be tall. In the absence of appropriate nutrition at critical times of growth, the genetic potential may not be realized.

**Box 7.5**

**Selected examples of recessive and dominant traits**

| Autosomal trait | Recessive trait |
|---|---|
| Brown eye colour | Blue or grey eye colour |
| Curly hair | Straight hair |
| Dark brown hair | All other colours |
| Near or far sight | Normal vision |
| Normal skin pigment | Albinism |
| Normal hearing | Deafness |
| Migraine headaches | Normal |
| A or B antigen (A, B, or AB blood group) | No A or B antigen (O blood group) |
| Rhesus antigen (Rh+ blood group) | No Rhesus antigen (Rh– blood group) |

**Fig. 7.12** ***Combination diagram to illustrate the genetic outcomes of crossing a homozygous male with brown eyes (carrying two dominant genes for brown eye colour, BB) and a homozygous female with blue eyes (carrying two recessive genes for blue eye colour, bb). All the offspring will be heterozygous, carrying one recessive gene and one dominant gene. All the children will have the phenotype of brown eye coloration.***

| PARENT | GENOTYPE | PHENOTYPE |
|---|---|---|
| Male | BB | Brown eyes |
| Female | bb | Blue eyes |

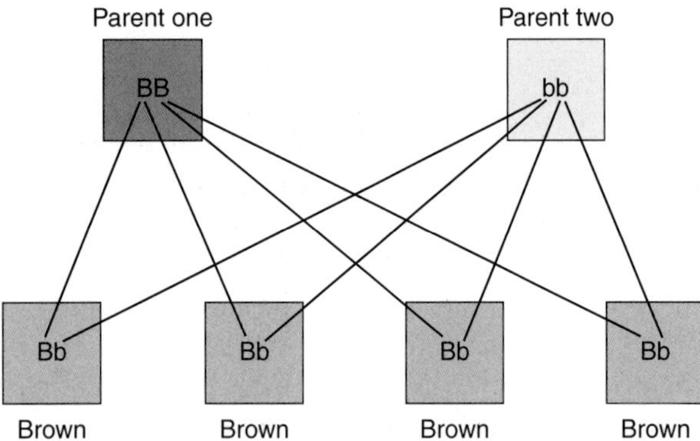


**Fig. 7.13** ***Punnett square.***

| | | Parent one Gametes | |
|---|---|---|---|
| | | **B** | **B** |
| **Parent two** Gametes | **b** | **Bb** | **Bb** |
| | **b** | **Bb** | **Bb** |

# Characteristics of different types of inheritance

## *Autosomal dominant inheritance*

The trait is expressed by a gene on an autosome and is expressed provided that at least one chromosome has the dominant gene. Each person expressing the trait usually has a parent with the trait (Fig. 7.14 shows a pedigree chart for a pattern of autosomal dominant inheritance; the symbols used in these charts are shown in Box 7.6). This means that a particular characteristic or disorder can be traced through several generations if it has little effect on survival. However, a trait occurring in a new generation may be the result of polygamic behaviour (illegitimacy) or a fresh mutation. Autosomal dominant traits also tend to be extremely variable in expression so they may be undetectable and appear to 'skip' a generation. For instance, polydactyly (an extra digit) may be manifest as a tiny pedicle, rather than an extra finger. Autosomal dominant disorders are often caused by defects in structural proteins.

If an affected person mates with an unaffected person, the chances of any child being affected are one in two (i.e. 50%). In the UK, the most common dominantly inherited traits are Huntington's disease and achondroplasia (Table 7.2). Huntington's disease (chorea) is usually not expressed until the third or fourth decade when the person affected is likely to have reproduced. The age at onset seems to depend on the sex of the person receiving the gene.

A complication occurs in the case of achondroplasia (dwarfism). Humans exhibit selective rather than

**Fig. 7.14** *Inheritance of a dominant trait.*

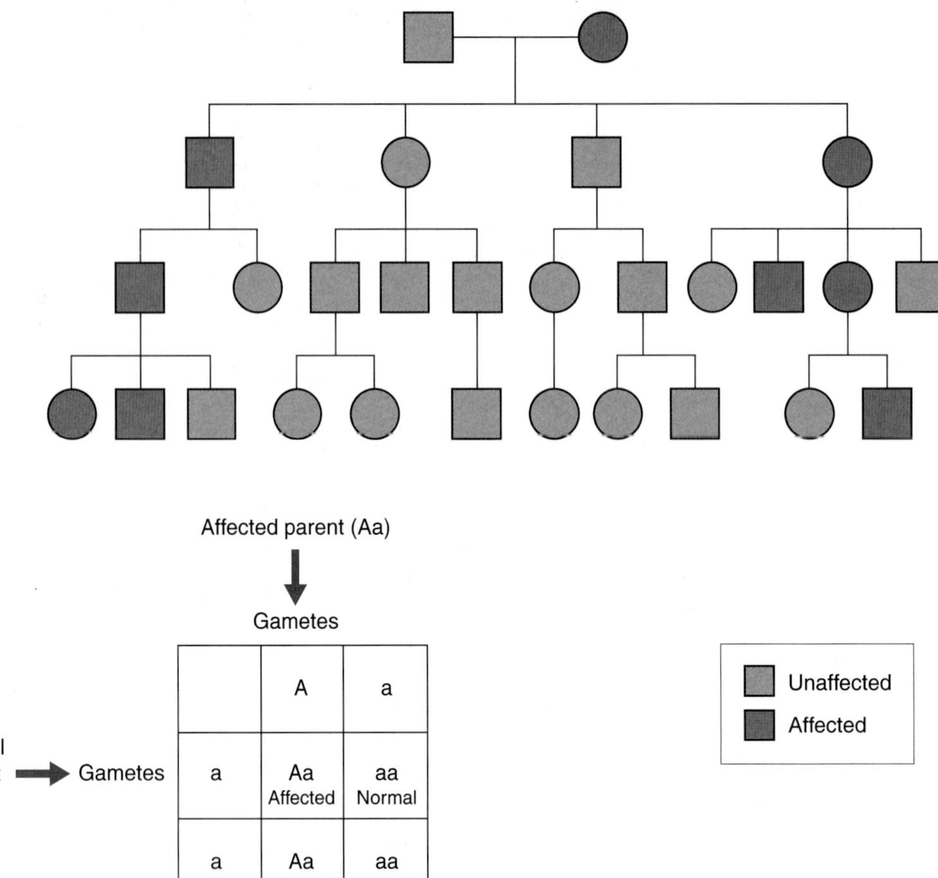


**Table 7.2** *Examples of autosomal dominant diseases*

| Trait | Incidence |
|---|---|
| Familial hypercholesterolaemia | 1/500 births |
| von Willebrand disease | 1/20–30 000 |
| Huntington's disease | 1/18 000 |
| Achondroplasia | 1/26 000 |

**Fig. 7.15** *Inheritance of achondroplasia.*

| | A | a |
|---|---|---|
| A | AA | Aa |
| a | Aa | aa |

Expected outcome might be 25% chance of child with normal height, but AA is lethal lung deformity so observed outcome is 2:1 chance of achondroplasia:normal height.

random mating, often being attracted to partners of similar height, intelligence and other physical attributes. In consequence, individuals with achondroplasia partner each other with a higher frequency than expected by chance. If two people with achondroplasia mate, there is an expected prediction of a one in four chance of a child having normal stature (Fig. 7.15). However, homozygosity (two genes for achondroplasia) results in the fetus having lethal respiratory problems, which are incompatible with survival. Hence the actual ratio of newborn children is one in three. (Arguably, achondroplasia could be viewed as a recessively inherited respiratory condition that confers dwarfism on the heterozygote.)

Box 7.6
Symbols used in pedigree charts

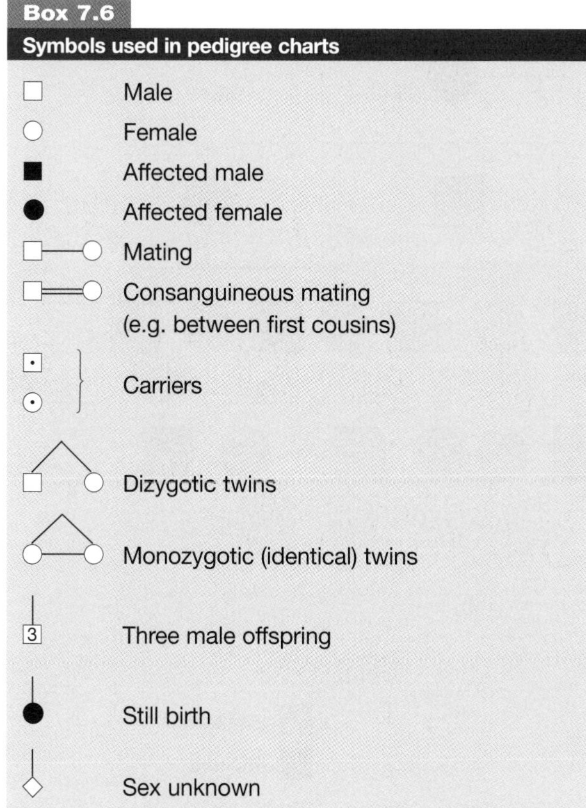

Male
Female
Affected male
Affected female
Mating
Consanguineous mating
(e.g. between first cousins)
Carriers
Dizygotic twins
Monozygotic (identical) twins
3
Three male offspring
Still birth
Sex unknown


## Autosomal recessive inheritance

As with autosomal dominant inheritance, this type of inheritance can affect both sexes equally. However, the recessive trait is expressed only if the gene is present on *both* alleles, which means it has been inherited from both parents. If the parents are heterozygotes, each carrying one recessive gene for the trait and one normal dominant gene, they express the dominant gene and are described as 'carriers' of the recessive gene. In some conditions, the carriers may exhibit mild signs of a disease or have an unusual level of certain biochemical markers that can be measured in genetic testing.

Most inherited enzyme disorders are recessive. Another characteristic of recessive disorders is that they show a variation in birth frequency among different populations (Table 7.3). It is suggested that the reason some recessively inherited disorders reach such a high incidence within a population is because advantages are conferred on the heterozygotes. For example, it is recognized that carriers of the gene for sickle haemoglobin (see Box 7.3), namely HbS or C, have a resistance to malaria falciparum, the most dangerous form of malaria (but not to other types). Obviously, such an advantage will selectively increase the number of people within the population who carry the gene. The incidence of malaria and the inheritance of other forms of altered haemoglobin, such as β-thalassaemia, can be mapped to the same parts of the world.

**Table 7.3** *Examples of recessively inherited diseases*

| Trait | Carrier frequency |
|---|---|
| β-thalassaemia | 1 in 6 Cypriots |
| Cystic fibrosis | 1 in 25 Northern Europeans |
| Phenylketonuria | 1 in 10 000 Europeans |
| Sickle cell anaemia | Varies amongst Mediterranean, Middle Eastern and Afro-Caribbean races |
| Tay–Sachs disease | 1 in 30 Ashkenazi Jews |

In the Caucasian population, the most common autosomal recessive condition is cystic fibrosis. The carrier rate within the population is about one in 25 people. This means that there is a one in 25 chance that any person might be heterozygous for (i.e. carry) the cystic fibrosis gene. The chance, therefore, of two carriers mating is one in 625 (25 × 25) (Fig. 7.16). If two heterozygous parents have children, there is a one in four chance that any child will be affected and a one in two chance that any child will be a carrier of the gene themselves. The livebirth rate of children with cystic fibrosis is about one in 2500 (625 × 4). Because of the relatively high incidence of the disease, parents who already have an affected child or those whose family history has a strong incidence of the disease will be offered genetic counselling. Carriers of the cystic fibrosis gene appear to have resistance to gastrointestinal conditions, tuberculosis and cholera, and to have increased fertility. Cystic fibrosis is a condition which has the potential to be treated by gene therapy (Box 7.7).

Box 7.7
Advances in gene therapy

Recent advances in gene therapy have led to techniques to insert normal genes into cells within which abnormal genes such as the cystic fibrosis gene are expressed. This is achieved by using a modified virus that acts as a vehicle by which the normal gene is carried into and thus incorporated into the genome. The altered virus is unable to replicate and so causes no harm to the recipient. The cells of the nasal passages and lining of the lungs are exposed to the virus in the form of an inhaled spray.

**Fig. 7.16** *Inheritance of cystic fibrosis, a recessive trait.*

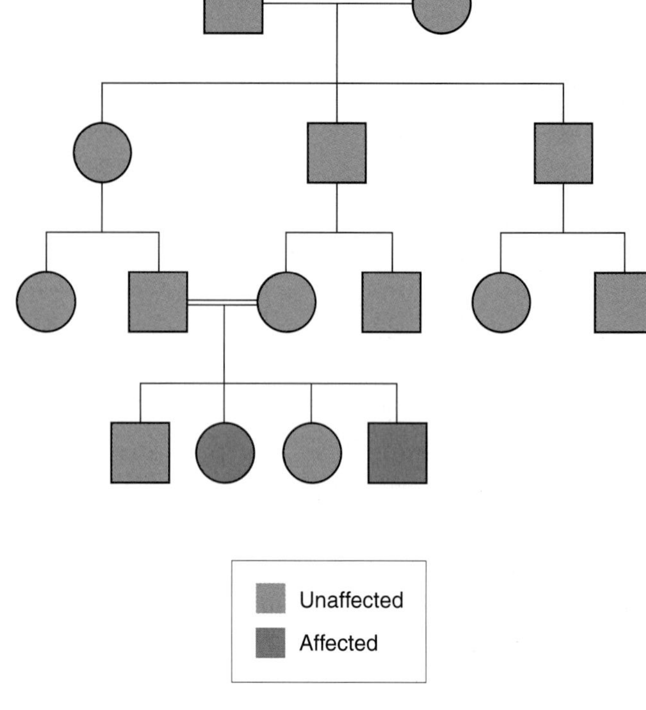

**Cystic fibrosis**

Carrier rate = $\frac{1}{25}$ **(Cc)**

Chance of two parents being carriers = $\frac{1}{25} \times \frac{1}{25} = \frac{1}{625}$

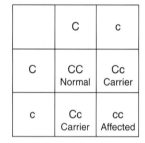

| | C | c |
|---|---|---|
| C | CC Normal | Cc Carrier |
| c | Cc Carrier | cc Affected |

Unaffected
Affected

Live birth rate approximately $\frac{1}{25} \times \frac{1}{25} \times \frac{1}{4} = \frac{1}{2500}$

## *Sex-linked inheritance*

The sex chromosomes not only determine the sex of the embryo but also have other structural genes. Very few genes appear to be carried on the Y chromosomes so sex-linked inheritance usually relates to X-linked inheritance. Most genes carried on the X chromosome are recessive. The effects of a recessive X-linked gene are usually masked in the female by the presence of the paired normal gene upon the other X chromosome. However, should such a woman carry an abnormal gene, she may pass it on to her sons. Males inherit only one of the paired X chromosomes, therefore if they acquire the abnormal gene on the X chromosome the disease will automatically be manifest because the Y chromosome lacks the corresponding allele of the other X chromosome that is found in the female. Also, if a female inherits two abnormal genes, one on each X chromosome, the condition is usually incompatible with life and the embryo is lost at a relatively early stage. X-linked recessive disorders therefore affect many more males than females. Very few sex-linked abnormalities are inherited as dominant traits which affect would both male and female offspring. One example is vitamin D-resistant rickets.

Most sex-linked diseases (Table 7.4) involve a female carrier partnered with a trait-free man (Fig. 7.17). There is a one in two chance that any male offspring will inherit and express the disorder and a one

**Table 7.4** *Examples of sex-linked recessive disorders*

| Trait | UK freq./10 000 males |
|---|---|
| Red–green colour blindness | 800 |
| Haemophilia A (factor VIII) | 2 |
| Haemophilia B (factor IX) | 0.3 |
| Duchenne muscular dystrophy | 3 |
| Fragile X syndrome | 5 |

Fig. 7.17 *Inheritance of a sex-linked trait.*

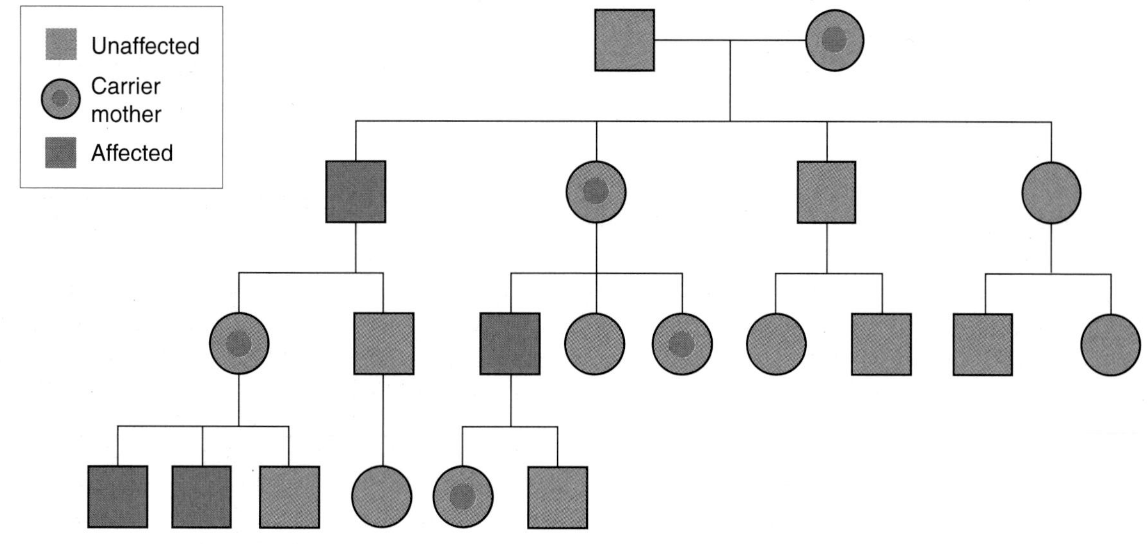


Carrier female ($X^oX$)

| Normal male (XY) | | $X^o$ | X |
|---|---|---|---|
| | X | $X^oX$ Carrier daughter | XX Normal daughter |
| | Y | $X^oY$ Affected son | XY Normal son |

Affected male ($X^oY$)

| Normal female | | $X^o$ | Y |
|---|---|---|---|
| | X | $X^oX$ Carrier daughter | XY |
| | X | $X^oX$ | XY |

in two chance that any female offspring will carry the trait. An affected man cannot pass the disorder to his sons because they will receive a Y chromosome only, but all of his daughters will be carriers of the disease.

The Y chromosome is small and contains very little active genetic coding. However, it does contain the *SRY* (sex-determining region of the Y chromosome) gene, which, when activated, influences the male form to develop (see Ch. 5). The male, however, still requires the presence of a X chromosome as this contains many genes that are vital for normal development to occur.

The female inherits two X chromosomes but evidence suggests that only one of the chromosomes is activated within the cell. On examination of the cell nucleus, one chromosome is always contracted, forming a characteristic Barr body at the outskirts of the nucleus. The number of Barr bodies is one of the tests used in determining the sex of a baby born with ambiguous genitalia. There are examples of mosaic phenotypes where a heterozygous woman has a mix of dominant and recessive expression. For instance, in X-linked ectodermal dysplasia, affected males have smooth skin with no sweat glands. Female carriers may have patches of normal skin interspersed with patches of dysplasic skin. Similarly, females who are heterozygous for ocular albinism may have a mosaic pattern of pigmentation in their irises. There

also seems to be some form of dosage compensation, as the inheritance of two X chromosomes does not result in twice the amount of proteins coded for by genes on the X chromosome. The explanation is that, early in embryonic development, a process called Lyonization occurs in which one of the X chromosomes is permanently inactivated (Box 7.8 and Fig. 7.18).

The three main types of inheritance are summarized in Box 7.9.

**Box 7.8**
**Lyonization**

X-chromosome deactivation or Lyonization (named after Dr Mary Lyon, who first proposed the hypothesis in 1961) occurs at approximately 15 days into the gestation. In humans, the cell mass at around this stage is approximately 5000 cells (Fig. 7.18). Once deactivated, all the daughter cells arising from this point carry the same deactivated chromosome. In some animals, such as marsupials, it is always the paternally derived X chromosome that is deactivated but within mammals it appears that either one of the pair can be deactivated. As the inactivation appears to be a random process, it is possible that the X chromosomes from one parent may be predominantly inactivated so the X chromosomes from the other parent will then be expressed. This could lead to the dominant proportion of expressed X chromosomes carrying a disorder that can be expressed. The deactivated chromosome appears as a sex chromatin body (Barr body) and is identified as it always divides late in mitosis. However, not all the chromosome is totally inactivated: the pseudoautosomal region of the short arm as well as other loci remain active to prevent the manifestation of Turner's syndrome in all normal genotypical women.

**Fig. 7.18** *Lyonization.*

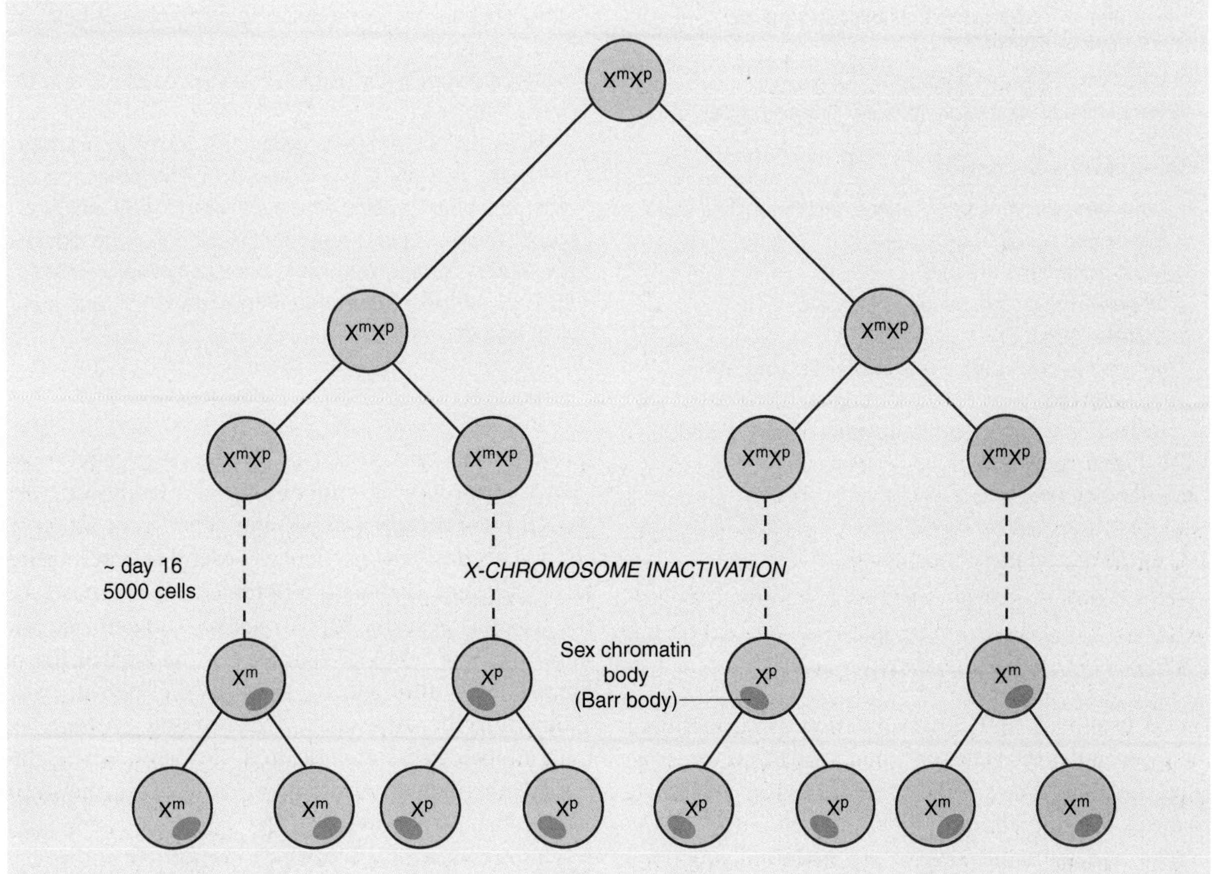

**Box 7.9**

**Characteristics of different types of inheritance**

### Autosomal dominant inheritance

- Effects are manifest in heterozygotes
- Affected person + unaffected person: half of offspring are affected
- Unaffected persons do not transmit condition
- Fresh mutation may produce abnormal genes
- An affected person usually has an affected parent
- Traits are often variably expressed and may not be penetrant (an individual can have the mutant gene but have a normal phenotype)
- Often structural, receptor or carrier proteins are affected and clinical effects tend to be less severe than those due to recessively inherited traits

### Autosomal recessive inheritance

- Effects are manifest in homozygotes
- Affected person receives genes from both parents
- Heterozygote = 'carrier'
- Heterozygote parents:
  - one in four chance that offspring will be affected
  - one in two chance that offspring will be carriers
  - one in four chance that offspring will be unaffected
- Variation in birth frequency
- Recessive traits usually result in enzyme defects

### Sex-linked inheritance

- Sex chromosomes carry genes *and* determine sex
- Sex linked = X linked
- Most conditions are rare
- Genes involved are usually recessive
- Female carrier:
  - one in two chance that male offspring will be affected
  - one in two chance that female offspring will also be carriers
- Affected male:
  - all sons will be normal
  - all daughters will be carriers

**Fig. 7.19** *Inheritance of ABO blood groups*

| PHENOTYPES OF PARENTS | | PHENOTYPES OF OFFSPRING POSSIBLE | IMPOSSIBLE |
|---|---|---|---|
| A | A | A, O | B, AB |
| A | B | A, B, AB, O | none |
| A | AB | A, B, AB | O |
| A | O | A, O | B, AB |
| B | B | B, O | A, AB |
| B | AB | A, B, AB | O |
| B | O | B, O | A, AB |
| AB | AB | A, B, AB | O |
| AB | O | A, B | AB, O |
| O | O | O | A, B, AB |

Antigens A and B are inherited as dominant traits whereas O is inherited as a recessive trait.

**Box 7.10**

**Erythrocyte surface antigens: blood group classifications**

The reason for the evolution of differing blood groups in humans remains a mystery except that at some point during evolutionary history they may have been advantageous to ensure overall survival of the population. Other animals do not have the same number or type of blood groups. The more common human blood cell antigens give rise to the blood groups A, B, AB and O (Table 7.5).

Other surface antigens commonly found in practice are Duffy, Rhesus D, C, E and Kell. The presence of other antigens explains why, even with closely matched blood, recipients can react to the blood of the donor. The Rhesus antigen, which is present in approximately 85% of the population, has implications for fetal survival (see Ch. 10).

## *Other types of inheritance*

Blood groups A and B are inherited as codominant genes, whereas the gene for blood group O is recessive (Fig. 7.19 and Box 7.10). Some disorders are inherited via the mitochondria. The mitochondria of the zygote and subsequent cells are maternally derived from the oocyte (see Ch. 6); therefore no paternal mitochondria are passed on to the next generation. Hence disorders of mitochondrial metabolism are passed from mother to child but never from father to child. This has been particularly useful in determining family lineage, such as the notable case of Anastasia, the Russian princess. DNA analysis showed that the mitochondrial DNA of members of the present Royal Family was different to that of the person who claimed to be Anastasia. Determining patterns of inheritance can be complicated, however, where different inherited disorders apparently cause the same effect, such as blindness.

The presence of 23 pairs of normal chromosomes indicates a normal karyotype (see Box 7.4).

**Table 7.5** *ABO blood groups*

| Blood type | A | B | AB | O |
|---|---|---|---|---|
| Antigen on RBC (agglutinogen) | A | B | A + B | None (universal donor) |
| Antibody in plasma (agglutinin) | b | a | None (universal recipient) | a + b |
| Can donate to | A and AB | B and AB | AB | All |
| Can receive from | A and O | B and O | All | O |
| Distribution in UK (%) | 42 | 9 | 3 | 46 |
| Genotype | AA, AO | BB, BO | AB | OO |
| Phenotype | A | B | AB | O |

RBC = red blood cell.

## Chromosomal abnormalities

Changes within the genetic message, for instance those due to mutation, may involve large parts of the chromosome (Box 7.11). If the changes can be seen by light microscopy, they are termed gross aberrations and can be detected from an examination of the karyotype. Chromosomal abnormalities can be classified as numerical or structural, affecting either the autosomes or the sex chromosomes. These types of abnormality are easier than a single gene abnormality to detect.

### *Numerical abnormalities*

The loss or gain of one or more chromosomes is described as aneuploidy (wrong number) whereas cells with the correct number of chromosomes are euploidic. Aneuploidy is usually due to non-disjunction in the formation of the gametes resulting in a zygote that does not have 46 chromosomes. Monosomy describes the loss of a complete chromosome and trisomy the addition of a single chromosome, as in Down's syndrome (trisomy 21) (see Table 7.1, p. 139). Monosomy and triploidy (an extra complete set of 23 chromosomes) are usually lethal. Abnormal numbers of sex chromosomes have a less serious effect on development; for instance a missing sex chromosome can result in a Turner's syndrome monosomy (45, X0).

**Box 7.11**

**Incidence of chromosomal abnormalities**

- Incidence of major chromosomal abnormality:
  - about 1 in 200 livebirths
  - about 1 in 20 perinatal deaths (stillbirths and early neonatal deaths)
  - about 1 in 2 early spontaneous abortions
- About 1 in 100 births: single-gene (unifactorial) disorder
- About 1 in 50 births: + major congenital abnormality

### Down's syndrome

Down's syndrome is the most common chromosomal anomaly at birth affecting one in 700 livebirths. The conception rate is much higher but it is associated with a high incidence of spontaneous abortion and stillbirth. Either the ovum or the sperm carries the extra chromosome 21. Although non-disjunction is associated with older maternal age, there is evidence to suggest that older men, perhaps because of a lower incidence of coitus, also have an increased rate of non-disjunction in their sperm formation. Affected children have typical stigmata of Down's syndrome (Box 7.12). Their life expectancy tends to be shorter because of an increased susceptibility to infection and congenital heart disease or leukaemia.

Over half of the conceptions with trisomy 21 fail, suggesting that the extra copy of chromosome 21 interferes with intrauterine development. Although males with Down's syndrome are infertile, females with Down's syndrome can reproduce; theoretically half the ova will have an extra copy of chromosome 21 but the effects on uterine development mean the livebirth rate does not correlate with the conception rate. Amniocentesis for cytogenetic screening is offered to all mothers over 35 years of age and the triple test is available to all women regardless of their age (see p. 154). Some women may also be offered ultrasonography screening.

**Box 7.12**

**Down's syndrome: clinical features**

- Slanting palpebral fissure; almond-shaped eyes
- A roundish head and flat facial profile
- Small nose
- Low-set ears
- Simian crease (single palmar crease) in 50% cases
- Folds of redundant skin around neck
- Clinodactyly (inwardly curved little finger) in 50% cases
- Usually mentally retarded with IQ < 50
- Congenital heart malformations occur in 40% of cases
- Prone to presenile dementia in fifth decade

About 4% of babies with Down's syndrome have 46, rather than 47, chromosomes. The extra chromosomal material from a chromosome 21 is attached to another chromosome (Robertsonian translocation—see Table 7.1). Usually, one of the parents is a carrier of Down's syndrome and has the translocation in a balanced form; 45 chromosomes with the extra copy of chromosome 21 attached to another chromosome (Fig. 7.20). This means that the translocation carrier is not directly affected but will produce a proportion of gametes with an unbalanced complement of chromosomes. There is frequently an associated history of recurrent spontaneous abortion due to lethal arrangements of chromosomes in the gametes.

Case study 7.1 looks at concerns related to Down's syndrome.

**Case study 7.1**

Josie is 48 years old and has four children between 14 and 24 years old. She attends the midwife's clinic in a state of shock as her doctor has just informed her she is 8 weeks' pregnant.

- What advice would the midwife need to give to Josie in relation to antenatal screening?

Josie attends her local maternity unit at 12 weeks' gestation for a nuchal translucency scan and is given an estimated risk of a one in six possibility of a Down's syndrome baby.

- What further investigations could be offered to Josie and how can the midwife best support her during this period of investigation?

**Fig. 7.20** *Robertsonian translocation.*

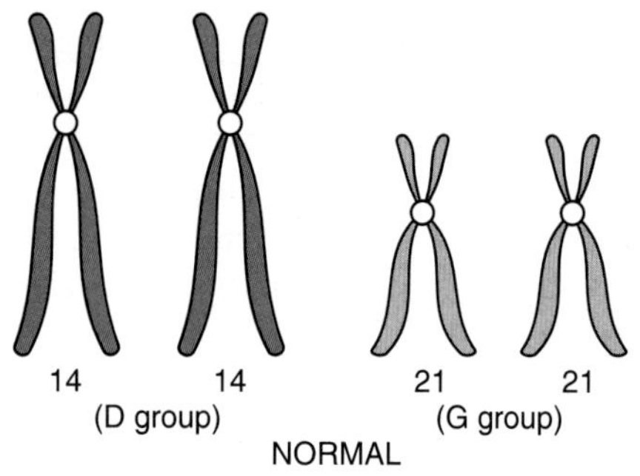


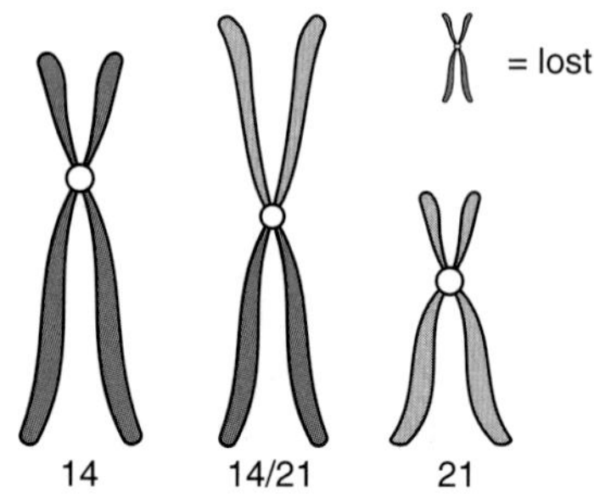


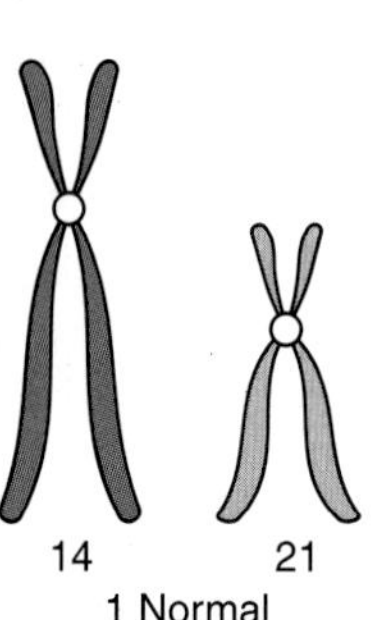


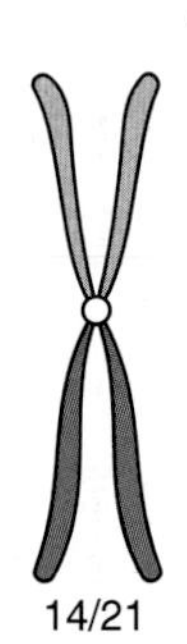


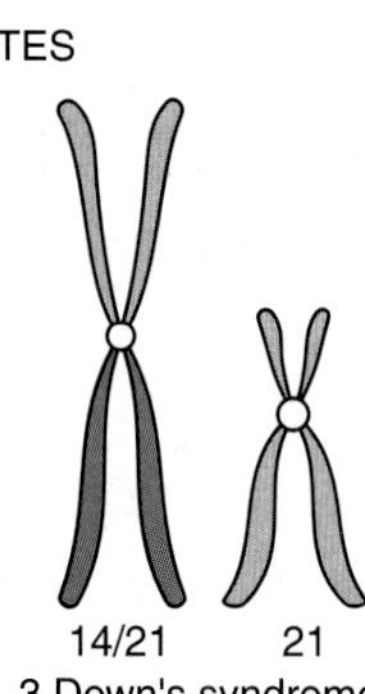


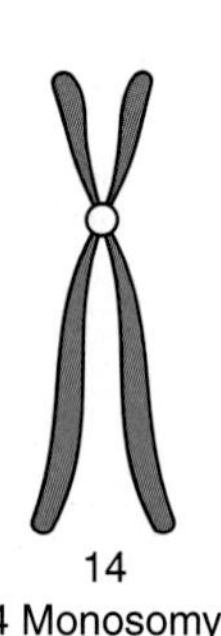

## Structural abnormalities

### Autosomal abnormalities

Structural chromosomal abnormalities include translocations, where material is exchanged between chromosomes, inversions, where a segments of the chromosome is rotated through 180°, and deletions, where segments of chromosomes are lost (Fig. 7.21). Cri du chat syndrome is associated with deletion of the short arm of chromosome 5. Deletions leave the affected chromosomes with fragile sites that adhere to each other, forming ring chromosomes. In inversions, a parent may have the correct amount of chromosomal material and therefore no clinical problem, but the chromosomes align inappropriately in meiosis so gamete formation is affected.

**Fig. 7.21** ***Gross chromosome aberrations: deletions, inversion, duplication, translocation.***

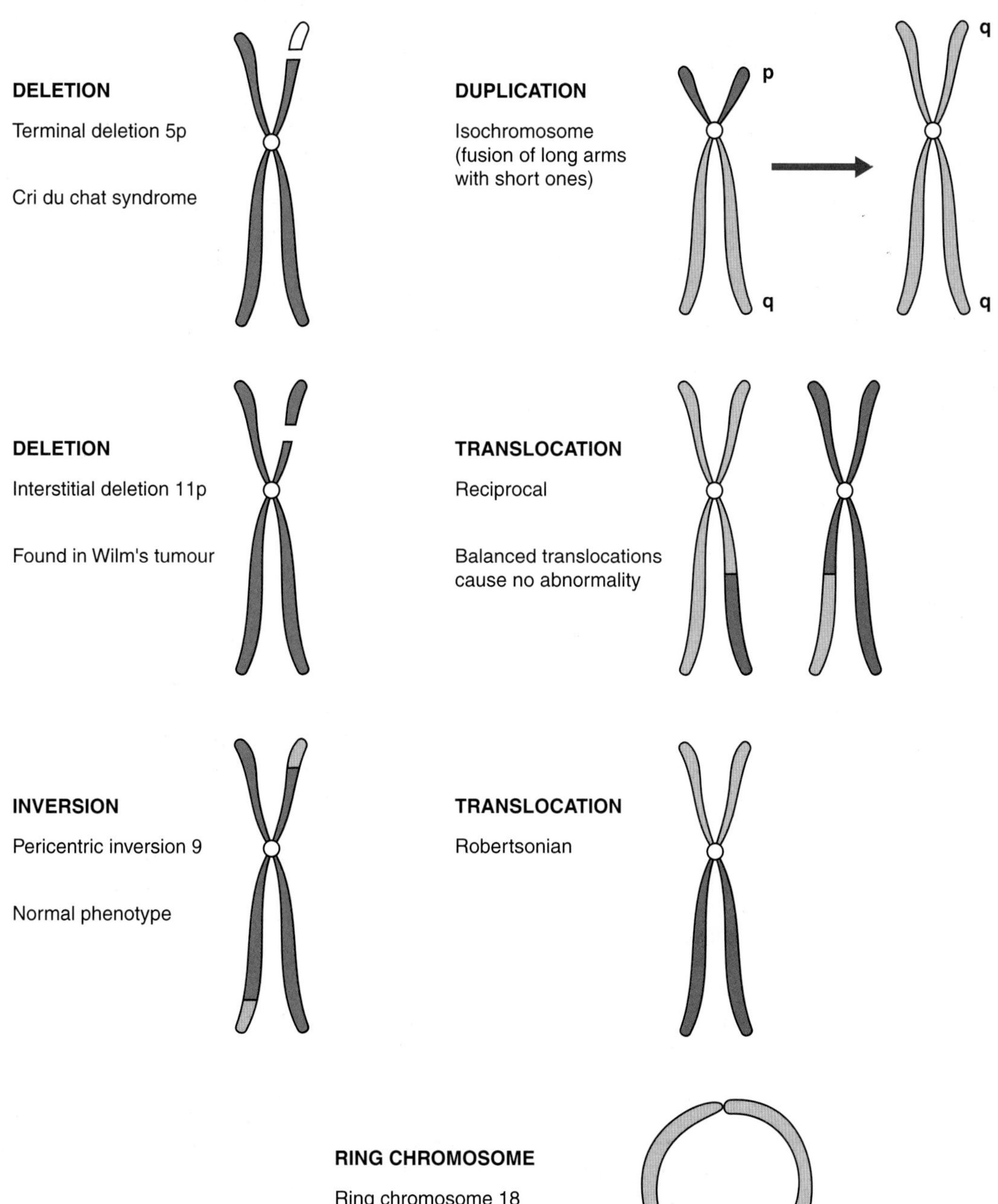

### Sex chromosome abnormalities

Sex chromosome anomalies are relatively common but produce fewer ill effects than autosomal anomalies. Generally, the greater the number of extra sex chromosomes the higher is the degree of mental retardation. Many sex chromosome anomalies affect reproductive performance (see Ch. 5).

An example of an X-chromosome abnormality is fragile X syndrome (Box 7.13).

**Box 7.13**
**Fragile X syndrome**

Fragile X syndrome is one of the commonest causes of mental retardation in males. It is inherited as an X-linked trait, affecting one in 1000 male babies. The fragile site on the X chromosome is on the long arm. Affected males often have a large head, prominent chin and ears and may develop large testes at puberty. A significant proportion of carrier women are mentally retarded.

## Genetic screening

The detection of abnormal genetic conditions such as cystic fibrosis (e.g. Case study 7.2) has been the focus of much ongoing research. There are three particular areas in which genetic investigation can be used to assess risk factors and confirm diagnosis of genetic disorder: parental screening, preimplantation screening and antenatal assessment.

**Case study 7.2**

Tania has a brother who was diagnosed as having cystic fibrosis some years ago. Tania has been identified as being a carrier. Tania presents herself at the midwife's clinic with an unplanned pregnancy at 8 weeks' gestation. Her partner, Paul, has no family history of cystic fibrosis.

- What reassurance and advice can the midwife give to Tania?
- What referrals should the midwife make and how should this be explained to Tania?

### *Parental screening*

Individuals from families with a known prevalent genetic disorder may be tested to confirm whether or not they carry the abnormal gene. The findings form the basis of genetic counselling in which both the risks of passing on the abnormal gene and the possible consequences for a child are discussed. Frequently, this follows the delivery of an affected baby, especially if there is no family history. The condition may have arisen by spontaneous mutation and so the chances of it reoccurring in subsequent pregnancies may be much smaller than if the parents were actually carrying the defective gene.

### *Preimplantation genetic screening*

With the development of in vitro fertilization techniques (see Ch. 6), it has become possible to detect some genetic abnormalities by removing one of the cells from the early cell mass and assessing its genetic content. While this is being done the cell mass is cryopreserved (frozen). If the cell is found to carry an abnormal gene, then the frozen embryo can be discarded; only normal cell masses are implanted into the uterine endometrium. Such an application has been used in an attempt to reduce the incidence of cystic fibrosis.

### *Antenatal assessment*

It is common throughout the UK for the screening for certain genetic disorders to be offered to all women. Currently two types of screening programmes are available: nuchal translucency (ultrasound) and the double/triple/Bart's test.

#### Nuchal translucency (NT)

At around 12 weeks' gestation, the nuchal fat pad at the back of the fetus's neck is measured using ultrasound assessment. NT increases with crown–rump length so the findings combined with maternal age and fetal size (crown–rump length) indicate a higher or lower risk of the fetus having Down's syndrome. The detection rate is about 83%. If the NT is raised, but the karyotype is normal, the fetus may be checked later for other physiological conditions such as cardiac abnormalities.

An increased NT (thicker fat pad) indicates an increased risk of a genetic or physical abnormality being present. Abnormal NT is also associated with other trisomies and fetal abnormalities (Souka et al 1998). It is not clear why such conditions result in a thicker NT but this may be related to oedema due to cardiac conditions, or failure of the neck lymphatic structures to develop at the right time, or both. Each case has to be assessed on an individual basis taking into consideration the maternal age and fetal size, although measurements less than 1.9 mm are probably normal, whereas those greater than 3 mm are probably abnormal.

### The Double/Triple/Bart's test

The risk of Down's syndrome can also be estimated by a combination of blood tests, such as the levels of hCG (which is usually raised in singleton Down's syndrome pregnancies) and alpha fetoprotein (which is usually low in a Down's syndrome pregnancy) at around 16 weeks in combination with maternal age (Table 7.6). These tests have various formats and are often referred to as Double, Triple or Bart's test, etc. Trisomy becomes more common with an increase in maternal age and is linked to an increasing failure of the division of the oocyte to be completed normally. The results from the biochemical indicators are combined with the maternal age risk and compared with normal values, adjusted for gestational age, to establish the likelihood ratio (probability or risk) of the pregnancy being affected.

### Ultrasound

All pregnant women are currently offered an ultrasound scan at approximately 20 weeks' gestation. The scan entails the detailed examination of the gross anatomical structures, such as internal organs, head, limbs and spine. Many physical abnormalities, such as cardiac defects and limb length, are markers which may indicate the presence of a genetic abnormality.

## *Amniocentesis and chorionic villus sampling*

Diagnosis of the above disorders can be confirmed only with more invasive procedures such as chorionic villus sampling (CVS) and amniocentesis (withdrawal of amniotic fluid) (Fig. 7.22). Both of these procedures enable the karyotype of the fetus to be examined, enabling fetal sexing, the identification of a trisomy or the presence of markers indicating the presence of abnormal alleles. Other invasive techniques are fetoscopy and cordiocentesis (fetal blood sampling) and biopsy. These procedures carry a slightly increased risk of procedure-related loss; however, the spontaneous abortion rate is higher in pregnancies with chromosomal abnormalities.

The fetal cells in the amniotic fluid or villus sample are grown in culture to produce enough cells for testing. The time taken for a result depends on the number of cells in the original sample and their growth rate, which can be affected by contamination with blood or maternal cells. The cell sample is greater in CVS so results are usually quicker. Occasionally, results can be complicated by chromosomal mosaicism where an individual has two or more cell lines, each with different chromosome numbers, derived from one zygote. For example, 1% of people with Down's syndrome are mosaics with both trisomic cells and normal cells; the clinical outcome is much better in these cases but if the abnormal cells are in the gonads there may be a high risk of producing abnormal gametes.

**Table 7.6** ***Combination test screening for chromosomal abnormalities***

| Indicator | Source | Rationale | Considerations |
|---|---|---|---|
| Alpha fetoprotein (AFP) | Amniotic fluid<br>Maternal serum (MSAFP—levels about 1000 times less than amniotic fluid) | MSAFP levels are reduced in pregnancies affected by trisomy 21 and other trisomies. AFP leaks from exposed capillaries into amniotic fluid in fetuses with NTD and some other malformations | The results are interpreted using appropriate standards for ethnic background: MSAFP is lower in Asian women and higher in Black women. Levels are reduced in mothers with insulin-dependent diabetes |
| Human chorionic gonadotrophin (hCG) | Maternal serum | Values are higher in trisomy 21 and lower in trisomy 18 | Free β-subunit may be measured |
| Unconjugated oestriol ($E_3$) | Maternal serum | Values are lower in trisomy 21 | |
| Pregnancy-associated plasma protein A (PAPP-A) | Maternal serum | Values are lower in trisomy 21 | PAPP-A increases with gestation. PAPP-A measurement may be used in first-trimester screening |

**Fig. 7.22** *A Amniocentesis; B transvaginal chorionic villus sampling (CVS). (Reproduced with permission from Brooker 1998.)*

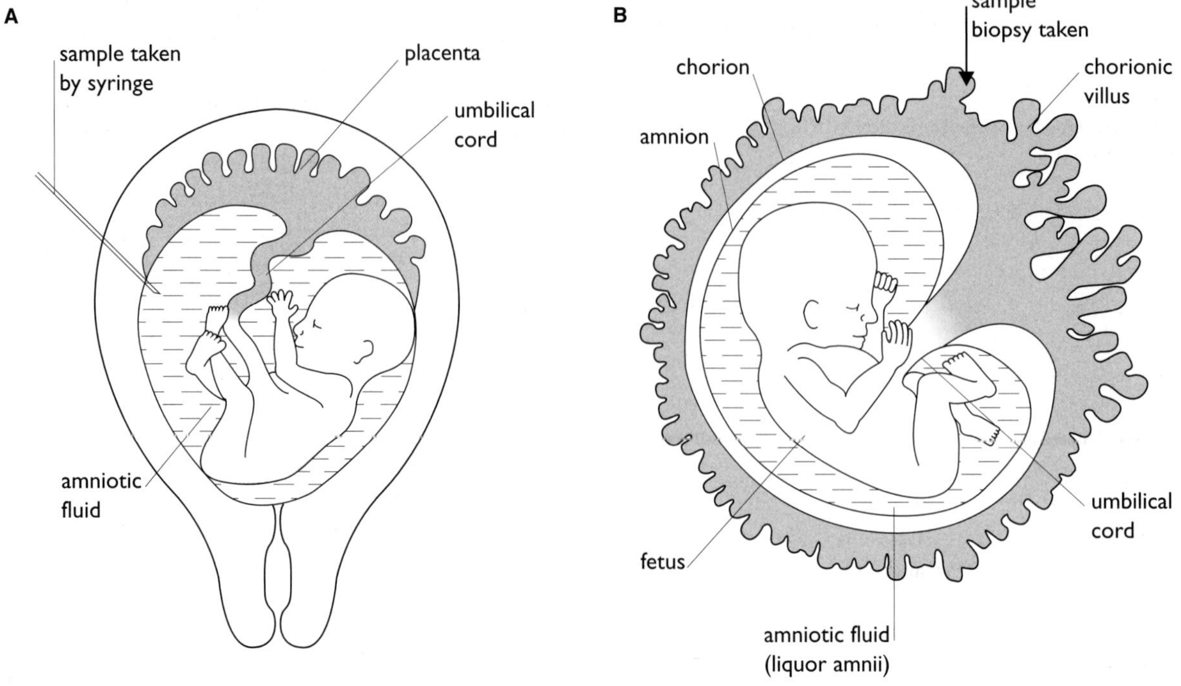


Table 7.7 summarizes the prenatal diagnostic procedures and Box 7.14 describes the techniques for molecular detection of abnormal genes.

# Evolution

Evolution is the study of genetic variation within populations and how this variation allows populations to evolve in response to changes within the environment in which they live. The variation of genes within a defined population is referred to as the gene pool. The work of Charles Darwin, illustrated by his book 'On the origin of the species by means of natural selection' (1859), was one of the earlier explorations of the theories of evolution.

As described earlier in this chapter, many disease processes have their aetiology in the physical expres-

**Table 7.7** *Prenatal diagnostic procedures*

| Procedure | Gestation at which test is performed (weeks) | Conditions screened for or diagnosed |
|---|---|---|
| *Non-invasive techniques* | | |
| NT measurement by ultrasound scan | 12 | Screen for trisomic conditions and other abnormalities |
| AFP test | 16 | Screen for neural tube defects |
| Triple/double/Bart's test | 16 | Screen for Down's syndrome |
| Ultrasound scan | 20 | Diagnosis of gross physical defects |
| *Invasive techniques* | | |
| CVS | 10–12 | Diagnosis of chromosomal abnormality |
| Amniocentesis | 16 | Diagnosis of chromosomal abnormality |
| Fetoscopy | | Diagnosis of chromosomal abnormality |
| Cordocentesis (removal of fetal blood from the umbilical cord) | | Diagnosis of metabolic disorders<br>Assessment of antibody status in haemolytic disease<br>Detection of fetal infection |
| Organ biopsy (liver, skin, etc.) | | Metabolic disorders<br>Hereditary disorders |

**Box 7.14**

**Molecular detection of abnormal genes**

Molecular genetics studies human variations and mutations at the level of the gene and is important for understanding and identifying genetic diseases. Application of molecular genetic methods allows DNA diagnosis from very small amounts of tissue.

**Fluorescent in situ hybridization (FISH)**

This involves the use of a genetic probe, which attaches to the target gene that it is designed to detect. The probe has a fluorescent label and so the abnormal gene can be visualized. FISH is used to identify microdeletions, aneuploidy and translocations.

**Polymerase chain reaction (PCR)**

A small fragment of DNA is selectively amplified (at least a million times) by enzymatic procedures to produce large quantities of the relevant restriction fragments. These fragments can then be visualized by electrophoresis through an agarose gel, which is stained with a fluorescent dye. PCR is used to identify fragile X syndrome, Huntington's disease and muscular dystrophy.

sion (phenotype) of an abnormal gene (genotype). They are normally recessive, so the effects of the abnormal gene are masked by the presence of a normal gene. The physical effects of recessive genes are only seen when there are two recessive genes present in the genome, for instance, in cystic fibrosis (see also in Case study 7.3, which looks at the Rhesus-negative blood type). Some abnormal genes may be partially expressed or modified by the presence of a normal gene. Many heterozygous, partially expressed genetic conditions may, in the right environment, impart a beneficial effect on the individual. An example is the sickle cell trait, HbA/HbS or HbA/HbC (see Box 7.3, p. 136). If one recessive gene is present the anaemia condition is expressed in a minor form. Whilst this can cause problems for individuals in periods of stress and physiological change, such as pregnancy, the symptoms are usually not life threatening; on the contrary, in the malaria zones of the world the sickle cell trait is beneficial to heterozygotes as it affords some protection from the malaria parasite. This is because entry of the parasite into the red blood cell causes the cell to die before the parasite has time to reproduce. In the major form of the disease when the individual inherits two abnormal genes, one from each parent, the haemoglobin configuration is abnormal. The erythrocytes are sickle shaped and fragile which leads to severe complications of blood cell lysis and coagulation. Hence, although the homozygous form has implications for the survival of the affected individual, the abnormal gene is maintained within the gene pool because its partial form confers advantage in the gene pool of the population by increasing resistance to malaria falciparum. The absence of the Duffy surface antigen, which is usually present on the erythrocyte cell membrane, also affords protection against malaria as the malarial parasite attaches itself to this particular antigen to enable it to enter the cell.

**Case study 7.3**

Jane is a 30-year-old woman expecting her second baby. Her first baby was born 3 years ago in rural Africa. She has now returned to this country at 36 weeks' gestation. The blood group results from her first antenatal visit show that Jane's blood group type is O, Rhesus negative.

- What are the implications of this?
- If it is known that her partner has the same blood group, what are the risks of the pregnancy being affected?
- If Jane's first baby was Rhesus positive, what risk is there to the current fetus and how does it depend on its own blood group?
- If a baby is affected by haemolytic disease of the newborn, what clinical symptoms are likely to be evident and how can they be treated?
- If the first baby had been born in England, how would Jane have been treated?

The environment is ever changing and so the process of evolution as a result continues to facilitate adaptation to such changes. The process of evolution itself may then complicate our own understanding of human physiological processes. More than one regulatory system may develop at different times within our evolutionary progression. Different prevailing environmental conditions would thus influence the evolution of changes within the regulation mechanisms to match the change within the environment. Human physiological processes can be described as being in two evolutionary states that are either progressing or declining. Our reproductive physiology may still be influenced by processes that evolved to cope with the Pleistocene environment, in which it is believed that the genus *Homo* first evolved, even though these may now be in a state of evolutionary decline. In contrast, it is believed that our physiological processes may be responding to 'younger' evolutionary influences and therefore be in a state of evolutionary progression.

Depending on the external (exogenous) and internal (endogenous) conditions present the response to either of these evolutionary types may still be initiated.

## Key points

- Genetics is a reductionist science that uses mathematical probability to predict the risk of inheriting certain characteristics, usually of medical relevance. Techniques such as combination diagrams and Punnett squares can be used to predict the probability of inheriting single-gene traits.
- DNA is the 'blueprint' of the organism, which is organized into chromosomes within the cell nuclei. A gene is a unit of a chromosome, or length of DNA, that codes for a particular instruction. Humans have 23 pairs of chromosomes: 22 pairs of autosomes and a pair of sex chromosomes—XX in females and XY in males.
- The structure of DNA facilitates its semiconservative replication prior to cell division, thus each cell of an organism has the same DNA.
- Mitosis is normal cell division producing daughter diploid cells with 23 pairs (i.e. 46) of chromosomes. Meiosis is a specific cell division in gamete formation that results in the number of chromosomes being reduced to 23 (the haploid number).
- DNA controls protein synthesis by acting as a template for the formation of mRNA (transcription); mRNA induces protein synthesis by directing the incorporation of amino acids into the protein (translation).
- There are accumulated errors in replicating DNA, which may manifest as mutations causing proteins with abnormal structure and function to be formed.
- A trait that is dominantly inherited is expressed if the individual has at least one copy of the gene, whereas a recessively inherited trait is expressed only if the individual inherits the gene from both parents. Sex-linked traits affect males more than females, who may be carriers.
- Chromosomal abnormalities may be numerical or structural and have serious clinical implications for those affected.
- Detection of fetal abnormalities is a routine part of antenatal care, which has developed screening programmes to assess risk and tests to confirm diagnosis.

### Application to practice

The focus of screening the fetus is based upon the detection of the abnormal. In many situations, this is explained by a genetic cause or dysfunction. Knowledge of this is essential for the midwife to be able to understand and explain what the tests actually involve and indicate.

It is important to realize that the genetic diversity of a population drives the process of evolution and adaptation to changes in the external environment.

Many genes are labelled as abnormal but they may be essential variants that may at least contribute to the survival of the population as a whole.

## Annotated further reading

Connor J M, Ferguson-Smith M A 1997 Essential medical genetics, 5th edn. Blackwell, Oxford

*A well-written text that introduces the basic principles and clinical applications of genetics with a focus on the molecular mechanisms involved in genetic disorders and diseases. Also covers the genetics of common diseases and cancer, prenatal screening and gene therapy.*

Kingston H M 1997 ABC of clinical genetics, 2nd edn (revised). BMJ, London

*A slim, well-illustrated volume targeted at clinicians which describes genetic mechanisms, diseases and diagnosis.*

Mueller R F, Young I D 1998 Emery's elements of medical genetics, 10th edn. Churchill Livingstone, New York

*A comprehensive textbook which is divided into three parts. Section A focuses on genetic principles, risk prediction and factors influencing inheritance. Section B covers medical aspects of genetics including genetic diseases and genetic factors in diseases. Section C deals with clinical applications including genetic counselling, ethical issues, screening and diagnosis.*

Riccardi V M 1997 The genetic approach to human disease. Oxford University Press, Oxford

*A clear and concise book which covers a variety of issues surrounding clinical genetics, including the ethical and moral aspects.*

Russell P J 1998 Genetics, 5th edn. Harper Collins, New York

*A weighty but clearly presented and well-organized genetics textbook covering fundamentals of genetics using a problem-solving approach. Includes experimental data, problems and worked examples.*

Suzuki D, Knudtson P 1990 Genethics: the clash between new genetics and human values. Harvard University Press, Boston

*A good review of the development of genetic engineering and gene manipulation with a balanced discussion of ethical issues.*

## References

Brooker C G 1998 Human structure and function, 2nd edn. C V Mosby, St Louis, pp 8, 20, 514

Darwin C 1859 On the origin of the species by means of natural selection. John Murray, London

Dawkins R 1989 The selfish gene, 2nd edn. Oxford University Press, Oxford

Dawkins R 1999 The extended phenotype: the long reach of the gene, revised edn. Oxford University Press, Oxford

Goodwin B 1997 Health and development: conception to birth. Open University, Milton Keynes

Jones S 1994 The language of the genes: biology, history and evolutionary future. Flamingo, London

Open University 1987 Inheritance and cell division. Unit 20 in: Science foundation course (S102). Open University, Milton Keynes, p 48

Open University 1988 DNA: molecular aspects of genetics. Unit 24 in: Science foundation course (S102). Open University, Milton Keynes, pp 14, 36

Souka A P, Snijders R J M, Novakov A, Soares W, Nicolaides K H 1998 Defects and syndromes in chromosomally normal fetuses with increased nuchal translucency thickness at 10–14 weeks of gestation. Ultrasound in Obstetrics and Gynecology 11:391–400

# 8 The placenta

## Learning objectives

- To describe the development of the placenta, membranes and umbilical cord.
- To understand the role of the placenta.
- To discuss how abnormal placental development might affect fetal development and the outcome of the pregnancy.
- To describe methods for monitoring placental function.
- To outline the development of the placenta in twin pregnancies.

## Introduction

The development of the placenta is critical for fetal survival because of the importance of the placenta in maternal–fetal transfer. It has a range of functional activities (Table 8.1), including complex synthetic capabilities, which are essential to the development of a normal term baby. The

**Table 8.1** ***Summary of placental functions***

| Function | Placental role |
|---|---|
| Respiration | Maternal oxyhaemoglobin dissociates in the intervillous spaces. $O_2$ diffuses through the walls of the villi where it binds to fetal haemoglobin forming fetal oxyhaemoglobin. Transfer is increased by the higher affinity of fetal haemoglobin for $O_2$ (see Ch. 15). The lower $CO_2$ level facilitates transfer of $CO_2$ in the reverse direction in pregnancy (see Ch. 11) |
| Nutrition | Active transport of glucose, iron and some vitamins and passive transport of other nutrients. The placenta can metabolize proteins, fats and carbohydrates into simple molecules. Fats cross the placenta with less ease and the fat-soluble vitamins (A, D, E and K) cross slowly. The placenta stores glycogen, which can be converted to glucose when required |
| Excretion | Waste products of metabolism, $CO_2$ and heat cross from the fetus to the mother |
| Protection | The placenta acts as a barrier against most bacteria (such as cocci and bacilli). However smaller microorganisms (such as the syphilis bacterium) and viruses (including rubella, varicella-zoster, cytomegalovirus, coxsackie and HIV) can cross the villi. The placenta transfers IgG antibodies (see Ch. 10) and Rhesus antibodies to the fetus. Drugs including teratogens (see Ch. 9), anaesthetics and carbon monoxide (from smoking) can cross the placenta |
| Endocrine role | Initially, the trophoblast produces hCG, which maintains the corpus luteum and its production of steroid hormones. From the 3rd month onwards, oestrogen and progesterone are produced in large quantities by the placenta. hPL is produced from the syncytiotrophoblast. The placenta also produces a broad range of other hormones including corticosteroids, ACTH, TSH, IGFs, prolactin, relaxin, endothelin and prostaglandins |
| Immunological role | The trophoblast has unique immunological properties that render it immunologically inert so a maternal antigenic response does not occur (see Ch. 10) |

placenta flourishes in an immunologically foreign environment and has an important role in the immunological acceptance of the fetal allograft (see Ch. 10). Essentially the placenta acts as a vascular parasite, depending on maternal blood for oxygen and nutrients. The structure of the placenta means that, although optimal diffusion gradients are established, maternal and fetal blood never actually mix.

The placenta and the chorion (outer membrane) are derived from the trophoblast layer of blastocyst cells (see Fig. 6.6, p. 118). Other extraembryonic tissues develop from the inner cell mass. These include the amnion (inner membrane), the yolk sac, the allantois (a largely vestigial structure in humans) and the extraembryonic mesoderm. The umbilical cord and the blood vessels of the placenta are derived from the extraembryonic mesoderm.

The placenta as seen at delivery is just the fetal component. The maternal component is the underlying placental bed and the uteroplacental circulation that vascularizes it. Abnormal placental function is strongly associated with fetal complications but study of the human placenta, particularly the maternal component, is not easy. Placentation in the human is unique, which means that observations from other species can be applied to humans only with caution. Placental reserve needs to exceed fetal requirements (otherwise the fetus could be compromised under conditions of hypoxia). It might be expected that placental size would increase in parallel with increased fetal size; however, the placental:fetal weight ratio actually decreases during gestation (Kingdom et al 1993). Instead, placental efficiency increases by increasing both the number of carrier proteins involved in the transport of substances across the placenta and the placental perfusion.

## Differentiation into cytotrophoblast and syncytiotrophoblast

There are two distinct cell layers in the blastocyst (see Ch. 6): the inner cell mass and the outer sphere of trophoblast cells. It is this outer layer that predominantly develops into placental tissue. The morula enters the uterus about 4 days after fertilization. It may float freely in the uterus before it hatches out of the protective zona pellucida (Kingdom & Sibley 1996). About 7 days after fertilization, the blastocyst hatches and comes into contact with the endometrium. The blastocyst orientates itself so that the embryonic pole implants first; this is the part of the blastocyst where the inner cell mass is located. Uterine contact stimulates the trophoblastic cells to undergo rapid mitosis and proliferate. Signals between the embryo and endometrium also cause endometrial changes, or decidualization, whereby the stromal cells under the endometrial epithelium accumulate lipid and glycogen and become known as decidual cells. The stroma thickens and blood flow increases. Decidualization promotes changes in the endometrium that make it receptive to implantation.

The trophoblast differentiates into two layers: the outer syncytiotrophoblast and the inner cytotrophoblastic layer. Some of the proliferative cells lose their cell membranes and coalesce to form a syncytium (a united mass of fused cellular material): the syncytiotrophoblast. Electron microscopy reveals the syncytiotrophoblast to be a mass of cytoplasm containing remnants of intercellular membrane, dispersed nuclei and a few intermediate cells. This syncytial organization of cells is unusual; other than the trophoblast, multinucleated cells are seen only in some tumour cells and inflammatory giant cells (Chard 1998). Interestingly, a range of tumour cells appear to secrete hCG (Iles & Chard 1991) but at lower concentrations than those characteristic of trophoblast cells.

The inner layer of cells, known as the cytotrophoblast, has large clear discrete cuboidal cells each with a single nucleus and a well-defined cell membrane. These cells have marked mitotic activity and DNA synthesis.

The syncytiotrophoblast increases in volume throughout the second week as cells detach from the proliferating layer of cytotrophoblast and fuse with the mass of syncytiotrophoblast. The syncytiotrophoblast secretes enzymes, which attack the endometrium, and hormones, which sustain the pregnancy. The syncytiotrophoblast is aggressively invasive; between 6 and 9 days' postfertilization the embryo becomes completely implanted into the endometrial stroma. The hydrolytic enzymes produced cause breakdown of the extracellular matrix between the cells of the endometrium thus eroding a pathway. The surface of the syncytiotrophoblast has tiny processes extending from it that penetrate between the endometrial cells, pulling the conceptus into the uterine wall. As implantation progresses, the expanding syncytiotrophoblast gradually envelops and encircles the blastocyst. The endometrial epithelium regenerates over the site of implantation, forming the decidua capsularis (Fig. 8.1). By 9 days, a thick layer of symmetrical syncytiotrophoblast within the endometrial wall encloses the entire blastocyst, apart from a small region at the embryonic pole. Implantation is complete by about 10 days after fertilization. A plug of a cellular material called the coagulation plug or operculum seals the small hole at the point of implantation (Fig. 8.2).

In the first week of development, as the free-floating embryo or conceptus moves towards the uterine cavity, propelled by the cilia movement and muscular contraction of the uterine tube, the cells can obtain nutrients and eliminate waste products by simple diffusion. Diffusion of oxygen and nutrients from the endometrium can continue to nourish the rapidly dividing embryo for only a short time, however. The increasing size of the mass of embryonic cells quickly makes diffusion inefficient and inadequate. Therefore, the uteroplacental circulation develops, providing a system in which the maternal and fetal circulation come into close contact to facilitate transfer of substances from one system to the other.

**Fig. 8.1** ***Regeneration of endometrium over the site of implantation.***

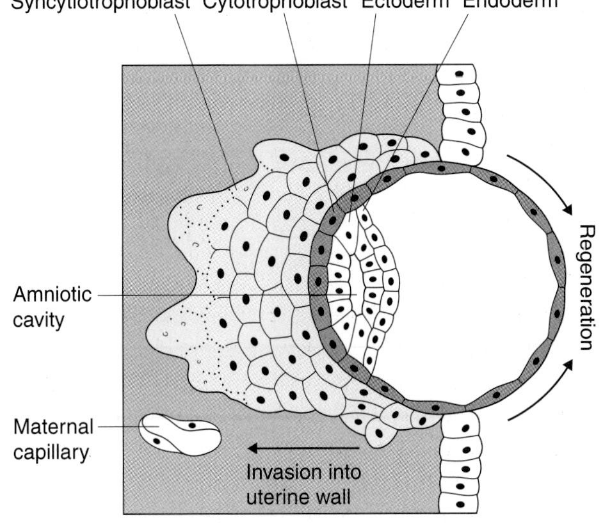


**Fig. 8.2** ***Implantation of blastocyst into the endometrial wall at 9 days postfertilization.***

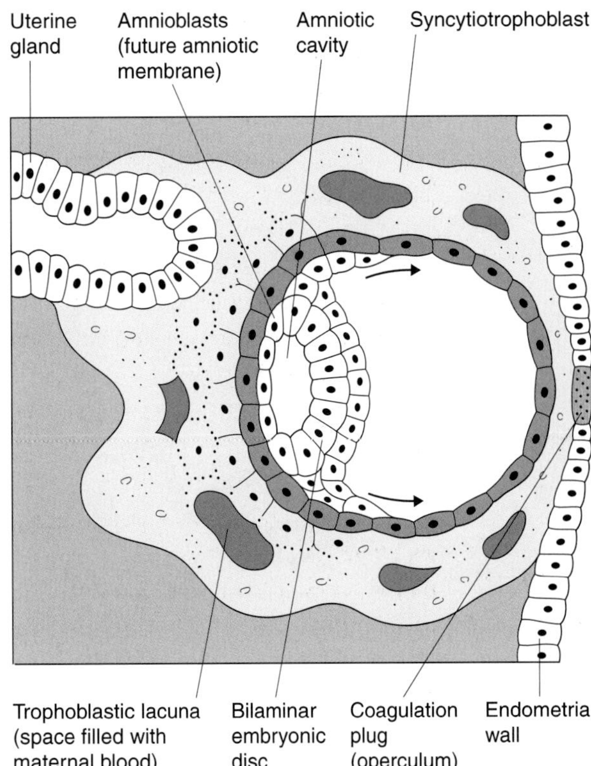


As the syncytiotrophoblast invades the uterine wall, it comes into contact with the maternal endometrial capillaries. Fragments of these are engulfed within the syncytiotrophoblast forming trophoblastic lacunae (literally 'little lakes'), which are the precursors of the intervillous spaces. As maternal blood vessels are progressively invaded, the lacunae fill with maternal blood. Maternal capillaries near the syncytiotrophoblast expand to form maternal sinusoids that rapidly anastomose with the trophoblastic lacunae. As this development continues, the lacunae become separated by columns of syncytiotrophoblast, or trabeculae, which effectively form a framework on which the villous tree develops. The trabecular columns project radially from the blastocyst. The cytotrophoblast at the core of the columns proliferates locally to form extensions, which grow into the columns of

Fig. 8.3 *Formation of extraembryonic mesoderm.*

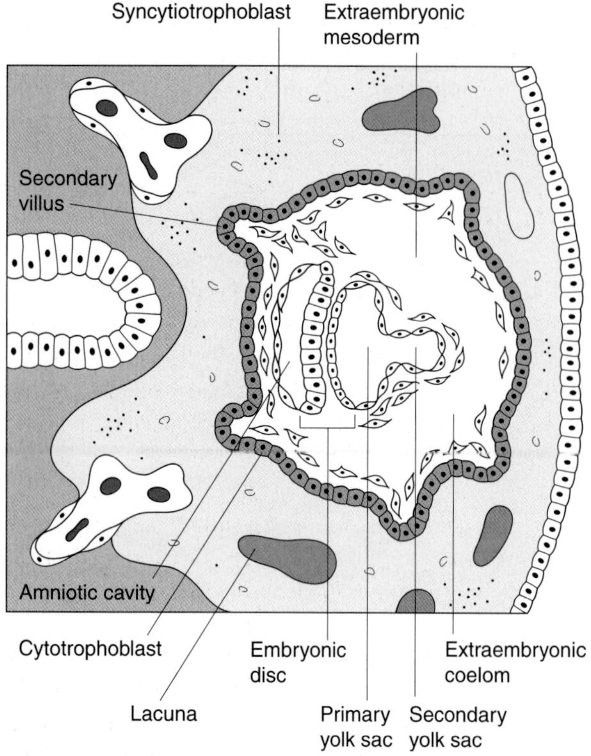


Fig. 8.4 *The stem villus: A primary (11–13 days); B secondary (16 days); C tertiary (21 days).*

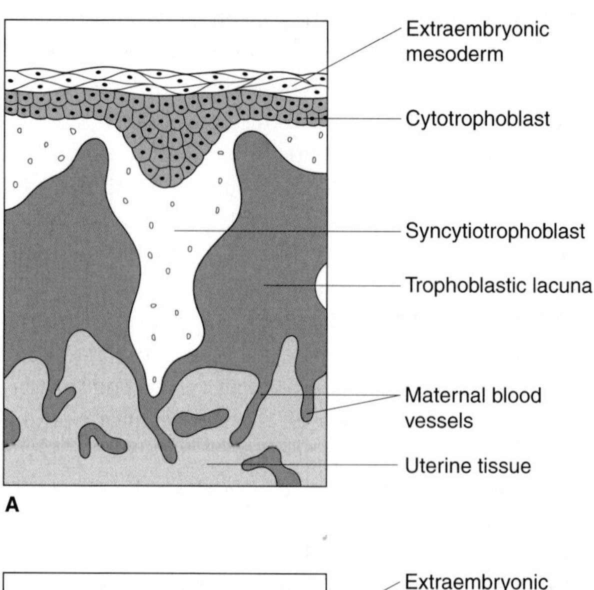


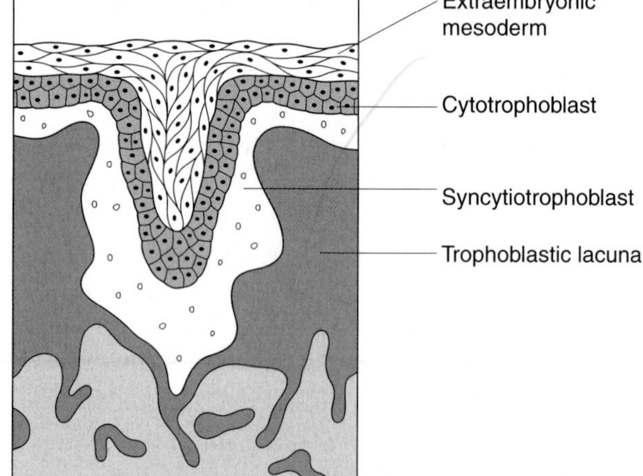


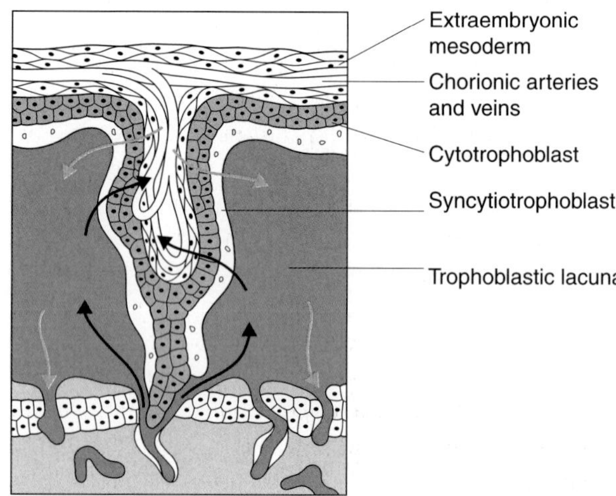


syncytiotrophoblast. The growth of these protrusions is induced by the newly formed extraembryonic mesoderm (Fig. 8.3). The result is the primary stem villus, an outgrowth of cytotrophoblast covered by syncytiotrophoblast, which penetrates into the blood-filled lacunae (Fig. 8.4).

## Extravillous cytotrophoblast and remodelling of the uterine vessels

### *Cytotrophoblast migration and invasion*

Some cytotrophoblast cells migrate beyond the leading edge of syncytiotrophoblast into the stroma, forming the extravillous cytotrophoblast. From about 12 days postfertilization, these cells invade the maternal capillaries and spiral arteries of the decidua. The extravillous cytotrophoblast cells initially block the lumen of the maternal vessels that have been invaded and subsequently replace the endothelium of these vessels. Plugging of the lumen of the invaded maternal blood vessels prevents bleeding and is achieved by day 14, which coincides with the expected date of the next menstrual period. If the maternal vessels are not plugged adequately during implantation and early development then vaginal bleeding may occur, which is associated with an increased risk of spontaneous miscarriage (sometimes haematomas can be seen on ultrasound investigation).

The lacunar spaces enclosed by the syncytiotrophoblast initially contain exudate from maternal vessels rather than blood. The developing placenta forms an effective barrier between the mother and developing embryo that persists up to 10 weeks' gestation when intervillous blood flow is established (Jauniaux et al 1992). It is at this time that peak hCG secretion occurs (Meuris et al 1995). Doppler ultrasound shows there is no intervillous blood flow in normal pregnancies before this period and $O_2$ electrodes have demonstrated that an oxygen gradient exists across the placenta and decidua (Hustin, Schaaps & Lambotte 1988). This means that embryogenesis occurs in a relatively hypoxic environment. In fact, maternal–placental blood flow has been observed in the first trimester in a number of non-viable pregnancies but it is not clear whether this is a cause of the pregnancy failure or an effect (Kingdom & Sibley 1996).

## Placental remodelling

Between the 4th and 16th week of gestation, villus growth and considerable remodelling of the placenta occur, including remarkable changes to the maternal blood vessels underlying the fetal placenta. In the early weeks, some of the cytotrophoblastic cells (described as extravillous cytotrophoblast) move from the tips of the anchoring villi to colonize the decidua and myometrium of the placental bed. It is this invasion of extravillous cytotrophoblast cells into the maternal blood vessels that promotes maternal recognition of the fetus and the subsequent production of blocking antibodies (see Ch. 10), which are important for the survival of the pregnancy. The extravillous cytotrophoblast cells are involved in the destruction of the endothelium of the maternal spiral arteries, which is completed by the end of the first trimester. After an apparent rest phase of a couple of weeks (weeks 14 to 16), there is a resurgence of the endovascular trophoblastic migration. The second wave of cytotrophoblast cells moves down the myometrial segments of the spiral arteries to their origin at the branching from the radial arteries. The syncytiotrophoblast cells are involved with the replacement of the endothelium, destruction of the musculoelastic tissue and a change in the vessel wall vasoresponsiveness. The result is conversion of the thick-walled muscular spiral arteries to dilated sac-like uteroplacental vessels that have low impedance to blood flow (Fig. 8.5). Insufficient remodelling of the spiral arteries is associated with pre-eclampsia (Box 8.1).

The remodelled vessels can passively dilate and accommodate a greatly increased blood flow but they are not responsive to vasoactive agents. The effect of this interaction between the trophoblastic cells and the maternal blood vessels is that a low-pressure, high-conductance vascular system is established, which provides an adequate maternal blood flow to the placenta and thus a plentiful provision of oxygen and nutrients to the fetus. The maternal uteroplacental circulatory system is mostly complete by mid gestation. In contrast, the fetal villous tree continues to branch and develop throughout the pregnancy, ensuring that the capacity of the placenta matches the growth of the fetus.

As the maternal cardiac output increases by about 40% (see Ch. 11), the net effect is to increase the uteroplacental blood flow by about 10-fold to over 500 ml/min (Kingdom & Sibley 1996). Doppler ultrasound can be used to monitor these changes in blood flow. Before pregnancy and in the first trimester, the

**Box 8.1**

**Pre-eclampsia**

One of the theories about the aetiology of pre-eclampsia is that it is due to partial failure of placentation resulting in inadequate blood flow to the placenta and fetus. In normal pregnancies, all spiral arteries in the placental bed are invaded by cytotrophoblast cells. In pre-eclampsia, it seems that only a proportion of the maternal vessels are invaded and that a significant number of vessels show complete absence of physiological changes. The second wave of arterial invasion may be the stage that is most compromised owing to the endovascular trophoblast failing to reach the intramyometrial portion of the vessels. This means that the spiral arteries are not completely transformed to uteroplacental vessels. Maternal uteroplacental blood flow is therefore restricted, which results in placental abnormalities and fetal complications such as IUGR. The effect is compounded by the persistence of vasoresponsiveness of the spiral arteries, which retain the ability to constrict and limit placental perfusion, like the spiral arteries of a non-pregnant uterus.

**Fig. 8.5** ***Conversion of spiral arteries into uteroplacental arteries. The maternal-spiral arteries have thick muscular walls and are responsive to vasoactive substances. They are remodelled by the trophoblastic cells in two waves, ultimately forming non-responsive dilated vessels. Where remodelling is inadequate, a proportion of the vessels retain the structure of preimplantation or partially remodelled vasoresponsive vessels.***



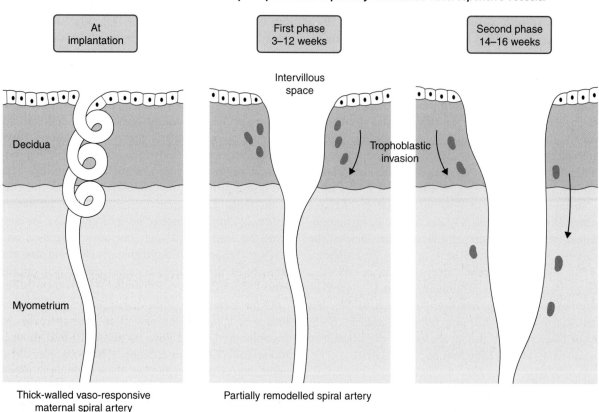

uterine arterial waveform has a low end-diastolic flow velocity and early dichrotic notch during diastole. By 18 to 20 weeks' gestation, successful trophoblastic invasion alters this pattern to one showing a high diastolic flow velocity and loss of the dichrotic notch (Adamson et al 1989). If the dichrotic notch and low end-diastolic velocity persist this indicates that the uterus still has high impedance to blood flow, which is predictive of intrauterine growth retardation (IUGR) and severe pre-eclampsia (Fig. 8.6).

**Fig. 8.6** ***Doppler ultrasound waveforms showing diastolic flow and dichrotic notch. (Reproduced with permission from Miller & Hanretty 1998.)***

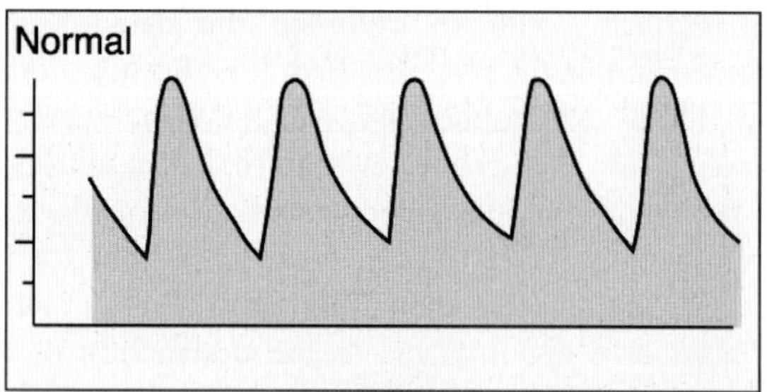


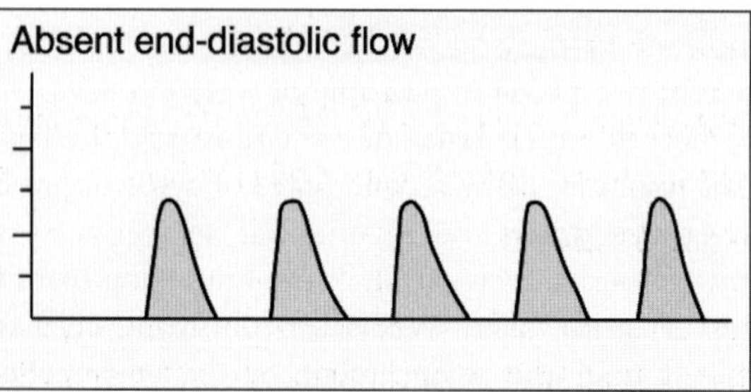


## Vascularization of the placental villi

Fetal blood cells are derived from blood islands in the extraembryonic mesoderm surrounding the yolk sac (see Ch. 9). The blood vessels that perfuse the placenta also develop in this tissue. In the 3rd week postfertilization, the extraembryonic mesoderm associated with the cytotrophoblast penetrates into the core of the

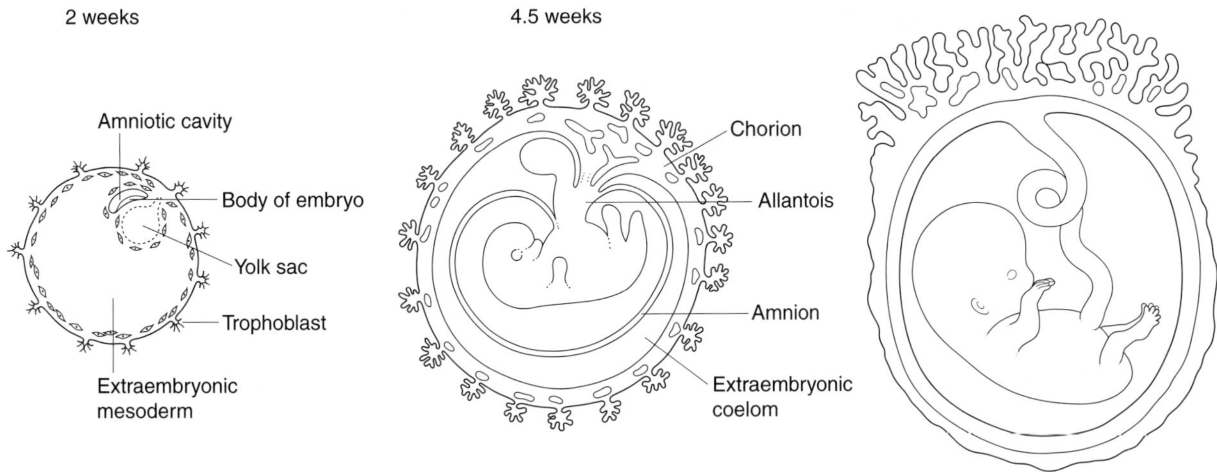


**Fig. 8.7** *Early villus formation occurs in a sphere-like organization around the whole of the enlarging conceptus; eventually most of the villi will degenerate leaving only the ovoid development of the fetal placenta.*

primary stem villi transforming them into secondary stem villi. This mesoderm develops into the blood vessels and connective tissue of the villi. It forms at the same time as the embryonic vasculature with which it will eventually connect. Haemangioblast cells (precursors of blood cells) appear and capillaries form. The linking of the blood vessels of the villi with the vessels of the embryo results in a circulating blood system so the villi begin to be perfused by the fetal circulation at about 28 days after fertilization. The fetal red blood cells containing embryonic haemoglobin allow $O_2$ transfer at low partial pressures of $O_2$ and low pH. The villi containing differentiated blood vessels are described as tertiary stem villi. By the end of the 4th week after fertilization, these villi cover the entire blastocyst surface forming a spherical shell of villi projecting outwards into the maternal tissue (Fig. 8.7). It is possible to remove a sample of the developing placental villi for genetic testing (Box 8.2). The placental barrier now effectively limits diffusion of gases, nutrients and waste materials. There are four layers: the endothelium of the villus capillary, the connective tissue in the villus core, a layer of cytotrophoblast and a layer of syncytiotrophoblast (Fig. 8.8).

**Box 8.2**

**Chorionic villus sampling (CVS)**

In the CVS procedure, 20–40 mg of placental tissue can be obtained from a villus for genetic diagnosis, for instance of trisomy 21 or a single-gene abnormality, such as cystic fibrosis or β-thalassaemia. After 10 weeks' gestation, the tissue can be extracted trans-abdominally by needle aspiration or transcervically using curved biopsy forceps. The collected trophoblast cells, which divide very rapidly, can be cultured for 24 hours and then the chromosome number can be determined (see Ch. 7). Because of the problems associated with mosaicism (see Ch. 7), a more accurate determination of chromosome number and structure is obtained by using fibroblast cells taken from the vascular core of the villus. These cells grow more slowly so they have to be cultured for 2 weeks before being stained and examined (which means the results of the test take longer). As fibroblast cells are derived from the mesoderm, they originate from the inner cell mass and are embryonic rather than the trophoblast-derived cells from the outer layers of the villus. Placental mosaicism is associated with increased fetal loss and IUGR. There is a 1–2% procedure-related loss in CVS, although it should be remembered that the procedure is being performed because there is already a concern about the pregnancy. Pregnancies associated with genetic abnormality have a much higher risk of spontaneous failure.

## Development of the discoid placenta and chorionic membrane

From the 4th week to the 16th week, the villus growth over the entire surface of the blastocyst is remodelled. Most of the villi orientated towards the uterine cavity degenerate and regress, leaving behind an area that develops into the typical placental structure and shape

Fig. 8.8 *Exchange of substances across the placenta occurs across a barrier consisting of four layers of tissue: syncytiotrophoblast, cytotrophoblast, mesoderm and fetal blood vessel wall. (Reproduced with permission from Miller & Hanretty 1998.)*

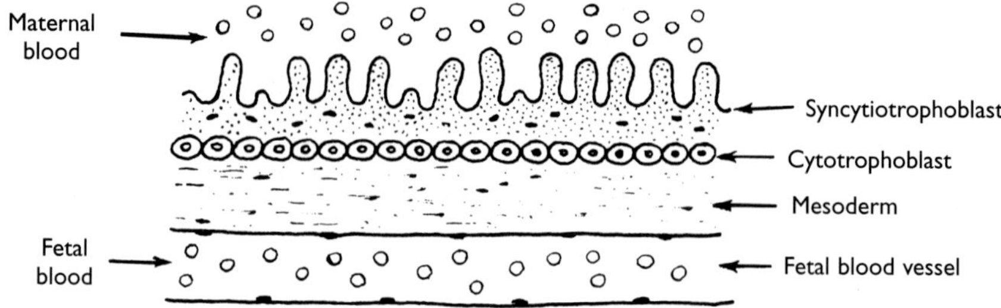


seen at delivery. As the embryo starts to enlarge, the uterine wall where it has implanted starts to protrude into the uterine cavity (Fig. 8.9). The protruding portion of the embryo is covered by the decidua capsularis (DC), a thin layer or capsule of endometrium. The layer of decidua under the embryonic pole of the embryo is the decidua basalis (DB). The remaining areas of the decidua are described as the decidua parietalis (DP).

In the 3rd month, as the fetus enlarges and grows to fill the uterus, the thin rim of decidua capsularis covering the bulge gradually thins and disappears so the chorion comes into contact with the decidua parietalis of the opposite wall of the uterus. Before the tropho-

Fig. 8.9 *Protrusion of the developing conceptus into the uterine cavity and formation of the decidua capsularis.*

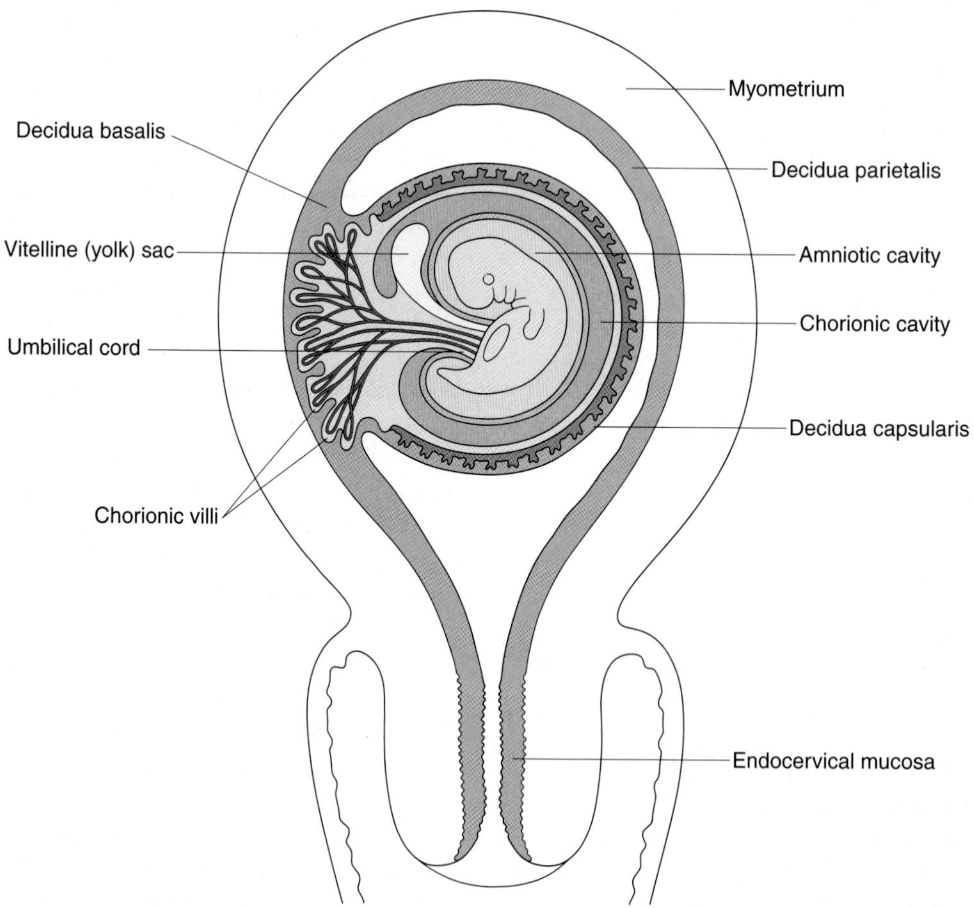

blastic shell comes into contact with the uterine wall on the opposite side, cells of fetal origin can enter the uterine cavity and can be collected by flushing or aspiration from the endocervical canal (Kingdom et al 1995). This is potentially a route of non-invasive prenatal diagnosis, particularly for newer testing procedures that require fewer cells. The size of the chorionic, or embryonic, sac can be used to determine the gestational age of the embryo.

The uterine cavity is obliterated by 12 weeks' gestation. The enlarging blastocyst compresses the trophoblastic layer, distal to the entry pole, and limits nutrient supply and further growth by the villi in this region of the decidua capsularis. The underlying villi slowly degenerate and regress so by the 5th month this region becomes devoid of villi and smoother. This flattened surface forms the chorion laeve, the uteroplacental membrane, which is also known as the chorionic membrane or bald chorion. Effectively the chorion is extraplacental trophoblast with similar immunological properties; it may also be an important source of hCG particularly in early pregnancy. The portion of the trophoblastic tissue associated with the decidua basalis implants further and receives a plentiful supply of nutrients so it continues growing. This area of the chorion, therefore, retains villi that proliferate and progressively arborize forming the chorion frondosum ('frondosus' is Latin for leaf), which ultimately develops into the definitive discoid fetal placenta. The placenta is a union between the chorion frondosum derived from the fertilized ovum and the decidua basalis (basal plate) formed from the maternal uterine wall. It is anatomically complete by the end of the first trimester but continues to grow throughout the pregnancy.

## Development of the amnion (inner membrane)

The amniotic cavity first appears at about day 7. The primitive ectoderm cells enclosing the cavity become flattened forming aminoblasts, cells which become the amniotic membrane. These cells secrete amniotic fluid, thus the embryo is enclosed in the fluid-filled amniotic sac. The outer surface of the amnioblast cell layer becomes covered with mesoderm. As the embryo expands, the amnion comes into contact with the chorion. The chorionic cells are lined with mesoderm cells on the inner side. When the amnion and chorion meet, the two layers of mesoderm loosely fuse.

### *Amniotic fluid*

Amniotic fluid has an important role in protecting the fetus, cushioning it from external impact and stresses. It also allows symmetrical fetal growth and movement, preventing fetal parts from adhering together or to the amnion. Amniotic fluid has bacteriostatic properties and is also important in maintaining a constant body temperature. In the first half of gestation, before skin keratinization takes place, fluid and electrolytes can diffuse freely across the skin (Abramovich 1981). Although the amnioblasts actively secrete amniotic fluid, the composition of the fluid at this time is similar to that of fetal tissue fluid. After 20 weeks, the skin becomes keratinized and transudation from maternal and fetal blood vessels contributes less to the amniotic fluid. Fetal urine and lung secretions are also important. Fetal swallowing and exchange across the amnion mean that turnover of fluid is rapid, particularly close to term. The fetus may swallow 20 ml of fluid per hour; the extra water crosses the gut, enters the fetal circulation and can then cross the placenta. By term, the normal volume of amniotic fluid is 500–1000 ml. Polyhydramnios is an excess amount of fluid (over 2000 ml), which is usually associated with multiple pregnancies or fetal swallowing problems. A deficiency of amniotic fluid (less than 500 ml) is classified as oligohydramnios, a condition often associated with impaired fetal renal function.

Amniotic fluid provides a useful tool to monitor fetal development and well-being. A small amount of amniotic fluid can be removed in amniocentesis for measurement and testing. Amniotic fluid contains many maternal and fetal proteins and fetal cells, which can be used for genetic testing (see Ch. 7). If the fetus has a neural tube defect (see Ch. 9), concentrations of alpha fetoprotein (derived from spinal fluid) in the amniotic fluid are very high. Levels of alpha fetoprotein are low in Down's syndrome (trisomy 21) and are measured as part of the triple test (see Ch. 7). It has been proposed that this could be due to the persistence of extraembryonic coelom or related to interferon receptor levels (Chard 1998).

## Growth and maturation of the placental villi

The placental villi continue to grow for most of the pregnancy. There is a widely held belief that the placenta ages during the pregnancy and that at term it is about to decline into functional senescence. Instead, the continuous morphological changes should perhaps be viewed as an increase in functional efficiency rather than ageing. Placental efficiency is favoured by the attenuated maternal:fetal barrier and reduced diffusion distance rather than by an increase in weight. Although the rate of placental growth does decline in the later part of gestation, this decrease in growth rate is not irreversible or inevitable. If the maternal environment becomes unfavourable, for instance because of maternal anaemia or increased altitude, fresh villus growth will ensue and the placenta will expand its surface area and continue branching past term. In all placentas, total placental DNA levels continue to increase linearly beyond the 40th week of gestation.

Later growth of the placenta (see Fig. 8.4, p. 162) can be divided into three stages. Earlier in pregnancy, the villi proliferate and form new generations of villi. Later on, more lateral branches develop and the layers forming the placental barrier become more refined. In the 9th week, the tertiary stem villi lengthen to form mesenchymal villi. These originate from the trophoblastic sprouts of the syncytiotrophoblast with a similar cross-section to the primary stem villi. By the 16th week, the terminal extensions of the tertiary stem villi reach their maximum length. At this stage, the villi are described as immature intermediate villi. The cells of the cytotrophoblast layer become more dispersed within the villi creating gaps in the cytotrophoblast layer of the villus wall. Near the end of the second trimester, the tertiary stem villi form numerous side-branches and are described as mature intermediate villi. The earliest mature intermediate villi finish forming by about week 32 and then begin to produce small nodule-like secondary branches characteristic of the terminal villi. This is the final structure of the placental villus tree. The terminal villi are not formed by active outgrowth of the syncytiotrophoblast but by coiled and folded villus capillaries that bulge against the villus wall and expand by unfurling. Two types of chorionic villi can be identified: deep villi anchor the placenta to the decidua basalis; shorter villi extend into the intervillous spaces and have a nutritive role.

The blood-filled intervillous space into which the villi project is formed from the trophoblastic lacunae that grow and coalesce. Therefore, the intervillous space is lined on both sides with syncytiotrophoblast. The maternal face of the placenta is the basal plate, which consists of syncytiotrophoblast lining plus a supporting layer of decidua basalis. The fetal side is formed of the layers of chorion of the chorion plate.

The functional unit within the placenta is the placentome, a villus tree arising from the chorionic plate within the intervillous space, which is perfused by a spiral artery. There are about 50–100 such units within the placenta. The villous tree has rami (major branches) and smaller ramuli. The terminal villi have little impedance to flow and therefore an increased fetoplacental flow; they are probably the major sites of nutrient and gaseous exchange in late gestation. The progressive development and branching of the placental tree structure is important for fetal growth and development. For instance, in IUGR pregnancies requiring elective preterm delivery, there are fewer terminal villi, which seem to have an abnormal extravillous cytotrophoblast structure.

The placenta is subdivided into cotyledons by wedge-like placental septa, which appear in the 3rd month. The placental (decidual) septa grow into the intervillous space from the maternal side of the placenta, separating the villi into 15–20 cotyledons. The placental septae do not fuse with the chorionic plate so maternal blood can flow freely from one cotyledon to another. This means that the villi are bathed in a lake of maternal blood which is constantly exchanging; this organization of placental perfusion is described as haemochorial.

## Placental blood flow

The fetal blood reaches the placental blood system via the two umbilical arteries which spiral around the umbilical vein (Fig. 8.10). On reaching the chorion, the vessels usually each supply half of the placenta. The arteries (which are vessels carrying blood away from the fetal heart and therefore carry deoxygenated blood) divide repeatedly to form a branching network of smaller arteries and capillaries running through the intervillous space. The fetal blood flow through the placenta is about 500 ml/min, propelled by the fetal heart. Smooth muscle fibres contracting in the villi may help to pump blood back from the placenta to the fetus.

The maternal blood enters the intervillous space via about 50–100 of the remodelled spiral arteries. There is a pressure gradient from the maternal arteries to the intervillous space to the maternal veins. The blood leaves the intervillous space via the endometrial veins. Most organs have a progressive decrease in arterial

**Fig. 8.10** *The umbilical cord and the circulation through the placenta.*

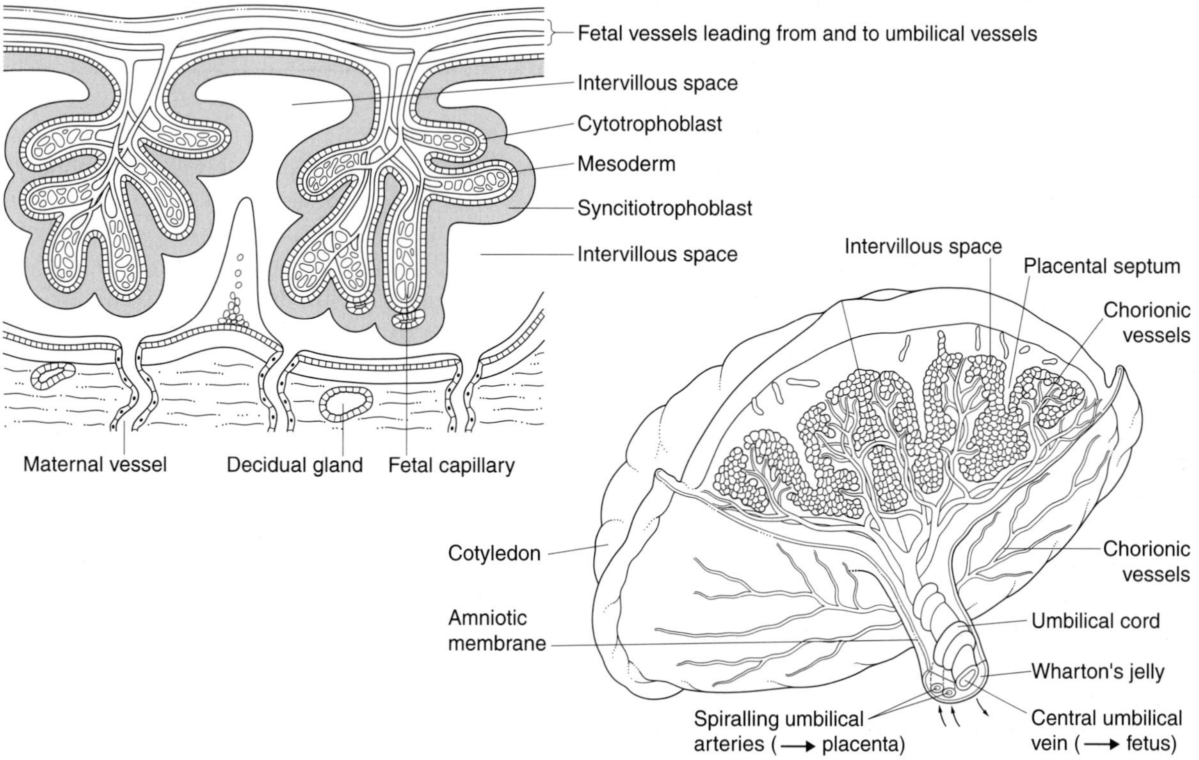

diameter as the blood nears its target tissue. In the uteroplacental vessels, the remodelled spiral arteries increase in diameter as the vessels approach the intervillous space. Therefore, the intervillous space is a low-pressure system; the blood gently flows through and washes over the fetal placental tissue. The placenta has little resistance to maternal blood flow and a high vascular conductance so there is little fall in pressure across the intervillous space. The main determinant of the rate of maternal blood flow is the vascular resistance in the myometrial arteries. Myometrial contractions can decrease or stop afferent blood flow to the intervillous space. This effect is probably due to the compression or occlusion of the veins draining this space. During a contraction, the space distends so the fetus is not totally deprived of oxygen.

## *Intrauterine growth retardation and 'placental insufficiency'*

Fetal hypoxia, IUGR or fetal death are often attributed to 'placental insufficiency'. A proportion of those babies with a low birth weight (less than 2.5 kg) probably failed to achieve their growth potential because placental transfer of oxygen and nutrients was inadequate. However, the fetal placenta is rarely insufficient. Like all essential organs, it has a considerable physiological reserve. It has been estimated that the placenta could lose 30–40% of its villi (and therefore surface area) without affecting its function.

Placental insufficiency really describes inadequate maternal uteroplacental blood flow, which is probably due to incomplete conversion of the spiral arteries during the early stages of pregnancy. Studies using radioisotopes have suggested that the uteroplacental perfusion is greatly reduced because of a failure of the trophoblast invasion into the myometrium and subsequent remodelling of the spiral arteries (Khong et al 1986). These structural studies indicate that there are fewer terminal villi and other placental abnormalities affecting blood vessels and membranes involved in diffusion. It is possible that some small-stem arterioles may be occluded by fetal platelets (Wilcox & Trudinger 1991). Measurement of abnormal oxygen and amino acid levels in the umbilical vein blood suggests a defect in placental transport mechanisms (Cetin et al 1990). However, it is not established whether these changes are causative or adaptive.

Compensatory mechanisms exist in the fetus, which result in redistribution of blood to the fetal brain at the expense of the lower body. This is supported by the finding that amniotic fluid volume is decreased presumably because blood flow to the kidneys is reduced (Kingdom & Sibley 1996). Substances that cause vasoconstriction, such as cocaine and alcohol, are implicated in preterm labour, possibly because they cause a decrease in blood flow to the placenta affecting uterine contractility and sensitivity.

Case study 8.1 details an example of a small baby.

**Case study 8.1**

Polly was diagnosed as carrying a small-for-dates baby. She spontaneously delivered Thomas at 39 weeks, and although he weighed only 2.4 kg, he appeared healthy and vigorous. The midwife noted that the third stage appeared complete but failed to identify that the placenta appeared significantly small.

- Do you think that there is any need to weigh placentae and to compare the placental and birth weights?
- Are there any situations where the weight and condition of the placenta may be used as a possible indicator for disease states in later life?

### Fetoplacental blood flow

Blood leaving the right atrium is diverted into the ductus arteriosus, into the aorta, and down to the lower body (see Ch. 15). At term, about 40–50% of the fetal cardiac output goes to the placenta via the umbilical arteries. Blood flow from the aorta to the umbilical arteries is high because the resistance to flow in these vessels is low compared with the systemic circulation of the lower body. The vessels of the fetoplacental circulation lack autonomic innervation (Reilly & Russell 1977) but a variety of substances can affect the smooth muscle of the stem villous arteries. Of particular importance are paracrine agents, which have a local effect on the fetoplacental circulation. Both prostacyclin and nitric oxide, which have vasodilatory and anticoagulant effects, are produced from the vessel endothelium. It is suggested that flow-mediated release of nitric oxide may have an important role (Learmont, Braude Poston 1994). Diffusion of nitric oxide into the intervillous space affecting maternal uteroplacental vessels may also be important (Myatt et al 1993). The heterogeneous cells of the placental vessel endothelium also produce endothelin-1 (a potent vasoconstrictor), substance P, serotonin, ATP, atrial natriuretic peptide and NPY (Cai et al 1993; Myatt, Brewer & Brockman 1992); whether these substances have a physiological role is yet to be established.

The fetus requires an adequate supply of blood to the placental bed via maternal arteries and normal delivery of fetal blood to a normally vascularized placenta. The fetus does not appear to have a mechanism to increase umbilical flow in response to hypoxia or volume depletion. It has a limited ability to increase cardiac output. Therefore, the fetus adapts to hypoxia or decreased nutrient availability by decreasing oxygen consumption and growth rate. The cardiac output is redistributed to the heart, brain and adrenal glands at the expense of the flow to the body and gut. Hypoxia and acidosis cause cerebral vasodilatation and constriction of the pulmonary and femoral vessels. Blood flow to the liver is high when oxygen and nutrients are plentiful but the hepatic circulation is bypassed if placental exchange is compromised.

It is hypothesized that perfusion of the placental vessels is controlled to match the maternal perfusion of the uteroplacental vessel in a similar way to the perfusion: ventilation matching in the neonatal or adult pulmonary system (see Ch. 1). If an area of the placenta is underperfused by the maternal blood flow, hypoxia ensues. The endothelium of the placental vessels responds by vasoconstricting (by decreasing nitric oxide synthesis and increasing endothelin-1 production) so fetoplacental blood flow is diverted to a better-perfused villous tree.

## Placental exchange

Many substances are transported from the maternal blood in the intervillous space to the fetal blood in the capillaries of the villi and vice versa. By term, most exchange occurs in the terminal villi, which have a high surface area and small diffusion distance—perhaps of only a few microns in some areas. The surface area of the placenta is calculated to be 5 $m^2$ at 28 weeks, increasing to about 11 $m^2$ at term (Carlson 1994). The precise mechanisms of placental transport for many substances are not clear. Diffusion depends on the concentration gradient, the placental permeability and the surface area. Lipophilic substances (soluble in lipid) are soluble in cell membranes so their transport depends on the concentration gradient and the relative rates of maternal and fetal blood flow. Diffusion of hydrophilic substances (soluble in aqueous solutions) is limited by the diffusion distance and the membranes of the placental barrier. The fetal capillary endothelium probably limits transport of large proteins (such as albumin, immunoglobulin G (IgG) and alpha fetoprotein). Transport studies of the syncytiotrophoblast suggest that it is much more permeable than was previously believed and probably offers a route continuous with, and containing, extracellular fluid (Kingdom & Sibley 1996), which allows the diffusion of large proteins. The transfer of substances across the placenta occurs in both directions, to and from the fetus.

There are specific transport proteins on the placental plasma membrane involved in the efficient transfer of metabolically important substances. Some of these proteins form channels and others act as shuttles. Glucose is carried by facilitated diffusion so it is transported in the direction of the existing concentration gradient (from mother to fetus). The transport mechanism can be saturated at high glucose concentrations but in the physiological range it is unsaturated. Some substances, such as certain amino acids and calcium, are transported by active transport against their electrochemical gradients. There are additional mechanisms for the transport of some very large molecules such as receptor-mediated pinocytosis for IgG (see Ch. 10). There is a net flux of water to the fetus, mostly across the placenta.

Steroid hormones cross the placenta but peptide hormones seem to be poorly transferred. Gas transfer occurs by diffusion and is probably limited by blood flow. As well as oxygen and carbon dioxide, the placenta permits diffusion of other gases such as carbon monoxide and inhalation anaesthetics.

## Placental hormone production

Placental hormones have a role in adjusting maternal physiology to provide the optimal environment for fetal development (see Ch. 11); however, roles for all of the placental products have not yet been elucidated. Concentrations of placental protein hormones are higher in the maternal blood than in the fetus because the fetal circulation limits the transfer of large molecules (Firth & Leach 1996). Conversely, levels of steroid hormones are about 10 times higher in the fetal circulation (Chard 1998). Although the levels of placental protein hormone fluctuate randomly, a true circadian rhythm of placental secretion has never been demonstrated (Chard 1998). This includes secretion of hCG, which is not higher in urine specimens collected in the morning (Kent, Kitau & Chard 1991).

The placenta has a broad endocrine capacity and diversity, producing many hormones that other endocrine organs also produce. The syncytiotrophoblast is probably the source of most placental products, although the cytotrophoblast may also produce hCG, hPL, inhibin, relaxin and placental releasing hormones (Chard 1998). The major steroids produced are progesterone and oestrogens (oestriol). The production of oestrogens requires both maternal and fetal precursors, so monitoring maternal oestrogen levels during the pregnancy is a useful indicator of fetal well-being. Cholesterol from maternal low-density lipoprotein (LDL) is mostly used as the precursor for steroid hormone production. Oestriol synthesis requires 16α-hydroxy-dehydroandrosterone sulphate derived from the fetal liver and adrenal gland. Most of the steroid hormones produced enter the mother's circulation, affecting her physiology (see Ch. 11).

### *hCG and steroids*

Initially hCG from the trophoblast rescues the corpus luteum from atresia (see Chs 4 and 6) thus maintaining the production of oestrogen and progesterone. Release of hCG from the trophoblast seems to begin about 7 days after fertilization (Chard 1998). However, levels of hCG and luteal steroid hormones are not directly related in normal pregnancies (Hamilton-Fairley & Johnson 1998). Hormone levels fall following in vitro fertilization despite increasing levels of hCG (Johnson et al 1993a). The relationship between hCG and steroid hormone production is stronger in anembryonic pregnancies (Johnson et al 1993b), where embryonic development has failed, suggesting that the embryo itself takes over the control of steroid hormone production by the corpus luteum. The corpus luteum becomes redundant at about 7 weeks after fertilization when steroid hormone production is taken over by the placenta. The change in site of production is described as the luteoplacental shift (Csapo & Pulkkinen 1978). Inadequate hormone production by the corpus luteum early in pregnancy before this shift, or insufficient placental development, is thought to be responsible for early miscarriages.

Human chorionic gonadotrophin can be detected in maternal blood about 10 days' postfertilization once implantation has occurred and secretions from the trophoblast can enter the maternal vessels. Dissociated α- and β-subunits of hCG, as well as the intact dimer (the complete hCG molecule formed of two subunits), are found (Kingdom & Sibley 1996). The concentration of α-subunits progressively increases throughout the pregnancy reaching maximal levels at about 36 weeks. The concentration of free β-subunits parallels the concentration of intact dimer, reaching a peak about 10 weeks after fertilization, and then declines to a plateau. It is thought that the cytotrophoblast produces α-subunits and the more differentiated syncytiotrophoblast produces both α- and β-subunits (Kingdom & Sibley 1996). Raised levels of β-subunits of hCG are associated with Down's syndrome (Spencer et al 1992). Levels of the hormone are also significantly higher in cases of severe pre-eclampsia (see Box 8.1, p. 163) and IUGR (Wenstrom et al 1994). The role of hCG in maintaining hormone production by the corpus luteum is clearly established. However, the peak of hCG production is reached after the function of the corpus luteum has already started to decline, suggesting other roles for the hormone. hCG levels appear to be associated with fetal testosterone production and so may be involved with male sexual differentiation (see Ch. 5).

### *hPL*

hPL is also a product of the syncytiotrophoblast. Levels of hPL increase during gestation and correlate well with placental mass. hPL affects maternal metabolism, erythropoietin activity, fetal growth, mammary gland development and ovarian function. However, there are reports of women with abnormally low or absent levels of hPL having completely normal pregnancies (Kingdom & Sibley 1996).

## The allantois and yolk sac

The allantois and yolk sac are semivestigial structures that have a more important role in other species, such as birds and reptiles, where the yolk sac is important in nutrition of the maternally isolated eggs and the allantois has a respiratory and excretory role. The allantois forms from a pocket of the hind gut embedded within the umbilical cord, which is incorporated into the developing urinary system. Blood cells develop in the wall of the allantois during weeks 3 to 5 and its blood vessels become the vessels of the umbilical cord. The yolk sac develops on the ventral side of the embryonic disc and is important in nutrition of the embryo whilst the uteroplacental circulation is forming. The primordial germ cells (see Ch. 5) and the blood islands develop in the tissue of the yolk sac. The yolk sac becomes thin and elongated and is incorporated into the umbilical cord and primitive gut. Its role in haematopoiesis is taken over by the liver in the 6th week of development.

## The placenta at term

The mature placenta is an oval/round disc about 18–20 cm across and 2–3 cm thick in the middle, petering out towards the edges. The margins of the placenta are continuous with the fetal membranes. On average, a placenta weighs about a sixth of the weight of the fetus, or 500 g. The amniotic membrane is smooth so the fetal aspect of the placenta appears shiny and grey. The maternal side is grooved and lobed with a dull red coloration, often flecked with blood clots. The chorion retains the ridged appearance owing to the regression of the early villi. The umbilical cord gets progressively longer with the duration of the pregnancy. At term, the umbilical cord is normally between 50 and 60 cm long. If the cord is abnormally short, it can cause bleeding problems. If it is long, it may prolapse through the cervix or entangle with the fetus, possibly forming knots that could impede fetal circulation during delivery, causing potentially fatal anoxia. Most umbilical cords are twisted but true knots occur in about 1% of births (Moore & Persaud 1998). The vessels of the cord, two arteries carrying blood from the fetus and one vein carrying blood to the fetus, are embedded in Wharton's jelly. This jelly is a connective tissue that protects the vessels of the cord. An abnormal number of cord vessels, such as a single umbilical artery, occur in about 1% of births and are associated with an increased frequency of fetal and chromosomal abnormalities, particularly of the cardiovascular system (Benirschke 1994).

## Examination of the placenta

Examination of the placenta, membranes and umbilical cord at delivery is an important responsibility of the attendant midwives. The vessel number in the cord is checked. There are usually two arteries and a vein.

If only two vessels are present, it signifies possible renal problems. Sometimes more vessels are present because the initial pair of veins has failed to fuse. Although an abnormality in the number of vessels is associated with congenital abnormalities, it is not clear whether the wrong number of vessels is a cause or an result of the abnormality.

The cord appearance is also examined. Macrosomic babies of diabetic mothers tend to have thick oedematous cords whereas thin delicate cords are associated with IUGR. The cord can be inserted into the placental bed in different ways. Insertion of the cord is usually central but it can be lateral. Abnormal insertion of the cord can create problems at delivery (Table 8.2). If the cord is ruptured, it indicates that there may have been some fetal blood loss during labour.

The membranes are easier to examine if the placenta is held up by the cord. Usually the two membranes hang down in a neat uniform way. The placenta is continuous with the chorion but the amnion should be able to be separated from the chorion up to the base of the cord. If the membranes are ragged and torn, some parts of the membrane may be retained in the uterus, which can impede uterine involution and staunching of blood loss.

A healthy placenta is normally round and uniform. An excessively large or oedematous placenta is associated with maternal diabetes, hydrops or cardiac abnormalities. The placenta is also examined for abnormal numbers of lobes (Table 8.2) or missing areas of the maternal surface, which could indicate that a lobe has been retained, potentially causing serious postpartum bleeding. Depending on whether

**Table 8.2** *Placental abnormalities*

| Condition | Description and cause |
|---|---|
| Abruptio placentae | Separation of normally situated placenta from site of implantation after 24th week of gestation, but before delivery of the fetus. More common in women with high parity and history of obstetric problems. May cause uterine tenderness and tetany, and variable bleeding. Complications may include disseminated intravascular coagulation (DIC), postpartum haemorrhage (PPH) and shock. It is essential to avoid vaginal examination until placenta previa has been excluded |
| Placenta previa | Abnormally implanted placenta, positioned partially or totally (over the os) in the lower segment, which obstructs normal delivery. More common in multigravidae, particularly those of high parity and with multiple pregnancy. Usually causes painless vaginal bleeding. Factors that cause damage and scarring of the endometrium increase risk. Possibly due to deficient decidua in fundus at implantation. The placenta is likely to be large and may have succenturiate lobes (see below) |
| Abnormal insertion of cord | Vasa previa is a rare condition that may occur with velamentous insertion of cord where some of the umbilical vessels cross the internal os. Velamentous insertion occurs in 1% of singleton pregnancies. The cord is attached to the membranes outside the placental boundary |
| Abnormal conformation of placenta | Placentation may be extrachorial, where the surface area of the chorionic plate is less than the basal (maternal) area. A circumarginate placenta has a flat ring at the transition from placenta to chorion. A circumvallate placenta has a raised rolled ring at the transition and is associated with increased incidence of growth retardation |
| Succenturiate (accessory) lobes | Variations in shape and number of lobes do not normally affect the outcome of the pregnancy. The placenta may have accessory lobes or be completely bi-lobed. This may cause problems in determining whether the placenta has been completely expelled at delivery |
| Hydatidiform mole and choriocarcinoma | Abnormal placental development where the embryo is absent or non-viable. Related to abnormal fertilization and survival of paternal chromosomes only (see Ch. 7). Hydatidiform mole is a non-invasive chorionic development and choriocarcinoma is a malignant tumour derived from trophoblast tissue, possibly from a hydatidiform mole. The villi are not vascularized in either case (as extraembryonic mesoderm is derived from the inner cell mass) |
| Abnormal adherence of chorionic villi | In placenta accreta, the villi adhere to the uterine wall, which has an abnormal decidual layer. In placenta percreta, the villi penetrate right through the myometrium to the perimetrium. The placenta fails to separate properly in the third stage of labour and maternal haemorrhage is likely |

twins are monozygotic or dizygotic, the placenta may be shared or regions fused (Box 8.3).

Case study 8.2 details an example of placental abnormality revealed by inspection.

**Case study 8.2**

Following what appeared to be a normal delivery, the midwife inspected the placenta and membranes. She discovered a hole in the membranes that had blood vessels leading to it, radiating out from the main body of the placenta.

- What do you think the midwife concluded from these findings?
- What care and observation will the woman require?
- How will this be explained to the woman and what information might she require?

**Box 8.3**

**The placenta in multiple pregnancies**

Dizygotic (non-identical) twins and monozygotic (identical) twins resulting from early splitting of the blastocyst prior to implantation can have separate placentas and membranes. However, if the two blastocysts implant in close proximity, the placentas and chorion may fuse. If monozygotic twins arise from division of the inner cell mass, they usually have separate amnions but share the placenta and chorion. The vascular systems within the placenta may remain separate but can fuse. If the vascular systems fuse within the placenta, twin-to-twin transfusion may occur where the twins have an unequal blood supply. This condition, which occurs in 5 20% of monozygotic twins with a shared placenta, can threaten the survival of both twins because the donor twin is anaemic and the recipient twin is polycythaemic and prone to heart failure.

**Key points**

- The placenta derives largely from the trophoblast layer of the embryo, which differentiates into two layers: the cytotrophoblast and the syncytiotrophoblast.
- The cytotrophoblast undergoes rapid mitosis and the syncytiotrophoblast aggressively digests and invades the maternal endometria wall.
- Fragments of maternal blood vessels are engulfed forming lacunae and a framework for villi development.
- Extravillous cytotrophoblast invades the maternal circulation resulting in remodelling of the spiral arteries.
- Extraembryonic mesoderm, originating from the inner cell mass, invades into the core of the villi and establishes the vasculature of the villi.
- The villi continue to grow and remodel throughout the pregnancy; the barrier to diffusion is reduced as fetal requirements increase.
- The placenta has specific transport mechanisms and a range of endocrine activities. It also has an important immunological role.
- Amniotic fluid, produced by the amniotic membrane, cushions and protects the fetus. It is also important in the development of the respiratory system.
- Inadequate maternal uteroplacental blood flow, described as placental insufficiency, is associated with the aetiology of pre-eclampsia and IUGR. Examination of the placenta is important in detecting any abnormality or retention of placental tissue.

**Application to practice**

The placenta has an important physiological role in supporting and maintaining pregnancy. Dysfunctioning of the placenta and its development result in abnormal conditions, which may be observed in pregnancy.

Knowledge of the gross anatomy and the variants in the placental structure is essential in the postnatal examination of the placenta and membranes.

## Annotated further reading

Benirschke K, Kaufmann P 2000 Pathology of the human placenta, 4th edn. Springer, New York

*A comprehensive reference text which covers the structure of the placenta at birth, types of placenta, early development and cellular details.*

Redman C W G, Sargent I L, Starkey P M (ed) 1993 The human placenta. Blackwell, Oxford
*A comprehensive review of the anatomy, physiology, pathology and immunology of the human placenta which links fundamental research to clinical practice.*

## References


Abramovich D R 1981 Interrelation of fetus and amniotic fluid. Obstetrics and Gynecology Annual 10:27–43

Adamson S L, Morrow R J, Bascom P A J, Mo L Y L, Ritchie J W K 1989 Effect of placental resistance, arterial diameter, and blood pressure on the uterine arterial waveform: a computer modeling approach. Ultrasound in Medicine and Biology 15:437–442

Benirschke K 1994 Obstetrically important lesions of the umbilical cord. Journal of Reproductive Medicine 39:226

Cai W Q, Bodin P, Sexton A, Loesch A, Burnstock, G 1993 Localization of neuropeptide Y and atrial natriuretic peptide in the endothelial cells of human umbilical blood vessels. Cell and Tissue Research 272:175–181

Carlson B M 1994 Human embryology and developmental biology. C V Mosby, St Louis

Cetin I, Corbetta C, Sereni L P et al 1990 Umbilical amino acid concentrations in normal and growth-retarded fetuses sampled in utero by cordocentesis. American Journal of Obstetrics and Gynecology 162:253–261

Chard T 1998 Placental metabolism. In: Chamberlain G, Broughton Pipkin F (eds) Clinical physiology in obstetris, 3rd edn. Blackwell, Oxford, pp 419–436

Csapo A I, Pulkkinen M 1978 Indispensability of the human corpus luteum in the maintenance of early pregnancy. Lutectomy evidence. Obstetrical and Gynecological Survey 33:69–81

Firth J A, Leach L 1996 Not trophoblast alone: a review of the contribution to the fetal microvasculature to transplacental exchange. Placenta 17:89

Hamilton-Fairley D, Johnson M R 1998 The ovary. In: Chamberlain G, Broughton Pipkin F (eds) Clinical physiology in obstetrics, 3rd edn. Blackwell, Oxford, pp 396–416

Hustin J, Schaaps J P, Lambotte R 1988 Anatomical studies of the uteroplacental vascularisation in the first trimester of pregnancy. Trophoblast Research 3:49–60

Iles R K, Chard T 1991 Human chorionic gonadotrophin expression by bladder cancers: biology and clinical potential. Journal of Urology 145:453

Jauniaux E, Jurkovic D, Campbell S, Hustin J 1992 Doppler ultrasonographic features of the developing placental circulation: correlation with anatomic findings. American Journal of Obstetrics and Gynecology 166:585

Johnson M R, Bolton V N, Riddle A F et al 1993a Interactions between the embryo and corpus-luteum. Human Reproduction 8: 1496–1501

Johnson M R, Riddle A F, Irvine R et al 1993b Corpus luteum failure in ectopic pregnancy. Human Reproduction 8:1491–1495

Kent A, Kitau M J, Chard T 1991 Absence of diurnal variation in urinary chorionic gonadotrophin excretion at 8–13 weeks gestation. British Journal of Obstetrics and Gynaecology 98:1180

Khong T Y, De Wolf F, Robertson W B, Brosens I 1986 Inadequate maternal vascular response to placentation in pregnancies complicated by pre-eclampsia and by small-for-gestational age infants. British Journal of Obstetrics and Gynaecology 93:1049–1059

Kingdom J, Sibley C 1996 The placenta. In: Hillier S G, Kitchener H C, Neilson J P (eds) Scientific essentials of reproductive medicine. W B Saunders, Philadelphia pp 312–318

Kingdom J C P, Awad H, Fleming J E E, Bowman A W 1993 Obstetrical determination of relative placental size. Placenta 14:A36

Kingdom J C P, Sherlock J, Rodeck C H, Adinolfi M 1995 Detection of trophoblast cells in transcervical samples collected by lavage and cytobrush. Obstetrics and Gynecology 86:283–288

Learmont J G, Braude P R, Poston L 1994 Flow induced dilation is modulated by nitric oxide in isolated human small fetoplacental arteries. Journal of Vascular Research 31 (suppl 1):26

Meuris S, Nagy A M, Delogne-Desnoeck J, Jurkovic D, Jauniaux E 1995 Temporal relationship between the human chorionic gonadotrophin peak and the establishment of the inter-villus blood flow in early pregnancy. Human Reproduction 10:947

Miller A W F, Hanretty K P 1998 Obstetrics illustrated, 5th edn. Churchill Livingstone, New York, pp 12, 99

Moore K L, Persaud T V N 1998 Before we are born: essentials of embryology and birth defects, 5th edn. W B Saunders, Philadelphia

Myatt L, Brewer A S, Brockman D E 1992 The comparative effects of big endothelin-1. endothelin-1, and endothelin-3 in the human fetal-placental circulation. American Journal of Obstetrics and Gynecology 167:1651–1656

Myatt L, Brockman D E, Eis A L W, Pollack J S 1993 Immunohistochemical localisation of nitric oxide synthase in the human placenta. Placenta 14:487–495

Reilly F D, Russell P T 1977 Neurohistochemical evidence supporting an absence of adrenergic and cholinergic innervation in the human placenta and umbilical cord. Anatomical Record 188:277–286

Spencer K, Coombes J, Mallard S A, Ward M A 1992 Free beta human chorionic gonadotrophin in Down's syndrome screening: a multicentre study of its role compared to other biochemical markers. Annals of Clinical Biochemistry 29:506–518

Wenstrom K D, Owen J, Boots L R, DuBard M B 1994 Elevated second trimester human chorionic gonadotropin levels in association with poor pregnancy outcome American Journal of Obstetrics and Gynecology 171:1038–1041

Wilcox G R, Trudinger B J 1991 Fetal platelet consumption: a feature of placental insufficiency. Obstetrics and Gynecology 77:616–621

# 9 Embryo development and fetal growth

## Learning objectives

- To describe the formation of the bilaminar and trilaminar embryonic discs in week 2 and week 3 of development.
- To outline the events involved in folding of the embryonic disc into the characteristic shape of the human embryo.
- To define key embryological terms: gastrulation, neurulation, primitive streak, somites and notochord.
- To outline events in development in the first 8 weeks.
- To describe characteristics of development of the fetal organ systems.
- To discuss factors affecting fetal growth and the implications these have for future health.
- To relate the timing of development with sensitive periods and to appreciate the developmental factors limiting survival of a preterm baby.

## Introduction

During pregnancy, the single cell of the zygote divides to produce six billion cells of the mature fetus. On average, an adult cell is the product of about 47 cell divisions from the zygote, at least 40 of which occur before birth. The first 3 weeks of development are described as the pre-embryonic period when the cells differentiate into germ layers from which all organs and tissues develop. This stage is similar in all sorts of animals, including *Drosophila* (fruit fly), nematodes, amphibians and birds as well as mammals. The embryonic stage lasts from weeks 4 to 8 in the human. During this time the organ systems are established and the embryo develops distinct human characteristics. The fetal stage, from week 9 to birth, is largely a period of growth, during which time the systems become more refined and mature, ready to function at birth. Fetal age is timed from fertilization whereas pregnancy is dated from the first day of the last normal menstrual period. This means that the timing of the pregnancy is 2 weeks more than the true fetal age. The average length of pregnancy is 280 days (40 weeks) when the fetus is 266 days old (38 weeks). Understanding fetal development is important in monitoring the well-being of the fetus. Pregnant women are also obviously interested in knowing how their baby is changing during the duration of the pregnancy. (The 1st week after fertilization is described in Chapter 6.)

## Week 2

By the end of the 1st week, the blastocyst has entered the uterine cavity, hatched out of the zona pellucida and started the process of implantation into the endometrial wall. Two types of cells are evident: the outer trophoblast (see Ch. 6) and the inner cell mass (or embryoblast). The inner cell mass gives rise to tissues of the embryo, and also contributes towards some of the extraembryonic membranes. At this stage, about day 7 after fertilization, the cells of the inner cell mass start to proliferate and differentiate rapidly. The inner cell mass becomes flattened into a bilaminar embryonic disc with the cells forming two distinct layers (Fig. 9.1). The cells adjacent to the blastocyst cavity appear distinctly cuboidal. These form the hypoblast or primary endoderm layer, which gives rise to the future gut and its derivatives. The upper layer of cells is formed of columnar epiblast cells, which will differentiate into the ectodermal layer. Some of the epiblast cells spread laterally to form the amniotic membrane that encloses the amniotic cavity. Cells from the hypoblast layer migrate to line the cytotrophoblast so the blastocyst cavity is also enclosed. This is the cavity that will become the primitive yolk sac. There are two waves of endoderm cell remodelling of the blastocyst cavity, which form the primary yolk sac and then the definitive yolk sac. The formation of the definitive yolk sac creates the chorionic cavity and the extraembryonic mesoderm, which gives rise to the vascular structures of the placenta (see Ch. 8). The bilaminar disc lies between two fluid-filled cavities: the amniotic cavity on the epiblast (ectoderm) side and the yolk sac cavity on the hypoblast (endoderm) side. At the end of the 2nd week, a region of endodermal cells starts to thicken and become columnar, forming the prochordal plate (Fig. 9.2). This marks the cranial region (head end) and is the site of the future mouth. The prochordal plate is also important in influencing further development of the cranial region.

By the 2nd week, according to the 'rule of twos' (Larsen 1993) the following have taken place:

- two germ layers have formed: the endoderm and ectoderm
- two trophoblastic layers have formed: cytotrophoblast and syncytiotrophoblast
- two waves of remodelling have occurred: that of the blastocyst into primary and then the definitive yolk sac
- two novel cavities have formed: the amniotic cavity and chorionic cavity
- two layers formed from the extraembryonic mesoderm.

**Fig. 9.1** ***Differentiation of the inner cell mass into the bilaminar disc: A 7 days; B 8 days; C 9 days. (Reproduced with permission from Fitzgerald & Fitzgerald 1994.)***

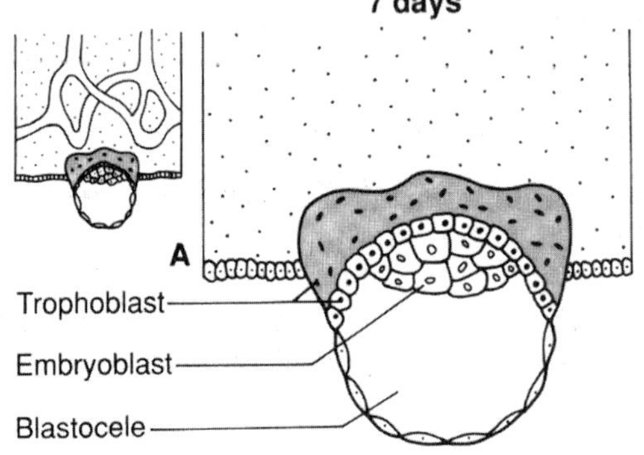


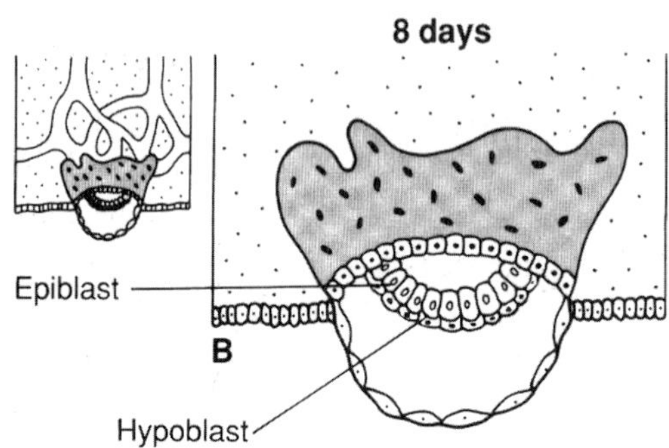


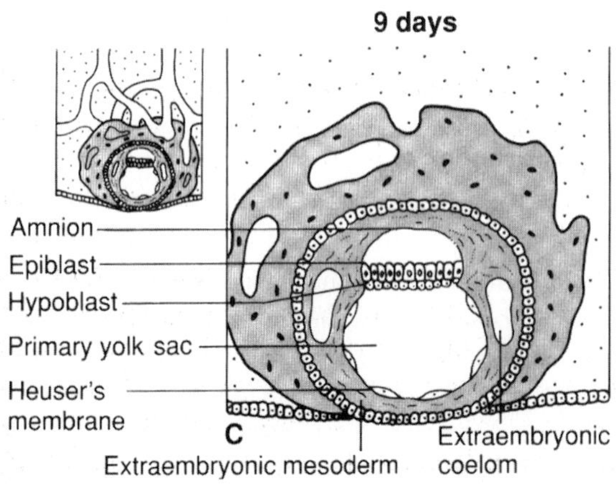


## Week 3

At this stage, when the woman may first realize she is pregnant, embryo development is rapid. A line of epiblast cells, starting from the caudal region (tail end) at the other side from the prochordal plate, undergoes very rapid cell division, forming the primitive streak in the midline (see Fig. 9.2). The cells of the primitive streak form a groove and then invaginate (move inwards) to spread between the epiblast and hypoblast layers. The bilaminar disc is, therefore, converted into a trilaminar disc consisting of three germ layers (ectoderm, mesoderm and endoderm), which give rise to specific tissues of the body (Fig. 9.3). The middle layer is the mesoderm, from which connective tissue, smooth

Fig. 9.2 *Formation of the prochordal plate (future mouth) and primitive streak on the bilaminar and trilaminar embryonic discs.*

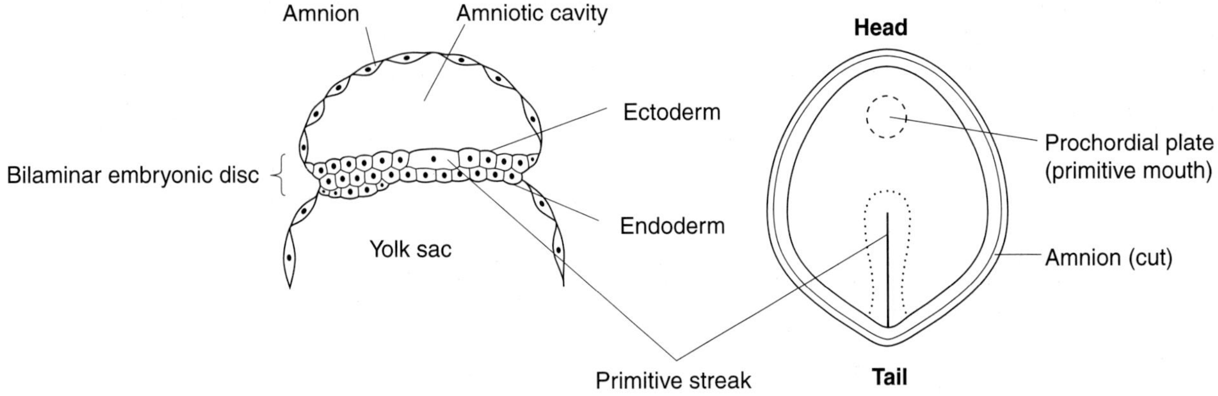


Fig. 9.3 *The invagination of cells of the primitive streak between the ectodermal and endodermal layers creates a trilaminar embryonic disc. (Reproduced with permission from Fitzgerald & Fitzgerald 1994.)*

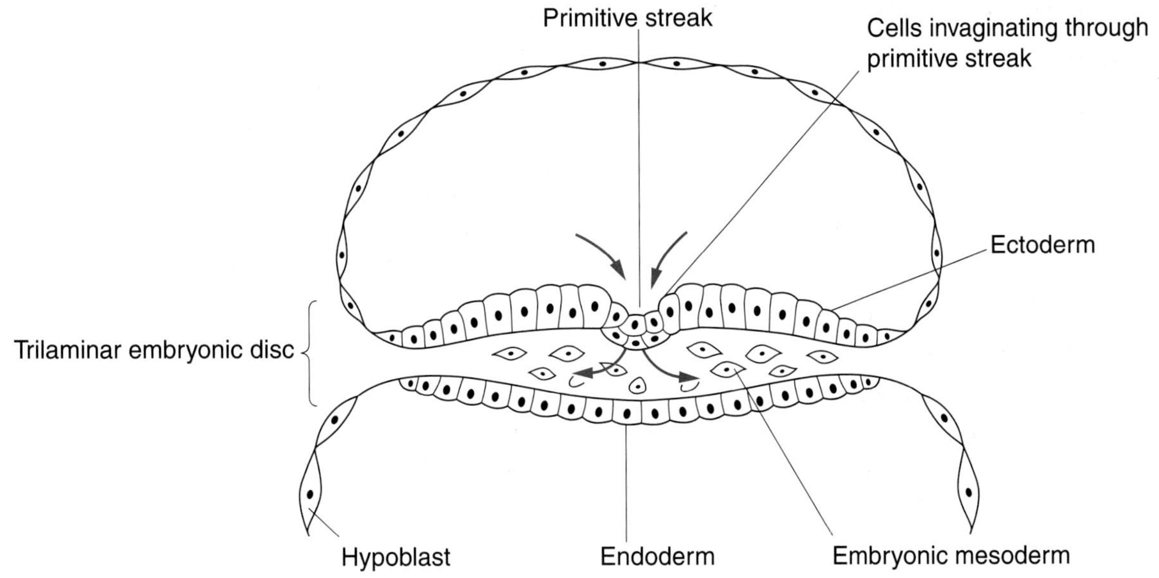


muscle, the cardiovascular system and blood, the skeleton, and the reproductive and endocrine systems develop (Fig. 9.4). The epiblast becomes the ectoderm, which will develop into the epidermis, central and peripheral nervous systems, and the retina. Therefore the ectoderm, which will give rise to the skin, is in contact with the amniotic cavity. The hypoblast becomes the endoderm, from which epithelial linings and some glandular structures will form. The three germ layers interact, generating signals that cause structural alterations and more complex interactions.

The endodermal prochordal plate is fused to the ectoderm forming the oropharyngeal membrane (future mouth). Below the primitive streak, there is another area of fusion between the ectoderm and endoderm; this is the cloacal membrane (the future anus). Some mesoderm cells migrate towards the prochordal plate forming a cord of adhesive cells (Fig. 9.5). This is the notochordal process, which develops a lumen forming the notochord canal. The notochord evolves into a cellular rod-like tube, which gives the trilaminar disc a degree of rigidity and

**Fig. 9.4** *The neural and surface ectoderm, the endoderm and the mesoderm will differentiate into future tissues of the body.*

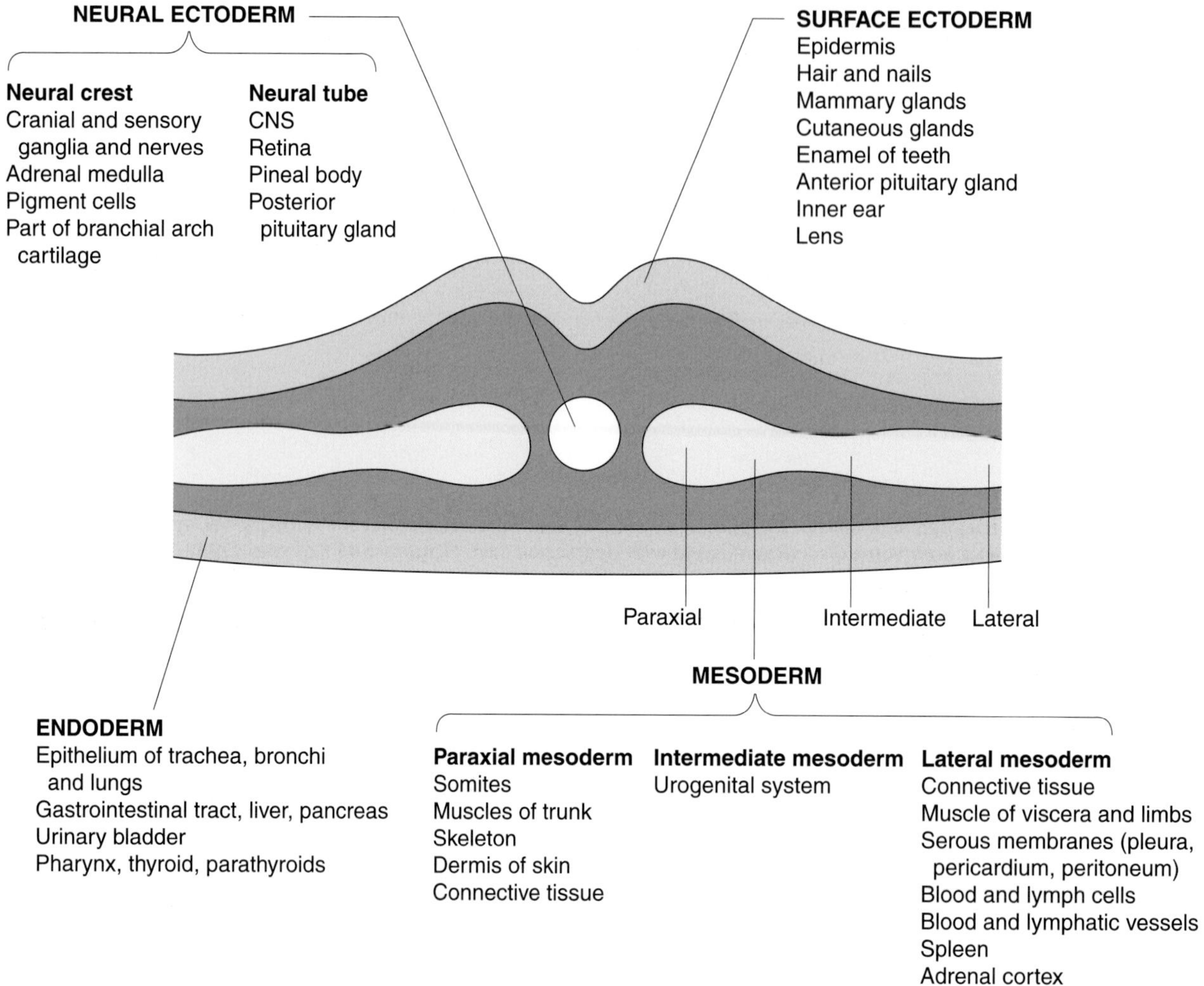


defines the central head–tail axis of the embryo. If identical twins are going to develop, there are two parallel notochords. If there are two notochords that cross, conjoined (Siamese) twins will result. The notochord establishes the development of the axial skeleton (bones of head and spinal cord) and the neural plate, which gives rise to the primitive nervous system. The vertebral column forms around the notochord and the notochord induces neurulation, the formation of the neural tube and early nervous system (see below). During the 3rd week, aggregates of mesoderm on either side of the notochord form pairs of bead-like blocks called somites, which direct the segmented structure of the body and induce the overlying ectoderm to form structures of the nervous system.

The formation of the primitive streak, the three germ layers, the prochordal plate and the notochord are described as gastrulation. Gastrulation marks the beginning of morphogenesis, the emergence and development of body form and structure. It begins with the appearance of the primitive streak at day 14. The primitive streak defines the time when experimental manipulation of human embryos is legally obliged to stop under the terms of the Human Fertilisation and Embryology Act of 1990. During the 3rd week of development, as well as gastrulation, the primitive nervous system and cardiovascular system begin to develop.

Box 9.1 is a summary of the events taking place in weeks 1 to 3.

Fig. 9.5 *Notochord formation: A 17 days; B 18 days. (Reproduced with permission from Goodwin 1997.)*

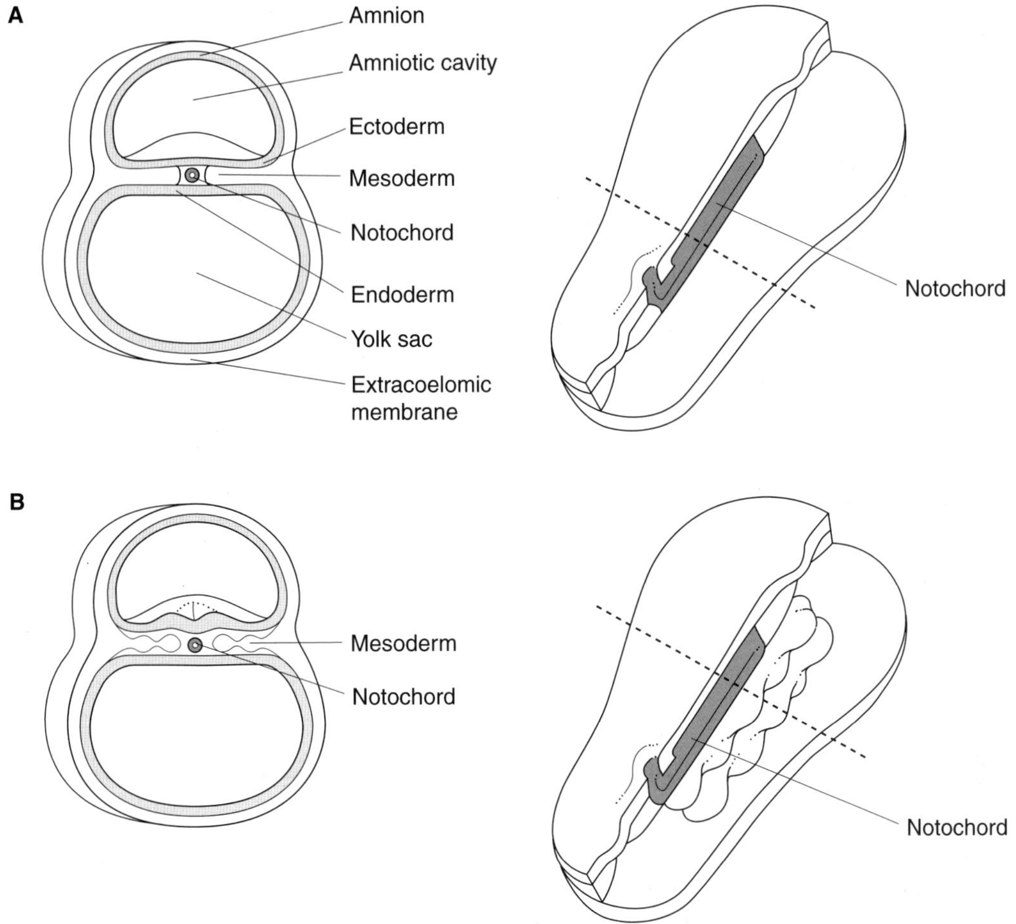


**Box 9.1**

**Summary of pre-embryonic period: weeks 1–3**

**Week 1: fertilization to produce zygote**

- Cleavage of zygote whilst travelling in uterine tube
- Cell division without increase in mass to form morula
- Fluid accumulation: hollow blastocyst formed
- 'Hatching' out of zona pellucida
- Blastocyst cells differentiate into trophoblast and inner cell mass
- Implantation in decidual wall

**Week 2: inner cell mass forms bilaminar embryonic disc of hypoblast and epiblast**

- Trophoblast differentiates into dividing cytotrophoblast and invasive syncytiotrophoblast (see Ch. 8)
- Lateral movement of cells from epiblast layer encloses yolk sac, forming the extraembryonic mesoderm
- Prochordal plate (mouth) develops at caudal end
- Day 14: primitive streak develops

**Week 3: gastrulation**

- Cells from primitive streak invaginate and migrate between the epiblast and the hypoblast forming the mesoderm
- Trilaminar disc of three germ layers: ectoderm (epiblast), mesoderm and ectoderm (hypoblast)
- Notochord forms, inducing development of the neural plate and giving axis of development
- Somites become evident
- Neurulation begins

## Weeks 4 to 8: organogenesis

During this period of embryonic development, the trilaminar disc folds into a C-shaped cylindrical embryo and all the major structures and organ systems are established. However, apart from the cardiovascular system, few of the systems function. Organogenesis, the development of the organ systems, is a critical period where the processes are susceptible to external influences that can cause disruption and subsequent serious congenital abnormalities. By the end of the 8th week, the embryo becomes known as the fetus and has a distinct human appearance (Fig. 9.6). Human development can be divided into three phases (Moore & Persaud 1998a):

- growth: cell division
- morphogenesis: development of form, which involves movement of sheets and masses of cells
- differentiation: maturation of cells forming tissues and organs capable of specialized function.

Fig. 9.6 *A 4-week-old and B 8-week-old fetus. (A reproduced with permission from Fitzgerald & Fitzgerald 1994.)*

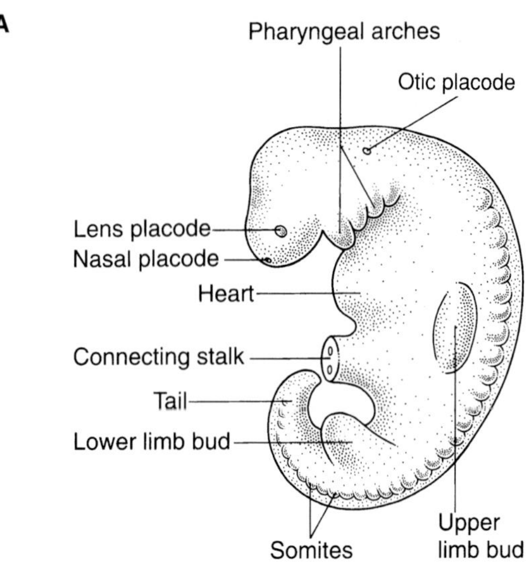


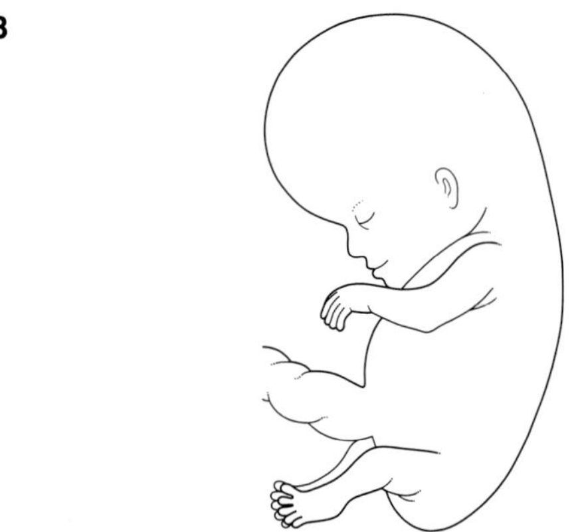


### Folding

The disc-like arrangement of the germ layers is converted into a recognizable vertebral embryo by folding in the 4th week of development. Folding is due to a differential rate in growth of the different parts of the embryo. The embryonic disc grows rapidly particularly in length, because of the growth of the brain and tail, so it has to fold. Although this is a momentous stage of development, relatively little is known about it. The yolk sac does not grow and, as the outer rim of the endoderm is attached to the yolk sac, the embryo becomes convex. Folding occurs at the cephalic (head) and lateral regions on day 22 and at the caudal (tail) end of the embryo on day 23 (Fig. 9.7). The cephalic, lateral and caudal edges of the embryonic disc are brought into apposition and the layers fuse along the midline, which converts the endoderm into the gut tube. Initially the foregut and the hindgut fuse, leaving the midgut open to the yolk sac. The folds cause a constriction between the embryo and yolk sac. The yolk sac gives rise to the primitive gut. The amnion expands, enveloping the connecting stalk and neck of the yolk sac, forming the umbilical cord. Folding is precisely coordinated and controlled by genes in the chromosomes. The developmental pattern involves synchronized tissue communication and interaction. Adjacent tissues induce changes in the movement and behaviour of neighbouring cells. Signals integrating genetic and environmental influences control cell proliferation, migration and apoptosis (Bard & Weddon 1996). These signals, which may be diffusible molecules or direct physical contact, direct the expression of particular genes in the responding cells (Moore & Persaud 1998b). Although all cells have the same DNA in their nuclei, depending on the signal received, some will express certain genes but not others. So, for instance, a skin cell expresses the genes that control the behaviour of a skin cell because they are switched on by the signals skin cells receive. A liver cell has the same genes as the skin cell but expresses different genes.

Fig. 9.7 *Folding of the embryonic disc into the fetal morphology: A 21 days; B 22 days; C 23 days; D 25 days. (Reproduced with permission from Goodwin 1997.)*

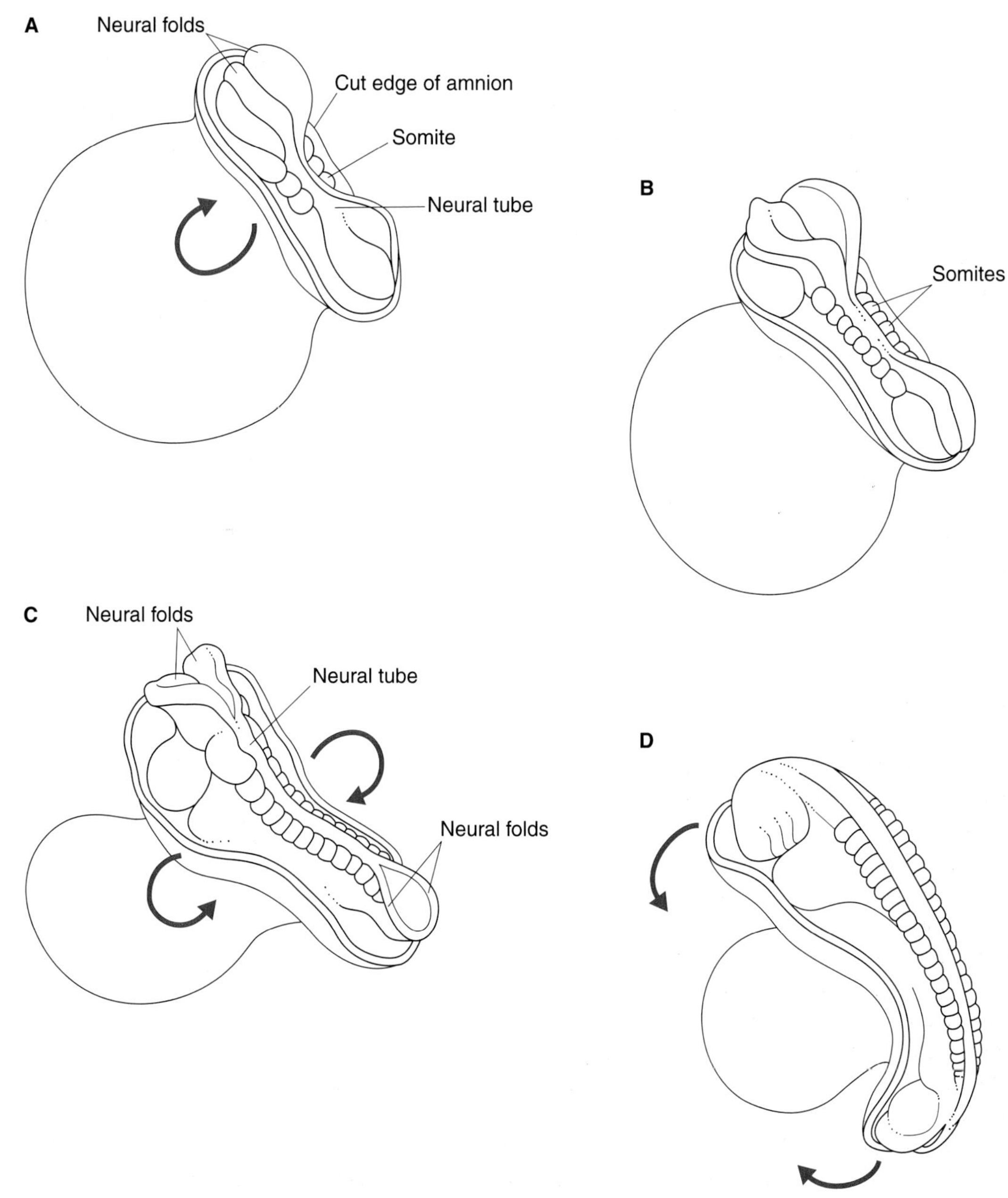


## *The organization of the basic body plan*

Techniques and concepts used to study molecular genetics (how the genetic code is expressed) in bacteria and *Drosophila* can be applied to mammalian embryogenesis, including human development. The DNA in the nucleus sets up a basic body plan, which establishes the pattern of the early embryo. The genes that control the basic body plan are the same in very diverse species. A highly conserved region of about 180 base pairs of DNA, known as the homeobox, is found in almost all species studied (Murtha, Leckman & Ruddle 1991). It codes for a protein that is a transcription factor (see Ch. 1), controlling the expression of genes. Other morphogenic agents, signals and growth factors activate the homeobox genes. There appear to be a series of three sequential steps in the conversion of the oval trilaminar embryonic disc into the cylindrical configuration with the endoderm on the inside, the ectoderm on the outside and the mesoderm in between (Fig. 9.8) (Carlson 1994). These steps result in segmentation of the embryo. Gap genes subdivide the embryo into broad regional domains. Pair-rule genes are involved in the formation of individual body segments and segment-polarity genes control the anterior–posterior organization of each segment (De Robertis, Oliver & Wright 1990). As the embryo develops, the segmental plan becomes less evident; remnants can be seen in the arrangement of the backbone and ribs and in the organisation of the spinal nerves.

**Fig. 9.8** ***Organization of the vertebrate body plan: three steps in the conversion.***

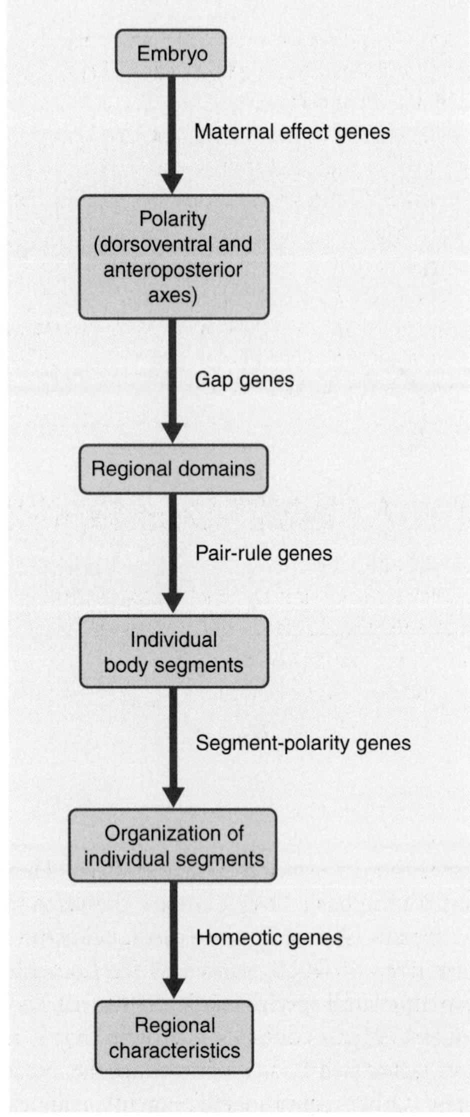


Box 9.2 is a summary of the events taking place in weeks 4 to 8.

## Ninth week to birth: fetal period

During this period, the body grows rapidly and the tissues and organs differentiate and mature (see below). The head growth rate becomes relatively slower so, by birth, the length of the head is about a quarter of the total length. Growth rate can be used to determine embryonic or fetal age (Box 9.3) and ultrasound examination can be used to examine developmental details (Box 9.4). With expert care, a fetus can be viable and may survive from 22 weeks.

Box 9.5 is a summary of the changes during the fetal period.

## Development of organ systems

### *The central nervous system*

Neurulation is the formation of the neural plate and neural folds and the closure of these folds to form the neural tube, which sinks into the body wall and differentiates into the brain and spinal cord. The neural tube is completed by the end of the 4th week. The developing notochord induces the overlying ectoderm to thicken forming the neural plate, a raised slipper-like plate of neuroepithelial cells. This will give rise to the central nervous system (brain and spinal cord) and other structures such as the retina. In the middle of the 3rd week, the neural groove appears in the centre of the neural plate (Fig. 9.9). To each side of the groove are neural folds, which enlarge at the cranial end as the start of the developing brain. Marked development of the brain is a characteristic of embryonic development in primates; human brain growth exceeds that of other species, continuing into adulthood. At the end of the 3rd week, the neural folds start to fuse forming the neural tube, which separates from the surface ectoderm. The neural crest cells, which detach from the lateral edges of the neural folds, give rise to the spinal ganglia and ganglia of the autonomic system as well as a number of other cell types (Box 9.6). The paraxial mesoderm, closest to the notochord and developing

**Box 9.2**

**Summary of embryonic period: weeks 4 to 8**

**4th week**

- Neural tube fusing but neuropores open at rostral (anterior) and caudal ends
- Folding produces characteristic C-shaped curved embryo
- Otic pits present (primitive ear)
- Optic vesicles formed
- Upper limb buds appear, then lower limb buds
- Three pairs of brachial arches present
- Beating heart prominent
- Forebrain prominent
- Attenuated tail
- Rudiments of organ systems established
- Rostral neuropore, then caudal neuropore, close
- Crown–rump length 4–6 mm

**5th week**

- Rapid brain development and head enlargement (cephalization)
- Facial prominences develop
- Upper limb buds become paddle-shaped
- Lower limb buds are flipper-like
- Mesonephric ridges denote position of mesonephric (interim) kidneys
- Crown–rump length 7–9 mm

**6th week**

- Joints of upper limbs differentiate
- Digital rays (fingers) of upper limbs evident
- External ear canal and auricle (pinna) formed
- Retinal pigment formed so eye is obvious
- Head very large, projects over heart prominence
- Reflex responses to touch
- Crown–rump length 11–14 mm

**7th week**

- Notches between digital rays partially separate future fingers
- Liver prominent
- Rapidly growing intestines hemiate out of small abdominal cavity into umbilical cord
- Crown–rump length 16–18 mm

**8th week**

- Digits of hand separated (but still webbed)
- Notches visible between digital rays of feet
- Stubby tail disappears
- Purposeful limb movements occur
- Ossification begins in lower limbs
- Head still disportionately large (about half of total embryo length)
- Eye lids closing
- Ears are characteristic shape but still low set
- External genitalia evident (but not distinct enough for sexual identification)
- Crown–rump length 27–31 mm

**Box 9.3**

**Estimation of embryonic/fetal age**

- Greatest length (GL) is used to measure embryos of about 3 weeks, which are straight
- Crown–rump length (CRL) is sitting height, used to measure older, curved embryos
- Carnegie embryonic staging system uses external characteristics to estimate developmental stage
- Number of somites
- Fetal head measurements, such as biparietal diameter (BPD) and head circumference
- Abdominal circumference
- Femur length and foot length

**Box 9.4**

**Ultrasound examination**

- Estimation of size and age of embryo
- Detection of congenital abnormality
- Evaluation of growth rate
- Investigation of uterine abnormality or ectopic pregnancy
- Guidance for CVS

neural tube, differentiates to form prominent paired blocks of tissue, or somites. The first somites appear from day 20. There are about 30 pairs of somites by day 30 increasing to a total of 44 pairs, but the cranial ones begin differentiation as new somites are added at the caudal end. The somites differentiate into sclerotomes, myotomes and dermatomes, which give rise to the axial skeletal bones, skeletal muscles and the dermis of the skin respectively. The number of somites

**Box 9.5**

**Summary of changes in the fetal period**

**9–12 weeks**

- Growth in body length and limbs accelerates
- Ears are low set, eyes are fused
- Primary ossification centres develop in skeleton, notably skull and long bones
- Intestines return to abdominal cavity and body wall fuses
- Erythropoiesis (formation of red blood cells) decreases in liver and begins in spleen
- Urine formation begins
- Fetal swallowing of amniotic fluid

**13–16 weeks**

- Rapid growth
- Coordinated limb movements (not felt by mother)
- Active ossification of skeleton
- Slow eye movements
- Ovaries differentiated and contain primordial follicles
- External genitalia recognizable
- Eyes and ears closer to normal positions

**17–20 weeks**

- Growth slows down
- Limbs reach mature proportions
- Fetal movements felt by mother ('quickening')
- Skin covered with protective layer of vernix caseosa, held in position by lanugo (downy hair)
- Brown fat deposited

**21–25 weeks**

- Fetus gains weight
- Skin wrinkled and translucent, appears red-pink
- Rapid eye movements begin
- Blink-startle responses to noise
- Surfactant secretion begins but respiratory system immature
- Fingernails are present
- May be viable if born prematurely

**26–29 weeks**

- Lungs capable of breathing air
- CNS can control breathing
- Eyes open
- Toenails visible
- Fat (3.5% body weight) deposited under skin so wrinkles smooth out
- Erythropoiesis moves from spleen to bone marrow

**30–34 weeks**

- Pupillary light reflex
- Skin pink and smooth, limbs chubby
- White fat is 8% of body weight
- From 32 weeks, survival is usual

**35–38 weeks**

- Firm grasp
- Orientates towards light
- Circumference of head and abdomen are approximately equal
- White fat is about 16% of body weight, 14 g fat gained per day
- Skin appears bluish-pink
- Term fetus is about 3400 g, crown–rump length is about 360 mm

**Box 9.6**

**Tissues arising from cells of the neural crest**

- Spinal ganglia
- Ganglia of the autonomic system
- Adrenal medulla
- Glial cells
- Schwann cells
- Melanocytes (pigmented)
- Pharyngeal arch cartilage
- Odontoblasts (of teeth)
- Pupillary and ciliary muscles of eye
- Dermis and hypodermis of neck and face

indicates the age of the embryo. The limbs carry with them the nerves from the somites from which they developed. The somatic pattern of development is important in understanding referred pain (see Ch. 13).

Neural tube defects (NTD) are one of the most common congenital abnormalities (see Ch. 12). Neurulation is very sensitive to disturbances such as teratogenic drugs or lack of folate, which is required for DNA synthesis of the rapidly dividing cells (see Ch. 7). Most neurons are formed between 10 and 18 weeks; this is therefore the critical window for brain development. Undernutrition or other insults in the first trimester often result in microcephaly (James & Stephenson 1998). In later gestation, undernutrition may result in blood flow being redistributed to the

**Fig. 9.9** ***The neural groove and neural tube fusion: A 21 days; B, C 23 days.***

A

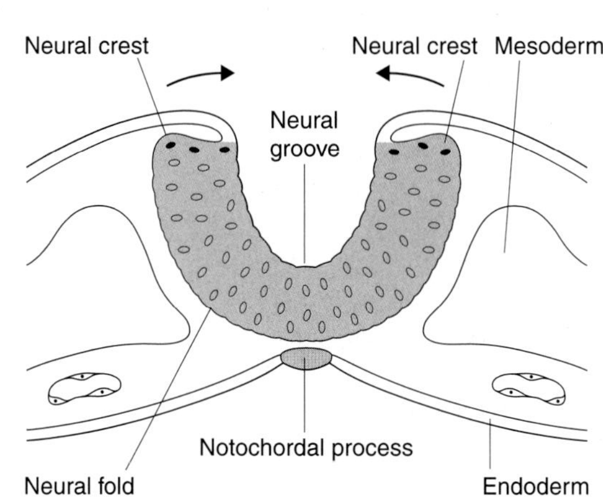


B

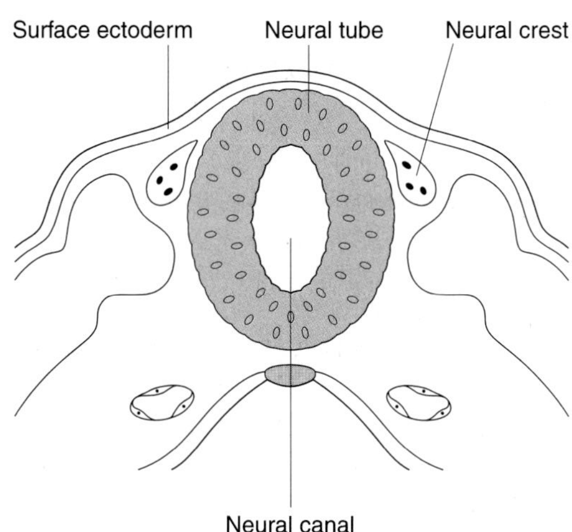

C

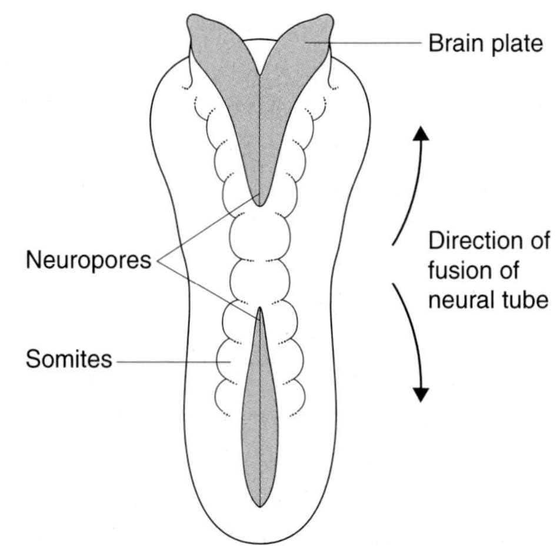


brain at the expense of other tissues. As brain size in humans is proportionately larger, the effects of protecting the brain from undernutrition may be exaggerated compared with other species (Barker 1998). Glial cells begin to develop at about 15 weeks. In the second half of pregnancy, the glial cells hypertrophy and the axons and dendrites undergo marked growth. This growth spurt continues until the second postnatal year (Dobbing & Sands 1979).

Fetal sensory organs develop around the middle of gestation. At 24 weeks, the fetus responds to noise. As gestation progresses, the fetus exhibits increased sensitivity and responds to an increased range of sound frequencies. Babies are thought to enjoy being carried and cuddled because they can hear sounds of their mother's heart and digestive system, which they became accustomed to in utero.

## *Gastrointestinal system*

The gut begins as a single tube running from mouth to anus. The mouth and anus are fused areas of endoderm and ectoderm (see above). The tube is therefore fixed at both ends so that when it grows it convolutes and loops (Fig. 9.10). Some parts of the tube dilate, such as the stomach and colon, and the gut rotates around other structures such as the developing liver. Between the 6th and 8th week of development, the proliferation of the epithelial cells lining the gut obliterates the lumen, which is then gradually recanalized. Early growth of the gut is extremely rapid so it extrudes into the amniotic cavity. If it is not withdrawn at about 10 weeks, the abdominal wall fails to close and the baby is born with exomphalos or gastroschisis. Normal fusion of the lateral body folds occurs at the linea nigra, the abdominal line that pigments in pregnancy (see Ch. 11). Normal growth of the gut depends on fetal swallowing. A fetus swallows about a third of the total volume of amniotic fluid per hour by the 16th week of development. Not only does amniotic fluid provide about 10% of the fetal protein requirements, but it also seems to be associated with effective development of the gastrointestinal mucosa, liver and pancreas and promotion of growth.

The digestive enzymes are present from about 24–28 weeks, with the exception of lactase (see Ch. 16). Peristaltic coordination of the fetal gut is evident from the 14th week of development. By 34 weeks there is coordination of sucking, swallowing and peristalsis. As the gut matures, it produces mucus, which will eventually be required to lubricate the

Fig. 9.10 *Convolution of the primitive gut. (Reproduced with permission from James & Stephenson 1998.)*

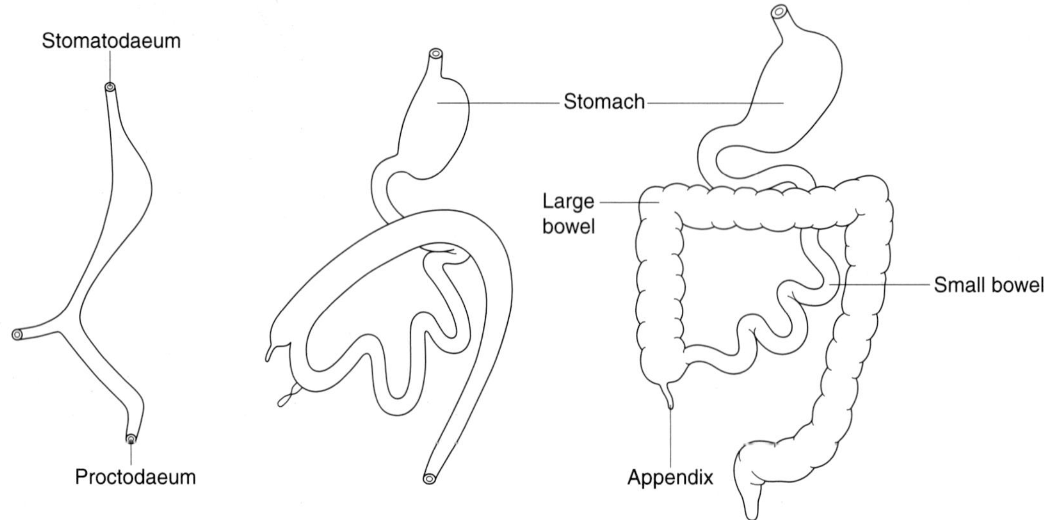


passage of food and faeces during transit. The mucus accumulates in the fetal gut as meconium. Adrenaline, produced in response to fetal distress, stimulates contractions of the gut, and can lead to meconium-stained amniotic fluid. The liver reaches metabolic maturity relatively late in gestation, storing glycogen in the last 9 weeks. Inadequate placental transfer of amino acids will affect tissues with high protein turnover, such as the liver (James & Stephenson 1998). It has been suggested (Bassett 1986) that fetal starvation results in protein catabolism to supply substrates for gluconeogenesis and placental requirements. As hepatic stores of glycogen and fat are mobilized in IUGR, the liver is the first organ affected so the head to abdomen ratio is an important indicator of IUGR.

Case study 9.1 is an example of developmental abnormality of the gut.

**Case study 9.1**

At 11 weeks of gestation, Julie has an ultrasound scan. She is asked to return for a further scan in 2 weeks as her unborn baby appears to have some gut tissue herniating into the umbilical cord. Julie seeks advice from her midwife.

- Is this normal?
- How might you reassure Julie that the ultrastenographer was just being cautious?
- If there were a pathological condition present, what two conditions are most likely?
- How would they be further investigated before Julie is advised upon the prognosis?

## The face

The face is formed between weeks 5 and 12 from the brachial arches. The nose grows downwards as a pillar of tissue (Fig. 9.11). The eyes, which are formed from a combination of nervous tissue and specialized ectoderm, are initially in a lateral position but move medially. The ears are initially low set. Below the nose, maxillary processes extend to form the floor of the nose and the roof of the mouth. The upper lip is formed from processes that extend to meet centrally. Inadequate fusion of the maxillary processes causes congenital malformations of the mouth, such as cleft lip or palate. Palatal fusion is complete by the 11th week.

## The skull

The skull develops from mesenchymal tissue around the brain. It is formed from the neurocranium, which protects the brain, and the viscerocranium, which forms the skeleton of the face. Each of these elements of the skull has membranous and cartilaginous components. Ossification is of the membrane rather than of cartilage and begins from the base of the skull (Larsen 1993).

The bones of the calvaria (cranial vault) have not completed development at birth. In the fetus, the flat bones of the calvaria are held together by soft fibrous sutures made of dense connective tissue, which allows some flexibility. The fetal head can mould to the shape of the maternal pelvis and distort as it passes through

Fig. 9.11 *Growth of the palate and nose between the 6th and 9th week. (Reproduced with permission from James & Stephenson 1998.)*

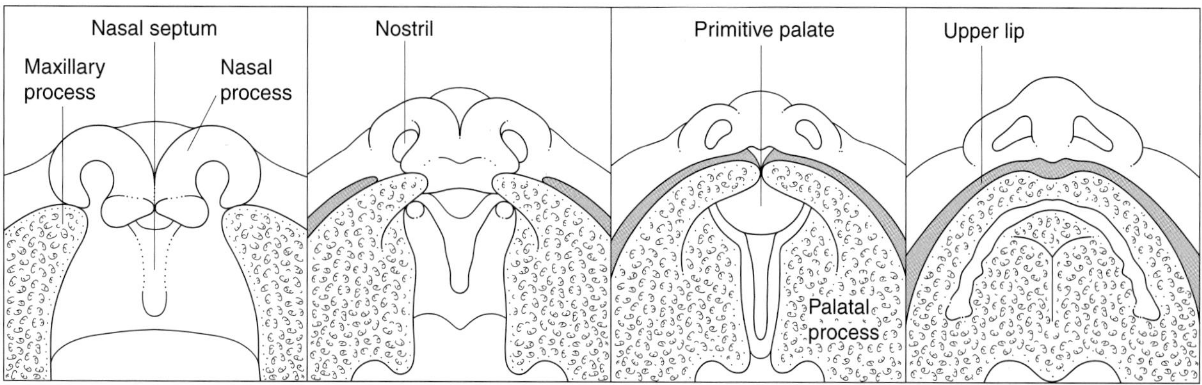


the birth canal. During delivery, the frontal bone becomes flat, the occipital bone is drawn out and the parietal bones overlap. The head usually returns to a normal shape a few days after delivery. Six large membranous fontanelles are formed where the sutures meet (see Ch. 13). The posterior fontanelles close at about 3 months after birth and the anterior ones close when the infant is about 18 months old. Raised intracranial pressure can be detected by palpating these fontanelles; a depression indicates dehydration.

The fetal skull is relatively large compared with the skeleton. The newborn skull has relatively thin bones compared with those in later life. The face is relatively small and has a characteristic neonatal roundish shape because the jaws are small. The paranasal sinuses (which give the individual shape of the face and resonance of the voice) are virtually absent and the facial bones are underdeveloped (Moore & Persaud 1998b). After birth, brain growth is rapid so the calvaria increase markedly during the first 2 years. The calvaria continue to grow until the child is about 16 years old; the skull bones then thicken.

## The cardiovascular system

This is one of the first systems to develop; its function is important extremely early in development, unlike some of the other systems that do not have to achieve full function until after birth. This is because as the embryo becomes larger diffusion is no longer adequate.

A few cells in the mesoderm of the yolk sac lose adherence and start to move, forming clusters called blood islands (Fig. 9.12). The haemocytoblasts, the precursors of blood cells, are nucleated and start to synthesize primitive forms of haemoglobin. The outer cells of the blood islands, angioblasts, develop characteristics of endothelial cells, the cells that line blood vessels. The blood islands fuse, forming vascular channels that eventually connect together forming identifiable routes. The organization of the routes across the yolk sac is similar to the geographical organization of river deltas where little streams meander and combine, taking the route of least resistance. Expansion and elastic resistance of the vessel walls, which become rhythmic generating a peristaltic pattern, propel the blood cells.

The primitive heart develops from a horseshoe area of embryonic mesoderm, anterior to the prochordal plate. It forms two tubes one on each side of the foregut, which fuse forming a single heart tube. The primitive atrium forms where the flow from the umbilical veins from the placenta joins with the blood vessels from the head, generating the greatest volume of blood. The swirling vortex of blood leaving the primitive atrium induces the development of the primitive ventricle, which becomes the main source of pumping activity. The characteristic shape of the heart is generated by the flow of blood cells within the vascular channels; this causes the heart tube to form an S-shaped loop that will eventually take on the configuration of the heart (Fig. 9.13). By 21 days after fertilization, the cells surrounding the heart have become differentiated as myocardial cells capable of eliciting an organized response so the heart, which consists of four chambers in series, begins beating.

The development of the outer layers of the vessel walls is stimulated by stress (Martyn & Greenwald 1997). In areas where there is more turbulence, the

**Fig. 9.12** ***Formation of the first blood vessels: A appearance of blood islands; B vessels at 24 days (A reproduced with permission from Fitzgerald & Fitzgerald 1994; B reproduced with permission from Goodwin 1997.)***

*(Fig. 9.12B, see opposite)*

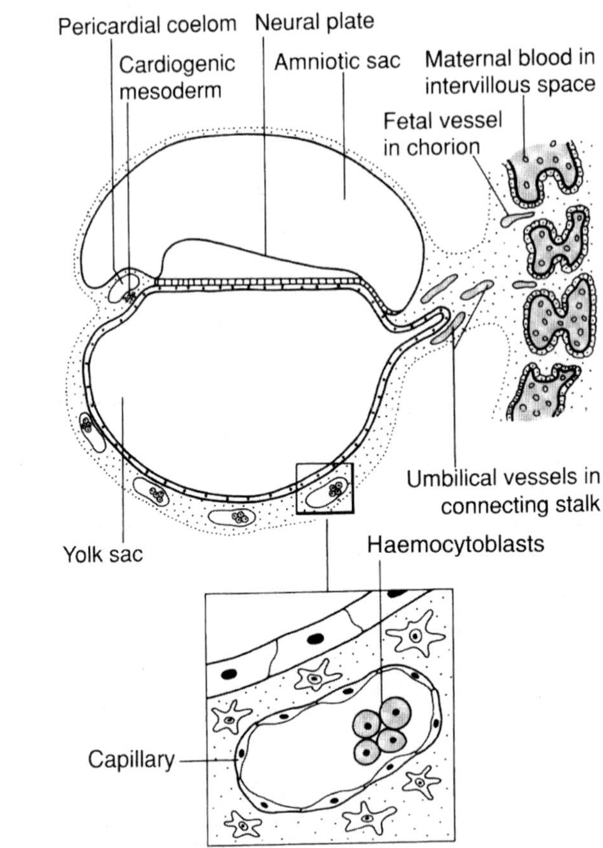


vessel wall responds by developing more elasticity. Therefore, the heart and arterial structures develop thicker and more elastic walls. The mature organization of the chambers of the heart is achieved by the ingrowth of the septa towards the central atrioventricular cushion in the centre (Fig. 9.13). The growth of the fetal heart partially depends on afterload. If afterload is increased by factors leading to peripheral vasoconstriction or high placental impedance, the likely outcome is a growth-restricted baby with an enlarged heart (Veille et al 1993). If the fetus receives less than adequate nutrition or oxygenation during its development then blood flow is diverted to the brain and heart. The decreased flow to the peripheral vessels results in the development of less elastic tissue, which is the hypothesis underlying the association of poor maternal nutrition with an increased risk of cardiovascular disease in adult life (Barker et al 1993). The initial response to impaired nutrition is to increase placental growth; if this is not adequate, blood flow is diverted to the brain. Therefore adults who were small at birth, but with relatively large placentas, have an increased risk of developing hypertension because less elastic tissue was established in their blood vessels during fetal development (Fig. 9.14).

## The respiratory system

The trachea and major bronchi develop as outpouches of the alimentary tract. The development depends on interaction between the endodermal bud from the developing foregut and the splanchnic mesoderm it invades at about day 22. The bud bifurcates between day 26 and 28. In the 5th week of development, three secondary buds develop on the right branch and two on the left; these are the primitive lobes of the lung. There are four stages in the development of the respiratory system: the embryonic phase from weeks 3 to 7, the pseudocanalicular phase from 7 to 16 weeks, the canalicular phase from 16 to 24 weeks and the terminal sac phase from 24 weeks until birth (Fig. 9.15).

**Fig. 9.12** ***Continued.***

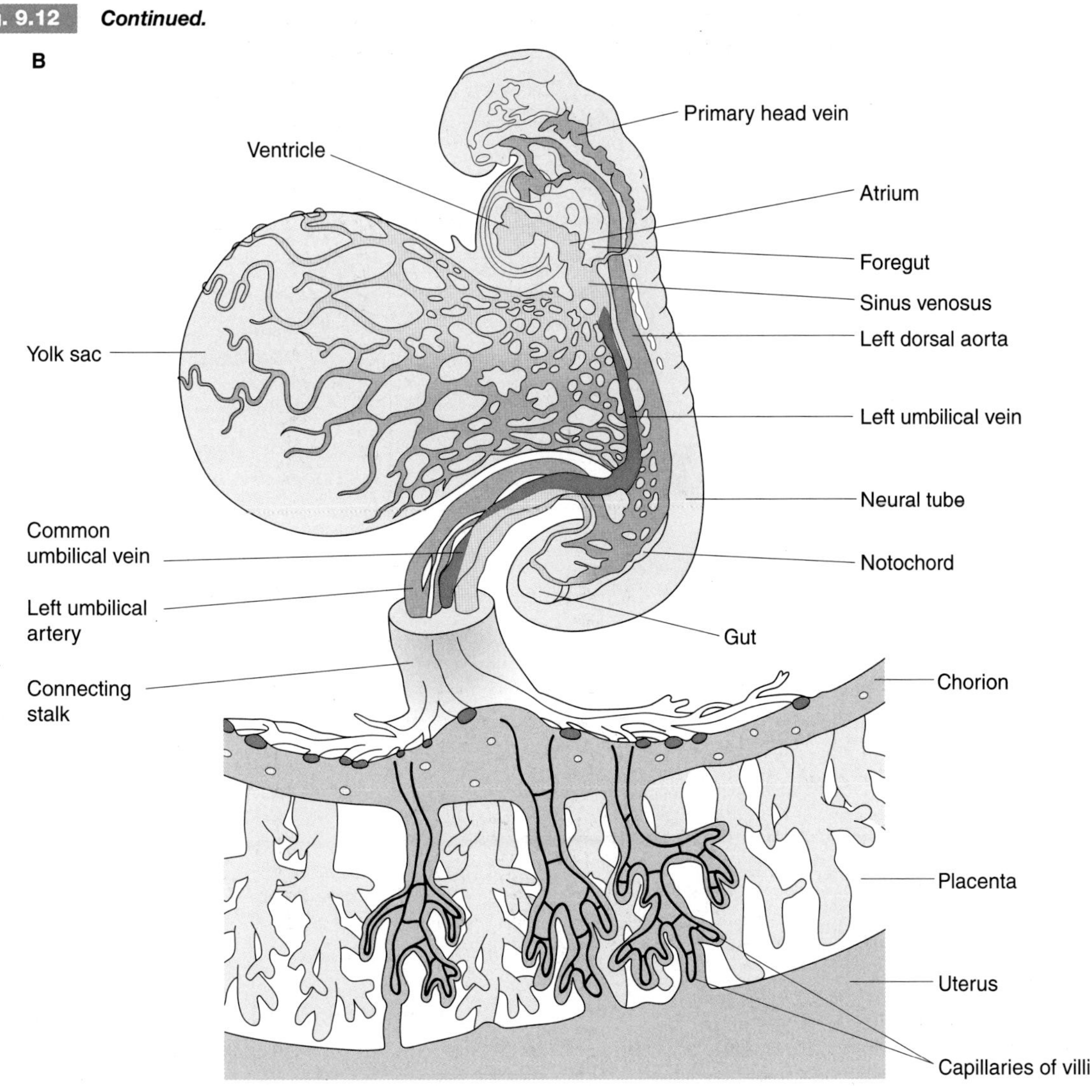


One of the most critical stages in development is the production of surfactant from the type II pneumocytes, allowing efficient inflation and gas exchange following birth and therefore postnatal survival. Although the cells can be identified about week 22, production of surfactant increases significantly after 30 weeks. The diaphragm starts to develop high in the neck and descends as the lungs and heart develop. This is the reason why diaphragmatic pain is often referred to the tip of the shoulder. If fetal breathing movements are limited, lung development is impaired (George et al 1987). Fetal lung volume establishes postnatal functional residual capacity. Decreased amniotic fluid volume causes decreased lung growth and expansion whereas tracheal occlusion, which prevents expulsion of lung fluid, can cause overgrowth of lung tissue (Nardo, Hooper & Harding 1998). At term, the infant has about 50 million alveoli, half the adult number; these continue to develop in the first 8 years of life (Reid 1979).

## *The urinary system*

The urinary and genital systems both develop from the intermediate mesoderm and are closely associated (see Ch. 5 for a description of genital development). During embryonic folding, urogenital ridges appear each side of the primitive aorta (Fig. 9.16). The nephrogenic ridge develops into the renal system of kidneys, ureters, bladder and urethra. Abnormalities of the kidneys and ureters affect 3–4% of newborn

Fig. 9.13 *Formation of the heart from bending of the cardiac tube (21 to 35 days), and formation of the heart chambers.*

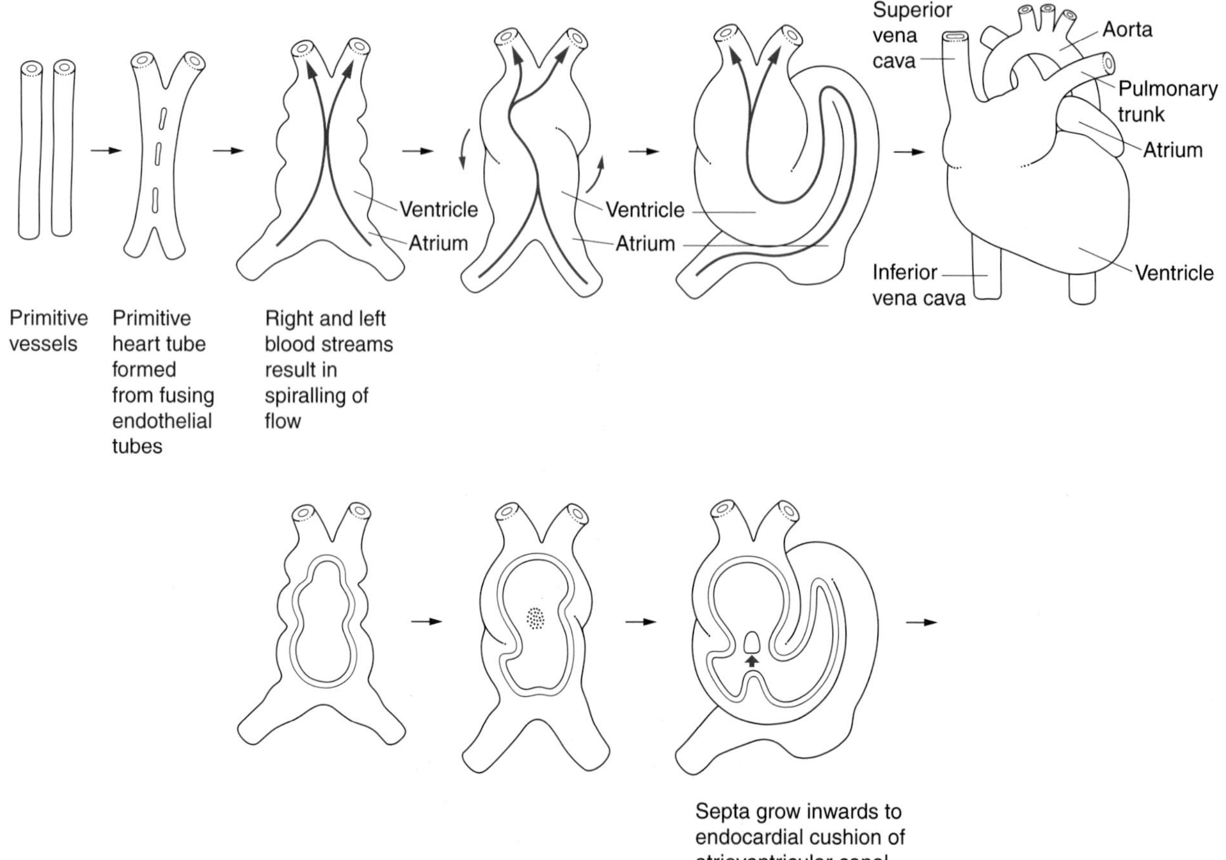


infants. Most of the abnormalities are harmless, such as variation in blood supply, abnormal position or shapes, and urinary tract duplications. However, unilateral renal agenesis (one kidney failing to develop) affects one in 1000 liveborn babies. Bilateral renal agenesis or Potter's syndrome (inadequate development of both kidneys) affects one in 3000 fetuses and is incompatible with life. It is usually associated with oligohydramnios. Three pairs of kidneys develop during fetal development: the pronephroi, the mesonephroi and the metanephroi (singular pronephros, mesonephros and metanephros). The pronephroi are transient non-functional structures that exist for only a few weeks. When they degenerate, their ducts are utilized in the next stage. The mesonephroi appear in the 4th week and function as intermediate kidneys until the end of the embryonic period, disgorging waste products into the remnants of the yolk sac. They degenerate and disappear in the 8th week, although parts of their structure persist as mesonephric or Wolffian ducts in males (see Ch. 5).

The permanent kidneys, or metanephroi, develop from the 5th week and begin to function about 4 weeks later. The kidneys start development in the pelvis and appear to migrate upwards. In fact, this observation is due to continued downward growth of the embryo. As the kidneys 'ascend' out of the pelvic area, new arteries at successively higher levels supply them. During fetal life, the kidney is subdivided into lobes, which disappear in infancy as the nephrons grow. The main increase in size is due to elongation of the proximal convoluted tubules and loops of Henle. Functional maturation of the kidneys occurs after birth.

Until 20 weeks' gestation, the skin is not keratinized so fluid can move through this semipermeable membrane. Essentially the outer barrier is the amnion. As the skin matures and lays down keratin, the rate of transudation decreases and the outer barrier of the fetus becomes the skin. The urine then becomes an important source of amniotic fluid. The fetus produces up to 600 ml of urine per day. Amniotic fluid is also

**Fig. 9.14** *The link between poor fetal nutrition and altered cardiovascular and placental development.*

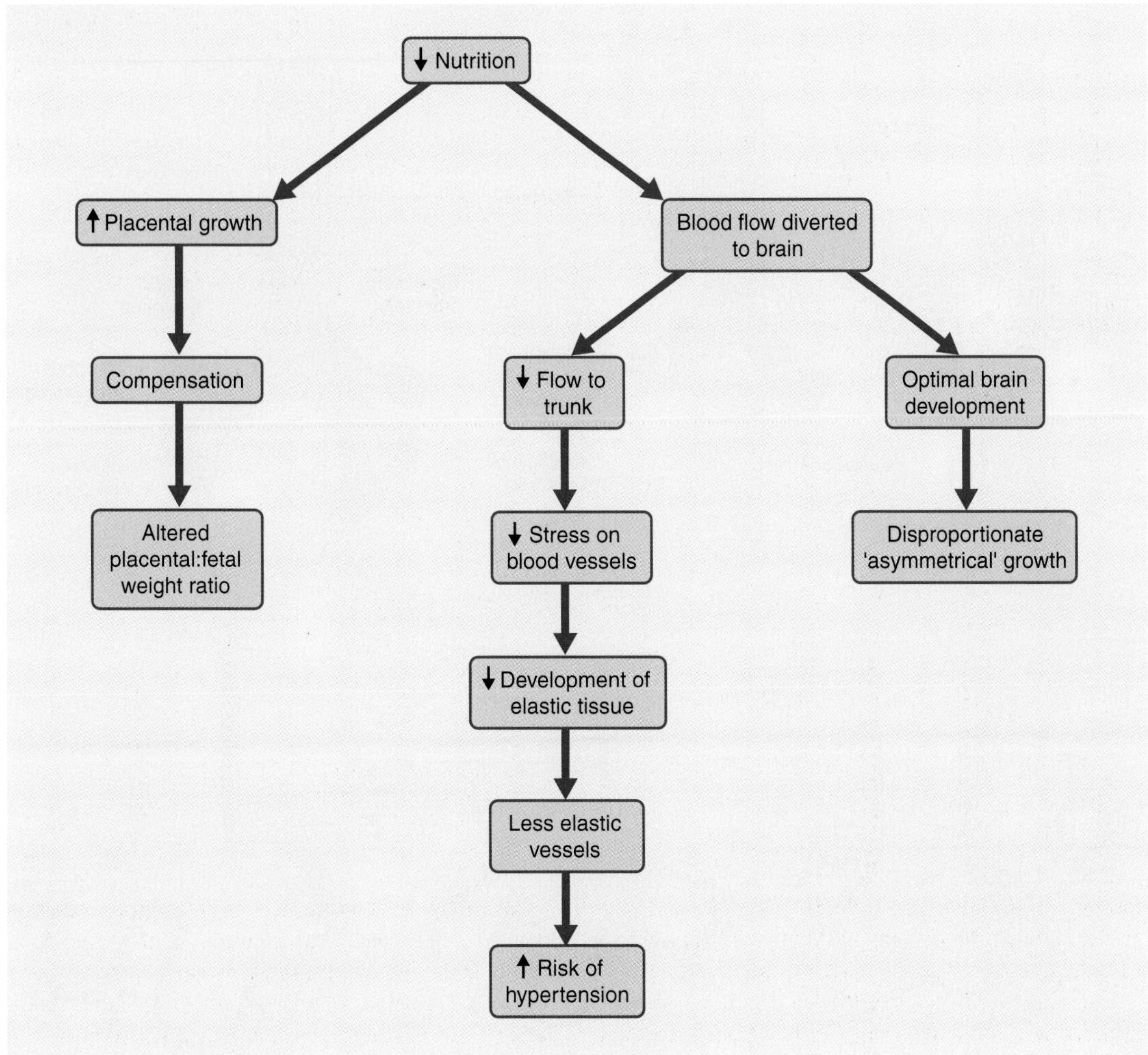


produced by the amniotic membrane and the fetal lungs. The fetus swallows most of the amniotic fluid; the rest diffuses through the amniotic membranes to the maternal circulation.

The epidermis of the skin develops from the ectoderm, which is colonized from melanocytes from the neural crest and Langerhans cells from the bone marrow. The dermis is derived from the embryonic mesoderm.

## *The muscles and limbs*

The first muscles to develop are the back muscles from the paired somites. Bone formation is closely associated with muscle growth and the nervous connections from the spinal cord. The limbs become evident as buds or bulges associated with particular somites in the 4th week of development. The limb buds are formed from migration of muscle cells from the myotomes. The cells form pairs of muscle masses. Adhesive cells form a compacted region between the two muscle masses, which differentiates into cartilage. Cartilage is stiff but flexible whereas bone is stronger but more brittle and able to fracture. Ossification, the conversion to bone structure, begins from about 8 weeks but is still not complete by birth. This preponderance of cartilage in the skeleton aids flexibility at delivery. The arms are slightly ahead of the legs in

**Fig. 9.15** *Respiratory system development: A pharyngeal pouches (4 weeks); B 32 days; C 35 days; D pseudocanalicular phase (17 weeks); E canalicular phase (17–26 weeks); F terminal sac phase (26 weeks).*

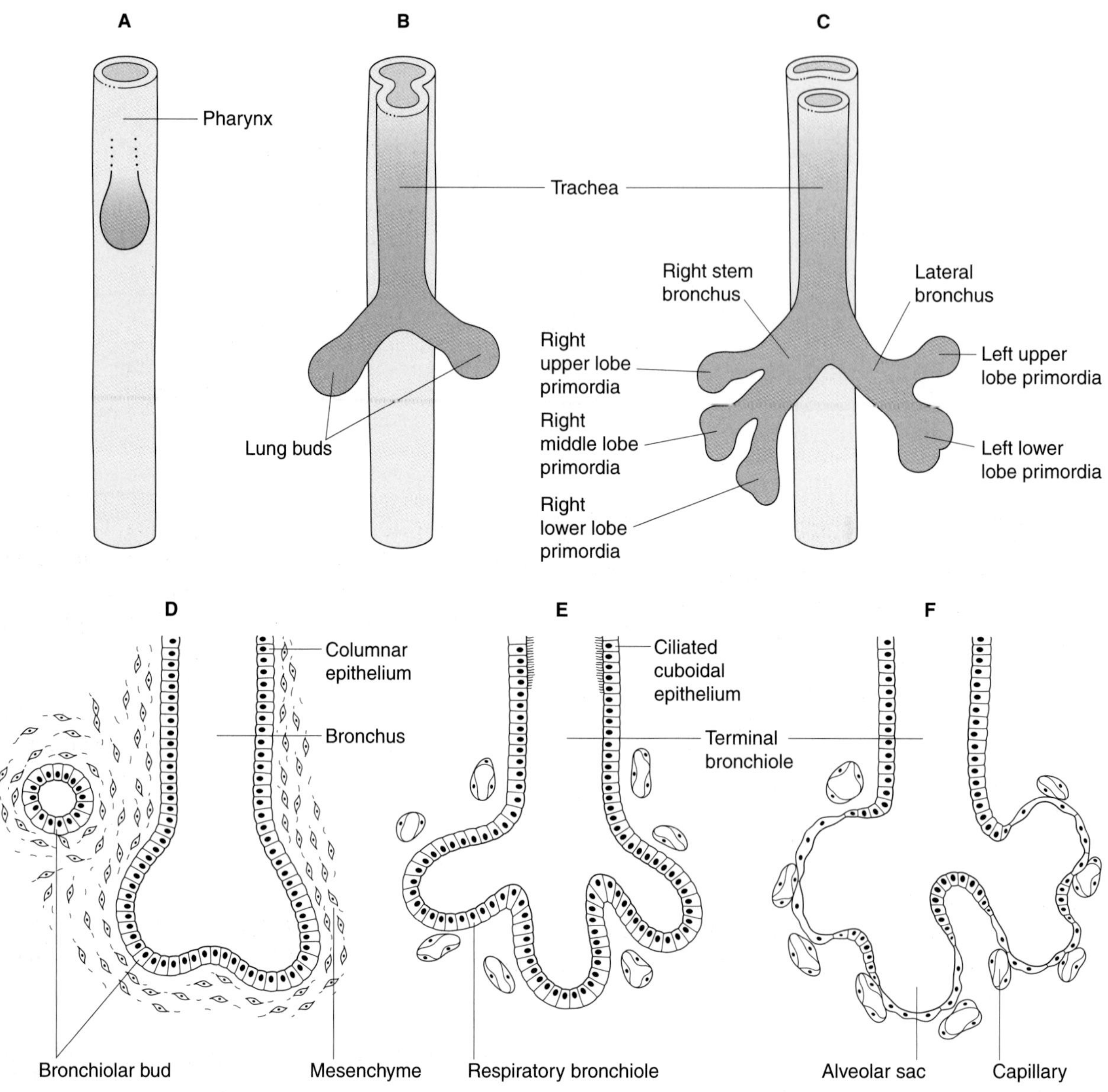


development because the fetal circulatory system gives an advantage to the upper body (see Ch. 15). Bones and muscles closest to the body develop first so the humerus and femur develop before the distal regions of the limbs. The differential timing of development means that drugs such as thalidomide affect different limbs and parts of the limbs depending on time of exposure of the fetus to the teratogens (Box 9.7). By 41 days, the fingers and toes develop from paddle-like plates. The sculpting of the digits is due to apoptosis of the tissue between the digital rays. A common minor congenital defect observed at birth is a failure of separation of the digits. By 9 weeks, the body skeleton is almost complete, although the skull bones are still forming.

## Fetal growth

At 4 weeks, the crown–rump length is about 4 mm and increases by 1 mm per day up to 30 mm (Beck 1996). Thereafter, between weeks 8 and 28, the growth increases markedly, to about 1.5 mm per day, so this period is recognized as the fetal growth period.

**Fig. 9.16** *The development of the renal system from the urogenital ridges.*

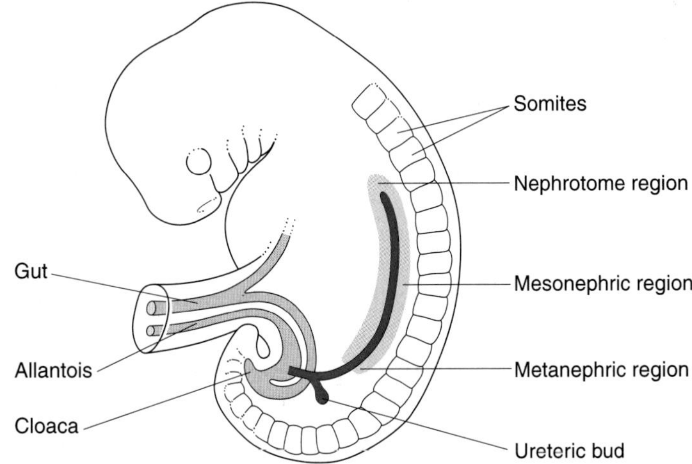


**Box 9.7**
**Thalidomide**

Thalidomide was marketed as 'Contergan' in 1957. Congenital malformations of the limbs and ears rose in parallel with sales of the drug with a lag of 7 to 8 months (Lenz 1962, McBride 1961). The drug was withdrawn in November 1961; 5850 infants were affected, of which 40% died, leaving 3900 survivors. Thalidomide disturbs cartilage formation and the establishment of the nerve connections to muscles. It is teratogenic 20 to 36 days after fertilization. Limb development begins at 24 days. Early exposure to thalidomide caused absence of arms; later exposure successively affected development of ears, legs and thumbs. Different species metabolize the drug differently; fetal development in the test species of rats and mice was not affected.

The organs and tissues continue to grow and mature. Although growth is most rapid during this period (compared with any other time in life), factors affecting growth may have their origins earlier. In fact, environmental insults regulating growth appear to last for several generations. Fetal growth is due to interaction between the genetic drive for growth and the nutritional supplies in pregnancy to support it, which involves a dynamic interaction between fetus, placenta and mother.

There are characteristic differences during the different phases of growth during development (James & Stephenson 1998). Growth in the first trimester is principally through increased cell number. In the second trimester, cell division continues albeit at a slower rate and the cells increase in size. In the third trimester, cell division slows further and the increase in cell size continues. Fat deposition, determined by nutrient availability and insulin levels, plays an important contribution in the final weight. There are 42 successive cell divisions between fertilization and birth, but only five more from birth to adult size (excluding mitotic cell division to replace dead cells).

A variety of factors affect fetal growth (Box 9.8).

## *Fetal factors*

Male offspring on average are heavier than females. The ovaries have limited capability to synthesize

**Box 9.8**
**Factors affecting fetal size**

- Fetal factors
- Maternal size (lean body mass)—maternal genetic effects
- Maternal weight gain and nutrition in pregnancy
- Maternal behavioural factors such as smoking, drug use
- Fetal oxygenation—affected by maternal anaemia, etc.
- Medical conditions such as hypertension, heart disease, infections
- Placental sufficiency affected by pre-eclampsia, uterine blood flow, etc.
- Growth hormones such as insulin and IGFs

steroid hormones whereas the testes produce testosterone, which has anabolic effects. Studies suggest that the Y chromosome positively promotes growth (James & Stephenson 1998). Multiple pregnancies tend to result in smaller babies, probably because of the limited haemodynamic support in late gestation although overcrowding is also implicated.

### Maternal size

The classic experiments on horses showing that the size of offspring of hybrid crosses between small Shetland ponies and large carthorses was most closely related to maternal size demonstrated that maternal size is a critical determinant of birth weight (Walton & Hammond 1938). However, final adult size is also affected by paternal genetics to different degrees in different species; in humans about 5% of the variability in size is attributed to paternal influences (Robinson & Owens 1996). In the recent past, pregnant women were asked for their shoe size, which correlates with their pelvic size, and their husband's hat size, which was found to be related to the size of the baby; the relationship of the two sizes was used to predict the likelihood of difficulties in delivery (Moore, Peters & Frame 1984). A small maternal size appears to impose a constraint on fetal growth, although factors such as immaturity, social circumstances, maternal behaviour (such as smoking and alcohol consumption), diseases and psychological stress all affect the outcome of the pregnancy. Shorter maternal stature is positively correlated with lower socioeconomic status, malnutrition, chronic disease, increased levels of stress and large family size. The cycle of deprivation tends to repeat, as there is a correlation between maternal height and birth weight and between birth weight and adult size, which is not solely due to genetic influences.

Half-siblings who share the same mother have similar birth weights (Gluckman & Harding 1994). The birth weights of babies born after ovum donation are more strongly related to the weight of the recipient mother than to that of the donor woman (Brooks et al 1995). These findings suggest that birth size is more strongly influenced by uterine environment than genetics.

### Growth hormones

It has been suggested that growth in children from fetus, through infancy and childhood to puberty follows a mathematical model on which three growth curves are imposed, forming a sigmoidal curve (Fig. 9.17) (Karlberg et al 1994). Phase 1, the infancy growth rate, begins in fetal life with a rapid deceleration until about 3 years old. This is the phase of growth that seems to be regulated by IGFs (see Ch. 4); the effect of poor nutrition on growth may be mediated by IGFs. The childhood phase begins in the 1st year of life and is due to the effect of growth hormone (GH, see Ch. 3) provided thyroid hormone secretion is normal. During this period most of the growth is localized in the lower body (particularly leg length) as the long bones are very sensitive to GH. Children who have deficiency of GH or who are encephalic have normal birth weight and early infant growth; the deficiency usually becomes apparent only after 6 months of age (Gluckman 1989). The final component of growth is the pubertal growth spurt, which is stimulated by the interaction of sex hormones with GH.

Although levels of GH in the fetus are high and GH receptors have been identified, the lack of impaired growth in GH-deficient fetuses or young infants suggests linear growth at this stage is almost independent of GH. Fetal growth seems to be controlled rather by IGFs and their receptors (Robinson & Owens 1996). IGFs are mitogens (i.e. they stimulate cell division and differentiation), and modulated by binding proteins, which control growth before and after birth (see Ch. 15). This mechanism can explain both the interaction of genetic drive and nutrient supply and the effects of maternal and paternal size. IGF-I increases the efficiency of the placenta so fetal weight increases without a corresponding increase in placental weight. Both IGF-I and IGF-II have anabolic effects via the type I receptor. IGF-II also binds to the type II receptor, which effectively competes with the type I receptor for available IGF-II. It is hypothesized that IGF-II is paternally imprinted; levels of IGF-II promote growth via the IGF-I receptor, whereas the type II receptor, which is maternally imprinted, limits or controls growth by 'mopping up' the free IGF-II (Harding & Johnston 1995). Fetal hyperinsulinaemia appears to inhibit the production of IGF-I-binding protein, thus lifting the restriction on IGF-I and contributing to macrosomia (Wang & Chard 1991). Nutrient availability may promote IGF-I levels and fetal growth. Thus, a balance can be achieved between paternal genes promoting growth and maternal genes restricting and regulating growth

Insulin itself has a growth-promoting effect in the fetus. Maternal hyperglycaemia causes increased

**Fig. 9.17** *Karlberg's model of growth: A sigmoidal curve from a combination of three growth curves; B the curve of weight increase; C the curve of increase in length. (Reproduced with permission from Karlberg et al 1994.)*

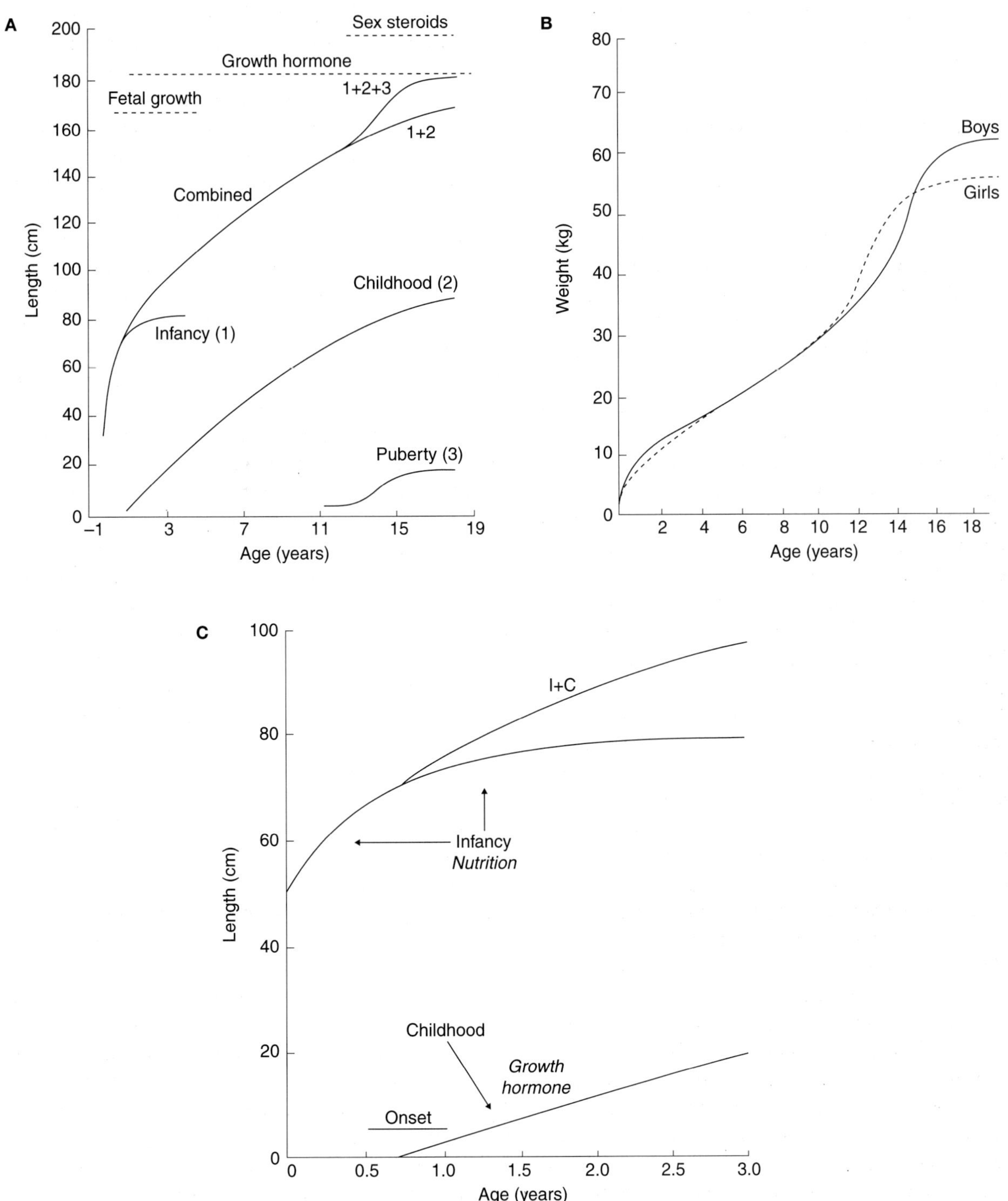


placental transfer of glucose to the fetus. The higher concentration of glucose stimulates the fetal pancreas to produce insulin, which facilitates cellular uptake of glucose, stimulating anabolic metabolism and fetal growth. Babies of diabetic mothers are often macrosomic owing to particularly large fat stores. Fetal insulin deficiency, which is rare, can occur with nutrient deprivation or pancreatic agenesis, and results in fetal growth retardation and decreased levels of body fat and muscle development (Robinson & Owens 1996).

## Maternal and paternal genes

It is suggested that there is a conflict between the maternal and paternal genes governing fetal size (Moore & Haig 1991). Paternal genes favour fetal growth and the transfer of nutrients to the parasitic fetus; if this happens at the expense of maternal health the male can choose a different mate. Maternal genes limit transfer to the fetus to optimize survival of the mother and her children. The father's birth weight influences placental size. Birth weights of mothers correlate with their children's birth weights and even with their grandchildren's birth weights, suggesting that the maternal constraint on fetal growth is set very early (Barker 1998). The paternal effect on the fetal growth trajectory is permitted by the lifting of the maternal constraint on growth. Therefore fetal growth rate responds to, and is appropriate for, the prevailing nutrient availability. Maternal constraint is also a mechanism for limiting fetal growth to maternal pelvis size.

## Maternal nutrition

Fetal growth is related to maternal size (reflecting nutrient level during her own fetal development), maternal body composition (which indicates nutrient supply), nutrient availability in pregnancy and placental efficiency. If periconceptual maternal nutrition sets the growth trajectory early in gestation, the fetal growth rate is more likely to be accommodated by nutrient availability when its demands are high in later gestation. The fetus is able to adapt metabolically to undernutrition in pregnancy by altering its growth rate and sparing nutrients for certain tissues, like the brain. This can lead to disproportionate organ development and fetal growth patterns; fetal adaptations to undernutrition tend to be permanent (Barker 1998).

Maternal nutrition stores correlate with birth weight. Pregnant women exposed to conditions of starvation during the famines during World War II were particularly susceptible to nutrient deficiency in the first half of their pregnancies. Not only was the size of their babies significantly smaller, but the prenatal growth of their grandchildren was also affected (Lumey 1992). Nutrient deprivation later in pregnancy affected birth weights, but the lengths of the neonates were not affected so much and the babies appeared to regain normal weights after birth. However, the metabolic adaptation in those fetuses exposed to nutrient deprivation late in gestation is associated with persistent insulin resistance and a marked trend to develop glucose intolerance and non-insulin-dependent diabetes mellitus (NIDDM) later in life (Phillips 1996).

In humans, dietary intervention studies have had disappointing results, producing improvement in fetal growth only in severely undernourished women (Rush 1989). Part of the problem may be the methodology and ensuring that supplements intended for pregnant women are not used as alternative sources of nutrition or to feed other members of the family. The timing of the nutritional supplements may also be important as fetal growth trajectories may be set before the nutritional status of the mother is improved by the intervention. Women experiencing marginal diets and seasonal famine for generations appear to have evolved strategies to conserve energy by suppressing metabolic rate and acquiring little fat during the pregnancy (Durnin 1987). The energy cost of pregnancy in affluent countries where food is plentiful may be met with little or no increase in energy intake, although economies in energy expenditure may offset the increased requirements (see Ch. 12). Prepregnant size (body fat levels) may direct the trajectory that sets fetal growth via leptin, the product of the *ob* gene (Rink 1994). Appropriate conditions during pregnancy can then fulfil the requirements required for this trajectory to be achieved. In experimental animals, the effect of moderate maternal malnutrition over a number of generations is decreased birth weight, which is maintained for a few further generations even when food supply is restored to a good level (Stewart et al 1980). A plentiful food supply imposed after generations of malnutrition in these animals is associated with obstructed labour and poor fetal outcome.

Maternal nutrition could also exert an effect on fetal growth even before fertilization. The nutritional support of follicular development prior to ovulation and fertilization may affect the growth trajectory of the embryo (see above). Nutrition of the embryo prior to implantation may be important, as demonstrated by IVF. Sheep and cattle embryos from IVF that are cultured for a few days before being replaced in the uterus grow into significantly larger fetuses (James & Stephenson 1998). It is not clear whether IVF affects human birth weight. However, some 'unexplained infertility' in humans appears to be related to an inadequately developed endometrial lining. Couples with a previous history of 'unexplained infertility' have a high rate of small-for-dates infants, which may be associated with poor conditions for implantation (Wang et al 1994).

## Maternal behaviour

Differences in birth weight across different socio-economic groups may be largely attributable to differences in cigarette smoking (Lumley et al 1985). The birth weight appears to fall by about 14 g multiplied by the average number of cigarettes smoked per day. Smoking is associated with a poorer diet and level of healthcare, although effects on oxygen transfer are probably compensated for by 2,3-BPG, which improves the efficiency of oxygen–haemoglobin dissociation (see Ch. 1). Smoking causes nicotine-induced vasoconstriction of the uterine vessels, carbon monoxide inhibits oxygen diffusion and cyanide affects enzyme systems (James & Stephenson 1998). Improving fetal oxygenation in conditions of maternal hypoxia has achieved an improved fetal outcome (Battaglia et al 1992) but there is a controversy about the effect of maternal iron deficiency on pregnancy outcome (Godfrey et al 1991). Alcohol consumption in excess of 40 ml per day is associated with effects on growth (Quellette et al 1977). The use of hard drugs, such as heroin and cocaine, in pregnancy is associated with low birth-weight babies but again it is difficult to dissociate the use of the drugs from the other variables. It is not clear whether caffeine, in either coffee or soft drinks, has an effect on fetal growth.

## Other factors affecting fetal growth

Medical complications of pregnancy or pre-existing diseases can affect fetal growth. Mild maternal hypertension does not restrict growth but severe hypertension is associated with low birth weight particularly if it is complicated with renal disease. Pre-eclampsia is a major cause of low birth weight; it has been suggested that IUGR of unknown cause may be due to undiagnosed pre-eclampsia (see Ch. 8). Severe respiratory and cardiovascular problems and chronic renal disease are also associated with growth retardation. Fetal growth retardation has also been observed in women with congenital uterine abnormalities.

Fetal malformations, especially those due to chromosomal abnormality, are strongly correlated with impaired growth rates. Trisomies and Turner's syndrome have a marked effect on birth weight (James & Stephenson 1998). CVS indicates that in 1–2% of conceptuses tested there is a degree of confined placental mosaicism (where one or more types of placental cells have nuclei with an abnormal number of chromosomes). Placental mosaicism is associated with an increased frequency of IUGR (Robinson & Owens 1996).

Maternal and fetal infections, such as rubella and cytomegalovirus, also detrimentally affect growth. It is not clear whether HIV affects fetal growth as coexisting problems cannot be dissociated. Placental supply of amino acids is close to the minimum required to support fetal protein synthesis. It is possible that the adverse circumstances limiting fetal growth do so by increasing levels of catabolic hormones, such as catecholamines, cortisol and β-endorphin (Robinson & Owens 1996) or by altering the expression of the receptor for IGF-II (Haig & Graham 1991).

## Complications associated with SGA

Babies who are small for gestational age (SGA) have an increased risk of perinatal complications (Box 9.9). Although some catch-up growth may occur postnatally, some of the effects of IUGR may be irreversible (Barker 1998).

Case study 9.2 details the example of a baby with low birth weight.

**Box 9.9**

**Complications associated with SGA**

- Intrapartum hypoxia
- Hypothermia
- Hypoglycaemia
- Necrotizing enterocolitis
- Polycythaemia
- Infection
- Pulmonary haemorrhage
- Sudden infant death syndrome
- Adult onset cardiovascular and metabolic disease

**Case study 9.2**

Razia gives birth to a healthy female infant at term. The baby appears healthy and chubby although she weighs only 2.6 kg.

- Is the midwife right to assume that Asian babies are normally smaller than Western babies?
- What reasons would you give to argue for or against this assumption?

## Key points

- During the 2nd week of development, the inner cell mass differentiates into the bilaminar disc, consisting of two germ layers: the epiblast and hypoblast. The definitive yolk sac is created and the amniotic and chorionic cavities are evident. The differentiated cells migrate and adhere and the genes are switched on and off.
- The embryonic period consists of cell growth (increased cell number and size), differentiation, organogenesis (organization of tissues into organs) and morphogenesis (development of shape). This is the period that is most susceptible to teratogens, which can cause major morphological abnormalities.
- Gastrulation is the major event of the 3rd week. It begins with the appearance of the primitive streak, results in the conversion of the bilaminar disc into a trilaminar disc, consisting of ectoderm, mesoderm and endoderm and establishes the axis for further embryonic development. The neural tube, precursor of the nervous system, and the somites also appear in the 3rd week.
- The trilaminar disc is converted into the characteristic vertebral structure by differential growth of the cell layers causing folding and fusion.
- Weeks 4–8 are the period of organogenesis, differentiation of the major organ systems.
- Fetal growth is influenced by genes and the environment, but limited by nutrient and oxygen supply. Paternal genes tend to favour fetal growth whereas maternal genes tend to constrain fetal growth to a growth trajectory that may be set by environmental influences prior to fertilization.
- The fetus can adapt to undernutrition by altering metabolism and blood flow to protect the brain, albeit at the expense of other organs.

### Application to practice

Understanding of fetal development is required in the explanation of congenital conditions.

Many things, some of which can be affected by advice and guidance of the midwife, for example in regards to smoking, affect fetal growth.

As pregnancy progresses, most women are keen to know how their baby is developing, so the midwife should be able to describe fetal development and growth in an appropriate way.

## Annotated further reading

Barker D J P 1998 Mothers, babies and health in later life, 2nd edn. Churchill Livingstone, New York

*Epidemiological studies link a number of adult diseases with fetal development. This book examines the evidence that fetal adaptation to undernutrition irreversibly alters anatomic, physiological and metabolic development, and links the fetal origins hypothesis to health policy.*

Carlson B M 1999 Human embryology and developmental biology, 2nd edn. C V Mosby, St Louis

*A well-illustrated textbook which covers the molecular basis of development, cellular aspects, developmental anatomy and the progression of development. Includes recent research findings, case studies, timeline information review questions and useful end-of-chapter summaries.*

Fitzgerald M J T, Fitzgerald M 1994 Human embryology: a human approach. Baillière Tindall, London

*This illustrated textbook provides students with an understanding of early human development and the aetiology of many congenital malformations.*

Larsen W J 1993 Human embryology. Churchill Livingstone, New York

*An up-to-date text which covers stages of human development in detail with timelines and sections on the interaction between genetics and human development. Links molecular aspects and experimental principles to clinical applications.*

McLachlan J 1994 Medical embryology. Addison-Wesley, New York

*This book describes human development, focusing on developmental mechanisms, providing a basis for the understanding for the aetiology of congenital defects. It includes evolutionary aspects, methods of monitoring development, prenatal diagnosis and the ethical problems which arise from the calculation of risk.*

Moore K L, Persaud T V N 1998 Before we are born: essentials of embryology and birth defects, 5th edn. WB Saunders, Philadelphia

*This book covers normal and abnormal human development week by week from fertilization through the development of the major organs and physiological systems to birth.*

Moore K L, Persaud T V N 1998 The developing human: clinically orientated embryology, 6th edn. WB Saunders, Philadelphia

*This book is a more detailed description of embryological development, targeted at clinicians, which covers new research findings and their clinical applications. It includes aspects of molecular biology, effects of teratogens and detection of fetal defects.*

## References


Bard J B L, Weddon S E 1996 The molecular basis of mammalian embryogenesis. In: Hillier S G, Kitchener H C, Neilson J P (eds) Scientific essentials of reproductive medicine. WB Saunders, Philadelphia, pp 261–273

Barker D J P 1998 Mothers, babies and health in later life, 2nd edn. Churchill Livingstone, New York

Barker D J P, Gluckman P D, Godfrey K M, Harding J E, Owens J A, Robinson J S 1993 Fetal nutrition and cardiovascular disease in adult life. Lancet 341:938–941

Bassett J 1986 Nutrition of the conceptus: aspects of its regulation. Proceedings of the Nutrition Society 45:1

Battaglia C, Artini P G, Dambrogio G, Galli P A, Sgre A, Genazzani A R 1992 Maternal hyperoxygenation in the treatment of intrauterine growth retardation. American Journal of Obstetrics and Gynecology 167:430–435

Beck F 1996 Human embryogenesis. In: Hillier S G, Kitchener H C, Neilson J P (eds) Scientific essentials of reproductive medicine. WB Saunders, Philadelphia, pp 274–281

Brooks A A, Johnson M R, Steer P J, Pawson M E, Abdalla H I 1995 Birth weight: nature or nurture? Early Human Development 42:29–35

Carlson B M 1994 Human embryology and developmental biology. CV Mosby, St Louis

De Robertis E M, Oliver G, Wright C V E 1990 Homeobox genes and the vertebrate body plan. Scientific American 263(1):46–52

Dobbing J, Sands J 1979 Comparative aspects of the brain-growth spurt. Early Human Development 311:79

Durnin J V G A 1987 Energy requirements of pregnancy: an integration of the longitudinal data from the five-country study. Lancet ii:1131–1133

Fitzgerald M J T, Fitzgerald M 1994 Human embryology, 1st edn. Baillière Tindall, London, pp 23, 241 37, 42

George D K, Cooney T P, Chiu B K, Thurlbeck W M 1987 Hypoplasia and immaturity of the terminal lung units (acinus) in congenital diaphragmatic hernia. American Review of Respiratory Disease 136:947–950

Gluckman P F 1989 Fetal growth: an endocrine perspective. Acta Paediatrica Scandinavica Suppl 349:21–25

Gluckman P F, Harding J E 1994 Nutritional and hormonal regulation of fetal growth: evolving concepts. Acta Paediatrica (suppl) 399:60

Godfrey K M, Redman C W, Barker D J, Osmond C 1991 The effect of maternal anaemia and iron deficiency on the ratio of fetal weight to placental weight. British Journal of Obstetrics and Gynaecology 98:886–891

Goodwin B 1997 Health and development: conception to birth. Open University, Milton Keynes, pp 203–205, 209

Haig D, Graham C 1991 Genomic imprinting and the strange case of the insulin like growth factor II receptor. Cell 64:1045–1046

Harding J E, Johnston B M 1995 Nutrition and fetal growth. Reproduction, Fertility and Development 7:539–547

James D K, Stephenson T 1998 Fetal nutrition and growth. In: Chamberlain G, Dewhurst J, Harvey D (eds) Clinical physiology in obstetrics, 3rd edn. Gower Medical, London, pp 467–497

Karlberg J, Jalil F, Lam B, Low L, Yeung C Y 1994 Linear growth retardation in relation to the three phases of growth. European Journal of Clinical Nutrition 48 (suppl 1):S25–S44

Larsen W J 1993 Human embryology. Churchill Livingstone, New York

Lenz W 1962 Thalidomide and congenital abnormalities. Lancet 1:45

Lumey L H 1992 Decreased birthweights in infants after maternal in utero exposure to the Dutch famine of 1944–1945. Paediatric Perinatal Epidemiology 6:240–253

Lumley J, Correy J F, Newman N M, Curran J T 1985 Cigarette smoking, alcohol consumption and fetal outcome in Tasmania 1981–82. Australian and New Zealand Journal of Obstetrics and Gynaecology 25(1):33–40

McBride W G 1961 Thalidomide and congenital abnormalities. Lancet 2:1358

Martyn C N, Greenwald S E 1997 Impaired synthesis of elastin in walls of aorta and large conduit arteries during early development as an initiating event in pathogenesis of systemic hypertension. Lancet 350:953–955

Moore T, Haig D 1991 Genomic imprinting in mammalian development: a parental tug of war. Trends in Genetics 7:45–49

Moore K L, Persaud T V N 1998a Before we are born: essentials of embryology and birth defects, 5th edn. WB Saunders, Philadelphia

Moore K L, Persaud T V N 1998b The developing human: clinically orientated embryology, 6th edn. WB Saunders, Philadelphia

Moore J, Peters A, Frame S 1984 The relevance of shoe size to obstetric outcome. In: Thomson A, Robinson S (eds) Research and the midwife: proceedings of conference held in the Great Hall, Sparshott House, Manchester Royal Infirmary, Nov 1983. Department of Nursing, University of Manchester, Manchester, pp 53–68

Murtha M T, Leckman J F, Ruddle F H 1991 Detection of homeobox genes in development and evolution. Proceedings of the National Academy of Sciences USA 88:10711–10715

Nardo L, Hooper S B, Harding R 1998 Stimulation of lung growth by tracheal obstruction in fetal sheep: relation to luminal pressure and lung liquid volume. Pediatric Research 43:184–190

Phillips D I W 1996 Insulin resistance as a programmed response to fetal undernutrition. Diabetologia 39:1119–1122

Quellette E M, Rosett H L, Rosman N P, Weiner L 1977 Adverse effects on offspring of maternal alcohol abuse during pregnancy. New England Journal of Medicine 297:528

Reid M 1979 The pulmonary circulation: remodeling in growth and disease. American Review of Respiratory Disease 199:531–546

Rink T J 1994 In search of a satiety factor. Nature 372:406–407

Robinson J S, Owens J A 1996 Control of fetal growth In: Hillier S G, Kitchener H C, Neilson J P (eds) Scientific essentials of reproductive medicine. WB Saunders, Philadelphia, pp 329–341

Rush D 1989 Effects of changes in protein and calorie intake during pregnancy on the growth of the human fetus. In: Chalmers I, Enkin M, Keirse M J N O (eds) Effective care in pregnancy and childbirth. Oxford University Press, Oxford, pp 284–291

Stewart R J C, Sheppard H, Preece R, Waterlow J C 1980 The effect of rehabilitation at different stages of development of rats marginally malnourished for ten to twelve generations. British Journal of Nutrition 43:403–411

Veille J C, Hanson R, Sivakoff M, Hoen H, Ben-Ami M 1993 Fetal cardiac size in normal, intrauterine growth retarded, and diabetic pregnancies. American Journal of Perinatology 10:275–279

Walton A, Hammond J 1938 The maternal effects on growth and conformation in Shire horse–Shetland pony crosses. Proceedings of the Royal Society of London B 125:311–335

Wang H, Chard T 1991 The role of insulin like growth factor-1 and insulin like growth factor binding protein-1 in the control of fetal growth. Journal of Endocrinology 132:11

Wang J X, Clark A M, Kirby C A et al 1994 The obstetric outcome of singleton pregnancies following in vitro fertilization/gamete intra-fallopian transfer. Human Reproduction 9:141–146

# 10 Overview of immunology

## Learning objectives

- To review the immune system, identifying the roles of innate and specific immunity.
- To recognize how pregnancy affects the maternal immune system.
- To outline the effects of HIV infection on the functioning of the immune system.
- To discuss the reasons why the fetus is not rejected.
- To appreciate the importance of placental transfer of immunoglobulins.
- To demonstrate an understanding of Rhesus incompatibility and how it is prophylactically treated.
- To appreciate the immunological immaturity of the neonate and why this is relevant to midwifery practice.
- To understand the principles of neonatal immunization.

## Introduction

Knowledge of the immune system is important in midwifery for several reasons. First, implantation and the nurture of an immunologically foreign fetus present some interesting questions as to the functioning of the immune system in pregnancy. Some causes of infertility may be related to the immunological rejection of the sperm or fetus. During pregnancy, the maternal immune system alters so the fetus is not attacked, but maternal defences against disease still function. Pregnant women have enhanced immunological responses to bacterial infections. However, they seem to develop increased susceptibility to viral infections and human immunodeficiency virus (HIV)-related problems may increase during pregnancy. Some immunology-related conditions improve during pregnancy and some conditions worsen. Maternal immune adaptations in pregnancy also seem to prepare for possible pathogenic contamination of the placental wound site, during the vulnerable period of the puerperium. Blood group incompatibility and the resulting immune response can compromise the well-being of the developing fetus. The neonate is born immunologically immature but receives some passive immunity, both during pregnancy and neonatally in breast milk.

The immune system is a complex network of specialized cells and chemical signals, which interact providing a defence against infectious organisms. A number of microorganisms are associated with the body. Some, described as commensals, exist within or on their host without causing any harm. Others are positively beneficial, or symbiotic, like those inhabiting the skin and the gut. However, some organisms, including microbes (bacteria, viruses, fungi) and larger organisms like tapeworms, are potentially damaging and are described as pathogens because they cause disease. The immune system of the human has evolved to detect and eradicate these pathogenic organisms. Pathogens are diverse and numerous and have a rapid rate of replication and therefore are constantly evolving their own mechanisms to combat the host's defence.

The role of the immune system becomes clearly evident when it is compromised such as in acquired immune deficiency syndrome (AIDS) when HIV causes breakdown of the immune system (Fig. 10.1). However, under less extreme conditions both infections and poor nutrition can overwhelm the immune system. To some extent, both the pregnant woman and the neonate are immunocompromised.

Fig. 10.1 *The effect of HIV on the helper T cell and other cells of the immune system.*

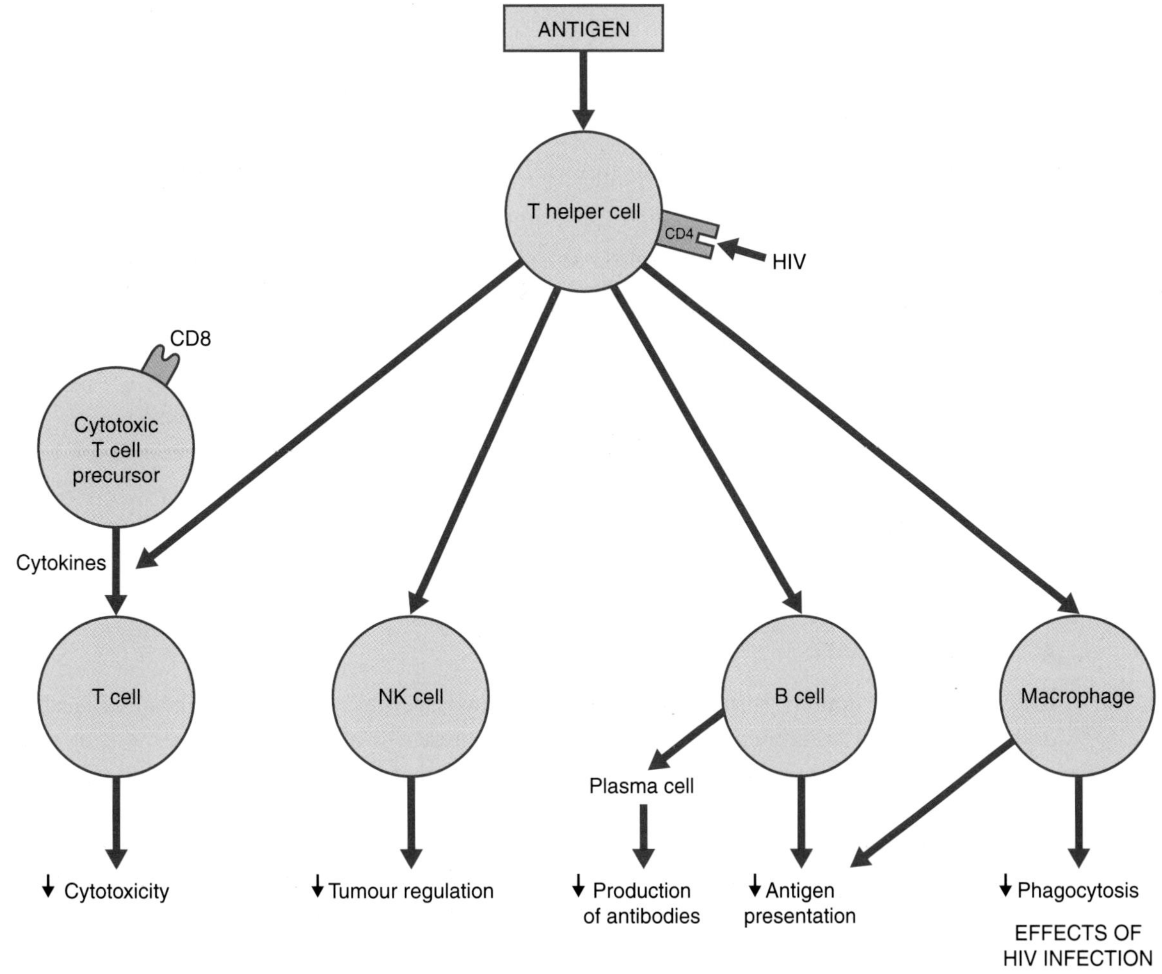


## The evolution of the immune system

The detection of the presence of pathogens initiates the immune response in the host, stimulating a cascade of interactions, which culminates in a counter-attack on the pathogen. There are two types of mechanisms. Innate (natural) immunity pre-exists in an organism before any contact with pathogens. Innate immunity occurs throughout the animal kingdom, occurring in mammals, birds, sponges and worms. It evolved early and is particularly effective against bacteria, probably the earliest form of life on earth. The second mechanism is adaptive immunity, a mechanism that adapts to the presence of pathogens and becomes more effective with each exposure. As organisms became more complex and colonized new habitats they were vulnerable to a broader range of more recently evolved pathogens such as viruses. Adaptive immunity occurs in organisms that evolved relatively recently such as mammals, birds and some fish. It has evolved in response to increased pressure on survival and augments innate immunity.

## Overview of the immune system

### *Innate immunity*

Innate immunity is inherent and does not require contact with a pathogen for responses to occur. The first line of defence can be considered to be the physical and chemical barriers of the respiratory, reproductive and gastrointestinal systems and skin (Brostoff et al 1991) (Fig. 10.2). Included in this first line of

**Fig. 10.2** ***The main physical and chemical barriers to infection (the 'first lines of defence'). (Reproduced with permission from Brostoff et al 1991.)***

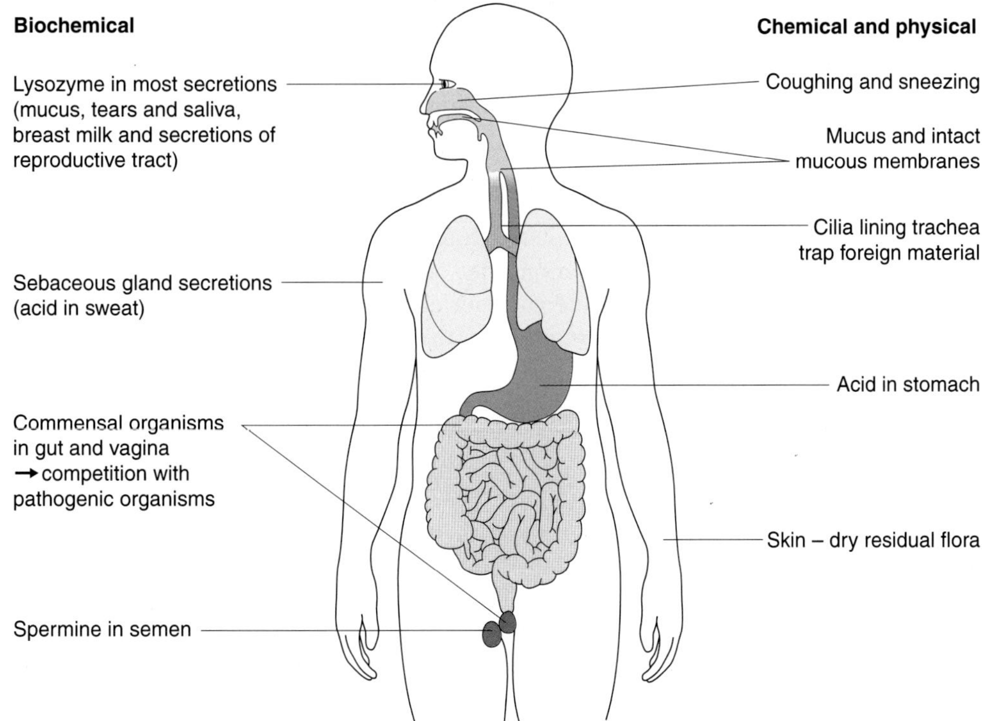


defence are chemical protective mechanisms (such as that provided by lysozyme), the complement system, interferons and phagocytotic activity of the white blood cells (Table 10.1).

## Lysozyme

Lysozyme is an enzyme that attacks the unique polysaccharide structure of bacterial cell walls. It is a component of body secretions such as blood, sweat, tears, nasal secretion, breast milk and the mucus secretions of the reproductive tract.

## Complement

Complement is a system involving as many as 30 interacting proteins and receptors. These form part of an amplification cascade of defence, responsible for

**Table 10.1** ***Defensive activity of the innate immune system***

| | |
|---|---|
| Phagocytosis | Neutrophils and macrophages adhere to the surface of the target organism. Adherence is enhanced by opsonins, which form a bridge between the pathogen and the phagocyte. The phagocytic cells produce pseudopodia facilitating the engulfing of the pathogen into a cellular vesicle. Lysosomes fuse with the phagosome and degrade it |
| Cytotoxicity | Eosinophils and NK cells adhere to targets (opsonins increase efficiency). Eosinophils secrete chemicals, which damage the target cell membrane, causing cell death, and an inflammatory response, which is particularly effective against parasites. NK cells attack body cells expressing viral proteins in their membranes and some tumour cells. The NK cells adhere and release perforin, which penetrates the cell membrane causing cell death |
| Inflammation | The sequence of events is that the trigger (such as a bacteria signal) stimulates vasodilation and increased blood flow and delivery of blood cells (redness, heat and pain). Vascular permeability (swelling) occurs, which increases exudation and extracellular fluid (oedema), phagocyte invasion, promotion of fibrin wall enclosing infection and tissue repair |

destroying bacteria. As in the blood coagulation cascade, the molecular components of the complement cascade exist in an inactive form that can be triggered and activated. The two main triggers are the classic pathway, which involves antibodies (or immunoglobulins), and the alternative pathway, where the complement cascade is activated by the unique composition of an organism's cell wall (activator surfaces). The outcome of complement activation is the formation of a cylindrical assembly of proteins that form a tube that perforates the surface of target cells. The perforation permits fluid to enter cells by osmosis so the bacterial cells swell and burst. The complement cascade stimulates the release of histamine and kinins from mast cells and enhances phagocytosis.

### Interferons

Interferons carry out non-specific defence against viruses. They are specialized proteins produced by cells that have been infected by a virus. Viruses replicate by 'hijacking' the mechanism of protein synthesis in the cells that have been infected. Therefore, the cell is diverted to make viral mRNA, which is translated into viral proteins and assembled as viral particles. Interferons interfere with the production of new proteins; they damage the viral mRNA and inhibit protein translation, not just in the infected cells but in neighbouring uninfected cells—subsequently creating a barrier around the viral infection, which prevents the viral replication.

### Leukocytes and lymphocytes

The cells of the immune system are leukocytes and lymphocytes. Although they are described as white blood cells, some of the cells spend very little time in the circulation whereas others never enter the vascular system at all. Blood cells derive from a single population of stem cells in the bone marrow. These precursor cells have the potential to divide extremely rapidly and can differentiate into several types of end cell. After radiation for cancer treatment, the destroyed stem cells have to be replaced by a bone marrow transplant; very few cells need to be transplanted for regeneration of a mature population of cells.

### Phagocytes

Neutrophils and macrophages are phagocytic white blood cells that can engulf and digest foreign cells and unwanted matter through the processes of phagocytosis, cytotoxicity and the generation of an inflammatory response. The cells that mediate the innate immunity are the granulocytes: neutrophils, monocytes, eosinophils and basophils. Neutrophils, also known as polymorphonuclear leukocytes, are the most numerous white blood cells, forming about 40–70% of the circulating white blood cells. On entering the circulation neutrophils, which have a lifespan of a few days, cease cell division. Neutrophils exhibit chemotactic behaviour, moving through a concentration gradient towards chemical messengers, such as those released from dividing bacteria or activated platelets, towards the site of infection. Neutrophils have multilobed nuclei, which aids diapedesis (the amoeboid movement of the cells through the gaps between the capillary endothelial cells). Neutrophils usually reach the site of infection and begin phagocytosis within about 90 minutes of the initial stimulation.

Adherence of the phagocyte to the target cell can be increased by opsonization. Opsonins are chemical tags that have specific binding sites for the phagocyte and the pathogen, thus increasing the efficiency of recognition and adherence of the phagocyte. Effectively, the opsonin acts as a bridge between the pathogen and the phagocyte, so promoting phagocytosis.

Monocytes circulate for a short time in the bloodstream and then migrate to tissues and organs where they differentiate into macrophages and exhibit characteristics specific to their host tissue. Less than 7% of circulating white blood cells are monocytes, but macrophages are abundantly distributed in the body tissues and are particularly dense around blood vessels, the gut walls, the genital tract and lungs. Monocytes are the largest white blood cell and have a characteristic horse-shaped nucleus. They are also phagocytes and have a longer lifespan than neutrophils. Circulating monocytes respond more slowly than neutrophils, reaching the site of infection within about 48 hours, but they have a greater capacity for phagocytosis, engulfing more material than neutrophils.

### Natural killer cells

The other cells involved in the non-specific innate immune responses are the large granular lymphocytes, such as the natural killer (NK) cells, which are extremely effective in destroying virus-infected cells.

## *Specific immunity*

The small lymphocytes have relatively little cytoplasm that has few organelles and no granules. Small lymphocytes include B lymphocytes, which are responsible for humoral immunity (antibody production), and T lymphocytes, which are responsible for cell-mediated immunity (see Ch. 1). These cells, constituting about a third of the circulating white blood cells, coordinate the adaptive immune response. Small lymphocytes also circulate in the lymphoid system and spend much of the time resident in the organs of the lymphoid system. The lymphoid system is the main site of the adaptive immune responses. Fluid leaks out of the blood capillaries into the intercellular spaces. Some of the fluid re-enters the blood capillary (see Ch. 1) but some enters the lymphatic capillaries. This lymph fluid, therefore, has a similar composition to plasma, except that the protein component of plasma is retained within the blood vessels so lymph fluid has a low protein content. Ultimately the lymph fluid is transported through lymph vessels to the thoracic duct and back into the bloodstream. The small lymphocytes burrow out of the small veins as they pass through the lymph nodes and so enter the lymphoid tissue. Each lymphocyte spends minutes in the bloodstream compared with hours residing in the lymphoid system.

### Antigen recognition

The cells of the immune system differentiate between self and non-self, identifying foreign cells and pathogens and attacking them. The surface of a pathogen is embedded with a unique combination of atoms and charges that can be recognized by the immune cells, almost like an insignia or signature of 'foreignness' or non-self. The whole cell that engenders an immune response is described as an antigen, although the antigenic cluster itself is called the epitope. The antigen *gen*erates an immune response against itself. Antigens are often the pathogenic cell itself but can also be substances secreted by pathogens, for instance bacterial toxins, or substances from non-pathogenic sources, such as plant pollens, resulting in allergic responses, or chemicals such as synthetic vaccines. Antigenicity depends on the ability of the host to identify the substance as an antigen; there are variations in individual responses.

Small lymphocytes have cell surface receptors that specifically recognize antigens presented on the surface of foreign cells and pathogens. Each small lymphocyte has a single type of specific antigen receptor, unlike the cells of the non-specific immune system, which have many different types of receptor on each cell. However, there are many types of small lymphocyte, thus as a population they can recognize and bind to a diverse range of antigens. There are over 100 million pathogenic epitopes. Each person has, at birth, a population of small lymphocytes consisting of clones, each of a few cells. A clone is a few identical small lymphocytes each of which have many copies of the same antigen receptor on its surface. The population of lymphocytes has the capability, described as its repertoire of receptors, to respond to a vast number of antigens, most of which are unlikely to be encountered in a lifetime. Initially the number of cells expressing cells for any particular antigen is small and this clone will remain small unless the antigen reacts. So one of the first steps in mounting an effective immune response is to expand the clone by increasing the number of cells expressing the same antigen.

There are far more antigen receptors than there are human genes encoded for by DNA (about 100 million epitopes and only 100 000 different human genes). It is hypothesized therefore that each antigen receptor site is coded for by five or six randomly selected genes. As there are several hundred possible genes involved, the random selection of a few genes that can be cut and spliced (somatic recombination) can produce enough combinations to make all the 100 million epitope-binding sites. However, in this random production of antigen receptors, some lymphocytes will possess receptors for the body's own antigens. In the fetal thymus, clonal deletion takes place, which results in the destruction of self-reactive T lymphocytes. Any T lymphocyte binding to specialized cells presenting self-epitopes on the surface will be stimulated to undergo apoptosis. Self-reactive B lymphocytes do not need to be destroyed because they require a signal from a T lymphocyte (helper T cell) before they can function. It is important that the immune system has self-tolerance and does not harm cells or molecules that are not recognized as antigenic otherwise the host would be damaged (as happens in autoimmune diseases).

## *Clonal selection and immunological memory*

The immune response to a second and subsequent exposure to the antigen is faster and more effective than the first exposure (Fig. 10.3). The primary adaptive response, on the first exposure, is slow to develop, perhaps taking 7–14 days, and then builds slowly to a peak about 2 weeks later. The time for the response to become evident is termed the 'incubation period'. Then symptoms become apparent until the immune response has become effective. The secondary adaptive response, when the host encounters the antigen subsequently, develops sooner, lasts longer and is more

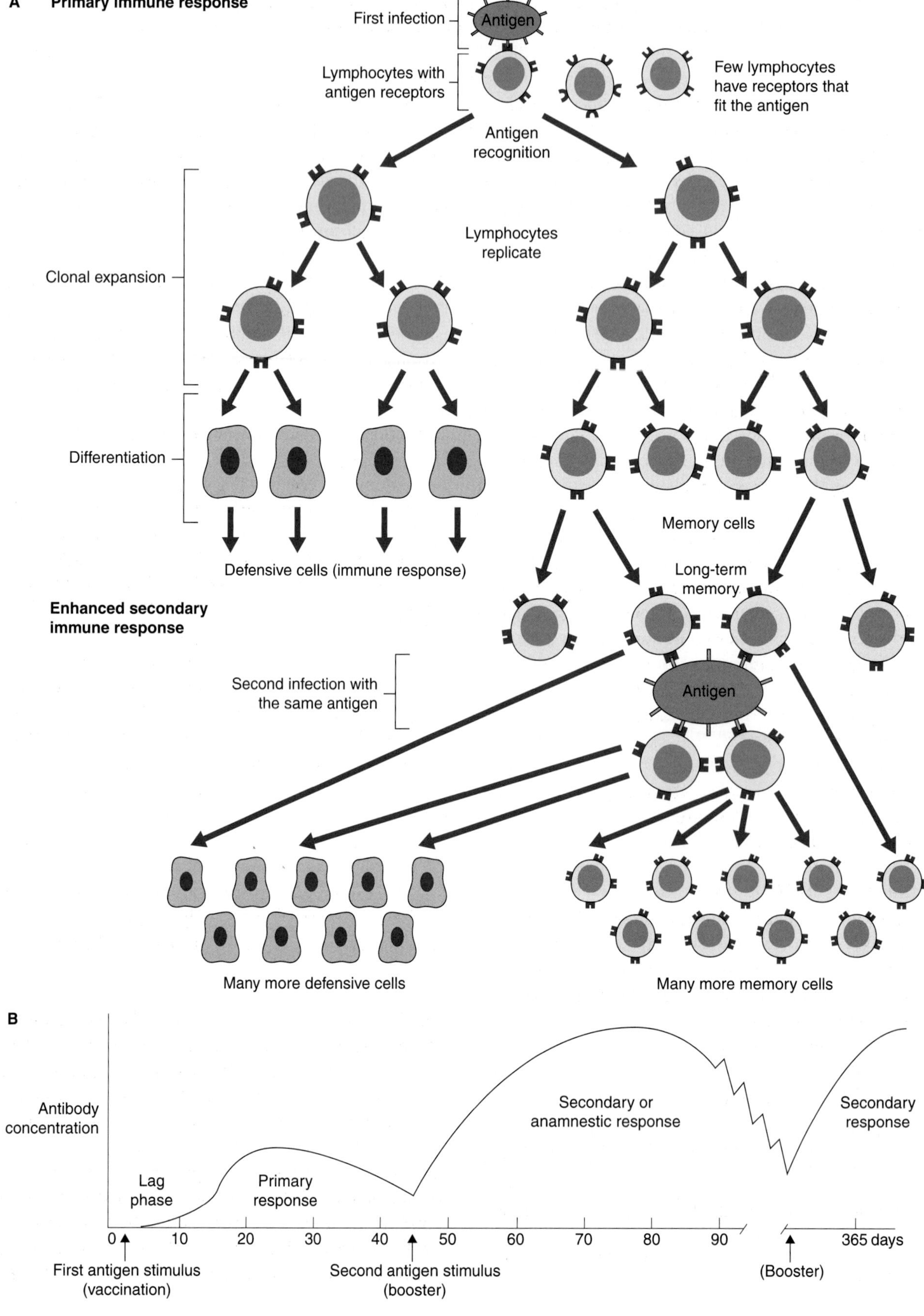
A Primary immune response
First infection
Antigen
Lymphocytes with antigen receptors
Few lymphocytes have receptors that fit the antigen
Antigen recognition
Lymphocytes replicate
Clonal expansion
Differentiation
Memory cells
Defensive cells (immune response)
Long-term memory
Enhanced secondary immune response
Second infection with the same antigen
Antigen
Many more defensive cells
Many more memory cells
B
Antibody concentration
Lag phase
Primary response
Secondary or anamnestic response
Secondary response
0
10
20
30
40
50
60
70
80
90
365 days
First antigen stimulus (vaccination)
Second antigen stimulus (booster)
(Booster)

Fig. 10.3 *A The enhanced secondary immune response after clonal expansion; B graph of antibody production following exposure to antigen. (A reproduced with permission from Stewart 1997.)*

effective so signs of infection or symptoms may be prevented. On first exposure, the small numbers of lymphocytes binding the antigen are stimulated to undergo rapid cell division. A single lymphocyte can divide fast enough to produce 64 000 daughter cells in 4 days. As the new cells, also bearing receptor sites specific to the stimulating antigen, are produced they mature and differentiate. Some members of the new population of lymphocytes are active in attacking the cells bearing the antigen. Others become memory cells, which have a long life and continue to circulate as a permanently enlarged clone of lymphocytes capable of recognizing specific antigens. Effectively, the initial immune response is boosted by repeated exposure.

Individuals have immunity to an antigen if their immune system can mount a fast and effective specific response to that antigen. The role of a vaccine is to stimulate the immune response and increase the clonal size without causing the illness. Effective vaccines can be in the form of killed whole organisms, harmless organisms, substances with similar epitopes, synthetic epitopes or inactivated toxins (Table 10.2). Some antigens are more effective at triggering clonal expansion, such as rubella (German measles) virus, which is highly antigenic; thus after primary exposure the host rarely acquires the infection again. Other pathogens, such as *Neisseria gonococcus* (causing gonorrhoea) and *Treponema pallidum* (causing syphilis), are only weakly antigenic; therefore there are no effective vaccines available.

### Passive immunity

Resistance to a specific pathogen, acquired by previous exposure or deliberate immunization resulting in clonal expansion, is active immunity. However, sometimes, the effect of infection can be disastrous before the immune system has time to mount a response. Passive immunization can overcome this by providing temporary resistance in the form of products from a donor source. Passive immunization causes destruction of the pathogenic cells without creating clonal expansion so its effects are not permanent. An individual who has no prior immunity but is exposed to antigens or a potentially dangerous disease is given antibodies. Examples include treatment following a bite from a rabid dog or anti-D immunization following potential exposure to Rhesus-incompatible antigens (see below). The transfer of placental antibodies to the fetus and consumption of antibodies in colostrum and breast milk by the neonate are also examples of passive immunity.

Case study 10.1 looks at an example of German measles exposure.

Table 10.2 *Types of acquired immunity*

| Active | | Passive | |
|---|---|---|---|
| Natural | Artificial | Natural | Artificial |
| Clinical or subclinical disease | Vaccines: dead or extract attenuated toxoids | Congenital (across placenta) Colostrum | Antiserum Antitoxin Gamma globulin |

**Case study 10.1**

Melanie is expecting her first baby. She attends the midwife's clinic at 11 weeks' gestation concerned over the welfare of her unborn baby. Her 3-year-old nephew, Michael, whom she sees regularly, has German measles.

- What factors would the midwife need to consider in advising Melanie over her concerns?
- Would there be any specific investigations to carry out?

## *Lymphocytes*

There are two types of lymphocytes: those that mature in the bone marrow, called B lymphocytes, and those that mature in the thymus, called T lymphocytes.

### B lymphocytes

On binding to an antigen, B lymphocytes undergo clonal expansion producing two types of daughter cells: memory cells and plasma cells. The plasma cells synthesize and secrete large amounts of antibodies (immunoglobulins), which are specialized glycoproteins. Antibodies enable other components of the immune system to attack the precise organism bearing the antigen fast and effectively. There are five classes of antibody (Table 10.3); these differ in the structure of the 'Y'-shape of the tail, which affects whether the antibodies bind in groups or singly (Fig. 10.4). The

**Table 10.3** *Classes of antibodies*

| Antibody | Role and characteristics |
|---|---|
| IgG | Most abundant antibody (85% circulating antibody), found in blood and all fluid compartments including cerebrospinal fluid. Produced in large amounts at secondary adaptive response, therefore represent 'history' of past exposure to pathogens. Long lasting. Can diffuse out of bloodstream to site of acute infection and can cross placenta. Act as powerful opsonins bridging phagocyte and target cell. Important in defence against bacteria and activation of the complement system via the classic pathway |
| IgM | IgM molecules join in groups of five 'IgM pentamers', therefore tend to aggregate antigens into a clump that is a target for phagocytes and NK cells. Large molecules so cannot diffuse out of bloodstream. Very powerful activators of complement, important in immune responses to bacteria. First antibody produced when the body is confronted by a new antigen |
| IgA | Mostly in secretions such as saliva, tears, sweat and breast milk, especially colostrum. Link in groups of two to three. Protects body by adhering to pathogen and preventing its adherence to body cavity. Cannot activate complement or cross placenta |
| IgE | Tail binds to receptor on mast cells so involved in acute inflammation, allergic responses and hypersensitivity. Binding sites for antigens on larger parasites such as worms and flukes. Some people have IgE for common harmless environmental proteins such as pollen, fur, house dust mite and penicillin |
| IgD | Rarely synthesized; little is known about its functions. Large, found only in blood. May be involved in antigen stimulation of B cells |

**Fig. 10.4** ***A B-cell surface immunoglobulins are receptors for antigens; B the antibody molecule is a hinge-like structure that allows binding to two antigens. (Reproduced with permission from Stewart 1997.)***

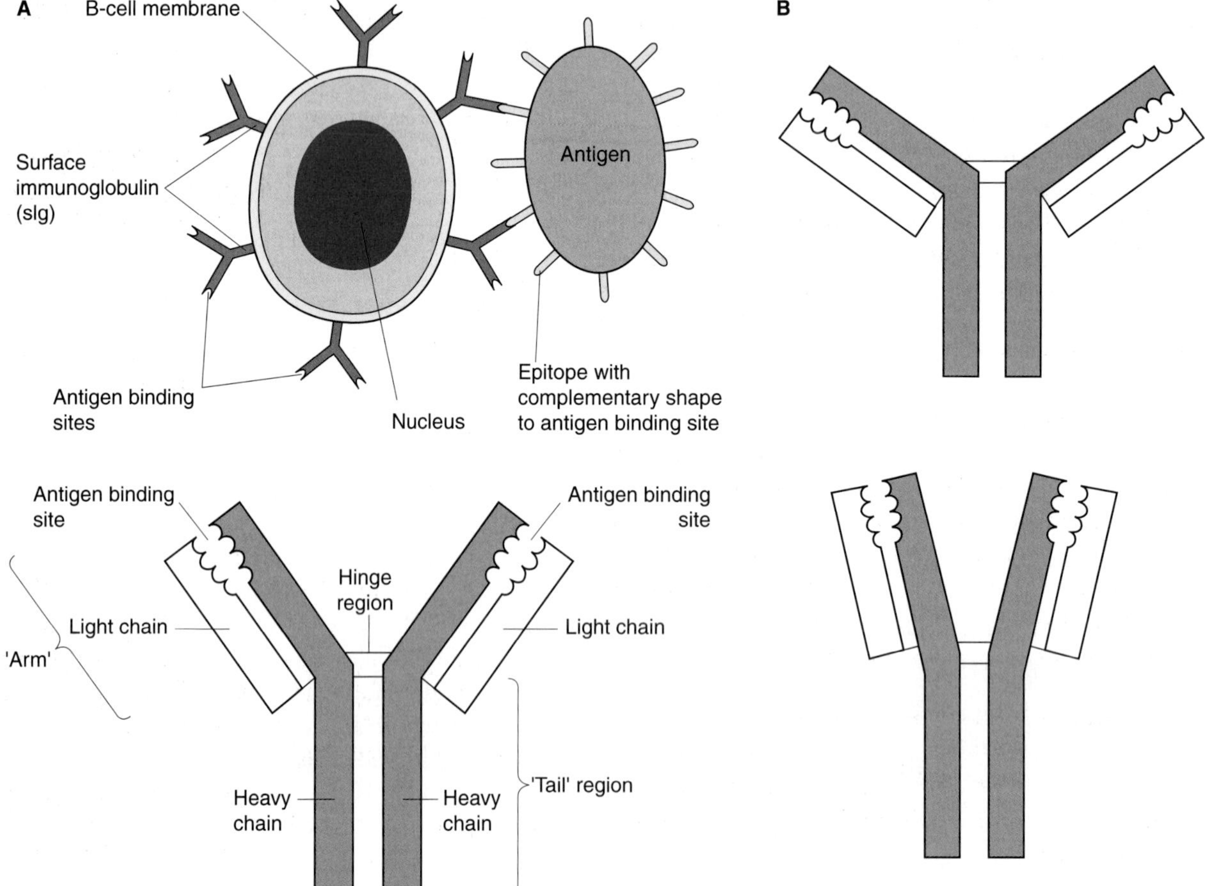

antigen receptor on B lymphocytes is a surface immunoglobulin (sIg) closely resembling the structure of the antibody-binding site that will bind to the same antigen. The binding of the B cell to the epitope is relatively straightforward in that the antigen is intact or native, whereas T lymphocytes bind only to processed antigens. However, antigen binding by a B lymphocyte usually requires helper T-cell activity before clonal expansion can take place.

## T lymphocytes

T lymphocytes stimulate other B and T lymphocytes and are involved in the response to viral infection, graft rejection and suppression of hypersensitivity reactions. There are three subsets of T lymphocytes: helper T cells, suppressor T cells and cytotoxic T cells. Molecules on the cell surface, which are involved in mediating cell function, can be identified using monoclonal antibodies and used to differentiate subpopulations of cells. The system of nomenclature is based on the cluster of differentiation (CD) system. Cytotoxic and suppressor cells express CD8 protein markers in the plasma membrane. Helper cells express CD4 proteins, and are sometimes called CD4 cells.

Helper T cells synthesize and secrete signalling molecules, such as cytokines, which are essential to activate and regulate other components of the immune system. Cytokines are soluble polypeptides with a short range and lifespan that are also synthesized by lymphocytes and macrophages. They can induce fever, stimulate lymphocytes, stimulate antigen expression and potentiate in the destruction of tumour cells. Cytokines include interleukins, interferons, TNF and some colony-stimulating factors. Helper T cells have an important role in stimulating antibody production by B lymphocytes and enhancing the activity of cytotoxic T lymphocytes.

The receptor for HIV is the CD4 protein expressed not only by T cells but also by macrophages and possibly other cells. HIV reduces the number of helper T cells by inducing apoptosis so none of the immune mechanisms work effectively. Infection of macrophages shifts the profile of cytokines produced, which contributes to wasting and acute respiratory distress syndrome. Macrophages can act as a reservoir of the virus.

Suppressor T cells limit the activity of the immune cells and prevent damage to the body's own cells. Cytotoxic cells produce toxic and perforating substances that kill any of the body's own cells that have been infected.

T lymphocytes have antigen receptors on their surface, formed of two peptide chains that contain the binding site for a specific epitope. However, the T lymphocyte cannot bind to an epitope unless it is has been processed and presented to the T lymphocyte by one of the host's own cells. Antigen-presenting cells (APCs) are B lymphocytes and phagocytic cells that bind the antigen and phagocytose it. The epitope fragments are displayed in the cleft of the major histocompatibility complex (MHC) molecule (Box 10.1) on the APC's surface (Fig. 10.5). Helper and suppressor T lymphocytes bind only to epitopes processed in this manner. Cytotoxic T cells recognize the epitopes of intercellular pathogens, such as viruses, that are incorporated into the cell membrane during cell replication of an infected cell harbouring the virus.

## Interaction of B and T lymphocytes

B lymphocytes and T lymphocytes interact (Fig. 10.6). The B lymphocyte binds to the native (intact) antigen via the surface immunoglobulin (sIg) receptors on its

**Fig. 10.5** ***Antigen processing by the APC. (Reproduced with permission from Stewart 1997.)***

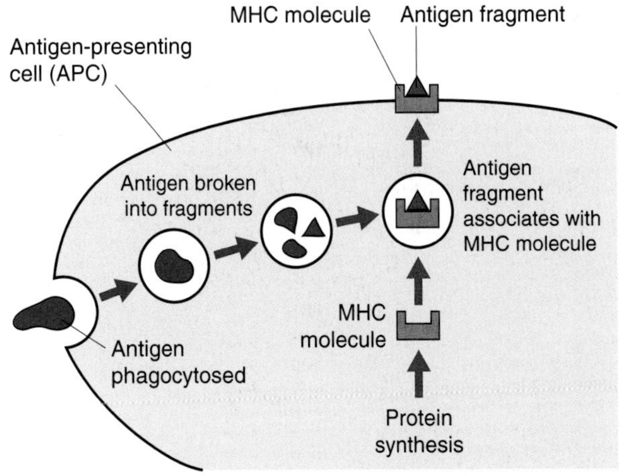


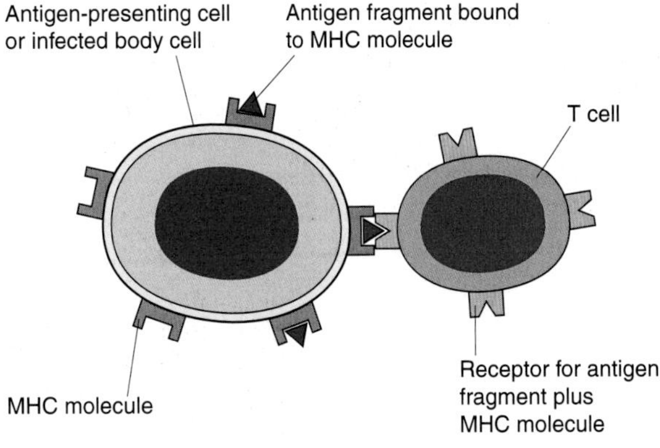

**Box 10.1**

**The major histocompatibility complex**

Each person has a unique configuration of MHC antigens or molecules on the surface of their cells (except monozygous twins who have identical MHC). MHC molecules are a marker of 'self' and are synonymous with human leukocyte antigen (HLA). MHC molecules present the antigens to T cells. There are different classes of MHC molecules, which present antigens with different effectiveness. MHC molecules restrict helper T cells to interact with immune cells that have already bound to the epitope for which the T cell also has an antigen receptor. It is these cells that are involved in rejection of transplanted tissue, as all MHC molecules are different. Tissue grafts have increased survival if there is some similarity in MHC structure between the donor and recipient (hence the need for tissue typing) and if drugs are used to suppress the immune response.

**Fig. 10.6** *The role of three different T cells and their interaction. (Reproduced with permission from Stewart 1997.)*

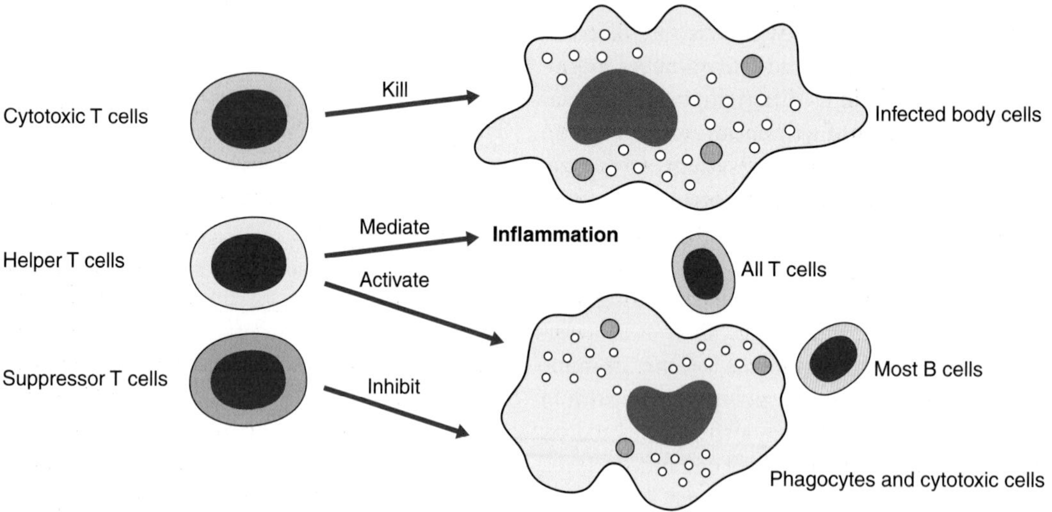


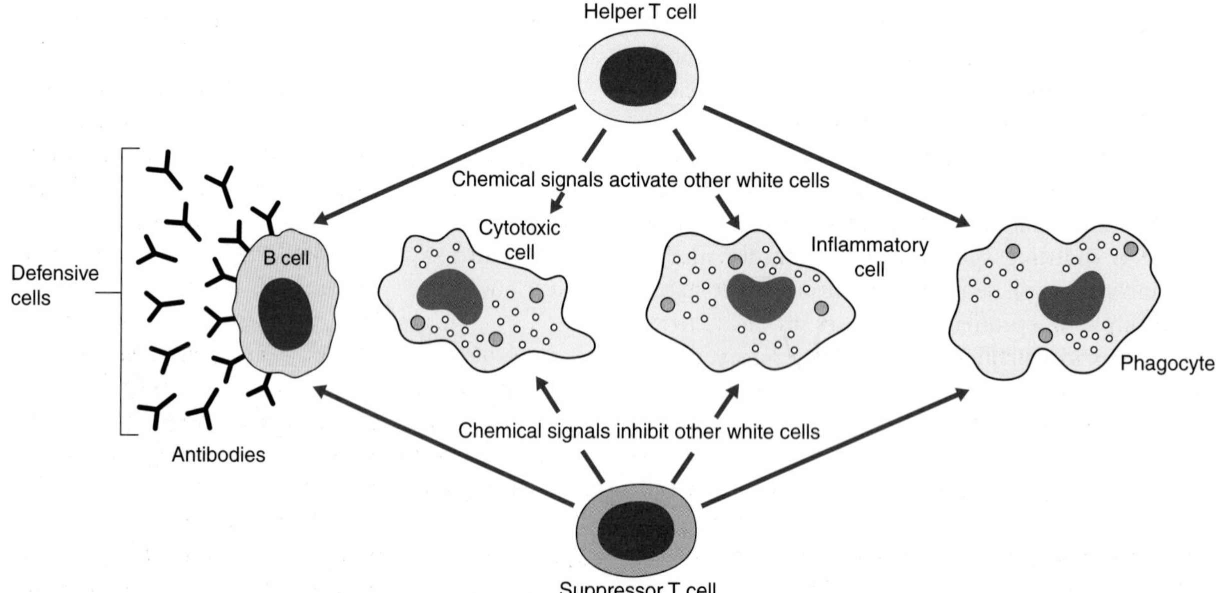

cell surface. The antigen is then internalized by the B lymphocyte and processed so fragments appear on its cell surface associated with the MHC molecule. In this form, the T lymphocytes can recognize it so helper T cells are activated, producing the signal that allows the B lymphocyte to start cell division and differentiation.

## Acceptance of the fetus

Humans are 'outbred'. The genetic diversity resulting from sexual reproduction means that the fetus is phenotypically unique and immunologically distinct from both of its parents. The fetus has a unique combination of histocompatibility antigens. The fetus is classified as an allograft: foreign tissue from the same species but with different antigenic make-up. There is a marked antigenic difference between the maternal tissues and the paternally inherited antigens expressed by the fetus. If tissue from the offspring is grafted on to its mother, a strong maternal immune response is mounted and the tissue is rejected. It seems surprising therefore that the mother does not reject the fetus because of its foreign antigens. Medawar (1953) proposed several possibilities to explain why the fetus is not rejected: as fetal tissue is antigenically immature it may not express normal antigens, the uterus may be a privileged site (or not in contact with fetal tissue), or pregnancy may affect the maternal immune system and normal immune responses.

### Fetal antigen expression

Fetal tissue does express antigens and immunocompetence from an early stage (Manyonda 1998). Major histocompatibility antigens, albeit in smaller amounts, are present on embryonic cells from the time of implantation throughout the pregnancy. Paternal antigens are apparent at the eight-cell stage of the cleavage and major histocompatibility antigens become present later in cell division. The zona pellucida and early trophoblast have glycoprotein coatings, which may limit the cell-mediated immune responses. Immunological problems are usually not a problem prior to implantation because the endometrium secretes immunosuppressive factors.

### The uterus as a privileged site

The mother and other individuals both reject grafts of fetal tissue because fetal tissue expresses antigens. Maternal responses to transplanted tissue remain competent in pregnancy; a pregnant mammal rejects tissue from the father of the fetus and tissue from the fetus grafted to areas other than the uterus. Some tissues, such as parts of the eye and brain, lack components required in immune responses or are not accessible to them (Niederkom 1990). These sites are immunologically privileged and can accept transplanted tissue with fewer problems. However, the uterus is not a privileged site as was suggested (Billingham 1964). The increased vascularization of the pregnant uterus allows efficient delivery of lymphocytes and other maternal immune cells so non-fetal allogenic tissue transplanted in the uterus is rejected (Beer & Billingham 1974). Maternal and placenta tissue are closely related and in intimate contact.

### The chorion and trophoblast as a barrier

The fetus is separated from the mother by the placenta and fetal membranes. It is suggested that the chorionic membranes are resistant to maternal rejection and can protect the fetus from maternal antibodies and immune cells. The placenta and chorion originate from cells derived from the fertilized zygote, which are therefore genetically and antigenically different to the maternal cells. Maternal blood bathes the chorionic villi (see Ch. 8) and is therefore in close contact with tissues derived from the zygote with non-maternal antigens. This means that maternal blood containing immunologically responsive cells is in apposition with the syncytiotrophoblast (outer layer of non-mitotic cells; see Ch. 8).

Some cytotrophoblast cells (the dividing cells underlying the syncytiotrophoblast) penetrate through the syncytiotrophoblast layer to form the cytotrophoblast columns, which anchor the villi to the maternal tissue. During implantation and placental development, other invasive trophoblast cells and fragments break away from the mass of placental tissue and enter the uterine veins and maternal venous system. It is this extravillous (non-villous) trophoblast that remodels the uterine spiral arteries to allow increased maternal blood flow to the intervillous space (see Ch. 8). This extravillous trophoblast layer of cells therefore makes extensive contact with the maternal tissue. Some of the cells breach the trophoblast and invade into the maternal blood system, forming minute emboli which lodge in the pulmonary circulation where they are destroyed.

However, even within the maternal circulation, the extravillous trophoblast cells do not appear to provoke a normal inflammatory or immune response (Johnson & Christmas 1996). So the trophoblast appears to provide an insulating barrier, protecting the fetus from the immunologically responsive maternal cells.

Some components of MHC are absent from trophoblast cells (Faulk & Temple 1976). The trophoblast cells do not express classic antigens, polymorphic class I or class II HLA, at all stages of gestation. Therefore, they are not recognized by cytotoxic T lymphocytes or anti-HLA antibodies (Hunt 1992). Non-trophoblastic placental cells, such as macrophages and stromal cells, do express fetal HLA antigens but are separated from the maternal cells by the HLA-negative trophoblastic barrier. Effectively, the trophoblastic tissue is presented to the mother's immune system as antigenically neutral. However, invasive extravillous cytotrophoblast cells do express a unique (non-classic) class 1 antigen, HLA-G, which is not found in adult tissues (Kovats et al 1990). It is suggested that the role of this antigen may be to mediate intercellular recognition and protect the cytotrophoblast from cytolysis by NK cells and cytotoxic T lymphocytes (Ljunggren & Karre 1990). NK cells recognize and lyse cells that are not recognized by T lymphocytes because they are deficient in class 1 HLA expression.

## The mother's immune response

The mother does respond immunologically to fetal antigens on the trophoblast or entering the maternal circulation. Both lymphocytes and antibodies that recognize fetal antigens are present in maternal blood in pregnancy. In fact, an immune reaction by the mother to the paternal histocompatibility antigen seems to be essential for a successful outcome of pregnancy. The maternal recognition of fetal antigens stimulates the generation of blocking antibodies (Johnson & Christmas 1996). The blocking antibodies mask the antigenic sites preventing maternal cells from binding to the antigens (Singal et al 1984). They could bind to fetal cells in the maternal circulation so they cannot interact with maternal lymphocytes and could cross the placenta to bind to antigenic sites.

It is suggested that a lack of maternal immune response to the fetus could be harmful. The success of fertility and pregnancy is enhanced when the parents are genetically dissimilar (a concept described as 'hybrid vigour'). The incidence of pregnancy where the parents are closely related, as in incest, is far less frequent, which favours heterozygosity within the population. A close relationship between the parents means that the fetal antigens will be more similar to the maternal antigens so the maternal immunological response will be less.

Conversely, embryo implantation into a surrogate mother, where the embryo is less related to the mother than in a normal implantation, has a higher success rate. It has been suggested that unexplained recurrent spontaneous abortion (RSA; more than three consecutive early pregnancy miscarriages) may be due to a failure of maternal immunological adaptation (Fraser, Grimes & Schulz 1993). Other known causes of RSA include chromosome and endocrine abnormalities, anatomical problems and infections of the mother's reproductive system. It was controversially hypothesized that increased similarities of antigens between parents (described as HLA parental sharing) would result in the fetus having a high degree of antigen similarities with its mother. The mother would then not produce such a strong immune response to fetal cells, with perhaps fewer blocking antibodies, which would prejudice the outcome of the pregnancy. However, immunotherapy treatment for RSA where women are immunized with paternal cells has not been successful (Fraser, Grimes & Schulz 1993).

Fetal lymphocytes inhibit replication of stimulated lymphocytes in both the mother and unrelated individuals. This may account for the increased number and increased severity of maternal viral infections, especially in the later part of gestation. Trophoblastic cells express high levels of three membrane-bound complement-regulatory proteins that thwart potential complement-mediated damage to the trophoblast by either the classic or alternative pathways (Rooney, Ogelesby & Alterson 1993).

The placenta is in contact with fluids containing high concentrations of progesterone, corticosteroids and hCG, which may act as local immunosuppressants and inhibit the effectiveness of immune cells. The uterine endometrium has extensive numbers of white blood cells, constituting up to a third of endometrial cells (Bulmer 1989). The macrophages are highly activated and secrete substantial amounts of interleukin and IgE, which may play a vital role in immunosuppression and rapid non-specific anti-inflammatory activity. T lymphocytes are present but B lymphocytes are uncommon. There are also numerous large neutrophil-like granular cells which appear similar to peripheral blood NK cells. These uterine large granular leukocytes (U-LGL) seem to be hormonally regulated as they occur in decidualized tissue in extrauterine ectopic pregnancies. They have low cytolytic activity and are probably not involved in removal of damaged embryonic cells or regulating trophoblastic invasion. However, they do produce cytokines, which may be important in immunosuppression and growth regulation. IgA, secreted from the cells lining the uterine tubes, may also be important in protecting the uterine environment.

## Effects of pregnancy on the immune system

The maternal immune response is affected by pregnancy. The number of white blood cells, particularly neutrophils, increases and the cells respond more readily to challenges. hCG stimulates neutrophil production and response (Barriga, Rodriguez & Ortega 1994). The high levels of oestrogen and progesterone decrease the number of helper T cells and increase the number of suppressor cells. Yeast infections increase in pregnancy, possibly because of the effect of oestrogen on the flora of the reproductive tract.

Local concentrations of corticosteroids around the fetus and placenta suppress phagocytic activity, especially in response to gram-negative bacteria. This means that pregnant women have a decreased ability to respond to gram-negative infections of the reproductive tract such as gonococcal infection (Gibbs & Sweet 1994) and *Escherichia coli*. Components of the complement cascade increase from the end of the first trimester so chemotaxis and opsonization are enhanced. Changes like this, which do not occur at the beginning of pregnancy, may be delayed to protect the fetus during implantation.

### NK cells and cytokines

NK-cell activity around the uterus is suppressed by local increased concentrations of prostaglandin $E_2$ (Daunter 1992). This suppression of NK cells may be important in preventing rejection of the fetus. However, maternal resistance to intracellular pathogens such as *Toxoplasma* and *Listeria* may also be reduced (Wegmann et al 1993). The relative proportions of cytokines change in pregnancy. The association between chorioamnionitis and premature rupture of membranes may be related to cytokine-mediated stimulation of proteolytic enzyme released from neutrophils.

Theoretically, the fetus could be perceived by the maternal immune system as a tumour. The conceptus may secret cytokines, which affect tissues locally, promoting trophoblast growth and fetal survival (Wegmann et al 1993). Concentrations of cytokines that attack tumours, such as TNF, and stimulate NK cell activity, such as interleukin-2, are suppressed. Local secretion of such cytokines may be important in protecting the fetus without compromising maternal immune function.

### Antibodies and B lymphocytes

The levels of most antibodies do not change during pregnancy. However, IgG concentrations may fall. This fall may be due to haemodilution, increased loss in urine or placental transfer of IgG in the third trimester and it can increase the risk of streptococcal infection. Fetal secretion of cytokines may suppress cell-mediated immunity and enhance humoral responsiveness (Wegmann et al 1993). Systemic lupus erythematosus (SLE), an autoimmune condition causing tissue damage in the joints and kidneys, has an increased 'flare-up' frequency in pregnancy, which may be related to enhanced activity of B lymphocytes. This enhanced responsiveness by B lymphocytes may compensate for decreased T lymphocyte activity. B lymphocytes may also produce blocking antibodies which protect the fetus from attack by maternal T lymphocytes.

### T lymphocytes

T lymphocytes are involved in graft rejection and could therefore pose a serious threat to the fetus. However, T-cell function is suppressed in pregnancy, especially in the first trimester (Nakamura et al 1993). Circulating numbers of T lymphocytes are lower and they have decreased ability to proliferate, to produce interleukin-2 and to kill foreign cells. Ratios of helper and suppressor cells change. Rheumatoid arthritis, a cell-mediated autoimmune disease, frequently goes into remission during pregnancy, because of the suppression of T lymphocytes. The amelioration of symptoms in pregnancy led to the identification of glucocorticoids as anti-inflammatory agents (Hench 1952). Hormonal changes in pregnancy may augment the suppression of T lymphocytes. As T lymphocytes are involved in the responses to viral infection, pregnant women are at increased risk of viral infections and may experience more severe viraemia.

### Susceptibility to infection

As maternal immune responses are suppressed in pregnancy, to favour acceptance of the fetus, a pregnant woman may have increased susceptibility to infection. Historically, pregnant women were observed to contract smallpox and poliomyelitis more readily. Today, viral hepatitis infections, particularly in developing countries, pose a major threat to pregnant women, who have 10 times the infection rate of non-pregnant women and experience higher morbidity and mortality rates. Women who lack immunity and are exposed to primary cytomegalovirus (CMV) have an increased susceptibility to infection in pregnancy, which is associated with fetal congenital abnormalities. Pregnant women have an increased susceptibility to listeriosis, influenza, varicella (chickenpox), herpes, rubella (German measles), hepatitis and human papillomavirus. In addition, a number of latent viral diseases and other infections may be of greater severity. These include malaria, tuberculosis (TB), Epstein–Barr virus and HIV-associated infections (Wegmann et al 1993), which can be reactivated in pregnancy. Pregnancy-induced suppression of helper T-cell numbers may be permanent so pregnancy can cause a progression of HIV-related disease. Pregnant women appear to have increased immunological responses to bacterial infection. However, increased incidences of urinary tract infections are probably related to anatomical changes rather than altered immunological responses.

## Fetal and neonatal passive immunity

The neonate's immune system is augmented by maternal transfer of immunoglobulins across the placenta to the fetus and in breast milk. The profile of immunoglobulins transported across the placenta and secreted into breast milk depends on specific transport mechanisms for the different classes of immunoglobulin (see Table 10.3). Maternal IgG crosses the placenta into the fetal circulation via a specific active transport mechanism, which is effective from around 20 weeks' gestation but markedly increases in activity from 34 weeks. The mother will produce an immune response to antigens she encounters by producing IgG, which can cross the placenta. Even if maternal levels of IgG are low they will be transported across the placenta. This means that the fetus will receive passive immunization against prevalent pathogens likely to be in the environment from birth. This passive immunity provides essential temporary protection postnatally until the neonate's own immune system matures and produces its own antibodies. Preterm babies are at risk of transient hypoglobulinaemia because they receive less IgG and they are born with immune systems that are less mature than a term infant's. Placental dysfunction limits the transfer of IgG, therefore SGA babies have lower levels of IgG. IgA, IgM and IgD do not cross the placenta but are supplied in high concentrations in the colostrum.

As well as beneficial IgG, potentially harmful IgG can cross the placenta. Maternal antibodies to fetal HLA will be generated as the maternal immune system encounters a few fetal cells. The maternal anti-fetal HLA antibodies will cross the placenta but do not cause any damage as they bind to non-trophoblastic cells in the placenta, which bear fetal HLA and can sequester maternal IgG (Johnson & Christmas 1996). In autoimmune diseases, however, pathogenic maternal antibodies can be transferred across the placenta. For instance, antiplatelet antibodies can cross the placenta into the fetus of a mother with autoimmune thrombocytopenic purpura (Johnson & Christmas 1996). The passive transfer of autoimmune antibodies may affect fetal growth and development and can potentially cause at least transient symptoms of the disease in the neonate. The resulting increased risk of haemorrhage in babies born to mothers with thrombocytopenia means that traumatic procedures, such as fetal blood sampling and instrumental delivery, are avoided.

### The Rhesus factor and Rhesus incompatibility

In the last trimester, the placental transfer of maternal IgG will include IgG antibodies directed against the fetus's own antigens. Most of these are thought to bind to non-trophoblastic cells bearing fetal antigens within the placental villous tissue so they do not reach the fetal circulation. However, antibodies to the Rhesus antigen can cause severe complications. People who express the Rhesus antigen on their own red blood cell surface do not make antibodies against the Rhesus antigen. These people are described as Rhesus positive (Fig. 10.7). A mother who is Rhesus negative does not have the Rhesus antigen on her own red blood cell

Fig. 10.7 ***A Rh-negative woman can be sensitized when red cells from Rh-positive fetus cross placenta into her circulation. B Response comes after delivery of first fetus but in subsequent pregnancies, maternal antibodies can cross placenta and damage fetus. C Anti-D gamma globulin given to mother immediately at delivery results in fetal Rh-positive cells not being recognised by maternal immune systems, so antibodies are not produced to endanger subsequent pregnancy.***

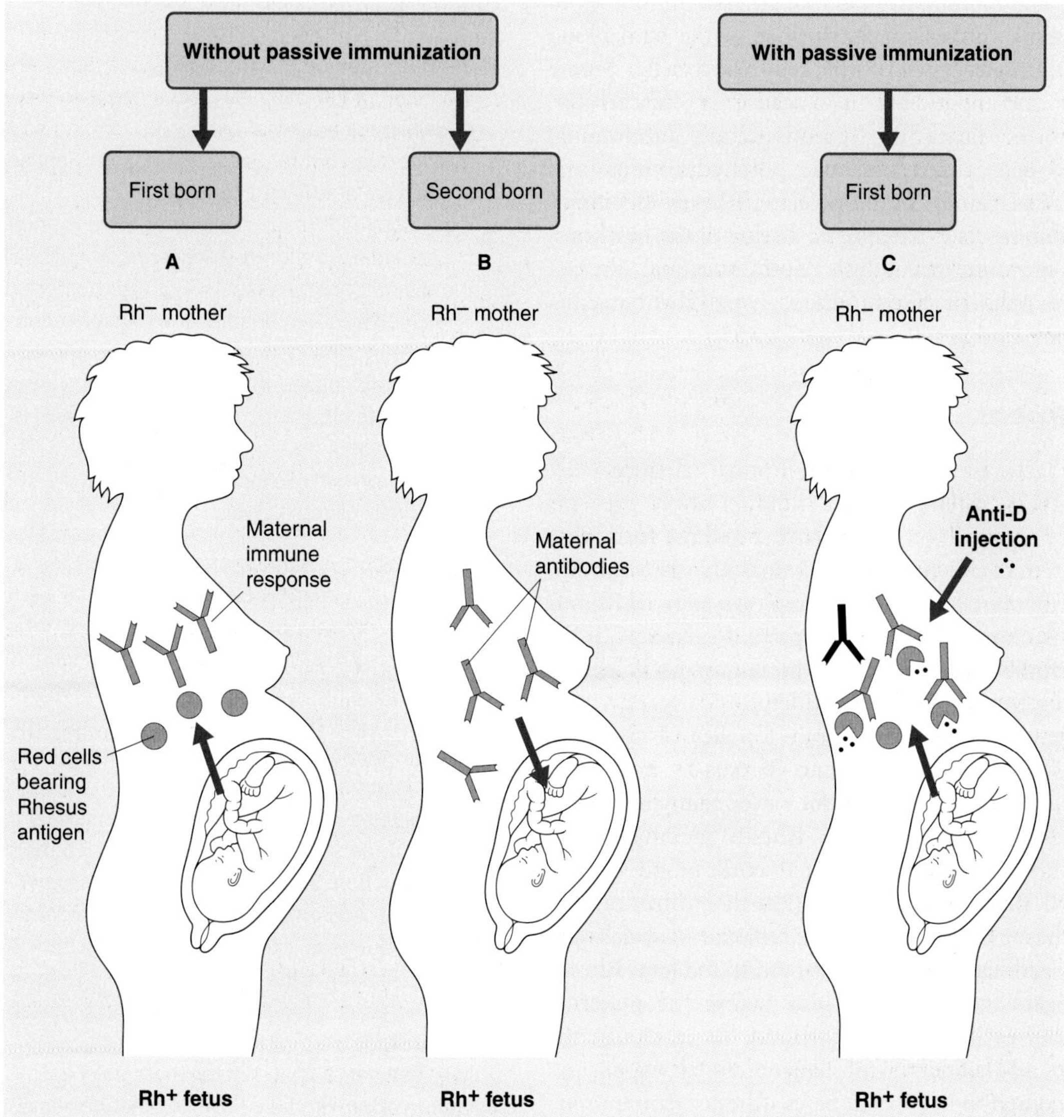


surface and her immune system has the capability of making Rhesus antibodies.

The Rhesus antibody is not preformed (existing from birth) like the antibodies of the ABO blood grouping system. Rhesus antibodies are produced if the immune system is given the opportunity to recognize the Rhesus antigen as a foreign protein. In practice, this means that a Rhesus-negative mother could produce antibodies to the Rhesus antigen (which would recognize and attack the red blood cell of a Rhesus-positive fetus) if her immune system encountered it. The immune response can be generated from exposure to red blood cells bearing the Rhesus antigen, for instance from transplacental leakage of Rhesus-positive fetal cells (following delivery or miscarriage) or in rare instances from a Rhesus-positive blood transfusion.

The occasion when Rhesus isoimmunization is most likely to occur is at the time of the third stage of labour. During placental separation, there is the potential for a small amount of fetal blood (perhaps half a millilitre) to cross into the maternal circulation. As this blood is Rhesus positive, it could stimulate the maternal immune cells to respond by clonal expansion, developing the capacity to produce large quantities of

IgG. Once a woman makes antibodies to Rhesus antigens, she is isoimmunized for life. These IgG antibodies can then be transported across the placenta to the fetal circulation late in gestation of a subsequent pregnancy. The binding of maternal Rhesus antibodies to the Rhesus antigen on the surface of the fetal blood cells stimulates lysis of the red blood cells. Severe Rhesus incompatibility is a cause of miscarriage, intrauterine death or hydrops fetalis (abdominal ascites, generalized oedema, polyhydramnios and enlarged placenta). In the neonate, Rhesus incompatibility can result in haemolytic disease of the newborn, where profound haemolysis causes anaemia, increasing the risks of heart failure, hyperbilirubinaemia (jaundice) and kernicterus (see Ch. 15).

## Treatment

Prophylactic treatment has been practised since 1967 (Box 10.2). Giving passive immunization prevents primary sensitization of the mother and the formation of cells that can produce IgG anti-Rhesus antibody. Although there is actually a complex system of Rhesus antigens, controlled by three pairs of genes (Cc, Dd and Ee), the Rhesus D antigen predominates in incompatibility between mother and fetus.

Most maternity units operate a policy of giving all Rhesus-negative women anti-Rhesus-D antiserum within 72 hours of delivery. However, many maternity units delay treatment until Rhesus incompatibility is confirmed from a umbilical cord blood sample (Box 10.3). If a small volume (less than 5 ml) of fetal blood has entered the maternal circulation at delivery, the exogenous antibodies will bind to the fetal Rhesus D antigen and cause cell lysis before the maternal lymphocytes have the opportunity to recognize the antigen and undergo subsequent clonal expansion. ABO compatibility exacerbates Rhesus isoimmuniz-

**Box 10.2**

**Prophylactic anti-D immunoglobulin treatment**

- Delivery of Rhesus-positive baby
- Spontaneous abortion
- Therapeutic termination of pregnancy
- Threatened abortion
- Antepartum haemorrhage
- Following external cephalic version of breech presentations
- Following CVS, amniocentesis or other invasive intrauterine procedure

**Box 10.3**

**Maternal and cord blood tests**

When a mother is Rhesus negative, a sample of the baby's blood is obtained from the umbilical cord. Two tests are performed:

1. the baby's blood group and Rhesus factor are identified; if the baby is Rhesus negative there is no possibility of maternal antibodies forming so the mother does not require anti-Rhesus-D antiserum (known as 'anti-D') administration
2. if the baby is Rhesus positive or there is another maternal/fetal antibody/antigen incompatibility then the direct Coombes test would also be performed. The Coombes test enables the differentiation between normal neonatal haemolysis and abnormal haemolysis caused through the action of maternal antigens. It is based on three variables and is positive when there is a reduced haemoglobin in conjunction with an increased reticulocyte count and raised bilirubin levels.

Maternal blood is also taken so that the Kleihauer test (Kleihauer, Hildergard & Betle 1957) can be performed. The test is based upon the resistance of fetal blood cells to be destroyed by acid (acid elution test). Not only does the test allow the presence of fetal erythrocytes to be detected but the amount of fetal blood transfused into the maternal circulation can be estimated as well. The test is not as accurate if there are maternal haemoglobinopathies present as abnormal maternal erythrocytes (such as sickle cell disease) are also resistant to acid destruction. The test may also be falsely negative if there is an A/B incompatibility as the maternal anti-A and/or B antigens quickly destroy the fetal erythrocytes, especially if the Kleihauer test is delayed, so it should be conducted within half an hour of delivery of the third stage.

It is estimated that a fetal–maternal blood transfer occurs in approximately 50% of pregnancies (Zipursky et al 1959). Usually the amount of blood is small, less than 0.5 ml. However, in 8% of pregnancies it may be in the range of 0.5–40 ml and in 1% it may well exceed 40 ml. In most cases 500 IU of anti-Rhesus-D antiserum is enough to eradicate the misplaced fetal erythrocytes. However, if a large transfusion is suspected then larger doses will be administered. If an exceptionally large transfusion is suspected following the administration of anti-Rhesus-D antiserum the Kleihauer test should be repeated and if fetal cells are still detected then further doses of anti-Rhesus-D antiserum would be administered.

ation so ABO incompatibility offers a degree of protection against Rhesus sensitization. If the fetal blood transfused is of a different ABO grouping, the existing natural maternal IgM anti-A or anti-B antigens will rapidly eliminate the fetal blood cells before an immune response can be mounted against the Rhesus-D antigen.

### *Other antibodies*

Most antibodies in the ABO system are IgM type so they do not cross the placenta. However, in successive ABO-incompatible pregnancies in group O mothers, a degree of neonatal haemolysis, causing mild neonatal jaundice, may occur. Haemolytic disease can potentially occur with other blood group incompatibilities such as Kell and Duffy. However, the density of these minor antigens on fetal red blood cells is so low that maternal IgG antibodies usually do not elicit a cytolytic effect.

## Vulnerability of the neonate

Neonates are born immunocompromised and are susceptible to infection. The natural flora colonizes and protects the external surfaces of the body, and those membranes that appear external but come into contact with external pathogens, such as the upper respiratory tract, gut and urinary system. The natural flora may protect by competing with pathogenic micro-organisms for resources or by altering the local environment making it less hospitable to pathogens. The fetus in the uterus is sterile because there is no route for colonization. Colonization takes about 6–8 weeks, which is similar to the time that NASA (North American Space Agency) astronauts, who are made bacteriologically sterile before a space flight, take for the resident flora of non-pathogenic bacteria to repopulate. As the bowel flora produces much of the body's vitamin K requirements, neonates have an increased risk of vitamin K deficiency until the resident flora is established. Colonization processes can be disrupted, for instance, by disinfectant swabs or antibiotic use. Colonization of the neonate begins at birth, with transfer of organisms from the mother's vagina, skin of her hands and breasts and the respiratory tracts of the baby's carers.

Neonatal skin is delicate and easily damaged, which can offer a route for opportunistic infection. The umbilical cord, which becomes necrotic, presents a locus for possible infection and offers a potential pathway to the liver. The neonatal defence mechanisms are further compromised by procedures, such as blood sampling or insertion of endotracheal or nasogastric tube or intravenous cannulas.

Infants have less efficient immune systems, especially if they are born prematurely or are small at birth. The cells of the immune system are immature and do not function as efficiently in early life; for instance, T lymphocytes have decreased responses and cytolytic function. The phagocytes exhibit decreased phagocytosis and bactericidal activity. Their function in severe illness, such as respiratory distress syndrome or meconium-aspiration pneumonia, is further limited. The complement cascade components at birth are 50–80% of the adult levels.

### *Active immunization*

The immature immune system of the neonate is supported by natural passive immunization from placental transfer of IgG and breast milk provision of IgA. It is also supported by programmes of deliberate immunization. Active immunization requires administration of an antigen in a form that is inactivated and does not produce a disease (Box 10.4). IgG levels start to increase by 3 months so immunization is delayed after birth. However, some protection is required before the immune system is mature. Therefore, immunization programmes are often started when the baby is 3 months old. At about this age, many babies receive the 'triple' vaccine, of pertussis, diphtheria and tetanus antigens presented appropriately. Diphtheria and tetanus elicit a strong antigenic responses despite the infant's immature immune system, whereas children are given further doses of pertussis vaccine. Live polio vaccine is given orally at the same time as the 'triple' vaccine. Although theoretically only one dose is required, there are at least three strains and the immune response may not be produced the first time. Measles vaccine is usually delayed until the infant is about a year old as maternal IgG, which is present for the first 6 to 9 months of life, tends to destroy the attenuated organisms of the vaccine before the infant's immune system has time to recognize and respond to them.

Immunization using viral vaccines may be ineffective if the individual has had a recent viral infection, such as a cold. Levels of interferon persist after a viral

**Box 10.4**
**Principles of immunization**

**Adjuvants**

For example, aluminium hydroxide or phosphate. Increases antigenic properties of a vaccine that would otherwise produce only a weak immune response, e.g. triple vaccine of diphtheria, tetanus and pertussis toxins

**Toxoid**

Bacterial exotoxin treated so it does not cause a disease but still stimulates the immune cells. Examples include treatment of diphtheria and tetanus toxin with formalin

**Killed vaccine**

Dead organisms such as pertussis, typhoid and paratyphoid. As with toxoid preparations, two or three doses and booster doses required as only a small number of antigens introduced each time

**Attenuated vaccines**

Live organisms that have been cultured to produce non-pathogenic strains. Very effective as organisms multiply within body mimicking a natural infection. Therefore only one dose is required for full immune response (lifetime immunity), e.g. smallpox, poliomyelitis, measles, rubella, TB

infection so the virus in the vaccine preparation may not be able to reach concentrations adequate to stimulate the immune system. Therefore, immunization may not be effective until 2–3 weeks after a viral infection. Oral doses of vaccines may be ineffective if their absorption is compromised, for instance with diarrhoea or vomiting. High levels of steroids suppress the immune response, so steroid therapy or overactive adrenals can limit the effectiveness of a live vaccine and compromise the immune response. Allergic reactions can occur, especially to vaccines prepared in tissue culture or containing whole cells. Problems with allergic reactions are often associated with vaccines grown in egg-based tissue culture preparations or where antibiotics are added. Obviously, a severe reaction to a vaccine precludes its further use. Administration of live vaccines is not recommended in pregnancy. Immunization programmes benefit the health of the population, unfortunately at the expense of the few individuals who may have an extreme reaction to a vaccine with irreversible effects.

## Other immunological aspects of pregnancy

Antisperm antibodies in either the male or female partner have been implicated in the causes of infertility (Manyonda 1998). Antisperm antibodies could inhibit spermatogenesis or fertilization. However, the Sertoli cell protects the developing sperm and seminiferous tubules from antibodies and suppressor T cells secrete immunosuppressive cytokines in the epididymis. Some are coated with glycoproteins and lactoferrin, which may be why some antigen sites are evident only after capacitance. Seminal fluid has potent immunosuppressive properties and can inhibit a range of immune responses (James & Hargreave 1988). The presence of antisperm antibodies in the secretions from the genital tracts, rather than in the blood, seems important particularly in male infertility. The risk of developing antisperm antibodies is increased with exposure to sperm that is excessive, as in prostitutes, or in an inappropriate site, as in homosexual men (Johnson & Christmas 1996). Generation of antisperm antibodies may reflect a lack of immunosuppressive factors in the seminal fluid.

Endometriosis, which is deposition of endometrial tissue at non-uterine sites, can be very painful if the tissue becomes inflamed. Severe endometriosis can cause infertility but many women have extrauterine endometrial tissue that neither causes pain nor affects fertility. The cause of endometriosis is not known but an autoimmune aetiology has been proposed.

Pre-eclampsia, inadequate placental development following inadequate remodelling of the spiral arteries, is also suggested to have an immune component (see Ch. 8). The incidence of pre-eclampsia is higher in first pregnancies and in subsequent pregnancies with a new partner, which suggests an immunological mechanism.

The effects of HIV and AIDS in pregnancy are detailed in Box 10.5 and Case study 10.2.

**Box 10.5**

**HIV and AIDS in pregnancy**

- HIV (human immunodeficiency virus) causes AIDS (acquired immunodeficiency disorder)
- HIV is a retrovirus, which invades cells expressing CD4, including helper T cells, monocytes and neural cells
- A retrovirus contains a single strand of RNA, which is incorporated into the host cell's DNA by an enzyme called reverse transcriptase
- When the infected cell is activated it will produce viral proteins, which can be released and infect other cells
- HIV infection causes decreased numbers of helper T cells, which affect the organization of all the immune responses so the risk of opportunistic and pathogenic infection increases
- In Britain, women usually acquire HIV from sexual exposure and intravenous drug use
- Pregnancy can mask some of the non-specific symptoms of HIV infection, such as fatigue, anaemia and dyspnoea
- HIV can remain latent for years (estimated to be an average 11 years) before AIDS becomes evident
- Progression to symptom development may be accelerated by pregnancy
- HIV can be transmitted to the baby via the placenta, from exchange of body fluids at birth or from the breast milk
- Mothers with HIV may be advised to breastfeed their babies if the risk of fatal malnutrition is considered to be higher than the risk of HIV infection

**Key points**

- Pregnancy enhances humoral immunity and suppresses cell-mediated immunity so responses to bacterial infection are enhanced but there may be increased susceptibility to viral infections.
- Histoincompatibility, such as the differences in fetal and maternal antigen expression, would normally lead to tissue rejection.
- The trophoblast cells lack classic HLA antigens, which prevent an antifetal response, but express HLA-G, which prevents non-specific cytolysis.
- Fetal cells entering the maternal circulation are important in the generation of blocking antibodies, which block any immune response that does occur.
- Maternal IgG is transferred to the fetus late in gestation, which provides the neonate with passive immunization during the period of immunological immaturity. Harmful antibodies against fetal antigens are sequestered by non-trophoblastic tissue in the placenta.
- The birth of a Rhesus-positive baby to a Rhesus-negative woman can initiate an immune response. Prophylactic administration of anti-Rhesus-D immunoglobulin is therefore given after possible or actual exposure.
- The neonate is immunocompromised at birth. Immunization programmes seek to address this lack of immunity.

**Case study 10.2**

Mary is 16 weeks' pregnant. She has no fixed abode and has not previously been seen by a health professional in relation to her pregnancy. Mary attends the local hospital antenatal clinic in a state of distress. She informs the midwife that she is an intravenous drug abuser and her best friend has just died from an AIDS-related illness.

- How prepared would you be, as the midwife, to counsel and advise Mary?
- What referrals and expert advice would you seek on her behalf?
- What considerations are needed in relation to the unborn child, in relation to both HIV transmission and Mary's general situation?

**Application to practice**

Pregnancy results in an alteration of the immune system, so normal non-pregnant white cell counts cannot be applied in pregnancy. An understanding of changes within the immune system will enable the midwife to explain the consequences of such changes to the pregnant women.

Midwives may be involved in the administration of some vaccines such as rubella and TB so an understanding of the immune system is required.

The interaction of the maternal immune system and the baby is an important aspect of lactation and breastfeeding.

## Annotated further reading

Brostoff J, Male D K 1994 Clinical immunology: an illustrated outline. C V Mosby, St Louis
*This book focuses on clinical aspects of immunology including disease mechanisms and diagnostic tests.*

Kassianos G C 1990 Immunization: precautions and contra-indications, 2nd edn. Blackwell, Oxford
*A useful reference source which covers immunization theory and mechanisms together with practical aspects. Each vaccine is considered separately with detailed notes about use, precautions and side-effects.*

Kirkwood E, Lewis C 1989 Understanding medical immunology, 2nd edn. John Wiley, Chichester
*A clear, well-illustrated introductory text which includes recent developments and an introduction to the immunological aspects of AIDS.*

Playfair J H L 1996 Immunology at a glance, 5th edn. Blackwell, Oxford
*Covers a wide range of immunological topics using clear, well-labelled diagrams to summarize and simplify the mechanisms of immunological processes together with succinct written explanations on facing pages.*

Roitt I M 1997 Essential immunology, 9th edn. Blackwell, Oxford
*A comprehensive and popular textbook which includes recent developments in immunology such as cellular signalling and hormonal regulation of the immune system.*

Staines N, Brostoff J, James A 1993 Introducing immunology, 2nd edn. C V Mosby, St Louis
*A small volume which introduces the basic concepts of immunology, with sections on immunity, hypersensitivity, interaction of nutrition and immunity, cancer and transplantation.*

## References


Barriga C, Rodriguez A B, Ortega E 1994 Increased phagocytic activity of polymorphonuclear leukocytes during pregnancy. European Journal of Obstetrics, Gynecology and Reproductive Biology 57:43–46

Beer A E, Billingham R E 1974 Host responses to intra-uterine tissue, cellular and fetal allografts. Journal of Reproduction and Fertility 21:49

Billingham R E 1964 Transplantation immunity and the materno-fetal relation. New England Journal of Medicine 270:720

Brostoff J, Scadding G K, Male D, Roitt I M 1991 Clinical immunology. Gower Medical, London

Bulmer J N 1989 Decidual cellular responses. Current Opinion in Immunology 1:1141–47

Daunter B 1992 Immunology of pregnancy: towards a unifying hypothesis. European Journal of Obstetrics, Gynecology and Reproduction Biology 43:81–95

Faulk W P, Temple A 1976 Distribution of b2-microglobulin and HLA in chorionic villi of human placentae. Nature 262:799

Fraser E J, Grimes D A, Schulz K F 1993 Immunization as therapy for recurrent spontaneous abortion: a review and meta-analysis. Obstetrics and Gynecology 82:854–859

Gibbs R S, Sweet R L 1994 Clinical disorders. In: Creasey R K, Resnik R (eds) Maternal-fetal medicine: principles and practice, 3rd edn. W B Saunders, Philadelphia, pp 639–703

Hench P S 1952 The reversibility of certain rheumatic and non-rheumatic conditions by the use of cortisone or of the pituitary adrenocorticotrophic hormone. Annals of Internal Medicine 36:1

Hunt J S 1992 Immunobiology of pregnancy. Current Opinion in Immunology 4:591 596

James K, Hargreave T B 1988 Immunosuppression by seminal plasma and its possible significance. Immunology Today 5:357

Johnson P M, Christmas S E 1996 Immunology in reproduction. In: Hillier S G, Kitchener H C, Neilson J P (eds) Scientific essentials of reproductive medicine. W B Saunders, Philadelphia, pp 284–291

Kleihauer E, Hildergard B, Bethe K 1957 Demonstration von fetlem Hamoglobin in den Erythrocyten eines Blutausstrichs. Klinische Wochenschrift 35:637

Kovats S, Main E K, Librach C, Stubblebine M, Fisher S J, DeMars R 1990 A class I antigen, HLA-G, expressed in human trophoblasts. Science 248:220–223

Ljunggren H-G, Karre K 1990 In search of the 'missing self': MHC molecules and natural killer cell recognition. Immunology Today 11:237–244

Manyonda I T 1998 The immune system. In: Chamberlain G, Broughton Pipkin F (eds) Clinical physiology in obstetrics, 3rd edn. Blackwell, Oxford, pp 129–163

Medawar P 1953 Some immunological and endocrinological problems raised by the evolution of viviparity in vertebrates. Symposium of the Society for Experimental Biology 11:320

Nakamura N, Miyazaki K, Kitano Y, Fujisaki S, Okamura H 1993 Suppression of cytotoxic T-lymphocyte activity during human pregnancy. Journal of Reproductive Immunology 23:119–130

Niederkom J Y 1990 Immune privilege and immune regulation in the eye. Advances in Immunology 48:191

Rooney I A, Ogelesby T J, Atkinson J P 1993 Complement in human reproduction: activation and control. Immunological Research 12:276–294

Singal D P, Butler L, Liao S-K, Lui K 1984 The fetus as an allograft: evidence for anti-idiotypic antibodies induced by pregnancy. American Journal of Reproductive Immunology 6:145

Staines N A, Brostoff J, James A 1993. Introducing immunology, 2nd edn. C V Mosby, St Louis

Stewart M 1997 Growing and responding. Open University, Milton Keynes, pp 185, 188–191, 193, 200

Wegmann T G, Lin H, Guilbert L, Mosmann T R 1993 Bi-directional cytokine interactions in the maternal–fetal relationship: is successful pregnancy a TH2 phenomenon? Immunology Today 15:15–18

Zipursky A, Hull A, White F D, Israels L G 1959 Foetal erythrocytes in the maternal circulation. Lancet 1:451

# 11 Physiological adaptation to pregnancy

## Learning objectives

- To outline the roles of hormones mediating the physiological adaptation to pregnancy.
- To describe cardiovascular adaptations to pregnancy.
- To discuss the need for iron supplementation in pregnancy.
- To describe the respiratory changes in pregnancy.
- To describe the gastrointestinal adaptations in pregnancy.
- To relate physiological changes with signs, symptoms and discomforts of pregnancy.

## Introduction

During the 279 days of an average pregnancy, maternal physiology changes remarkably to support the development of the fetus and to prepare the mother for labour and lactation. The changes begin in the luteal phase of the menstrual cycle, before fertilization and implantation, as progesterone secretion from the corpus luteum is initiated. If fertilization is successful, levels of progesterone and oestrogen progressively increase. Together, they orchestrate many of the changes to the maternal physiology in pregnancy.

## Endocrine changes in pregnancy

The physiological changes of pregnancy are controlled by an alteration in hormone secretion. The trophoblastic cells produce hCG, which stimulates secretion from the corpus luteum, increasing ovarian steroid hormone production. As the placenta develops, it also produces oestrogen and progesterone. However, placental endocrine function is much broader as the placenta synthesizes a range of hormones and releasing factors that are similar to those originating from the hypothalamus and other maternal endocrine organs (see Ch. 8). Placental products may reach both the maternal and fetal circulation, thus regulating maternal physiology and fetal development.

### Steroid hormones

Progesterone levels increase gradually at first (Fig. 11.1). There is little change in progesterone concentration between the 5th and 10th week, but after the 10th week the levels increase more markedly (Tulchinsky & Hobel 1973). By the end of the first trimester, levels of progesterone are 50% higher than luteal levels and by term the levels have increased three-fold. The syncytiotrophoblast uses maternal cholesterol as a substrate for progesterone synthesis. Placental production of progesterone is adequate by 5–6 weeks. A primate pregnancy can survive ovariectomy (oophorectomy, removal of ovaries), although the corpus luteum is essential in other mammalian pregnancies (Lutjen et al 1984). Human corpus luteal production of 17α-hydroxyprogesterone decreases from 6 to 9 weeks as placental production increases. Measurement of progesterone metabolites indicates placental function.

The primary oestrogen of pregnancy is oestriol. Early in pregnancy, oestrone and oestradiol levels increase but oestriol levels do not begin to rise until the 9th week when the fetal adrenal glands begin to synthesize the precursor dehydroepiandrosterone sulphate (DHEAS) for placental production of oestriol. Maternal and placental steroids are conjugated in the

Fig. 11.1 *Increasing concentrations of oestrogen and progesterone during pregnancy.*

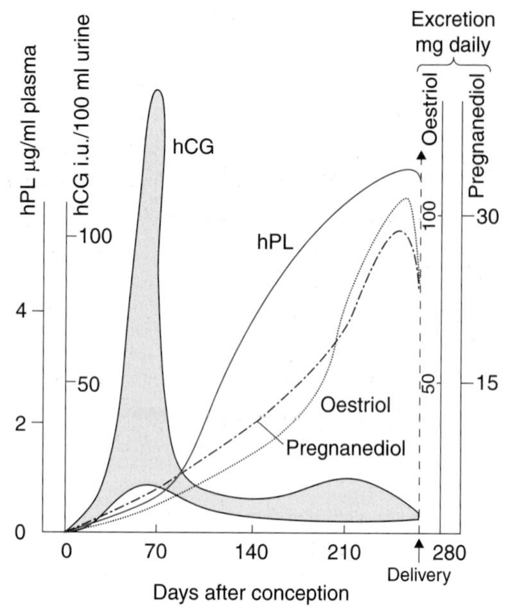


fetal liver and adrenal glands into water-soluble and thus biologically inactive forms (so the fetus is protected from the effect of the steroids' precursors). As the 16-hydroxyl precursor originates only from the fetal liver, oestriol is an indicator of fetal well-being. In 'at risk' pregnancies, decreased oestriol may indicate fetal distress and be used as an indicator for a need to induce premature delivery, although as an index of placental function and fetal well-being it has largely been replaced by Doppler investigation and biophysical profiling. Oestriol measurement is part of the Bart's (triple) test for Down's syndrome (see Ch. 7). Oestrone and oestriol levels increase about 100 times and oestradiol levels about 1000 times during the course of the pregnancy (Tulchinsky & Hobel 1973). The oestrogens have growth-stimulatory properties, markedly promoting the growth of the endometrium. They also stimulate fluid retention and increase the ability of connective tissue to retain water, affecting its composition.

## Human chorionic gonadotrophin

hCG is produced initially by the outer cells of the blastocyst. These cells differentiate into trophoblast cells and subsequently into the placenta. The syncytiotrophoblast, which evolves from the trophoblast (see Ch. 8), continues to produce hCG. It is secreted, and can be detected, before implantation in vaginal secretions. Usually hCG can be detected in maternal blood 8–10 days after fertilization (see Fig. 11.1). When the lacunae begin to be formed by the invading syncytiotrophoblast, the hormone can then diffuse into the maternal blood. Measurable urine values are present 2 weeks after fertilization. The presence of hCG confirms successful fertilization as, apart from very rare production by certain gut tumours, it is not produced by other tissues (Iles & Chard 1991). hCG is produced by hydatidiform moles (see Ch. 8); following evacuation of a molar pregnancy, urinalysis for the presence of hCG is continued for 2 years to exclude choriocarcinoma.

Production of hCG is maximal at 60–90 days and then falls to a low level that is maintained throughout the pregnancy. Persistently low levels of hCG are associated with abnormal placental development or ectopic pregnancy. hCG has a very similar structure to that of LH and acts on LH receptors, prolonging the life of the corpus luteum. If hCG is given to non-pregnant women, the corpus luteum is maintained and progesterone secretion rises. Alternatively antibodies to hCG given to a pregnant woman cause the corpus luteum to regress. hCG, rather than LH, is used to induce ovulation in fertility treatment. By 4 to 5 weeks, the placenta and fetus are synthesizing significant amounts of steroid hormones and can assume endocrine control of the pregnancy. hCG has thyroid hormone-stimulating properties, affecting appetite and fat deposition, and also affects thirst and the release of ADH (Davison et al 1988). It also promotes myometrial growth and inhibits myometrial contractility (Kornyei, Lei & Rao 1993).

The effects of hCG are summarized in Box 11.1.

## Human placental lactogen

As hCG levels fall, there is increased secretion of hPL. The levels of hPL increase in parallel with the size of the placenta and correlate well with fetal and placental weight. hPL has properties similar to growth hormone and prolactin, being lactogenic and stimulating growth of both maternal and fetal tissues. hPL appears to protect the fetus from rejection and low levels of hPL are associated with pregnancy failure and spontaneous abortion. hPL is antagonistic to insulin, resulting in raised plasma glucose levels. This diabetogenic effect of pregnancy adjusts glucose and fat metabolism to the advantage of the fetus (see below).

**Box 11.1**
**Effects of human chorionic gonadotrophin**

- Luteotrophic effect on corpus luteum that maintains synthesis and secretion of oestrogen and progesterone
- Stimulates placental progesterone production
- May be responsible for nausea and vomiting
- Stimulates maternal thyroid gland; increases appetite and fat deposition
- Increases sensitivity to glucose
- Decreases osmotic threshold for thirst and release of ADH
- Suppresses maternal lymphocyte activity
- Promotes myometrial growth
- Inhibits myometrial contractility
- Modulates trophoblastic invasion
- Affects fetal nervous tissue development
- Affects male sexual differentiation and stimulates fetal testes to produce testosterone
- Stimulates fetal adrenal glands to increase production of corticosteroids

### *Relaxin*

Relaxin can be isolated from the corpus luteum. It may be synthesized in the ovaries and stored in the placenta. Levels of relaxin are highest in the first trimester. Relaxin has a role in the softening of elastic ligaments of pelvic bones and has been used clinically in cervical ripening during induction of labour (see Ch. 13). The precise role of relaxin during pregnancy is not clear but it appears to inhibit uterine activity early in pregnancy. The softening and relaxation of the pelvic ligaments allow mobilization and growth of the uterus into the abdomen. Sometimes women experience low-back pain in pregnancy, which is associated with the stretching of these ligaments.

### *Adrenal and pituitary hormones*

The adrenal gland increases in both size and activity in pregnancy. Oestrogen stimulates adrenal cortisol production by inhibiting the metabolism of cortisol and increasing the synthesis of cortisol-binding protein (transcortin). Progesterone increases tissue resistance to cortisol by competing at the receptor level and binding to the cortisol-binding protein; this also results in an increase in cortisol production. Cortisol secretion is regulated by corticotrophin-releasing hormone from the hypothalamus, which affects the release of ACTH, MSH and β-endorphin from the anterior pituitary gland. ACTH stimulates the adrenal gland production of cortisol. Cortisol levels increase in response to stress, including increased cardiac output and decreased fasting glucose levels in the second trimester of pregnancy. Both CRH and ACTH are also produced by the placenta as well as the maternal hypothalamic–pituitary axis; the placental hormones are subject to different feedback control mechanisms and may be important in initiating labour (see Ch. 13).

The increase in circulating levels of cortisol has a positive effect on certain conditions, such as rheumatoid arthritis and eczema. This observation led to the clinical use of exogenous cortisol as a treatment for these conditions. Both progesterone and oestrogen act synergistically to increase mineralocorticoid production. Adrenal synthesis of androgens, oestrogen, progesterone and cholesterol increases in pregnancy.

The pituitary gland markedly enlarges in pregnancy. Much of the increase is due to increased number and activity of cells of the anterior pituitary gland. The gonadotrophs decrease in number as the raised oestrogen concentration inhibits release of FSH and LH, which are barely detectable for most of the pregnancy. However, under the influence of progesterone and oestrogen, the prolactin-secreting cells increase from 10% of the cell population to 50%. Prolactin levels increase progressively through the pregnancy to values 20 times higher than the prepregnant level. Production of adrenocorticotrophic hormone increases, resulting in increased adrenal activity. MSH synthesis also increases so pigment dispersal is increased in melanocytes, resulting in deeper pigmentation (Ances & Pomerantz 1974). Pregnant women frequently observe that they tan more deeply or develop irregular pigmented patches. Towards the second half of pregnancy, oxytocin production from the posterior pituitary increases.

### *Thyroid hormones*

Oestrogen, hCG and altered hepatic and renal function cause levels of $T_3$, $T_4$ and thyroid-binding globulin (TBG) to change. Oestrogen stimulates hepatic synthesis of TBG by 50–100 times resulting in increased total amounts of $T_3$ and $T_4$, although free concentrations remain within normal physiological limits. hCG has mild TSH activity so it stimulates both the production of $T_4$ and the deiodination of $T_4$ to $T_3$

in the peripheral tissues. Pregnancy mimics hyperthyroidism in a number of respects, for instance by increasing body temperature, and stimulating appetite and feelings of fatigue. In 70% of pregnant women, the thyroid gland enlarges because thyroid activity increases and renal iodine loss is increased. Ancient Egyptians used the observation of pregnancy-induced goitre (thyroid gland hypertrophy) as confirmation of pregnancy (Glinoer & Lemone 1992). The thyroid gland hypertrophies as it attempts to increase uptake of iodine for hormone synthesis. Nowadays, with better diets and iodine supplementation of table salt, unless women are at the threshold of iodine deficiency, goitre is rare in pregnancy. Basal metabolic rate increases by 20–25% from the 4th month of pregnancy but much of the increase is related to the increased surface area of the mother and the increased work she has to do maintaining maternal and fetal tissue requirements. Nausea and vomiting have been linked not only to the changes in hCG (see above) but also directly to the rise in free $T_4$.

## The reproductive system

### The blood vessels

The vasculature of the uterus undergoes a number of remarkable and unique changes during pregnancy. Uterine blood flow increases; the vessel diameter increases and vascular resistance falls. These changes accommodate the increased blood flow to the placenta, which is maintained under conditions of low blood pressure. The coursing of blood through the enlarged tortuous arteries produces a uterine 'souffle', which may be heard through a stethoscope or with a sonicaid.

### The uterus

The uterus increases in size and changes shape (see Chs 2 and 13). The endometrium thickens into the decidua. The three layers of the myometrium become clearly defined as the uterine muscle undergoes initial hyperplasia (development of new fibres) and subsequent hypertrophy (increase in length and thickness of existing muscle fibres). As the pregnancy progresses, the timing and speed of the myometrial action potentials change and the muscle cells increase their content of contractile proteins, gap junctions, sarcoplasmic reticulum and mitochondria.

In early pregnancy, the uterine isthmus increases from about 7 to 25 mm (Fig. 11.2). From 32 to 34 weeks, the isthmus forms the lower uterine segment (LUS). As effacement commences (at approximately 36 weeks), the external os is incorporated into the LUS (see Ch. 13). The blastocyst usually implants in the fundus (upper part) of the uterus. By 12 weeks, the fetus fills the uterine cavity and the fundus can just be palpated (felt) at the pelvic brim. As the uterus expands during pregnancy, it loses its anteverted and anteflexed configuration and becomes erect, tilting and then rotating to the right under the pressure of the descending colon.

The uterus is never completely quiescent and exhibits low-frequency activity throughout the pregnancy. Braxton–Hicks contractions are painless contractions that are measurable from the first trimester of the pregnancy. These contractions do not dilate the cervix but assist in the circulation of blood to the placenta. The contractions are usually irregular and weak, unsynchronized and multifocal in origin. The uterine ligaments soften and thicken under the influence of oestrogen, resulting in increased mobility and capacity of the pelvis.

**Fig. 11.2** *The uterine isthmus increases from about 7 to 25 mm in the early part of pregnancy. (Reproduced with permission from Miller & Hanretty 1998.)*

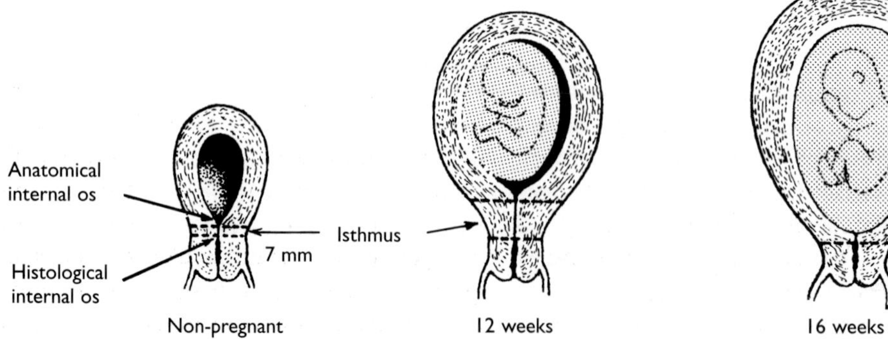

### The cervix

The cervix increases in width during the pregnancy. Oestrogen increases the blood supply to the cervix resulting in a lilac coloration and softer tissue texture. The cervical mucosa proliferates and the glands become more complex and secrete thickened mucus, which forms a plug or operculum protecting the cervix from ascending infection. The plug is held laterally by projections of thickened mucus in the mouths of the mucus-secreting glands. It is this plug that is released as 'the show' at the onset of labour when the cervix starts to be drawn up to form the lower uterine segment.

### The vagina

Blood flow to the vagina increases likewise resulting in softer vaginal tissue which is more distensible. The lilac coloration of the vagina and cervix was traditionally recognized as being an indicator of pregnancy (described as Jacquemier's sign). The increased blood flow means that the pulsating of the uterine arteries can be felt through the lateral fornices (Osiander's sign). Venous engorgement results in increased vascular transudation, which together with the increased cervical mucus production results in an increased vaginal discharge. The vaginal discharge has a low pH (because of the effect of raised oestrogen levels on the vaginal flora) and is white with an inoffensive odour. Oestrogen also stimulates the vaginal epithelial cell division so the cells acquire a distinctly boat-shaped appearance (which should not be mistaken for carcinoma cells). Early in pregnancy, the hypertrophied corpus luteum, which is about 3–5 cm long, distends from the ovarian surface; this may be palpated in some women or visualized during endoscopic examination in women undergoing egg retrieval for IVF.

### The breasts

In early pregnancy, vascularization of the breasts increases. This tends to result in a marbled appearance of the skin owing to the marked dilation of the superficial veins. The breasts may feel sensitive and tingle because of the engorgement of blood. (Changes to the breast in pregnancy are described in more detail in Ch. 16.)

The signs of pregnancy are summarized in Box 11.2.

**Box 11.2**

**Signs of pregnancy**

- Amenorrhoea
- Softening of vagina and cervix
- Increased blood flow to vagina and cervix causing lilac coloration (Jacquemier's sign)
- Pulsating of uterine arteries (Osiander's sign)
- Tingling and sensitive breasts with dilated superficial veins marbling surface
- Nausea and vomiting, possible changes in taste
- Increased frequency of urination as uterus compresses bladder
- Increased pigmentation of skin
- Bleeding gums
- Tiredness
- Increased appetite and thirst

## The cardiovascular system

The most notable physiological changes occur in the cardiovascular system in preparation for the increased demands of maternal and fetal tissues (Fig. 11.3). These changes are caused both indirectly by hormones and directly by mechanical effects. Heart disease affects less than 1% of pregnancies and causes 10 deaths per million in England and Wales, but symptoms of heart disease (such as breathlessness, palpitations, fainting and oedema) are present in over 90% of pregnant women (de Swiet & Fidler 1981). Superimposed on a pre-existing cardiac disease state, pregnancy may be dangerous and even potentially fatal. Measurement of cardiovascular system parameters is technically difficult and notoriously variable. Measurements obviously have to be indirect and are very sensitive to changes such as emotion, exertion and posture. In the research literature, there are many inconsistencies, some of which reflect differences in standardization of conditions (de Swiet 1998a).

### Blood volume

Total blood volume increases by 30–50%, more in multiple pregnancies (Brown & Gallery 1994). The rise correlates well with birth weight and, as it begins early in pregnancy, the mechanism of these early changes in the cardiovascular system is thought to be hormonally driven. It has been disputed whether the increase in volume (sodium and fluid retention)

**Fig. 11.3** *The changed distribution of blood flow in pregnancy.*

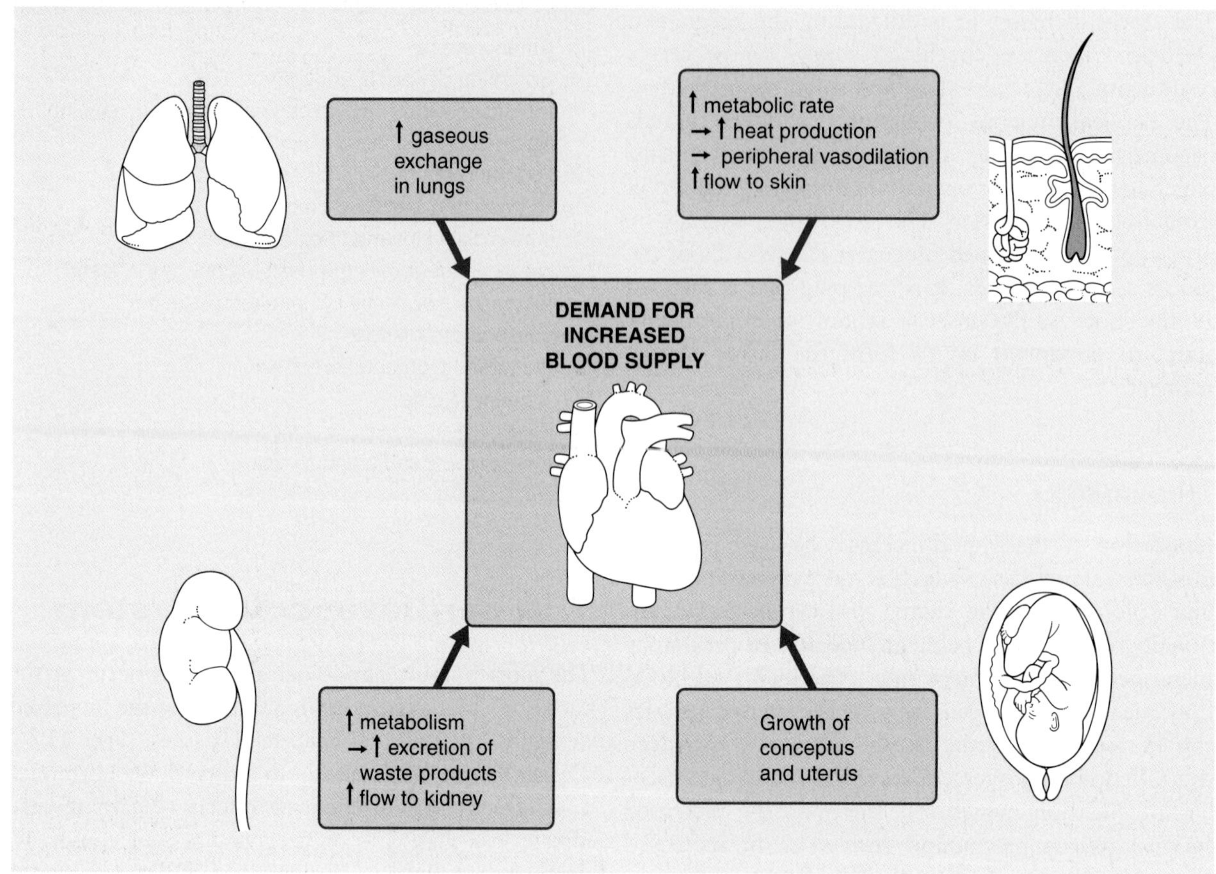


precedes the increased vascular space ('overfill' hypothesis) or whether the changes are stimulated by relative hypovolaemia (increased vascular capacity), known as the 'underfill' hypothesis (Scrier 1992). The arguments for the 'underfill' hypothesis are supported by the observation that blood pressure falls before plasma volume expands (Duvekot et al 1993). Often in early pregnancy women feel faint, suggesting that the physiological compensation of the underfill has yet to occur.

Oestrogen stimulates angiogenesis (formation of new blood vessels and vascular beds) and increases the blood flow to the tissues. Oestrogen affects the distribution of collagen in the tunica media of the large vessel walls, increasing venous distensibility. Oestrogen also stimulates endothelium-dependent vasodilatation, by increasing synthesis of nitric oxide (a potent vasodilator) and vasodilatory prostaglandins and inhibiting the release of endothelin-I (a vasoconstrictor). Production of both prostacyclin ($PGI_2$) and nitric oxide increases in pregnancy (Morris, Eaton & Dekker 1996). Current interest focuses on the role of these messengers in placental blood flow, particularly effects on spiral artery remodelling (see Ch. 8), but they may also play a part in maternal vessel changes elsewhere.

Progesterone relaxes vascular smooth muscle causing vasodilatation and decreased peripheral resistance. Therefore, the circulatory system increases its capacity and is relatively underfilled. Both progesterone and oestrogen increase water retention by affecting the renin–angiotensin system (RAS). Oestrogen increases hepatic angiotensinogen production. This results in a rise in angiotensin II, which increases renal fluid resorption and stimulates the production of aldosterone. These components of the RAS may mediate the oestrogen-stimulated angiogenesis and increased cell growth and division. The alterations in RAS are some of the earliest hormonal responses to pregnancy. During the menstrual cycle, the hormones of the RAS peak at ovulation; if conception occurs the levels do not fall (Sundsfjord & Aakvaag 1973).

Progesterone stimulates a 10-fold increase in the amount of circulating aldosterone. Progesterone is antagonistic to aldosterone but some progesterone is converted to deoxycorticosterone (DOC), which has mild aldosterone-like properties. Progesterone augments its effects on the circulatory volume by resetting the thirst centres in the hypothalamus and increasing thirst. Progesterone also lowers the sodium threshold for the RAS and blocks the vasopressive activity of angiotensin II in pregnancy (Gant et al 1973). The net result of the changes in oestrogen and progesterone is an increase in vascular resistance followed by increased sodium and water retention and expansion of the circulating volume (Fig. 11.4).

## Cardiac output

Blood volume and cardiac output increase in parallel (Fig. 11.5). Cardiac output increases by 30–50%, an

**Fig. 11.4** *The likely pathways for blood volume increase in pregnancy.*

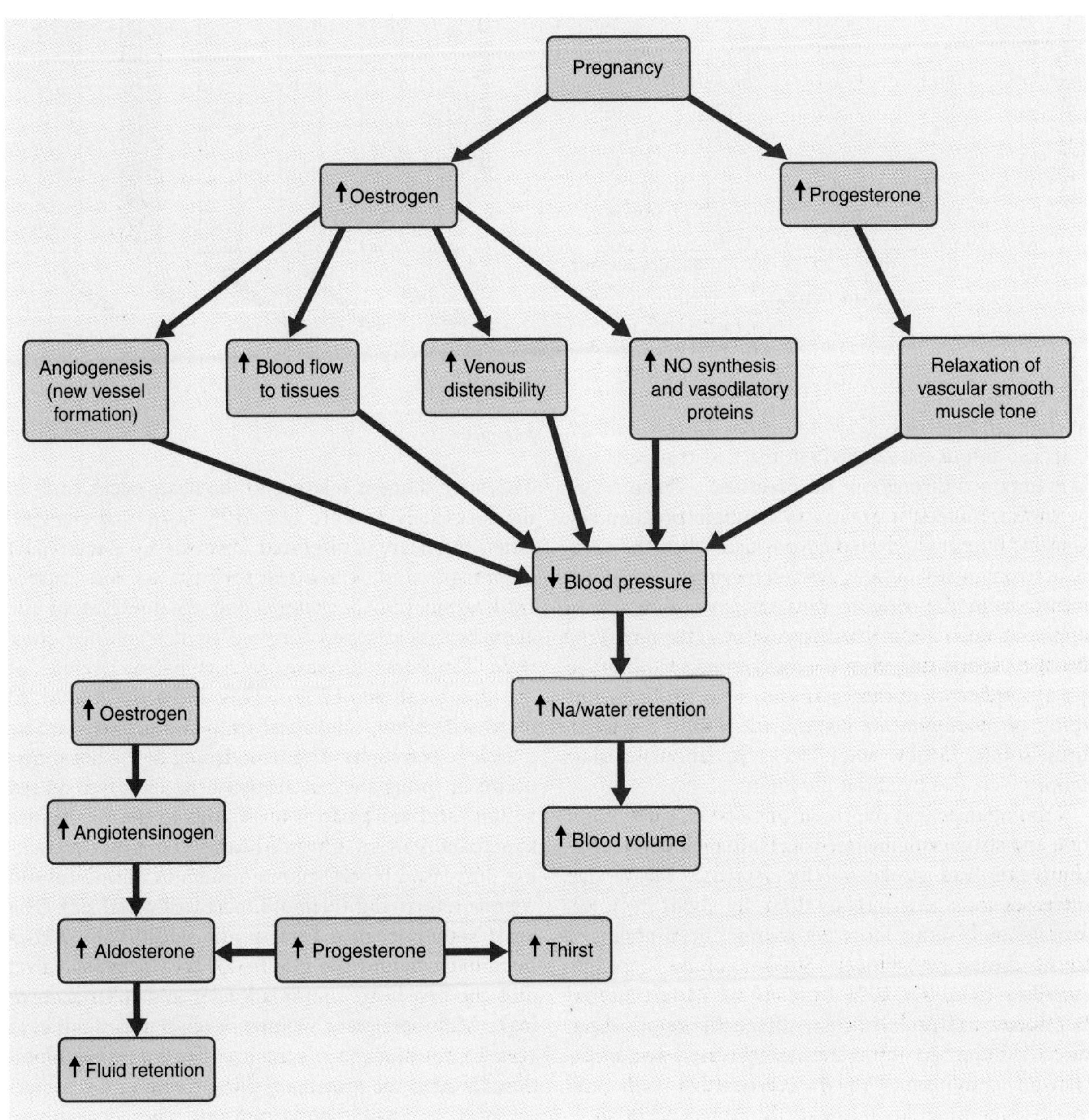

**Fig. 11.5** *The parallel increase in A blood volume and B cardiac output during pregnancy. Blood volume is increased up to 40%, thus increasing the load on the heart. (Reproduced with permission from Chamberlain, Dewhurst & Harvey 1991. B after Whitfield C R (ed) 1986 Dewhurst's textbook of obstetrics and gynaecology for postgraduates, 4th edn. Blackwell Scientific, Oxford.)*

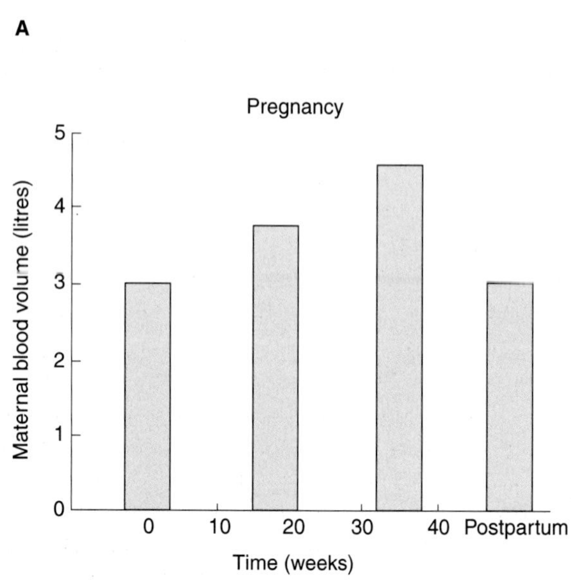


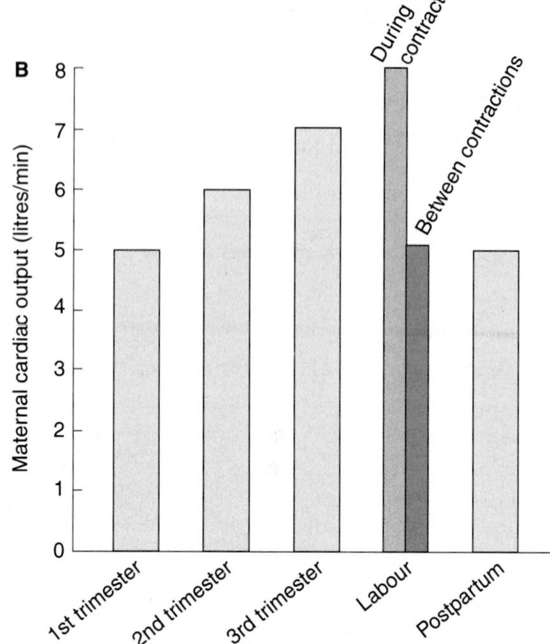


average increase of 1.5 l/min from 4.5 to 6 l/min. Cardiac output rises quickly in the first trimester and is maintained throughout the pregnancy. The increase in cardiac output is greater in multiple pregnancies. Cardiac output is affected by posture; when the pregnant woman lies supine, her uterus impedes venous return from the inferior vena cava resulting in an apparent decrease in cardiac output. The measured drop in cardiac output in the third trimester, observed by a number of researchers, was most probably the result of measurements being made with the woman lying supine (Mabie et al 1994). In labour, cardiac output increases by about 2.0 l/min.

Cardiac output is the result of two variables: heart rate and stroke volume (see Ch. 1). In pregnancy, both heart rate and stroke volume increase. Heart rate increases soon after implantation, by about 20% (an average of 15 beats more per minute) from about 70 to 85 beats per minute. Stroke volume typically increases by about 10% from 64 to 71 ml. Steroid hormones and prolactin may affect the myocardium directly. Oestrogen stimulates an increased accumulation of components of the myocardial cells and increases contractility (Duvekot & Peeters 1998).

## Heart

The early changes relating to the heart occur early in the pregnancy and are caused by hormonal changes. Later, the heart is displaced upwards by elevation of diaphragm and is rotated forward so the electrocardiogram (ECG) changes and the location of the apex beat is directed forward to the anterior chest wall. The heart increases in size by an average of 70–80 ml (about 12%). This increase is due to increased filling and oestrogen-stimulated cardiac muscle hypertrophy. The remodelling of the heart that occurs in pregnancy in response to increased blood volume and workload is analogous to the ventricular hypertrophy of an athlete's heart in continuous training. Increased blood volume results in an increase in venous return and therefore increased atrial size. The heart sounds change because the mitral valve closes marginally before the closure of the tricuspid valve; thus the first heart sound is louder and splits accordingly. Many pregnant women develop non-significant systolic murmurs in pregnancy. The increased blood flow through the mammary blood vessels may be perceived as a possible heart murmur. The net result of increased contractility, increased venous return, cardiac hypertrophy, decreased peripheral resistance and increased heart rate is increased cardiac output.

### Arteriovenous difference

Increased cardiac output exceeds increased oxygen consumption (especially early in pregnancy when cardiac output increases considerably and oxygen consumption is relatively low) so more oxygen is returned to the heart from venous circulation compared with prepregnant values and the arteriovenous (AV) difference is smaller. The AV difference is 34 ml in mid pregnancy rising towards term but is always less than the non-pregnant values of about 45 ml (de Swiet 1998a). The higher return of oxygen to the heart suggests that the commonly measured decrease in haemoglobin concentration is not physiologically inadequate and the relatively small increase in total haemoglobin (oxygen-carrying capacity) is more than sufficient to compensate for increased oxygen requirements. This supports the argument that the term 'physiological anaemia' is inappropriate (see below). The increased AV difference, especially early in the pregnancy before increased oxygen consumption, means that early fetal development and organogenesis occur in an environment which is well-oxygenated despite the maternal spiral arteries not connecting with the intervillous spaces in the early part of pregnancy (see Ch. 8).

### Blood pressure

Normal pregnancy has relatively little effect on arterial blood pressure. Despite increased cardiac output and increased vascular capacitance, there is relatively little change in systolic pressure in pregnancy. However, diastolic blood pressure is lower in the first two trimesters and returns to prepregnant values in the third trimester. Both the development of new vascular beds and the relaxation of peripheral tone by progesterone result in decreased resistance to flow. This is augmented by a change in the profile of prostaglandins produced. The levels of prostaglandin $E_2$ and prostacyclin, which stimulate vasodilation, rise early in pregnancy. Nitric oxide (formerly known as endothelium-derived relaxing factor, EDRF) also appears to play an important vasodilatory role (Palmer, Ferrige & Moncada 1987). The most important stimulator for nitric oxide production is flow rate, particularly if it is pulsatile (Pohl et al 1986). The increased difference between diastolic and systolic blood pressure means that for much of the pregnancy the pulse pressure is increased. Hypotension, particularly in early pregnancy, has been associated with fatigue, headaches and dizziness, which many women experience.

Blood pressure in pregnancy is affected by posture in normotensive women (Wichman, Ryden & Wichman 1984). Their blood pressure is higher when sitting and falls on lying, especially lying on one side. Effects on venous pressure are relatively dramatic compared with the effects on arterial pressure. As there are no valves between the return from the femoral veins to the vena cava and heart, venous pressure in the legs is similar to the pressure in the heart so if a pregnant woman lies horizontally the venous return falls if the flow is obstructed. Lying supine results in the uterus and its contents compressing the great vessels, particularly the thinner-walled inferior vena cava and the iliac veins, thus decreasing venous return. (The aorta is compressed as well but to a lesser degree because it has a much thicker vessel wall.) Return of blood to the heart can also be impeded by the pressure of the fetal head on the iliac veins and by hydrodynamic obstruction due to outflow of blood from the uterine vessels. Most women experience a drop in blood pressure greater than 10% when they lie down; for some of these women this fall is extreme, reaching up to 50%. The effect of assuming the lithotomy position in labour is to decrease cardiac output significantly (Carbonne et al 1996).

In late pregnancy, most women experience oedema of the lower extremities (e.g. Case study 11.1) owing to the combined effects of progesterone relaxing the vascular tone, the impeding of the venous return by the gravid uterus and gravitational forces. The peripheral circulatory volume is increased by 500–600 ml per limb (de Swiet 1998a). Oedema is further increased in

**Case study 11.1**

It is the height of summer and Kathy, 38 weeks' pregnant, informs her midwife she feels fat and sluggish and cannot cope with the hot weather. Kathy's ankles are visibly swollen.

- Is the midwife right to assume that this is normal?
- What indicators would the midwife be able to use in an assessment to reassure Kathy that all was well?
- What factors may alert the midwife to suspect that all was not well?

**Fig. 11.6** *The effect of increased venous pressure leading to increased incidence of varicose veins of the legs, vulva and haemorrhoids. A, normal vein with normal vascular tone; B, varicose vein: the effects of progesterone on muscle tone cause incomplete valve closure, allowing the back-flow of blood.*

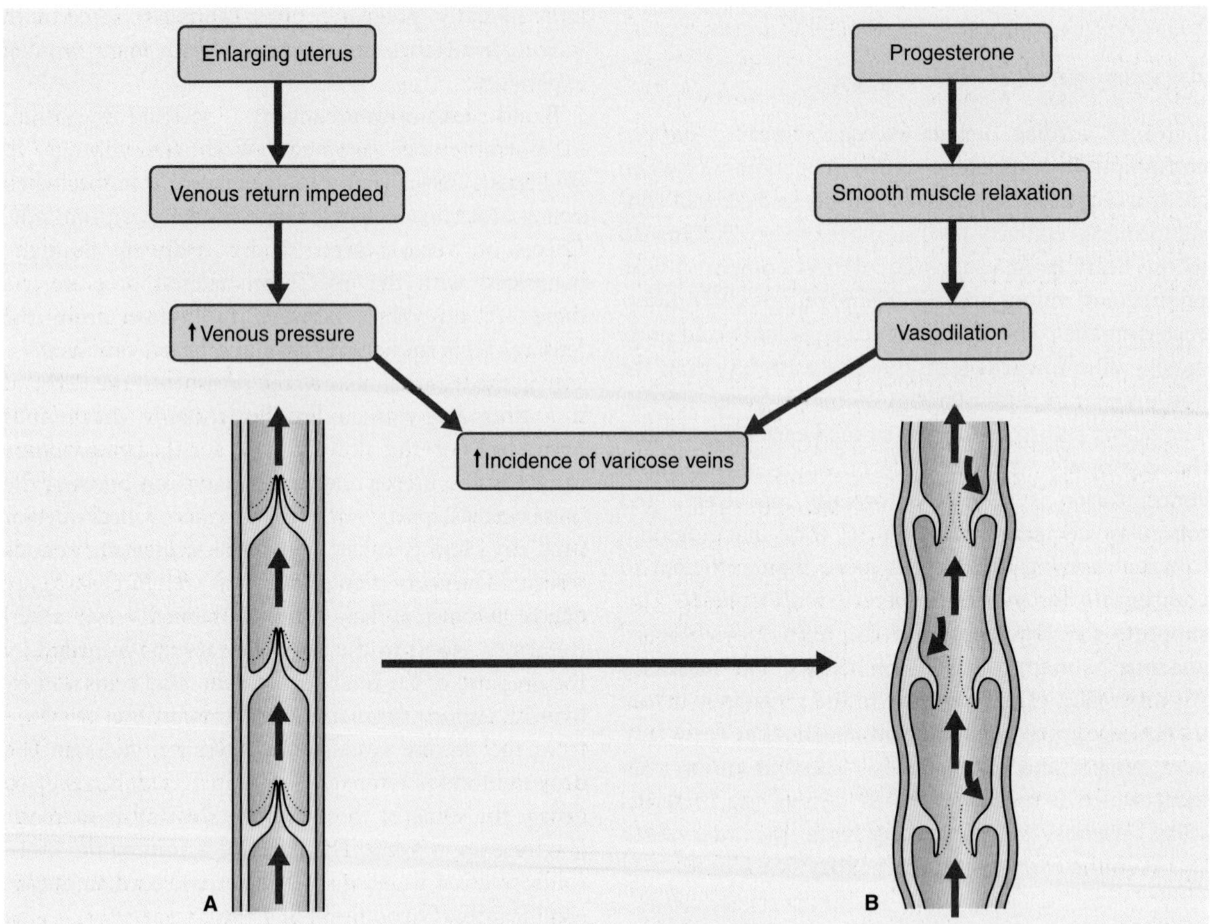


hypertensive women. Water drunk by the pregnant woman appears as increased leg volume and the expected diuresis is delayed until she lies down, resulting in increased nocturia. Blood pressure is higher on the side of placental implantation and oedema may also be more marked in the leg on the side of placental implantation (de Swiet 1998a). The effect of increased venous pressure is to increase the incidence and severity of varicose veins of the legs, vulva and haemorrhoids (Fig. 11.6).

The tendency to develop oedema is also affected by the concentration of plasma proteins (see Box 11.3). The increment in plasma volume is not matched by an increase in plasma protein synthesis so there is decreased plasma colloidal pressure. This, together with the increased venous pressure, means there is an increase in fluid loss from the capillaries. There is no evidence for a physiological increase in capillary permeability.

**Box 11.3**

**Oedema and hypertension**

The pressures in right ventricle, pulmonary arteries and pulmonary capillaries do not change but cardiac output increases. The higher pulmonary blood flow therefore has to be absorbed by decreased pulmonary resistance and dilatation of the pulmonary vascular bed so the volume of pulmonary circulation increases to match the increased cardiac output. Conditions where pulmonary resistance is increased and fixed have a poor maternal prognosis such as Eisenmenger's syndrome, which has a 50% mortality rate. Exercise presents an increased demand on the cardiovascular system (see Box 11.4).

The effects of exercise on the cardiovascular system are summarized in Box 11.4.

**Box 11.4**
**Exercise in pregnancy**

Exercise affects maternal physiology because there is a hormonal response, weight is redistributed and heat is generated. Many women experience very good physical health especially early in pregnancy. However, the question is whether the adaptive response to exercise compromises fetal oxygenation and well-being. The ability to increase cardiac output in response to exercise progressively declines throughout pregnancy. Theoretically redistribution of weight could affect the venous return and blood could be preferentially circulated to the skeletal muscles and to the skin for heat dissipation. Studies on animals suggest that uterine blood flow can be decreased substantially before fetal oxygen uptake or temperature regulation is compromised. It has been reported that over a third of the female medal winners in the 1956 Russian Olympic team were pregnant and the cardiovascular changes were responsible for their performance (de Swiet 1998a). In practice, moderate exercise in normal healthy pregnancy is encouraged as maternal and fetal health seem to benefit. However, pregnant women are advised to avoid jumping and jerky movements because of joint instability. Vigorous exercise is not recommended during hot humid weather or if the mother has a fever. It is suggested that heart rate should not exceed 140 beats per minute, strenuous exercise should be done for less than 15 minutes at a time and a pregnant woman should not allow herself to become breathless. A pregnant woman should stop physical exercise if pain, vaginal bleeding or dizziness is experienced or there are known risk factors.

### *Distribution of blood flow*

Oestrogen increases blood flow to all tissues (Rosenfeld 1980) but the distribution of flow is affected by posture. Venous tone is affected by progesterone. The increased venous distensibility results in an increased incidence of varicose veins, venous thrombosis and thromboembolism. The uterus is the central target of the increased circulatory flow during pregnancy but distribution of flow to the kidneys, skin and lungs increases as well. It is difficult to distinguish between blood flow to the increasing uterine tissue mass and that going specifically to supply the placenta because the uterine vessels are complex and inaccessible. Arteriovenous shunts in the uterine vasculature have been identified; these allow a short circuit of the placental site after delivery of the placenta, rather than being important in increased flow during pregnancy. The increased flow to the uterus is about 500 ml/min more than that to the non-pregnant uterus but changes in uterine flow occur relatively late in pregnancy (de Swiet 1998a).

Blood flow to the kidneys increases by about 400 ml/min from early pregnancy (Dunlop 1980), facilitating elimination of waste products. Vasodilatory prostaglandins are implicated in the peripheral vasodilation, which is particularly evident in the vessels of the breasts, hands and face. Oestrogen and progesterone depress the normal response to angiotensin-II and oestrogen abrogates the vasoconstriction mediated by the sympathetic nervous system. Distribution of blood to the skin is greatly increased (by about 500 ml/min) expediting heat loss. It is common for pregnant women to complain of being hot. Pregnant women usually have warm hands and feet and often complain that midwives' hands are cold. This vasodilatory effect is enhanced in smokers (Ashton 1975). Blood flow to the hands increases about sevenfold giving a very marked increase in skin temperature. The resulting peripheral vasodilation causes the capillaries to dilate and stimulates angiogenesis, and may give rise to the development of vascular spiders and palmar erythema. The increased flow means there is a decreased tendency to arteriolar spasm, therefore conditions such as Raynaud's syndrome are abolished.

The increased blood flow to the skin stimulates the growth of nails and hair. The ratio of actively growing hair to resting (prior to falling out) hair is altered from 85 : 15 to 95 : 5 (de Swiet 1998a). When this ratio returns to normal in the puerperium, vast amounts of hair can be lost. Mammary blood flow also increases (see Ch. 16). Coronary blood flow probably increases, reflecting the increased workload of the left ventricle, but it is thought that hepatic and cerebral blood flow do not significantly increase (de Swiet 1998a)

In evolutionary terms, heat dissipation from the mucous membranes had been very important in mammals (this is best illustrated by dogs panting to lose heat). The increased flow to the mucous membranes in pregnancy can result in an increased congestion of the mucosa, which is demonstrated by an increased incidence of sinusitis, nosebleeds and snoring in pregnancy. It is suggested that elimination of waste products by the kidneys and heat by the skin is best fulfilled by an increased plasma volume rather than an increase in whole blood, which demonstrates the importance of the apparent physiological anaemia.

## *Haematological changes*

The changes in maternal blood volume and composition increase the efficiency of the transplacental circulation and exchange mechanisms, thus benefiting fetal development. The haematological changes are also part of a maternal adaptive response that protects maternal homeostasis, including the ability to tolerate a sudden blood loss and to cope with placental separation. Thus, even women who have a degree of iron deficiency prior to pregnancy are protected from some decrease in haemoglobin levels at delivery. However, the adaptive responses to pregnancy potentiate the risks of iron-deficiency anaemia, thromboembolism and other clotting problems.

### Plasma volume and blood cell mass/number

Pregnancy is a state of hypervolaemia (see above). Blood volume increases in healthy pregnant women by about $1\frac{1}{2}$ litres (30–50% with a range of individual variation). Plasma volume increases initially rapidly from about 6 weeks' gestation and then the rate of increase becomes slower (Chesley 1972). The 50% increase in plasma volume is not matched by increased red blood cell mass and plasma protein production so there is a haemodilution (an apparent decrease) in haemoglobin and plasma protein concentration. Red blood cell mass increases by about 18–20% in women who do not take iron supplements and by about 30% in women supplemented with iron (Hytten 1985). The differences in plasma volume and red blood cell mass are accentuated by differential timing of the increases. Red blood cell mass begins to expand in the second trimester and the rate peaks in the third trimester. Oestrogen, prolactin and hPL all increase erythropoietin release and red blood cell production; however, red blood cell mass correlates best with hPL levels. The maternal RAS may be involved; angiotensinogen competes for the erythropoietin receptors and may be a precursor of erythropoietin. Maternal production of fetal haemoglobin is also increased in pregnancy (Pembrey, Weatherall & Clegg 1973).

The increase in blood volume is higher in multigravidae and women who are obese, have multiple pregnancies or where the pregnancy is prolonged. The increment in plasma volume is positively correlated with birth weight and placental weight; pregnancies resulting in recurrent abortions, stillborn and low birth-weight babies are associated with an abnormally low increase in plasma volume.

There is no reason for the relationship between plasma volume and blood cell mass, which are controlled by different mechanisms, to be retained throughout the pregnancy. The role of plasma is to fill the vascular space, maintaining the blood pressure, and to dissipate heat. Calculations suggest that the hypervolaemia is adequate to fill the increased vascular space of the pregnant uterus and the enlarged vascular beds of the breasts, muscles, kidneys and skin and to provide a reservoir against the pooling of blood in the lower extremities. It will also decrease the effect of the haemoglobin lost in bleeding at delivery. The decreased viscosity of the blood lessens the resistance to flow and therefore the cardiac effort required to propel the blood. Observation of a prepregnant or increased haemoglobin level (rather than a lower level seen in healthy pregnancies) may therefore represent an unsatisfactory increase in plasma volume rather than a true increase in haemoglobin concentration. Levels of haemoglobin are at their lowest between 16 and 22 weeks. The assertion that a degree of haemodilution is normal and a requisite adaptation to pregnancy, rather than indicating pathological anaemia, is supported by the increased arteriovenous difference (see above).

Most of the increase in blood cell mass is in the form of red blood cells. An initial depression of erythropoietin levels occurs, but progesterone, prolactin and hPL all stimulate erythropoietin synthesis and so accelerate red blood cell production. These influences result in mild hyperplasia of the bone marrow and an increased reticulocyte count. The function of red blood cells is oxygen transport; therefore red blood cell mass will increase physiologically at high altitude and decrease with prolonged bed rest. In pregnancy, the increment in red blood cells should reflect the need for more oxygen; the estimated increased requirement to supply the increased maternal tissues and conceptus is 15.0–16.5%, which is slightly lower than the measured rise of 18%.

The increased red blood cell number is due to raised erythropoietin levels. Levels of 2,3–DPG increase so the oxygen–haemoglobin dissociation curve shifts to the right (see Ch. 1) thus facilitating oxygen unloading at the tissues. Red blood cells become more spherical in appearance because plasma colloid pressure falls so more water crosses the erythrocyte membrane by osmosis.

### Iron status

If iron stores can be demonstrated not to be depleted, it would suggest that the decreased haemoglobin concentration cannot be attributed to iron deficiency. In pregnancy, the most accurate and appropriate method of determining iron status and anaemia seems to be measurement of serum ferritin levels (Jacobs et al 1972). Serum ferritin, the major iron storage protein, becomes depleted before clinical indicators reveal anaemia. Serum ferritin is stable, is not affected by recent ingestion of iron and quantitatively reflects iron stores, particularly in the lower range. Serum ferritin levels of less than 50 g/l in early pregnancy indicate a need for iron supplementation and levels above 80 g/l are probably adequate to protect the woman from iron depletion. However, routine iron supplementation in pregnancy, of apparently healthy women with no apparent iron deficiency, results in red blood cells increasing by 30% rather than by 18% in unsupplemented women (Letsky 1998). One method of assessing anaemia in non-pregnant subjects is by observing an increased red blood cell mass in response to increased iron supplementation (Yip & Dallman 1996).

The need for routine iron supplementation in pregnancy is a controversial area. Letsky (1998) argues strongly that clinical indicators of anaemia are not sensitive enough to demonstrate iron deficiency in practice. Iron depletion causes a reduction in mean blood cell volume (MCV). However, increased erythropoiesis results in a higher proportion of young larger red blood cells, which tends to mask the effect of iron deficiency on cell volume even with established anaemia (Thompson 1988).

Although the amenorrhoea of pregnancy helps to conserve iron stores and absorption of dietary iron increases, the requirement of iron in pregnancy can probably be met only if the woman has good iron stores prior to conception. Letsky argues that, although pregnancy is a physiological state, many women enter pregnancy with insufficient iron stores to supply the high requirements particularly of the third trimester. Active transport of iron across the placenta is maximal in the last 4 weeks of pregnancy. The inadequacy of dietary iron may be related to a trend to move towards diets having a lower proportion of meat and fish and a lower intake of haem iron (Finch & Heubers 1982). Although most of the body's iron is associated with haemoglobin, iron is also a component of the electron transport chain. Tissue enzyme malfunction occurs in the first stages of iron deficiency before significant anaemia is apparent. Introduction of iron supplements induces a feeling of increased well-being before the increased red blood cell production occurs (Addy 1986). Subclinical degrees of iron deficiency may adversely affect maternal exercise tolerance, cerebral function and well-being (Letsky 1998). Offspring of iron-deficient mothers may have reduced iron stores and are at risk of infantile anaemia, which may affect their mental and motor development. Maternal iron-deficiency anaemia correlates with high placental fetal weight, suggesting fetal growth is impaired (see Ch. 9). Low birth weight and high placental fetal weight have been associated with hypertension in adult life (Godfrey et al 1991) so iron-deficiency anaemia in pregnancy may have long-lasting and far-reaching effects.

## *Haemostasis*

Bleeding time in pregnancy decreases by about 30% because the ratio of clotting and fibrinolytic factors alters. There is an increase in fibrinogen and other clotting factors and a decrease in fibrinolytic substances. The number of platelets decreases slightly towards term but generally remains within the non-pregnant range. This response is variable; there may be increased platelet turnover and low-grade platelet activation (an increased number of aggregated platelets) as the pregnancy progresses, resulting in a larger proportion of younger platelets with increased volume. Low-grade chronic intravascular coagulation in the uteroplacental circulation may be part of the normal physiological response to pregnancy. Platelet count is further decreased in pregnancies with fetal growth retardation, and even in mild pre-eclampsia the lifespan of platelets is reduced.

Synthesis of antithrombin III (the main physiological inhibitor of thrombin and factor Xa) increases in pregnancy in parallel with the increased plasma volume. Levels decrease in delivery (thus increasing the tendency to thrombosis) and increase 1 week postpartum. There is a general increase in clotting factors, particularly in late pregnancy, as demonstrated in Von Willebrand's syndrome (an inherited clotting disorder), which improves with pregnancy. The change in amounts of clotting factors seems to be compensatory in preparation for labour. The hypercoagulability is optimal in labour, meeting the demands of placental separation. At delivery, total blood loss can be as much as 500 ml. The normal blood flow of 500–800 ml/min is staunched within seconds (aided by myometrial contraction, which decreases blood flow and rapidly closes spiral arteries). A fibrin mesh then rapidly covers the placental site as 5–10% of the

**Table 11.1** *Summary of haematological changes in pregnancy*

| | Change in pregnancy | Notes |
|---|---|---|
| Plasma volume | Increases by about 50% from 2600 ml to 3900 ml | More in second and subsequent pregnancies; correlates with birth weight |
| Red blood cell mass | Increases by about 18% | Increase is greater with iron supplementation (to 30%) |
| Neutrophil count | Both cell number and metabolic activity increase | Initial increase occurs early in pregnancy and is similar to the response to other physiological stresses |
| Plasma proteins | Decrease | Decreased osmotic pressure predisposes to oedema |
| Clotting factors | Increase | Fibrinolytic factors decrease |
| Platelet count | Slight fall | Coagulability increases |

total circulating fibrinogen is deposited. Fibrinolytic activity decreases in pregnancy and remains low in labour. It returns to normal within an hour of delivery; the placenta produces inhibitors that block fibrinolysis.

Table 11.1 summarizes the haematological changes in pregnancy.

## The respiratory system

Maternal respiratory effort has to be increased in pregnancy to meet the increased metabolic demands of the maternal and fetal tissues. By the end of the pregnancy, 16–20% more oxygen is consumed. The respiratory system is also affected by the expanding uterine volume. In terms of physiological reserve, the stress put on the respiratory system by pregnancy is small compared with the increases that can be measured on exercise (Table 11.2). This contrasts with the much larger proportion of the cardiovascular physiological reserve required in pregnancy. The clinical implication of this is that patients with respiratory disease are much less likely to deteriorate in pregnancy than are those with cardiac disease.

### Anatomy

Early in pregnancy, and therefore not secondary to pressure from the uterus, the diaphragm is displaced upwards by 4 cm (de Swiet 1998b) (Fig. 11.7). The respiratory excursion of the diaphragm increases and there is an increased flaring of the lower ribs (increasing the substernal angle from 68° in early pregnancy to 103° in late pregnancy) (Thomson & Cohen 1938). This compensatory increase in the diameter of the thorax by about 2 cm (the circumference of the chest increases by about 15 cm) means that the volume of the thoracic cavity is about the same as that in prepregnancy. The diaphragm performs the major work of respiration; the breathing is thoracic rather than abdominal. Hormonal influences cause the muscles and cartilage in the thoracic region to relax so the chest broadens. The subsequent decrease in chest wall compliance means the thoracic wall can move further inwards so there is less trapped air and the residual volume decreases. These anatomical changes probably do not completely reverse after the pregnancy (indeed it is said that the increased flaring of the rib cage is beneficial to opera singers after pregnancy).

**Table 11.2** *Pregnancy and physiological reserve*

| Parameter | Normal | Pregnancy | % increase | Exercise | % increase |
|---|---|---|---|---|---|
| Minute volume | 7.5 l/min | 10.5 l/min | 40 | 80 l/min | 1000 |
| Oxygen consumption | 220 ml/min | 255 ml/min | 16 | | |
| Cardiac output | 4.5 l/min | 6 l/min | 30 | 12 l/min | |

**Fig. 11.7** ***Displacement of the diaphragm in pregnancy: the ribcage in pregnancy (light) and the non-pregnancy state (dark), showing the increased subcostal angle, the increased transverse diameter and the raised diaphragm in pregnancy.***

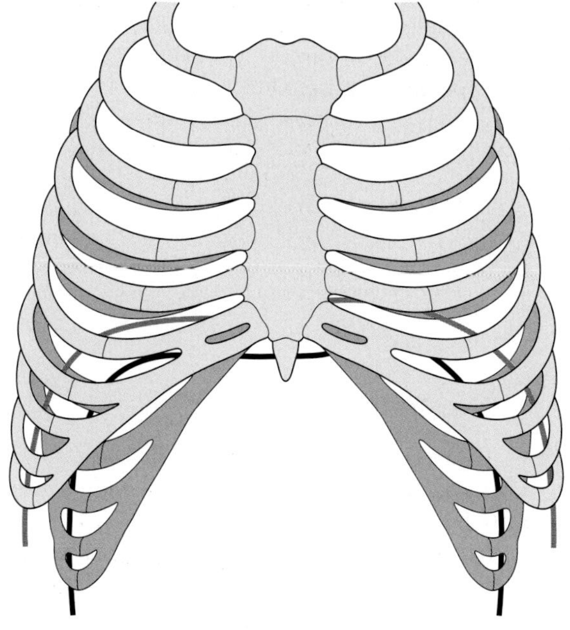

Progesterone lowers the sensitivity of the peripheral and central chemoreceptors for carbon dioxide (Skatrud, Dempsey & Kaiser 1978). This means that respiratory drive is stimulated at lower carbon dioxide levels so pregnant women breathe more deeply. As progesterone increases during the pregnancy, the increased responsiveness to $PCO_2$ results in an increased tidal volume and therefore minute volume (Table 11.3). So hyperventilation (increased tidal volume) is normal is pregnancy. Oxygen consumption increases but arterial oxygen pressure does not change.

In pregnancy, the respiratory rate is unchanged but minute ventilation increases by 40% because tidal volume increases; this is apparent as early as 7 weeks. This hyperventilation exceeds the increased oxygen consumption. Efficiency of alveolar gas exchange is much more efficient when tidal volume is increased rather than respiratory rate (Fig. 11.8). Alveolar ventilation is further enhanced by the decrease in residual volume. About 150 ml of an inspired breath remains in the upper airways where no gas exchange takes place (this is known as the anatomical dead space). Although the dead space increases by about 60 ml in pregnancy because of dilatation of the smaller bronchioles, the net alveolar ventilation is increased. The increased tidal volume means that the functional residual capacity is reduced, thus an increased volume of fresh air mixes with a much smaller residual volume of air remaining in the lungs. Alveolar ventilation in pregnancy is thus increased by about 70% resulting in increased efficiency of mixing of gases, which facilitates gas exchange because the diffusion gradient is bigger. The increased gradient of carbon dioxide concentrations between maternal and fetal blood aids transfer of carbon dioxide across the placenta and may be particularly important in adverse circumstances. Progesterone increases carbonic anhydrase levels in red blood cells (see Ch. 1) thus further increasing the efficiency of carbon dioxide transfer.

Maternal partial pressures of oxygen increase slightly (from 95–100 to 101–106 mmHg) and levels of carbon dioxide decrease (from 35–40 mmHg to 26–34 mmHg). The small increase in $PO_2$ has little effect on haemoglobin saturation. Posture, however, affects alveolar oxygen levels; a supine position in late pregnancy results in a lower alveolar oxygen pressure than a sitting position. This change in alveolar oxygenation is probably not significant for the fetus although it may be compensatory at high altitude. Air travel is associated with increased dyspnoea and respiratory rate. The decreased level of carbon dioxide in pregnancy results in a mild respiratory alkalosis. The change in pH affects levels of circulatory cations such as sodium, potassium and calcium, aiding transfer across the placenta and increasing provision for fetal growth. Metabolic compensation by increased renal excretion of bicarbonate ions occurs. The resulting fall in serum bicarbonate causes maternal pH levels to increase to the upper end of the normal physiological range, from 7.40 to 7.45. Maternal ability to compensate further for metabolic acidosis is therefore limited, which may create problems in prolonged labour or where there is inadequate tissue perfusion (see Ch. 13).

Progesterone has a local effect on the smooth muscle tone of the airways and the pulmonary blood vessels. Diffusion capacity is the ease with which gases can cross the pulmonary membranes. In early pregnancy, diffusion capacity decreases probably because of the effects of oestrogen on the composition of the mucopolysaccharides of the capillary walls, which increases diffusion distance (de Swiet 1998b). This effect may last for months after delivery. Increased water retention in the pulmonary tissues also results in

**Table 11.3** *Lung volumes and capacities*

| Parameter | Definition | Normal range | Change in pregnancy |
|---|---|---|---|
| Tidal volume (TV) | Volume of a normal breath at rest | 500 ml | Increases by 150–200 ml (25–40%)<br>75% increase occurs within first trimester |
| Respiratory rate (RR) | Number of breaths per minute | 12 breaths/min | Unchanged/slightly increased to 15 breaths/min |
| Minute volume (MV) | Total air taken in 1 minute of respiration (= TV × RR) | 6000 ml/min<br>6.5 l/min | Increased by about 40%<br>10 l/min |
| Inspiratory reserve volume (IRV) | Volume of air that can be inspired above the resting tidal volume | 3100 ml | Unchanged |
| Expiratory reserve volume (ERV) | Volume of gas that can be expired in addition to the tidal volume | 1200 ml | Reduces progressively from early pregnancy to about 1100 ml |
| Residual volume (RV) | Volume of gas remaining in the lungs after a maximal expiration | 1200 ml | Decrease progressively |
| Total lung capacity (TLC) | Maximum volume of the lungs (= TV + IRV + ERV + dead space) | 6000 ml | Unchanged |
| Vital capacity (VC) | Total volume of gas that can be moved in and out of the lungs (= TLC – residual volume) | 4800 ml | Increased 100–200 ml in late pregnancy? (not apparent in obese women)<br>???unchanged |
| Inspiratory capacity | Total inspiratory ability of the lungs (= IRC + TV) | 2200 ml | Increased about 2500 ml at term |
| Functional residual capacity (FRC) | Volume of gas remaining in the lungs after a resting breath (= ERV + RV) | 2800 ml | Decreases progressively to 2300 ml—increases mixing efficiency |
| Residual volume (RV) | Volume of gas remaining after a maximal expiration (= FRC – ERV) | 2400 ml | |
| Physiological dead space | | | Increases by ~ 60 ml |
| Alveolar ventilation | Difference between TV and volume of physiological dead space | | Increased |

a decrease in diffusion capacity. There is an increased closing volume suggesting that the calibre of the small airways is decreased; this may be due to increased lung fluid. The decreased efficiency of pulmonary gas transfer is partially compensated for by progesterone-induced relaxation of bronchiole smooth muscle, which decreases airway resistance. The decreased airway resistance means that air flow is increased. Prostaglandins also affect bronchiole smooth muscle. Prostaglandin $F_{2\alpha}$, which increases throughout the pregnancy, is a smooth muscle constrictor; prostaglandins $E_1$ and $E_2$, which increase in the third trimester, are smooth muscle dilators. How they affect respiratory efficiency in pregnancy is not clear, although when prostaglandin $F_{2\alpha}$ is used to induce a therapeutic abortion it can cause asthma in susceptible women (Kreisman, van de Weil & Mitchell 1975). The work of breathing is probably unchanged as the

Fig. 11.8 *A Alteration in alveolar gas exchange during pregnancy and B its mechanisms.*

A

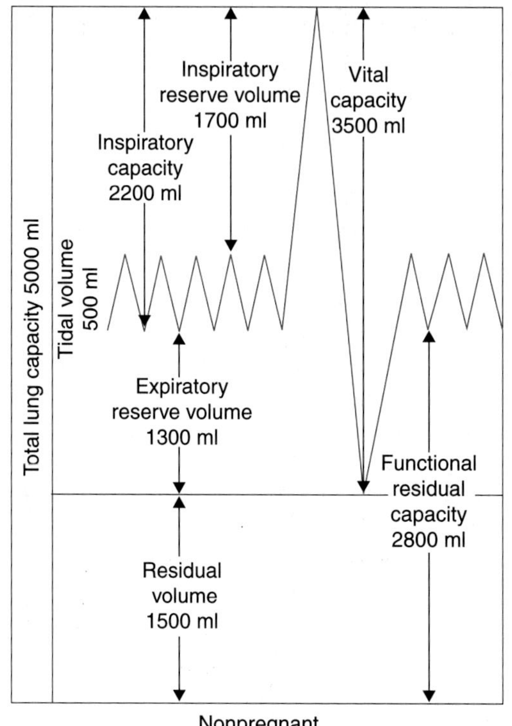


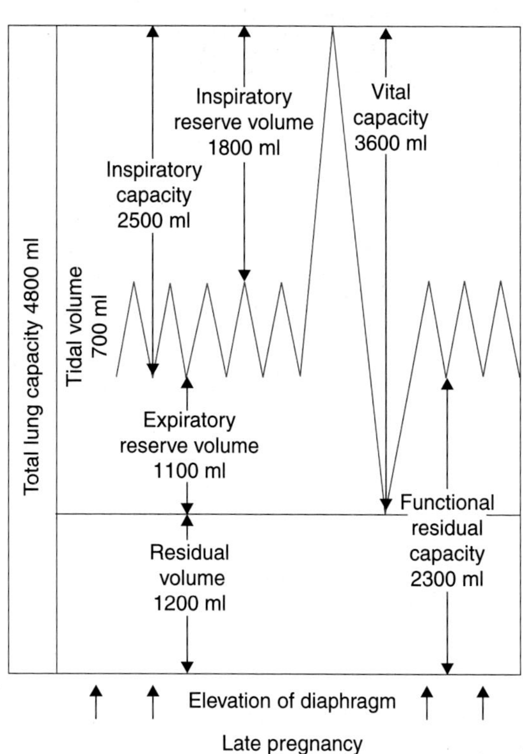


B

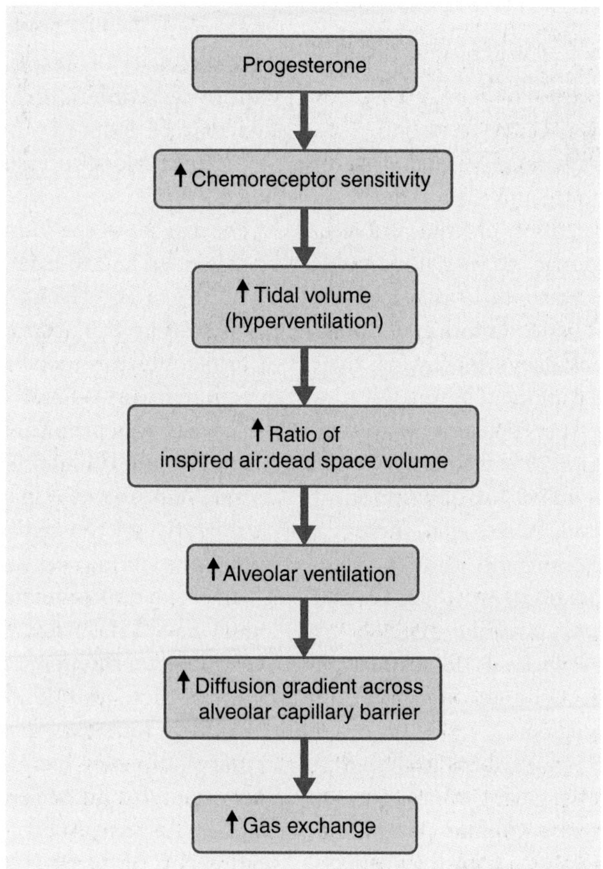

decreased airway resistance compensates for the congestion in the bronchial wall capillaries.

Many pregnant women experience dyspnoea, causing discomfort and anxiety, often early in pregnancy before there are changes in intra-abdominal pressure. This correlates well with $P_{CO_2}$ and may be due to hyperventilation (de Swiet 1998b). Capillaries in the upper respiratory tract become engorged, which can create difficulties in breathing via the nose and aggravate respiratory infections. Laryngeal changes and oedema of the vocal cords caused by vascular dilation can promote hoarseness and deepening of the voice, and a persistent cough. In severe cases, these changes in laryngeal thickening may cause complications should endotracheal intubation be necessary, for instance in anaesthesia. Forced expiratory volume over 1 second and peak flow rate are not usually affected in pregnancy.

In labour, pain causes an increase in tidal volume and respiratory rate (these effects are abolished by effective epidural anaesthesia). In the second stage, muscle demands result in metabolic acidosis (increased lactate and pyruvate production); this is countered to a degree by the respiratory alkalosis from hyperventilation (Blackburn & Loper 1992).

## The renal system

During pregnancy, the kidneys increase excretion of waste products in response to the increase in maternal and fetal metabolism, and retention of fluid and electrolytes is altered in response to cardiovascular changes. It is generally accepted that the increased circulating blood volume and haemodilution in pregnancy are achieved by the kidneys increasing their tubular reabsorption rate of sodium. The retention of sodium is stimulated by deoxycorticosterone derived from progesterone. Fluid retention is facilitated by the action of angiotensin II (see above for description of the renin–angiotensin system). Oestrogen increases both angiotensinogen production and renin production. ADH secretion tends to occur at lower plasma osmolality during pregnancy, possibly affected by human chorionic gonadotrophin levels (Blackburn & Loper 1992). Likewise, the osmotic threshold for thirst decreases from early pregnancy.

The gross anatomy of the renal system is altered in pregnancy. The kidneys enlarge owing to an increase in renal blood flow and vascular volume. Alterations in both prolactin and prostaglandin levels have effects on renal blood flow (Baylis & Davison 1998). The increased renal blood flow results in an increased glomerular filtration rate (GFR) from early pregnancy. The increased GFR results in more sodium, glucose and amino acids in the filtrate; however, tubular reabsorption also increases so most of the increased sodium load is reabsorbed. The sodium retention results in water accumulation.

The tendency to become insulin resistant in the latter part of pregnancy results in increased blood glucose. This, together with the increased GFR, results in increased glucose concentration of the filtrate, which can exceed the maximum capacity for glucose reabsorption in the tubules causing some glucose to be present in the urine (glucosuria). This does not necessarily indicate diabetes. Likewise mild proteinuria is common and benign in pregnancy, although with coexisting hypertension it can indicate complications of pre-eclampsia.

There is a cumulative retention of sodium and potassium especially in the last trimester when fetal demands for sodium are high. Urinary excretion of calcium increases but free calcium levels remain stable as dietary absorption of calcium increases (see p. 245). Acid–base balance is also altered in pregnancy (Baylis & Davison 1998). Hydrogen ions fall slightly primarily because of respiratory alkalaemia associated with hyperventilation. Although systemic blood pressure may be reduced, autoregulation (local control of glomerular blood pressure) maintains optimal renal function.

The calyces of the kidneys and the ureters appear to be distended and to lose some of their peristaltic activity in pregnancy. The ureters elongate and become tortuous so they can accommodate an increased volume of urine, which is associated with an increased risk of infection. It was generally accepted that this dilation of the ureters was primarily due to the action of progesterone on smooth muscle. However, the ovarian arteries and veins increase in size and compress the ureters, particularly on the right side where the vessels cross over the ureter almost at right angles, whereas on the left they run approximately parallel to the ureter. This, together with the stress imposed on the ureters by the expanding uterus upon the pelvic brim, explains the extent of these morphological changes.

Bladder function is also affected in pregnancy. Urinary frequency increases early in pregnancy as the growing uterus in the pelvic cavity puts pressure on the bladder. At term, when engagement occurs, the presenting part of the fetus increases stress on the bladder.

In the second trimester, the bladder is displaced upwards so urinary frequency is closer to prepregnant levels. Bladder tone decreases during pregnancy so capacity increases and may be up to a litre by term. The decreased bladder tone and displacement of the ureters by the enlarging uterus can affect competence of the vesicoureteral sphincters (valves created by the normal oblique angle of entry of the ureters into the bladder wall become compromised as the entry of the ureters tends to be perpendicular). The result is possible reflux of urine from the bladder into the ureters, which increases the chance of a urinary infection.

The walls of the bladder become more oedematous and hyperaemic, which increases the vulnerability to infection and trauma. The relatively lax walls of the bladder may also result in incomplete emptying of urine. This urinary stasis increases the risk of a urinary tract infection as the urine, which is richer in glucose and amino acids in pregnancy, remains in the bladder allowing the usually harmless number of bacteria in the urine to reach pathological levels. Women with urinary tract infections are thought to be at increased risk of premature labour. As the pregnancy progresses the effect of posture on renal functional becomes exacerbated. The structural changes of the renal system persist into the puerperium (see Ch. 14) and women who have experienced a urinary tract infection during pregnancy are at increased risk of recurrent infection in the puerperium.

Case study 11.2 details an example of a urogenital tract infection.

**Case study 11.2**

Penny is expecting her second child at 24 weeks' gestation and presents herself at the maternity day assessment unit. Two days previously, Penny noticed her frequency of micturition had dramatically increased. Since then she has felt lower central abdominal pain radiating from the groin round to the right side of her back. The midwife suspects that Penny may have a urinary tract infection (UTI). A provisional diagnosis is made on ward-based urinalysis that indicates the presence of leukocytes and nitrites.

- What are the significance of these findings and why do they indicate the presence of an infection?

The midwife instructs Penny on how to provide a midstream specimen of urine (MSU) and requests that the duty doctor examine Penny. Penny is prescribed a course of antibiotics with the proviso that this may be changed if the laboratory tests indicate that the antibiotic is inappropriate.

- How could the midwife describe to Penny the reasons why the UTI has occurred?
- What else besides taking the antibiotics could the midwife advise her in doing to a) help resolve the infection now and b) avoid further infection in the future?
- What are the risks and possible consequences if the infection is not treated?

## The gastrointestinal system

Maternal nutrition is very important in the outcome of pregnancy but disturbances of gastrointestinal function are the most common cause of complaints in pregnancy (Fig. 11.9). Over 50% of women experience an increased appetite (and consequent increased consumption of food) and even more an increased thirst. hCG affects the hypothalamus decreasing the osmotic threshold for thirst. The changes are most marked in the first half of pregnancy; subsequently they may decline although some persist, albeit to a lesser extent. Surveys have measured an increased intake of food and drink in pregnant women although not all of them are conscious of these changes (Hytten 1991). Changes in maternal appetite do not directly reflect changes in fetal growth or maternal metabolism. Appetite tends to be increased in early pregnancy. In advanced pregnancy, both appetite and the capacity for food intake decline owing to upward gastric displacement and pressure from the gravid uterus. A pregnant woman can compensate for her limited capacity by increasing the frequency of consumption of small meals and snacks. Oestrogen suppresses appetite but progesterone stimulates it, causing a shift in the central control of energy balance. Decreased plasma glucose and amino acid levels, which are secondary to increased responsiveness to insulin, also stimulate appetite. Cyclical patterns of appetite are also observed during the menstrual cycle. Thirst is increased; progesterone resets the thirst threshold by 10 mOsm so plasma osmolarity falls. Increased angiotensin and prolactin levels are also dipsogenic.

### Food crawings and aversions

Changes in food habits can be deliberate, for instance avoiding fried or fatty foods that are considered less

Fig. 11.9 *Gastrointestinal function in pregnancy.*

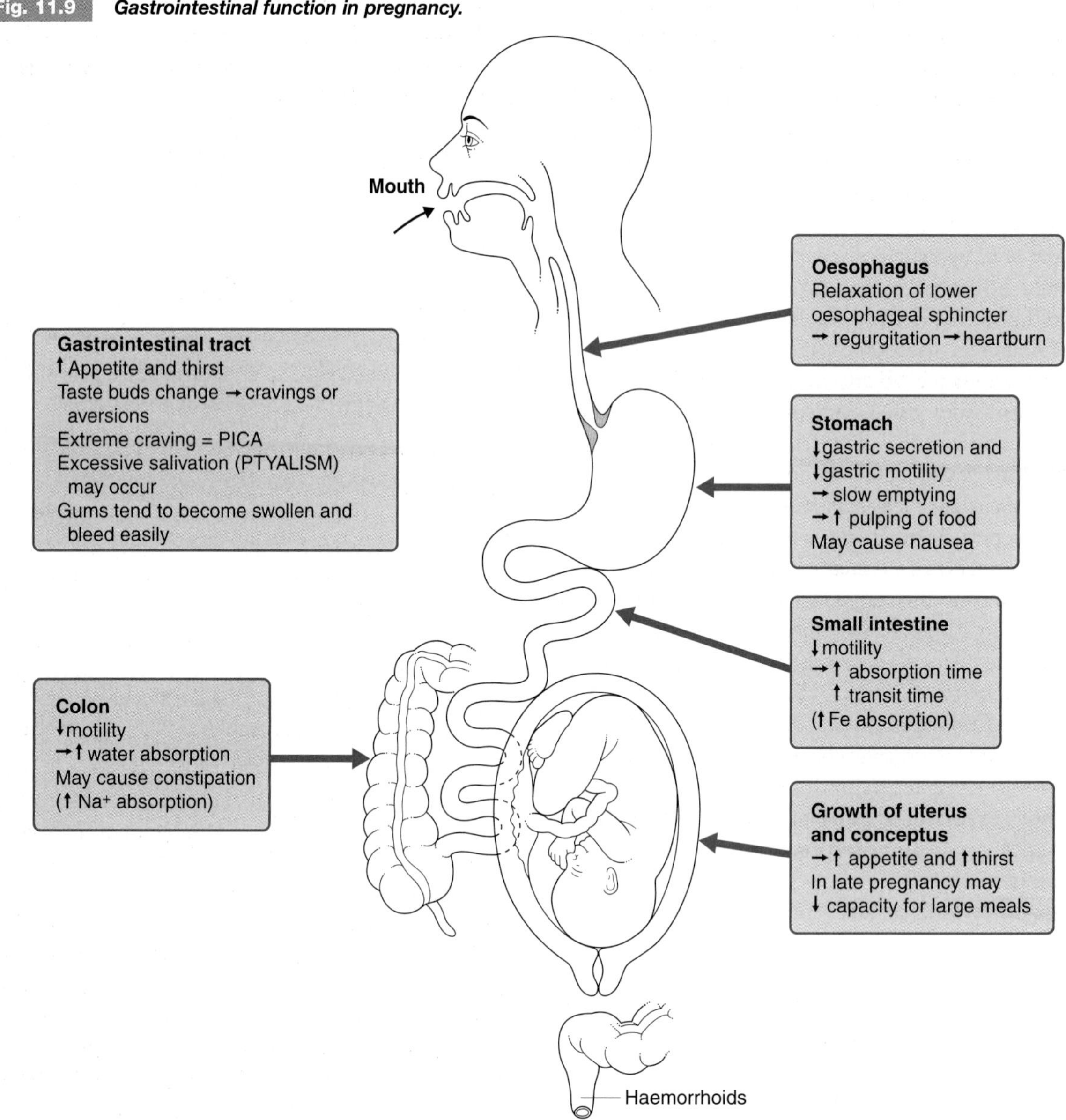


healthy. Two-thirds of pregnant women express marked food preferences as cravings or aversions. The commonest cravings are for fruit and highly flavoured foods such as pickles, kippers and cheese. It is suggested that the sensitivity of the taste buds is dulled in pregnancy (Bowen 1992) so highly seasoned foods are more appreciated. Common aversions are to tea and coffee, fried foods and eggs and to alcohol and smoking. Pica, an extreme craving usually for a non-nutritious substance, has been identified for coal, soap, disinfectant, toothpaste, mothballs and ice. Usually pica does not affect either maternal or fetal health. In the southern states of America, there seems to be a social tradition of Black women eating laundry starch, chalk and clay. The sense of taste may be dulled in pregnancy so the threshold for all taste sensations is increased. Sense of smell may be enhanced; pregnant women are especially sensitive to noxious smells such as nicotine and coffee. The changes in taste and smell appear to reflect secretion of hCG.

## Nausea and vomiting in pregnancy

Between 50 and 90% of pregnant women experience nausea and vomiting in pregnancy (NVP), usually in the first trimester although 20% of women experience

NVP throughout gestation. It may be the first physical manifestation of pregnancy. NVP is more common in Westernized urban populations and is affected by ethnicity, occupational status and maternal age. The peak of NVP is usually about 8–12 weeks; symptoms usually resolve by mid pregnancy. Although about 50% of women suffering from NVP are affected to a greater extent in the morning, some women experience nausea and vomiting in the evening, in a biphasic pattern or throughout the day.

There are several theories about the causes of NVP. Serum hCG peaks in the first trimester but the relationship between NVP and hCG secretion is not clearly established. The effects of progesterone on gastric smooth muscle tone, particularly those on upper gastrointestinal tract motility, the patency of the lower oesophageal sphincter and delayed gastric emptying, suggest a possible role for steroid hormones. NVP is usually conservatively treated with rest and reassurance and advice to consume frequent small meals rich in easily digested carbohydrate and low in fat. Meat and strong smells may aggravate NVP. Although NVP may have a socioeconomic impact, it is considered to be favourable prognostic sign and is associated with a positive outcome of pregnancy. Intractable nausea and vomiting causing dehydration, electrolyte imbalances, metabolic disturbances and nutritional deficiencies is known as hyperemesis gravidarum.

### Mouth

Gums often become hyperaemic, oedematous and spongy. This is because of the effects of oestrogen on blood flow and connective tissue consistency. Gums therefore bleed more easily and are more sensitive to abrasive food and vigorous tooth brushing. Gingivitis and periodontal disease occur in a large proportion of pregnant women and are more extreme with increased maternal age and parity and where there are pre-existing dental problems. Contrary to folklore belief that a tooth is lost for every baby, there is no evidence of demineralization of dentine resulting from pregnancy as fetal calcium stores are drawn from maternal body stores (skeleton) and not from maternal teeth (Blackburn & Loper 1992). However, there is an increase in the number of caries treated during pregnancy. This may be because gum changes result in an increased awareness of dental problems and many women receive free dental care in pregnancy. Pregnancy influences on the salivary glands result in a more acidic pH of the saliva, but the volume produced does not usually change. In rare instances, excessive production of saliva, termed ptyalism or ptyalorrhoea, may occur. It can occur in isolation or in association with hyperemesis gravidarum, where swallowing of saliva induces extreme nausea and vomiting in an affected woman.

### Oesophagus

Heartburn, a painful retrosternal burning sensation, is common in pregnancy, affecting 30–70% women. The effects of progesterone on the tone of the lower oesophageal sphincter mean its competence is impaired and regurgitation of gastric acid is more likely. Similar changes occur during the menstrual cycle and in women taking combined oral contraceptive pills. These changes are associated with increased progesterone levels. The risk of a hiatus hernia is increased; the sphincter is displaced and becomes intrathoracic instead of straddling the diaphragm. This usually begins in the second trimester and worsens as the pregnancy progresses. It is due to progesterone-induced relaxation of the lower oesophageal sphincter and a change in pressure gradients across the stomach. The enlarging uterus causes distortion of the stomach and changes the angle of entry of the oesophagus. Because the patency of the pyloric sphincter may also be impaired, both alkaline and acidic secretions may reflux into the oesophagus.

Heartburn is increased with multiple pregnancies, polyhydramnios, obesity and excessive bending over. Alcohol, chocolate and coffee all act directly on the lower oesophageal sphincter, reducing the muscle tone and exacerbating heartburn. Gastric reflux can be limited by advising more frequent intake of smaller meals, the avoidance of seasoned food, and of postural influences such as lying horizontally or bending forwards. Antacid preparations are associated with a number of undesirable side-effects: aluminium salts may cause diarrhoea, magnesium salts are associated with constipation, phosphorus may affect the calcium/phosphorus balance and exacerbate cramp, sodium may affect water balance and long-term use of antacids is associated with malabsorption, particularly of drugs and dietary minerals.

### Stomach

Studies on gastric secretion in pregnancy are not conclusive but suggest acid secretion tends to decrease, which may explain why remission of symptoms of a peptic ulcer is not an uncommon event. Secretion of pepsin also falls; this is probably secondary to the decreased acid secretion. Studies have shown that gastric tone and motility markedly decrease in pregnancy. Thus in advanced pregnancy the stomach drapes loosely over the uterine fundus. This tends to delay gastric emptying especially following ingestion of solid foods. The delay of chyme released from the stomach may increase the likelihood of heartburn and nausea and can result in delayed absorption of glucose.

### *Intestine and colon*

Progesterone-induced relaxation of smooth muscle decreases gut tone and motility and thus transit time in the gut increases, with potentially beneficial effects on absorption (Parry, Shields & Turnbull 1980). Duodenal villi hypertrophy and increase in height, which expands absorption capacity. Improved absorption of several nutrients, such as iron and calcium, has been measured (Hytten 1991); the increased absorption of iron in late pregnancy coincides with raised placental uptake and decreased maternal stores. However, progesterone may inhibit transport mechanisms for other nutrients such as the B group of vitamins.

The relaxation of the smooth muscle in the colon leads to increased water absorption and increases the incidence of constipation (Case study 11.3). The raised levels of angiotensin and aldosterone also increase sodium and water absorption from the colon in pregnancy. As the enlarging uterus compresses the colon, many women experience increased flatulence.

### *Liver and gall bladder*

Progesterone affects the smooth muscle tone of the gall bladder resulting in flaccidity, increased bile volume storage and decreased emptying rate. Water resorption by the gall bladder epithelium cells is decreased so the bile is more dilute and contains less cholesterol. There is a tendency to retain bile salts resulting in the formation of cholesterol-based gallstones in pregnancy. Cholestasis is a condition often observed in late pregnancy where women complain of itchy and irritable skin because bile salts are deposited in the skin.

In many species, pregnancy-induced liver enlargement results from increased circulation. In humans, however, morphological changes appear to result from hepatic displacement by the gravid uterus rather than an actual growth increase. Increased glycogen and triacylglyceride storage occurs in the hepatic cells. The raised level of oestrogen affects hepatic synthesis of plasma proteins, enzymes and lipids. The most marked changes are the fall in albumin (which is exaggerated by haemodilution), increase in fibrinogen (see above) and increased cholesterol synthesis. Synthesis of many binding proteins involved with placental transport of nutrients increases.

**Case study 11.3**

Josie is 14 weeks pregnant and is suffering from constipation. She is a vegetarian and normally consumes a high-fibre diet.

- What physiological changes may account for her constipation?
- What advice could the midwife give to help alleviate this problem?

## The skin and appearance

A number of changes can be observed in the appearance of a pregnant woman (Box 11.5). The increase in MSH means that there is an increase in skin pigmentation. The nipple and the areola darken early in pregnancy. A dark line develops from the navel to pubis; this is the linea nigra showing the embryonic folding and fusion line of the abdomen. Facial chloasma—mottled pigmentation usually in the shape of a butterfly mask ('mask of pregnancy') around the eyes and forehead—is common. Freckles and recent scars may darken; many women tan more deeply in pregnancy.

## The skeleton and joints

The weight of the gravid uterus changes the woman's centre of gravity altering the angle of inclination of the pelvic brim to the horizontal plane. The lumbar spine is naturally anteriorly convex, but this curve is exaggerated by the combined effects of progesterone, relaxin and the weight of the uterus on the intravertebral discs. The resulting lordosis of the spine compensates for the shift in the centre of gravity. By the end of pregnancy, many women adopt a typical posture where they stand and walk with their backs arched and the shoulders held backwards. Lordosis is

**Box 11.5**

**Top-to-toe observation of a pregnant woman**

- Hair—thicker and glossier
- Face—may have chloasma and/or oedema
- Hands—warm, may develop vascular spiders and palmar erythema
- Skin—warm, well-vascularized, hyperpigmentation (related to MSH production)
- Skin conditions, such as eczema, may improve
- Abdominal wall—pigmentation of linea nigra, lax abdominal muscles, striae gravidarum may be seen (related to cortisol production)
- Pruritus (localized itching usually of abdomen)—occurs in about 20% pregnant women in third trimester but earlier in pregnancy it may be a sign of pruritus gravidarum (intrahepatic cholestasis of pregnancy due to raised bile acids), which is associated with premature delivery, fetal distress and perinatal mortality
- Breasts—dilation of superficial veins, pigmentation of nipples and areola
- Legs—oedema may be evident around ankles; varicose veins may develop
- Posture and gait—lordosis, changed centre of gravity (related to effects of hormones on cartilage and connective tissue)

increased by poor posture generally, obesity, skeletal disorders, tuberculosis and by wearing high-heeled shoes. Oestrogen and relaxin affect the composition of the cartilage and connective tissue of pelvic joints, which soften in preparation for labour. The symphysis pubis and sacroiliac joints become more mobile and flexible so the pelvis becomes wider resulting in a rolling unstable movement and waddling gait when walking. Pregnant women may, therefore, experience muscle and ligament strain and discomfort or pain. The incidence of backache increases particularly after the 5th month. Some women experience severe back pain, often with peak intensity at night.

Occasionally in late pregnancy the symphysis pubis may separate. This condition, described as diastasis, can cause the pregnant woman great discomfort when walking or when her legs are abducted. The lower back is also affected by breast changes, stretching of the round ligament and decreased tone of abdominal muscles. In the third trimester, pressure of the uterus stretching or compressing nerves and blood vessels can result in numbness and tingling of extremities. Leg cramps, especially of the calf and thigh muscles, are common in the second half of pregnancy. They may be related to calcium/phosphorus metabolism and increased neuromuscular irritability. Raised phosphate levels are implicated and reducing dietary intake of milk is often beneficial. About 10% of pregnant women experience restless legs syndrome 10–20 minutes after getting into bed; the cause is unknown but is possibly associated with anaemia (Blackburn & Loper 1992).

## *Calcium metabolism*

There is increased turnover of calcium early in pregnancy with increased bone resorption and decreased bone volume. Maternal calcium metabolism changes to facilitate calcium transport to the fetus. The placenta actively transports calcium from the maternal blood. Placental calcium concentrations are higher than maternal levels so the fetus is protected if maternal concentrations fall. Placental efficiency is much greater than the absorptive capability of a fetus's gastrointestinal tract; thus a baby born prematurely with immature gut function cannot absorb calcium efficiently and remains undermineralized. In the last 10 weeks of gestation, the fetus obtains 18 g of calcium and 10 g of phosphorus from the maternal circulation, which is equivalent to 80% of the mother's normal dietary calcium in that period. However, the 25–30 g of calcium accumulated by the fetus represents a very small fraction of the total maternal calcium.

hPL and prolactin stimulate vitamin D synthesis, which increases absorption of calcium. Gastrointestinal absorption of vitamin D increases throughout the pregnancy. hPL increases bone reabsorption of calcium. Oestrogen stimulates parathyroid hormone secretion, which increases calcium absorption, decreases urinary losses and increases release of calcium from bone. Calcitonin secretion is also increased: calcitonin inhibits mineral release from the maternal skeleton but allows the actions of parathyroid hormone on the gut and kidney. Maternal serum calcium levels fall progressively in pregnancy. Levels are related to haemodilution of albumin and increased urinary losses and transport across the placenta. Urinary excretion of calcium decreases after 36 weeks, which augments dietary sources of calcium.

Homeostasis, mediated by maternal hormones, means that the maternal skeleton is conserved. If dietary calcium is adequate, there is no marked change in maternal skeletal mass or bone density. There is no evidence that high parity is associated with increased fractures in later life. Calcium supplements tend to reduce blood pressure by a small amount and may be useful in the treatment of pre-eclampsia. Calcium requirements in pregnancy are probably overestimated; clinical deficiency is rarely observed. However, a low vitamin D intake in pregnancy and little exposure to sunlight is associated with osteomalacia, as demonstrated by Asian women in UK who have lower plasma calcium and an increased incidence of maternal osteomalacia and neonatal rickets.

## Vision

The changed hormonal profile of pregnancy influences the maternal nervous system. In the third trimester, mild corneal oedema is common; fluid is retained and the cornea becomes slightly thicker, which affects refraction. Tear composition changes; levels of lysozyme alter and tears often become greasy. This, together with altered corneal sensitivity, may cause blurring or intolerance to contact lenses. Progesterone, relaxin and hCG affect intraocular pressure, which can fall (which will improve glaucoma). Unless they experience problems, it is wise for pregnant women to delay new prescriptions for spectacles. Women with pre-eclampsia and retinal oedema, and those with diabetes, are particularly prone to visual complications.

## The nose

The nasal mucosa becomes hyperaemic and congested in pregnancy, causing nasal stuffiness and obstruction. This seems to be oestrogen related and may interfere with sleep and sense of smell. It is associated with congestion of the Eustachian tubes (often described as blocked ears), which may cause mild hearing loss.

## Sleep

Sleep patterns change in pregnancy. An increased desire for sleep and napping in the first trimester has been observed (Brunner et al 1994). It is suggested that progesterone affects neuronal activity in the brain reducing the level of excitory neurotransmitters (Smith 1991). Oestrogen enhances this effect by increasing the number of receptors for progesterone. The amount of rapid eye movement (REM) sleep increases from 25 weeks, peaking at 33–36 weeks. Stage 4 non-REM sleep (deep sleep) decreases. It is this state that appears important for tissue repair and recovery from fatigue. In the second half of pregnancy, women tend to sleep less as they frequently are disturbed by nocturia, dyspnoea, heartburn, nasal congestion, muscle aches, stress and anxiety and fetal activity.

## Carbohydrate metabolism

Maternal metabolism changes in pregnancy to meet increased maternal needs, including the accumulation of maternal energy stores in readiness for labour and lactation, and to facilitate fetal growth and development (Fig. 11.10). Pregnancy is primarily anabolic; food intake and appetite increase and activity decreases. Pregnancy has been described as a 'state of accelerated starvation' (Frienkel et al 1972) because there is an increased tendency to become ketotic.

### *Early pregnancy*

Metabolism in the first half of pregnancy is predominantly anabolic with synthesis of new maternal tissues including deposition of maternal fat. Early in the pregnancy, there is an increased response to insulin so fasting blood glucose levels are lower than normal. The tissues exhibit increased sensitivity to insulin so there is increased uptake of nutrients and synthesis of macromolecules by cells. As the pregnancy progresses, most women develop insulin resistance so levels of glucose and amino acids in the blood rise, thus increasing the availability of substrates required by the fetus and placental uptake.

In the first half of pregnancy, increased insulin is produced in response to glucose. Early in pregnancy, the changes in metabolism are orchestrated by the raised levels of oestrogen and progesterone. Oestrogen stimulates pancreatic β-cell growth (hyperplasia and hypertrophy) and therefore insulin secretion. It also enhances glucose utilization in peripheral tissues and increases plasma cortisol. So the net effect is to decrease fasting glucose levels, improve glucose tolerance and increase glycogen storage. Hepatic metabolism of insulin may also be altered. Lowered glucose levels between meals increase the tendency to become ketotic. Placental transfer of amino acids, increased hepatic gluconeogenesis (conversion of amino acids,

**Fig. 11.10** *Changes in maternal carbohydrate handling during pregnancy.*

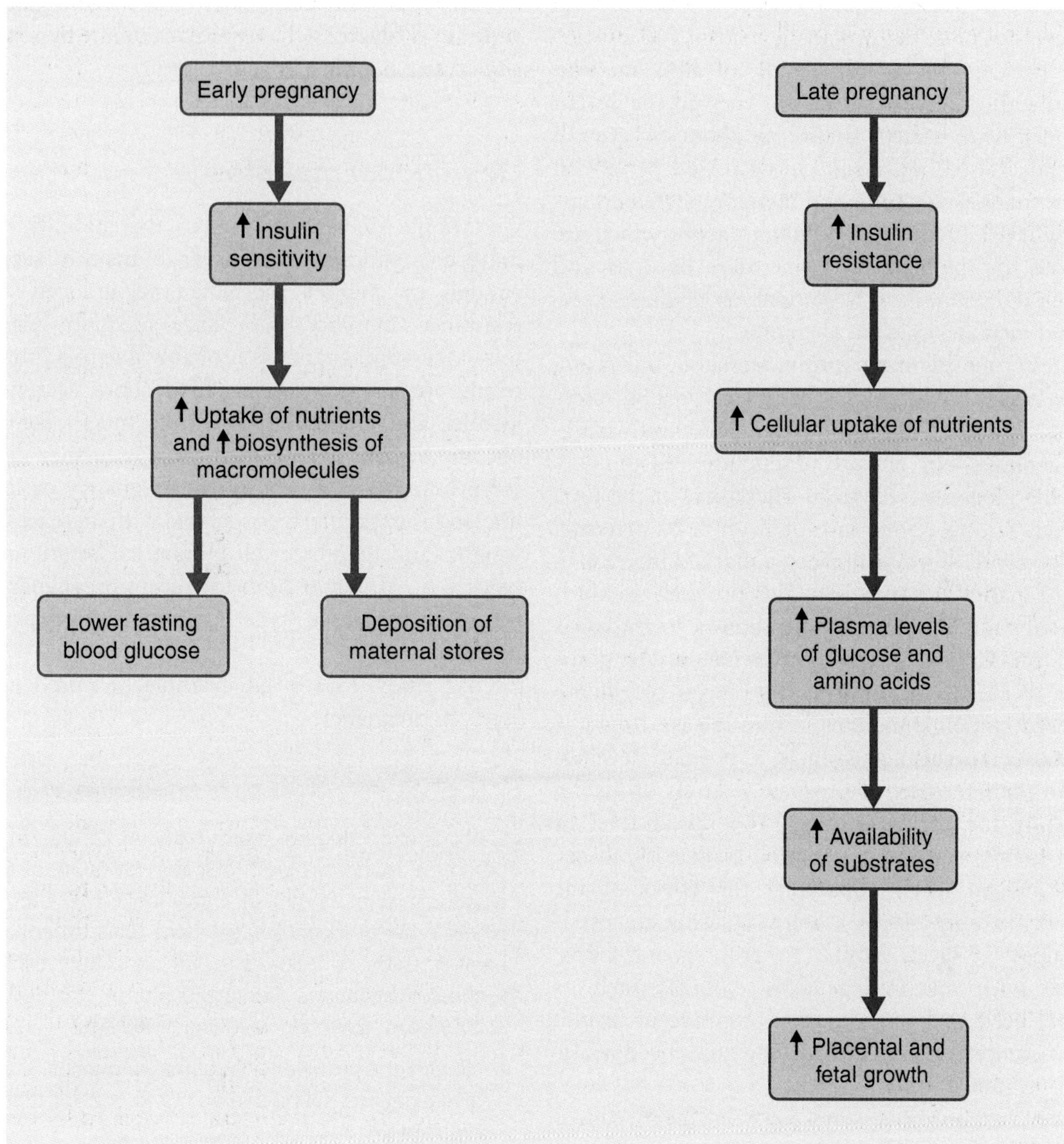


particularly alanine, to glucose) and raised insulin levels, which stimulate cellular uptake, together result in lowered maternal levels of amino acids. During the first two trimesters, the progressive increment in insulin levels, augmented by progesterone and cortisol, stimulates hepatic lipogenesis (triacylglyceride synthesis and storage) and suppresses lipolysis (fat breakdown). An increase in the numbers of insulin receptors on the adipocytes means there is enhanced removal of triglycerides from circulation. Increased fat storage in early pregnancy results in hypertrophy of adipose cells. During fasting, ketogenesis is increased as the triglycerides are utilized.

### *Late pregnancy*

As the pregnancy progresses, the fetal placental unit grows and levels of placental hormones, which are antagonistic to insulin, increase. Therefore maternal tissues exhibit decreased sensitivity, or resistance, to insulin, which means that insulin is less effective at stimulating glucose uptake. Pregnancy-induced insulin resistance affects adipocytes to a lesser degree. The dominant effect in the third trimester is related to the high levels of hPL, but prolactin, cortisol and progesterone are also involved. Levels of hPL increase markedly after 20 weeks. hPL is a very potent insulin antagonist with effects similar to those of growth hormone. Raised hPL results in decreased peripheral tissue responses to insulin and therefore increased circulating levels of glucose and amino acids, which are available for the fetus. hPL increases lipolysis and nitrogen retention, decreases urinary potassium excretion and increases calcium excretion.

Progesterone augments insulin secretion, increasing fasting levels, but decreases peripheral insulin effectiveness. Cortisol inhibits glucose uptake and oxidation, increases liver glucose production and possibly augments glucagon secretion. Therefore, in the final trimester, fasting results in mobilization of maternal triacylglyceride stores leading to a marked increase in levels of maternal fatty acids. This provides an alternative substrate for maternal metabolism so glucose is spared for CNS and fetal requirements. As tissue uptake of glucose is suppressed so levels of glucose are raised, which stimulates insulin release from the pancreas. Hyperinsulinaemia is a normal development in the later part of pregnancy; levels of insulin double by the third trimester. The raised level of insulin is important in stimulating protein synthesis. Raised insulin levels counteract the effect of the antagonistic hormones so maternal plasma glucose is maintained at levels similar to prepregnant levels. Women with insulin-dependent diabetes mellitus (IDDM) need to have a marked increase in insulin dose to compensate for the pregnancy-induced resistance to insulin.

In the postabsorptive states between meals, gluconeogenesis and fat mobilization provide substrates for maternal metabolism and placental transfer. Maternal cells metabolize the increased ketones and free fatty acids, thus sparing glucose and amino acids for placental uptake. As blood sugar increases in the pregnancy, it can exceed the transport maxima of the nephrons (i.e. the capacity to reabsorb the glucose from the glomerular filtrate) so some glucose is excreted in the urine. A degree of glucosuria is normal in pregnancy. As renal absorption of glucose is limited (so there are increased losses) and hepatic gluconeogenesis is decreased, hypoglycaemia, hypoalaninaemia, and hypoinsulinaemia result.

## *Gestational diabetes*

Gestational diabetes is due to the inability of the maternal pancreas to increase insulin secretion enough to counter the pregnancy-induced insulin resistance. Inability to produce adequate insulin at this stage of pregnancy is probably due to a limitation of the pancreatic β-cells. Inadequate secretion of insulin, and altered carbohydrate metabolism, may become evident again when there is further demand for insulin, as in a subsequent pregnancy or in later life, and is particularly associated with increased body weight (and therefore cell number). Gestational diabetes is a risk factor both for future pregnancies and for maturity onset (type 2, non-insulin-dependent) diabetes.

Case study 11.4 is an example of raised glucose levels in pregnancy.

**Case study 11.4**

Cathy is expecting her fourth baby. At 28 weeks' gestation, a random blood glucose revealed a blood glucose level of 11 mmol/l. Cathy looks well and, as in all her other pregnancies, says she feels exceptionally healthy. Cathy is referred to the consultant clinic for further investigations. Her previous baby was delivered at 37 weeks' gestation weighing 4.960 kg.

- What is the provisional diagnosis and what investigations will be carried out to confirm this diagnosis?
- What physiological interactions between the mother and fetus are occurring that could explain this phenomenon?
- How can the midwife best explain these to Cathy and what advice should she be given?
- What are the possible consequences for Cathy and her baby if no further investigations are carried out and no treatment advised?

## Key points

- The physiological adaptation to pregnancy is mediated by the increase of steroid hormone secretion. Steroid hormones are initially produced from the corpus luteum under the influence of hCG and subsequently from the placenta.
- The maternal endocrine system is affected by the increase in steroid hormones so other hormones augment the effects of oestrogen and progesterone. For instance, secretion of MSH and cortisol increases in pregnancy, affecting skin pigmentation and improving some pathological conditions such as eczema.
- Generally early physiological changes in pregnancy are regulated by hormonal changes, whereas later changes may be due to structural effects of the enlarging uterus.
- Reproductive system: under the influence of oestrogen, the uterus increases in size and vascularization, and spontaneous uterine contractions are suppressed. The breasts undergo development in preparation for lactation.
- Cardiovascular system: physiological changes are particularly marked in this system, meeting the increased demands of the maternal and fetal tissues. The vascular system expands as progesterone stimulates vasodilation of the vascular smooth muscle and oestrogen stimulates angiogenesis and increased blood flow. The RAS responds to the underfilled vascular system by increasing sodium and water retention; thus blood volume increases by about 40%. Plasma expansion is greater than blood cell increase leading to overall haemodilution.
- Cardiac output increases early in pregnancy, initially as a result of increased heart rate, which is subsequently followed by increased stroke volume. Myocontractility is increased throughout pregnancy, which stimulates a degree of ventricular hypertrophy.
- Blood pressure decreases in early pregnancy, reaching a minimum in mid pregnancy, and then returns close to prepregnant values towards term. The effects of posture on blood pressure are marked in pregnancy.
- The dilution of plasma proteins increases the formation of oedema. The ratio of clotting factors changes so bleeding time decreases.
- Respiratory system: excursion of the diaphragm alters as the rib cage flares increasing the efficiency of inspiration. Progesterone affects the sensitivity of the chemoreceptors, which increases respiratory drive. Therefore, hyperventilation is normal in pregnancy and results in lower circulating carbon dioxide levels and higher concentrations of cations, which facilitate exchange across the placenta.
- Gastrointestinal system: progesterone stimulates appetite and thirst and affects the sensitivity of the taste buds. Progesterone also affects the smooth muscle of the gut, which alters motility and transit time. This can result in increased efficiency of absorption but may also cause nausea and constipation. Decreased tone of lower oesophageal sphincter may result in reflux and heartburn.
- Skin: the increase in MSH levels results in increased pigmentation of the nipple and areola, the linea nigra and possibly chloasma. Increased blood flow to the skin, which is important in heat regulation, affects growth of hair and nails and may cause congestion of the mucous membranes.
- Skeleton: posture is affected by changed weight distribution and altered composition of the cartilage and connective tissue resulting in an exaggerated curvature of the spine.
- Metabolism: maternal metabolism is affected by altered thyroid hormone secretion and altered responses to insulin. In the first half of pregnancy, increased sensitivity to insulin favours deposition of maternal fat stores. In the second half of pregnancy, insulin resistance results in raised levels of substrates in the maternal plasma, which favour placental transport and fetal growth.

## Application to practice

Women experience many changes within their bodies and naturally will seek explanations and reassurance from the midwife as the changes occur. The midwife should use her knowledge of the physiological changes to aid her in assessing whether the pregnancy is progressing normally.

## Annotated further reading

Blackburn S T, Loper D L 1992 Maternal, fetal, and neonatal physiology: a clinical perspective. W B Saunders, Philadelphia

*An in-depth description of physiological adaptation to pregnancy and consequent development of the fetus and neonate that draws from physiological research studies. The chapters are clearly organized by physiological systems and link physiological concepts to clinical applications including the assessment and management of low- and high-risk pregnancies.*

Chamberlain G 1995 Turnbull's obstetrics, 2nd edn. Churchill Livingstone, New York

*A comprehensive textbook with a medical approach to obstetric principles and practice and the development of clinical protocols.*

Chamberlain G, Broughton Pipkin F 1998 Clinical physiology in obstetrics, 3rd edn. Blackwell, Oxford

*Comprehensively describes the physiological changes in pregnancy and relates recent research findings to practical considerations in the care of pregnant women.*

Creasy R K, Resnik R 1998 Maternal–fetal medicine: principles and practice, 4th edn. W B Saunders, Philadelphia

*Covers all disciplines pertinent to obstetricians including genetics and genetic testing, fetal and placental growth and development, epidemiology, immunology, physiological adaptation to pregnancy as well as clinical applications and medical complications in pregnancy.*

Davis D C 1996 The discomforts of pregnancy. Journal of Obstetrics and Gynecology and Neonatal Nursing 25:73–81

*A short paper which summarizes the minor complications and discomforts of pregnancy, relating them to the underlying physiological changes.*

## References


Addy D P 1986 Happiness is: iron. British Medical Journal 292:969

Ances I G, Pomerantz S H 1974 Serum concentrations of B-melanocyte stimulating hormone in pregnancy. American Journal of Obstetrics and Gynecology 87:275–280

Ashton H 1975 Cigarette smoking in pregnancy: differences in the peripheral circulation between smokers and nonsmokers. British Journal of Obstetrics and Gynaecology 82:868

Baylis C, Davison J M 1998 The urinary system. In: Chamberlain G, Broughton Pipkin F (eds) Clinical physiology in obstetrics, 3rd edn. Blackwell, Oxford, pp 263–307

Blackburn S T, Loper D L 1992 Maternal, fetal, and neonatal physiology: a clinical perspective. W B Saunders, Philadelphia

Bowen D J 1992 Taste and food preference changes across the course of pregnancy. Appetite 19:233–242

Brown M A, Gallery E D M 1994 Volume homeostasis in normal pregnancy and pre-eclampsia: physiology and clinical implications. Baillière's Clinics in Obstetrics and Gynaecology 8:287–310

Brunner D P, Münch M, Biedermann K, Huch R, Huch A, Borbély A A 1994 Changes in sleep and sleep electroencephalogram during pregnancy. Sleep 17(7):576–582

Carbonne B, Benachi A, Léveque M L, Cabrol D, Papiernik E 1996 Maternal position during labor: effects on fetal oxygen saturation measured by pulse oximetry. Obstetrics and Gynecology 88:797–800

Chamberlain G, Dewhurst J, Harvey D 1991 Illustrated textbook of obstetrics. Gower Medical (Mosby), London, p 104

Chesley L C 1972 Plasma and red cell volumes during pregnancy. American Journal of Obstetrics and Gynecology 12:440

Davison J M, Shiells E A Philips P R et al 1988 Serial evaluation of vasopressin release and thirst in pregnancy: the role of chorion gonadotrophin in the osmoregulatory changes of gestation. Journal of Clinical Investigation 81:798–801

de Swiet M 1998a The cardiovascular system. In: Chamberlain G, Broughton Pipkin F (eds) Clinical physiology in obstetrics, 3rd edn. Blackwell, Oxford, pp 33–70

de Swiet M 1998b The respiratory system. In: Chamberlain G, Broughton Pipkin F (eds) Clinical physiology in obstetrics, 3rd edn. Blackwell, Oxford, pp 111–128

de Swiet M, Fidler J 1981 Heart disease in pregnancy: some controversies. Journal of the Royal College of Physicians of London 15:183–186

Dunlop W 1980 Serial changes in renal haemodynamics during normal human pregnancy. Journal of Obstetrics and Gynaecology 88:1

Duvekot J J, Peeters L L H 1998 Very early changes in cardiovascular physiology. In: Chamberlain G, Broughton Pipkin F (eds) Clinical physiology in obstetrics, 3rd edn. Blackwell, Oxford, pp 3–32

Finch C A, Heubers H 1982 Perspectives in iron metabolism. New England Journal of Medicine 306:1520

Frienkel N, Metzger B E, Nitzan M et al 1972 'Accelerated starvation' and mechanisms for the conservation of maternal nitrogen during pregnancy. Israel Journal of Medical Science 8:426

Gant N F, Daley G L, Chand S, Whalley P J, MacDonald P C 1973 A study of angiotensin II pressor response throughout primigravid pregnancy. Journal of Clinical Investigation 52:2682

Glinoer D, Lemone M 1992 Goiter and pregnancy: a new insight into an old problem. Thyroid 2:65–70

Godfrey K M, Redman C W G, Barker D J P, Osmond C 1991 The effect of maternal anaemia and iron deficiency on the ratio of fetal weight to placental weight. British Journal of Obstetrics and Gynaecology 98:886

Hytten F 1985 Blood volume changes in normal pregnancy. Clinics in Haematology 14(3):601–612

Hytten F 1991 The alimentary system. In: Hytten F, Chamberlain G (eds) Clinical physiology in obstetrics, 2nd edn. Blackwell, Oxford, pp 137–149

Iles R K, Chard T 1991 Human chorionic gonadotrophin expression by bladder cancers: biology and clinical potential. Journal of Urology 145(3):481–489

Jacobs A, Miller F, Worwod M, Beamish M R, Wardrop C A 1972 Ferritin in serum of normal subjects and patients with iron deficiency and iron overload. British Medical Journal 4:206

Kornyei J L, Lei Z M, Rao C V 1993 Human myometrial smooth muscle cells are a novel target of direct regulation by human chorionic gonadotrophin. Biology of Reproduction 49:1149–1157

Kreisman H, Van de Weil W, Mitchell C A 1975 Respiratory function during prostaglandin-induced labor. American Review of Respiratory Disease 111:564–566

Letsky E 1998 The haematological system. In: Chamberlain G, Broughton Pipkin F (eds) Clinical physiology in obstetrics, 3rd edn. Blackwell, Oxford, pp 71–110

Lutjen P, Trounson A, Leeton J, Findlay J, Wood C, Renou P 1984 The establishment and maintenance of pregnancy using in vitro fertilization and embryo donation in a patient with primary ovarian failure. Nature 307:174–175

Mabie W C, DiSessa T G, Crocker L G, Sibai B M, Arheart K L 1994 A longitudinal study of cardiac output in normal human pregnancy. American Journal of Obstetrics and Gynecology 170:849

Miller A W F, Hanretty K P 1998 Obstetrics illustrated, 5th edn. Churchill Livingstone, New York, p 34

Morris N H, Eaton B M, Dekker G 1996 Nitric oxide, the endothelium, pregnancy and pre-eclampsia. British Journal of Obstetrics and Gynaecology 103:4

Palmer R M J, Ferrige A G, Moncada S 1987 Nitric oxide release accounts for the biological activity of endothelium-derived relaxing factor. Nature 327:524

Parry E, Shields R, Turnbull A C 1980 The effect of pregnancy on the colonic absorption of sodium, potassium and water. Journal of Obstetrics and Gynaecology 77:616–619

Pembrey M E, Weatherall D J, Clegg J B 1973 Maternal synthesis of haemoglobin F in pregnancy. Lancet i:1350

Pohl U, Busse R, Kuon E, Basenge F 1986 Pulsatile perfusion stimulates the release of endothelial autocoids. Journal of Applied Cardiology 1:215

Rosenfeld C R 1980 Responses of reproductive and nonreproductive tissues to 17β-estradiol during ovine puerperium. American Journal of Physiology 239:E333

Scrier R W 1992 A unifying hypothesis of body fluid volume regulation. Journal of the Royal College of Physicians of London 26:295

Skatrud J B, Dempsey J A, Kaiser D G 1978 Ventilatory response to medroxyprogesterone acetate in normal subjects: time course and mechanism. Journal of Applied Physiology 44:939

Smith S S 1991 Progesterone administration attenuates excitory amino acid responses of cerebellar Purkinje cells. Neuroscience 42:309–320

Sundsfjord J A, Aakvaag A 1973 Variations in plasma aldosterone and plasma renin activity throughout the menstrual cycle, with special reference to the pre-ovulatory period. Acta Endocrinologia (Copenhagen) 73:499

Sweet B, Tiran D 1996 Mayes midwifery, 12th edn. Baillière Tindall, London, p 131

Thompson W G 1988 Comparison of tests for diagnosis of iron depletion in pregnancy. American Journal of Obstetrics and Gynecology 159:1132

Thomson K J, Cohen M E 1938 Studies on the circulation in pregnancy II: vital capacity observations in normal pregnant women. Surgery, Gynecology and Obstetrics 66:591–597

Tulchinsky D, Hobel C J 1973 Plasma human chorionic gonadotropin, estrone, estradiol, estriol, progesterone, and 17-hydroxyprogesterone in human pregnancy. III. Early normal pregnancy. American Journal of Obstetrics and Gynecology 117:884

Wichman K, Ryden G, Wichman G 1984 The influence of different positions and Korotkoff sounds on the blood pressure measurements in pregnancy. Acta Obstetrica et Gynecologia Scandinavica (suppl) 118:25

Yip R, Dallman P R 1996 Iron. In: Ziegter E E, Filer L J (eds) Present knowledge in nutrition, 7th edn. ILSI, Washington DC, pp 277–292

# 12 Maternal nutrition and health

## Learning objectives

- To review nutritional requirements and explain the role of the main nutrient groups in human health.
- To identify how and why nutrient requirements might change during pregnancy.
- To describe how the fetus adapts to low nutrient levels.
- To relate undernutrition to outcome of pregnancy.
- To discuss other factors that may affect weight gain in pregnancy and birth weight.

## Introduction

It is common for pregnancy to affect a woman's sense of well-being. Some aspects of health may be affected positively and others negatively. The role of nutrition, both before and after pregnancy, is important for the health of both the mother and fetus.

## Overview of nutrition

Growth, development and optimal health rely on good nutrition and an adequate quality and quantity of nutrients for the cells. However, diet is influenced by many factors including wealth, religion, culture, and geographical and social factors. The insoluble macromolecules of food must be digested into soluble and absorbable subunits (see Ch. 1). The major components of the diet, or macronutrients, are carbohydrates, proteins and fats. Essential micronutrients are vitamins and minerals. Water is also an essential part of the diet.

### *Carbohydrates*

Carbohydrates are the major energy source in the majority of human diets, but the amount and type of carbohydrate consumed varies amongst different population groups. With increased affluence in the Western world, there is a tendency to increase the proportion of fat in the diet at the expense of carbohydrate. There are two major types of carbohydrate: polysaccharides and simple sugars (monosaccharides and disaccharides).

Monosaccharides, such as glucose, fructose and galactose, are not usually consumed in high quantities although they do occur in fruit. The major source of carbohydrate in the diet is starch from plant sources, plus some glycogen from animal liver and muscle. Dietary disaccharides include sucrose (table sugar), lactose (in milk) and maltose, which occurs in malt, beer and some sprouting seeds. Most starchy foods are high in carbohydrate and low in fat. Many are rich in indigestible non-starch polysaccharides (NSP or 'fibre'), which are associated with lower cholesterol levels, lower blood sugar levels and decreased incidence of gut diseases.

### *Proteins*

Proteins are made up of 20 types of amino acids linked together by peptide bonds. Essential amino acids are those that cannot be synthesized from others and, therefore, are required in the diet (Table 12.1). There are conditions, where requirement is high or there is limited ability to interconvert amino acids, that result in an amino acid that can usually be synthesized from an essential amino acid being required in the diet. These amino acids are described as being conditionally essential, for instance in premature babies with immature enzyme function or under conditions of stress. Protein quality depends on the proportion of dietary

**Table 12.1** *Amino acids*

| Essential amino acids | Conditionally essential amino acids | Non-essential amino acids |
|---|---|---|
| Lysine | Cysteine | Alanine |
| Threonine | Tyrosine | Glutamic acid |
| Histidine | Arginine | Aspartic acid |
| Isoleucine | Citrulline* | Glycine |
| Leucine | Taurine* | Serine |
| Methionine | Carnitine | Proline |
| Phenylalanine | | Glutamine |
| Tryptophan | | Asparagine |
| Valine | | |

* Conditionally essential or essential only at certain ages or in certain conditions.

protein that is absorbed across the gut (digestibility) and the ratio of the essential amino acids in the protein. A protein that is absorbed completely and utilized completely because the essential amino acids are in the optimum proportion for synthesis of new proteins is described as a high-quality protein, with a net protein utilization (NPU) value of 1.0 or 100%. Human milk and whole egg have NPUs of 1.0, whereas the overall protein availability in the Western diet is typically 0.7. The NPU of diets dependent on poor-quality proteins, such as those based on cassava (made from tapioca root), can be as low as 0.5.

In the absence of alternative sources of energy, protein can be metabolized as an energy source. Excess protein in the diet will also be used as metabolic fuel. An adult is usually in nitrogen balance: protein intake is equal to protein breakdown so nitrogen in the diet is equal to excreted levels of nitrogen. Under conditions of growth and protein synthesis, there is a net accumulation of protein, and hence nitrogen, which is described as a state of positive nitrogen balance (Hytten & Cheyne 1969). States of growth, including pregnancy, result in positive nitrogen balance. Negative nitrogen balance usually indicates tissue breakdown or nutrient deficiency resulting in energy generation from protein sources. Illness and trauma cause negative nitrogen balance, although it also occurs with reduced activity and decreasing muscle mass and during uterine involution (see Ch. 13).

## Fat

Fat is used for energy requirements. There is also a requirement for essential long-chain fatty acids, which cannot be synthesized by the body. These are the precursors of prostaglandins and leukotrienes. Fat also provides the vehicle for absorption of fat-soluble vitamins. Most fat is present in the diet as triglycerides; a triglyceride is a glycerol molecule with three fatty acids (Fig. 12.1). The fatty acids can be saturated, where the carbon atoms are fully occupied by hydrogen atoms, or unsaturated, where there are double bonds between some of the carbon atoms. The body handles fatty acids differently depending on their length and the degree of saturation (Fig. 12.1c). Fats in foods are formed of triglycerides containing a combination of different fatty acids, but are described by the predominant type. For instance, olive oil is particularly rich in monounsaturated fatty acids (with single double bonds).

Saturated fats are likely to be solid at room temperature and are usually of animal origin, although coconut and palm oils and cocoa butter are saturated. Saturated fats become rancid very slowly so they store well. Unsaturated fats are usually liquid at room temperature and mostly of plant origin. The C=C double bond is not very stable so it breaks down easily and the fat becomes rancid. In food processing, unsaturated vegetable oils are hydrogenated (have hydrogen atoms added to saturate the C=C bonds), which makes the fat harder and extends the shelf life. Unsaturated fatty acids from all vegetable and most animal sources adopt a cis configuration. Positional isomerism, where the fatty acid has the same length and number and position of double bonds, but the atoms lie in different positions, is described as a trans configuration (Fig. 12.2). Hydrogenation and heating can convert the cis bonds to the trans-isomer. Trans fatty acids are implicated in increased risk of myocardial infarction and other cardiovascular problems.

## Vitamins

Vitamins are organic substances required in small amounts for metabolism, growth and maintenance. Vitamins do not provide sources of energy but act as regulators of metabolic processes. They can be divided into water-soluble (Table 12.2) and fat-soluble vitamins (Table 12.3). The fat-soluble vitamins are more stable than water-soluble vitamins

**Fig. 12.1** ***Structure of fats: A a saturated fatty acid; B a triglyceride; C the fatty acid cycle.***

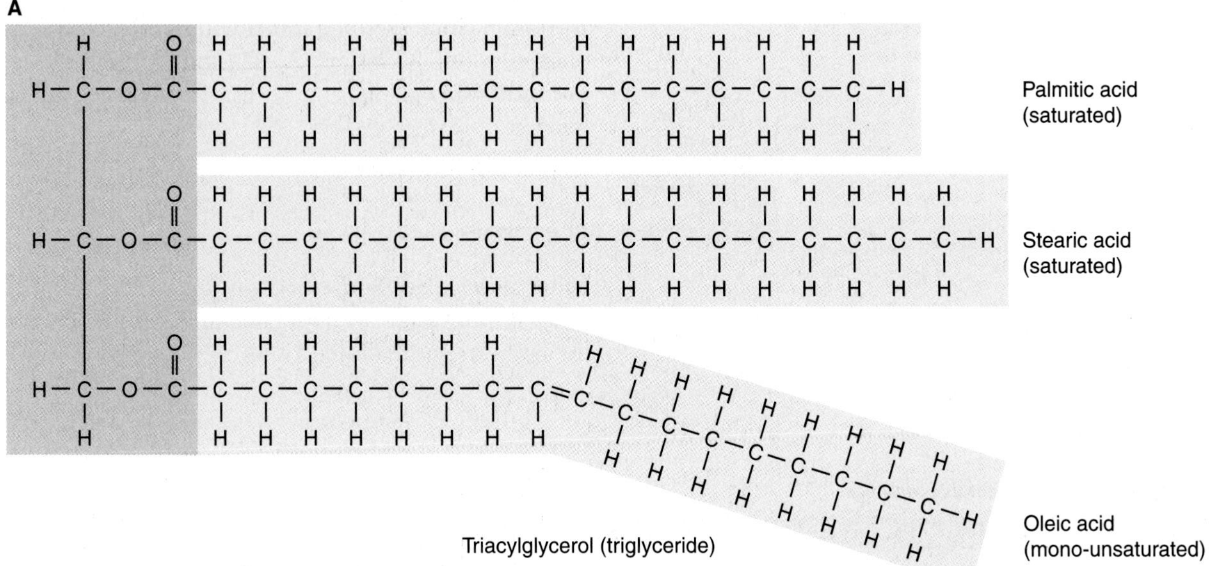


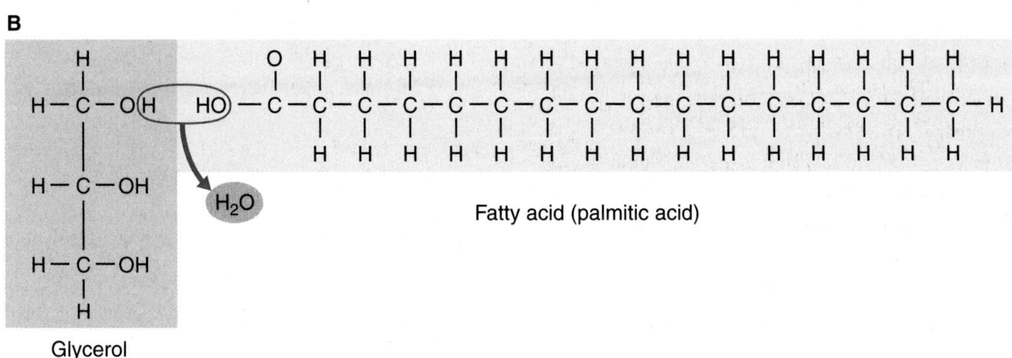


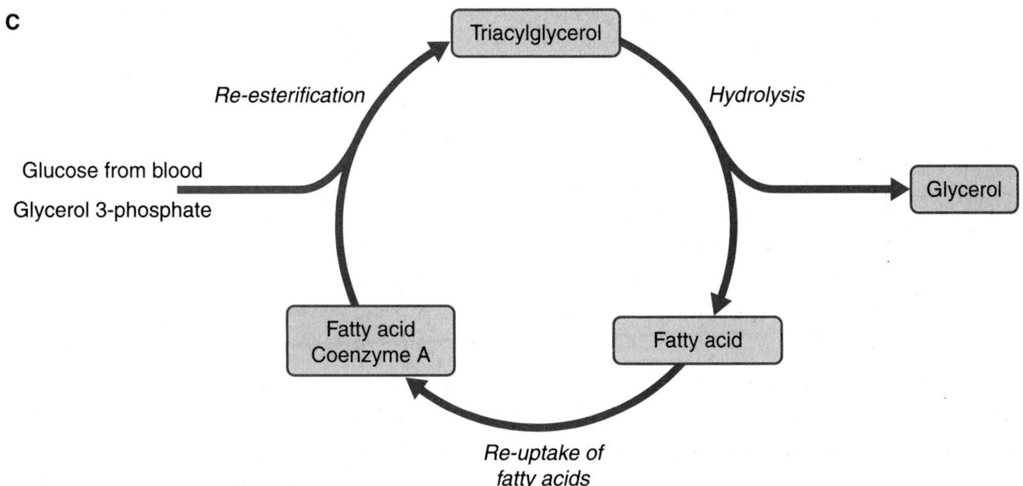

**Fig. 12.2** *A Cis- and B trans-isomerism of fatty acids.*

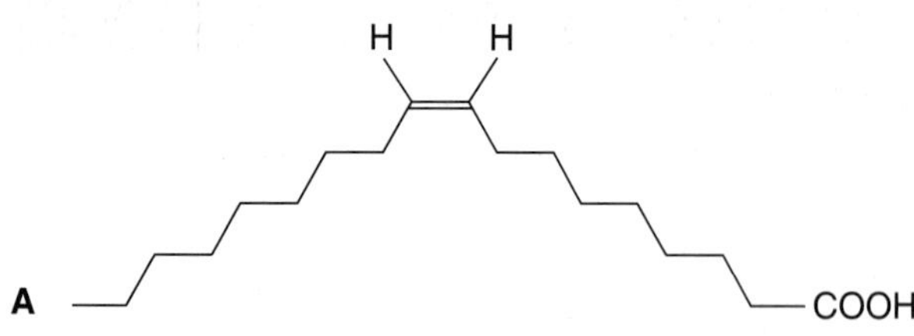


and are stored in the body. As B vitamins function as coenzymes in energy metabolism, requirement for B vitamins increases in parallel with increased energy consumption. Vitamins A, C and E function as antioxidants protecting cells from free-radical damage.

## *Minerals*

Minerals regulate body function and are essential to good health. They are inorganic and become part of the body structure (Table 12.4).

**Table 12.2** *Water-soluble vitamins*

| Vitamin | Role | Source |
|---|---|---|
| Thiamin ($B_1$) | Carbohydrate metabolism | Pork, wheat germ, yeast |
| Riboflavin ($B_2$) | Protein metabolism | Offal, milk, grains, legumes, eggs, vegetables |
| Niacin ($B_3$) | Production of energy from glucose; synthesis of fatty acids | Meat, nuts, legumes |
| Pyridoxine ($B_6$) | Synthesis and catabolism of amino acids; synthesis of antibodies and neurotransmitters | Pork, offal, grains, legumes, potatoes, bananas |
| Cyanocobalamine ($B_{12}$) | Reactions preceding use of folic acid in DNA synthesis | Animal and dairy products, eggs, yeast |
| Folate | Formation of DNA | Liver, green leafy vegetables, kidney beans, oranges, melon |
| Pantothenic acid | Metabolism; synthesis of acetylcholine | Liver, egg yolk, milk, dried and spouting beans |
| Biotin | Synthesis of fatty acids, amino acids and purines (required for DNA and RNA) | Offal, egg yolk, tomatoes |
| C | Collagen formation, tissue formation and integrity, antioxidant, iron absorption | Citrus fruit, tomatoes, other fruit and vegetables |

**Table 12.3** *Fat-soluble vitamins*

| Vitamin | Role | Source |
|---|---|---|
| A | Visual perception (rhodopsin synthesis); growth of epithelial tissue and bones, antioxidant | Liver, kidney, egg yolk |
| D | Hormone involved in bone mineralization and calcium homeostasis | Synthesized in skin, fish oils |
| E | Tissue growth + integrity of cell membranes; antioxidant | Vegetable oils, grains, milk, eggs, fish, meat |
| K | Synthesis of blood-clotting factors; bone metabolism | Gut flora, liver, green leafy vegetables |

**Table 12.4** *Minerals*

| Mineral | Function | Dietary source |
|---|---|---|
| Sodium (Na) | Extracellular ion essential for the generation of action potentials; required in the active transport of small molecules into the cell | Table salt (NaCl) |
| Potassium (K) | Intracellular ion essential for the generation of action potentials; utilized by the cell to maintain ion concentration gradients | Meat, milk, fruits, vegetables |
| Calcium (Ca) | Bone and teeth structural component; essential for blood clotting, muscle contraction and nerve impulse conduction | Dairy products, fortified flour, cereals, green vegetables |
| Chlorine (Cl) | Cation in body fluids; gastric acid excretions | Salt (NaCl) |
| Phosphorus (P) | Structural component of bones and teeth; essential for formation of ATP for energy storage | Meat, dairy products cereals, bread |
| Magnesium (Mg) | Required by some enzyme activities; present in cells, body fluids and bone | Vegetables, milk, cereals, bread |
| Iron (Fe) | Transfer of oxygen in haemoglobin molecule; oxidation processes; electron transfer chain | Meat, vegetables, flour |
| Zinc | Enzyme activity; growth and development of the immune system; spermatogenesis; tissue growth | Oysters, steak, crab meat, red meat, milk products |
| Iodide | Thyroid hormones | Seafood sea salt |
| Copper | Constituent of enzymes; energy production and release | Legumes, grains, nuts and seeds, offal |
| Manganese | Synthesis of urea; conversion of pyruvate in TCA cycle | Plant products |
| Fluoride | Essential to reduce decay in bone and tooth tissues | Fluoridated drinking water |
| Chromium | Carbohydrate and lipid metabolism | Unrefined foods, brewers yeast, whole grains and nuts |
| Selenium | Antioxidant; catalyst for the production of thyroid hormone | Liver, shellfish, fish meat |

## Preconceptual nutritional status

The sensitivity of the hypothalamus to environmental influences, such as nutrient availability, was probably of immense importance in promoting pregnancy in seasons when the fetus and infant had optimal chances of survival. Weight loss affects cyclical ovarian function in women. Anorexia nervosa disrupts the hypothalamic–pituitary–ovarian axis (see Ch. 4) and may cause amenorrhoea. Amenorrhoea related to inadequate nutrient intake is often reported in ballet dancers, competitive runners and other athletes (Frisch 1990). It not only affects ovulatory cycle but can result in low levels of oestrogens, which reduces bone density and predisposes to osteoporosis. It has been suggested that the menarche depended on women reaching a 'critical weight' (Frisch & McArthur 1974). However, low body weight is not always associated with amenorrhoea (Franks & Robinson 1996). Conversely, dieting and nutrient restriction can suppress normal reproductive cycles in women of normal body weight (Pirke et al 1985).

A minimal level of nutrient intake and fuel metabolism seem to be required to maintain reproductive functions, particularly the pulse generating secretion of GnRH (see Ch. 4). Fluctuations in body fat can also disturb the transport and metabolism of the steroid-hormones, which are fat soluble. Nutrient deficiency may itself suppress appetite. Studies in animals suggest optimal pregnancy outcome may depend on long-term nutritional status rather than a period of 'flushing', or short-term good-quality diet (Wynn & Wynn 1991).

Although restricted nutrient intake can suppress reproductive function, excess energy intake may also be disruptive. Obesity also affects conception rate. Polycystic ovary syndrome (PCOS), which is often associated with anovulation (see Ch. 6), disrupts glucose–insulin homeostasis. The symptoms and effects of PCOS on reproduction are more severe with increased body weight. In PCOS, increased obesity disrupts normal production of steroid hormones and affects carbohydrate handling. Disruption of ovulation is associated with insulin resistance and hyperinsulinaemia (Franks & Robinson 1996).

A woman's weight, particularly if it is related to her height, indicates her nutritional status to some degree. Weight loss and nutrient fluctuation caused by self-imposed dieting, affecting reproductive function, may be the cause of infertility in a large proportion of the women seeking fertility treatment. It has been suggested that nearly 80% of women attending infertility clinics can be classified as underweight (Wynn & Wynn 1991). Maternal nutritional status can be assessed by calculation of body mass index (BMI) (Box 12.1). A BMI of about 24 kg/m$^2$ seems optimal for women planning pregnancy. A BMI less than 20 kg/m$^2$ is not associated with good fertility or pregnancy outcome.

Maternal protein intake affects gonadotrophin secretion and ovulatory maturation (Wynn & Wynn 1991). Both diets with abnormally high and those with very low protein concentrations affect the menstrual cycle and fertility. It is possible that high-protein diets may cause one of the coenzymes involved in protein metabolism to become limiting. It is also suggested that low levels of B vitamins depress pituitary hormone secretion. Both embryonic development, especially early in gestation, and follicular development involve a rapid rate of protein synthesis and cell division, which are associated with a high energy and nutrient requirement. Preconceptual nutrient deficiency may retard development of the follicle and corpus luteum, affecting subsequent embryonic growth, even if the level of deficiency is not adequate to cause infertility. Excess intakes of some nutrients may increase mutation rate. Nutrient deficiency also affects male fertility, by altering DNA synthesis and rates of cell division. Selenium availability may be an important factor in male fertility.

Whether the mother enters pregnancy with high nutritional stores may affect the outcome of the pregnancy. Placental size in humans appears to be governed by genetic growth potential, anoxia and nutrient availability. In sheep, a period of poor nutrition early in gestation increases placental size, presumably as an adaptive mechanism to increase nutrient extraction (McCrabb, Egan & Hosking 1992). Provided this nutrient restriction is transient and the sheep are then returned to richer pasture, the increase in placental size is associated with an increase in lamb birth weight. In humans, a increased placental:fetal weight

**Box 12.1**

**The body mass index**

Body mass index is used to indicate nutritional status and risk factors associated with obesity. It is a ratio of weight (measured in kilograms) for height (measured in metres squared).

Calculation:

$$\text{BMI} = \frac{\text{weight}}{\text{height}^2} \left\{ \frac{\text{kg}}{\text{m}^2} \right\}$$

Interpretation:

| Grade | BMI* | Definition |
|---|---|---|
| — | <20 | Underweight |
| 0 | 20–24.9 | Desirable weight |
| I | 25–29.9 | Overweight |
| II | 30–39.9 | Mild obesity |
| III | 40 | Severe obesity |

* Normal: 19.8–26.0

A healthy shape is considered to be that usually associated with a BMI of 20–25 kg/m$^2$. Waist circumference and waist to height ratios are also used as indicators of healthy shape. A waist circumference of less than 80 cm is considered healthy in women and less than 94 cm in adult men, with waist circumferences above 88 cm and 102 cm respectively indicating risk. A waist: height ratio of less than 0.5 is also considered healthy with a ratio greater than 0.6 indicating risk to health.

ratio is associated with poorer outcome and long-term health prognosis (Barker 1998). However, larger babies have larger placentas but in proportion to their birth weight. Morning sickness may produce a period of poor nutrition in early pregnancy, which could stimulate placental growth. Provided the woman entered pregnancy with good nutrient stores and the effects on nutrient consumption were limited, nausea in pregnancy could therefore promote placental enlargement and positively affect the fetal growth trajectory. Interpregnancy interval may be important to allow replenishment of maternal stores especially vitamins such as folate.

Case study 12.1 looks at an example of nutritional status in pregnancy.

**Case study 12.1**

Fiona informs the midwife at the booking appointment that she has a healthy balanced diet.

- How can the midwife assess that this is an accurate statement?

**Box 12.2**
**Food safety**

**Listeriosis:**

- Caused by: bacterium *Listeria monocytogenes*
- Possible effects: miscarriage, stillbirth and neonatal death, brain damage
- Sources: soil, soft cheeses, poultry, cook–chill food
- **Note**: bacteria can multiply at low temperatures

**Salmonellosis**

- Caused by: *Salmonella*
- Possible effects: maternal high fever, vomiting, diarrhoea and dehydration associated with food poisoning may increase the risk of preterm labour or miscarriage
- Source: raw meat, poultry and eggs
- **Note**: survives in soft boiled eggs and mayonnaise

**Toxoplasmosis**

- Caused by: *Toxoplasma gondii*
- Possible effects: congenital mental retardation or blindness, neonatal convulsions
- Sources: soil, raw meat, cat's faeces, goat's milk

## Non-nutritional factors affecting reproductive function

Food can provide nutrition but it is also the source of a number of maternal infections (Box 12.2). Pregnant women are advised to be particularly careful about food hygiene. Although nutrient intake and weight gain are associated with clear effects on birth weight, a number of other factors have been shown to affect fetal size and growth potential (Box 12.3).

**Box 12.3**
**Factors affecting weight gain in pregnancy or birth weight**

- Maternal diet before and during pregnancy
- Maternal size, particularly lean body mass
- Age (younger women tend to gain more weight but pregnancy in adolescents is associated with an increased likelihood of a low birth-weight baby)
- Birth order (first babies tend to be slightly smaller)
- Parity (multigravidae tend to gain less weight)
- Fetal sex (male babies tend to be an average of 150 g heavier)
- Nicotine (both smoking and tobacco chewing are associated with decreased birth weight)
- Alcohol (regular alcohol consumption is associated with lower birth weight)
- Hypoxia (high altitude and chronic maternal anaemia depress birth weight)

Age affects cell proliferation and gamete formation. Some diseases accelerate premature ageing of the germ cells. These include diabetes, parental gene mutation, multiple sclerosis, ulcerative colitis and Crohn's disease (Wynn & Wynn 1991). Smoking, drugs, alcohol and radiation all affect cell division. Viruses are mutagenic and have long been associated with abnormal fetal development. Sexually transmitted diseases (STDs) can cause pelvic inflammatory disease, which may affect fertility and pregnancy outcome. Diseases caused by larger organisms, such as syphilis and gonorrhoea, are relatively easy to diagnose and treat. However, STDs caused by smaller microorganisms, such as chlamydia, papilloma, HIV, herpes and mycoplasmas, are difficult to eradicate. STD prevalence is associated with increased mobility of the population.

# Nutritional requirements in pregnancy

## Energy requirements

The nutritional costs of pregnancy can be calculated by estimating the cost of the new maternal tissues and the tissues of the conceptus (fetus, placenta, membranes and other tissues), the 'capital gains', and the metabolic costs of maintaining these growing tissues, the 'running costs' (Campbell-Brown & Hytten 1998). Tissue accrued accounts for about 50 000 kcal and increased metabolism accounts for about 36 000 kcal bringing the total specific cost of pregnancy to about 80 000 kcal (Fig. 12.3). As more studies about nutritional requirements during pregnancy are performed, the recommended daily allowances of energy and other nutrients have progressively decreased. However, recommended allowances are intended to be a standard against which the nutritional status of a population, rather than an individual person, can be assessed.

Energy requirements during the pregnancy are highest in the middle (from 10 to 30 weeks) when maternal fat stores are being assimilated. During the last 10 weeks of the pregnancy, the rapid growth of the fetus has a high energy requirement but the rate of maternal fat storage is decreased. In effect, the increased nutrition requirements of the pregnancy are spread fairly evenly over the later three-quarters of the pregnancy. The daily increase in energy requirement is calculated to be about 300 kcal over the final three-quarters of pregnancy (Campbell-Brown & Hytten 1998). This is calculated from the total cost of the pregnancy, estimated to be 80 000 kcal divided by 270 days of pregnancy. The actual energy consumed in pregnancy by women 'eating to appetite' (with free access to food) is about 200 kcal extra per day, less than the theoretical expected cost of the pregnancy. Many women, including those in developing countries and the poorer parts of affluent countries, successfully reproduce supported by energy intakes far below the recommended level.

Some of the additional energy requirements of pregnancy can be met by increased efficiency of maternal metabolism and decreased energy expenditure (Durnin 1987). The additional requirements are a relatively small proportion (about 25%) of the average total energy requirements for a non-pregnant woman. Thus decreased activity can make up a considerable proportion of the extra requirement. Decreased energy expenditure in the second and third trimesters of pregnancy has been observed in the Five Country Study of pregnant women (Lawrence et al 1987), which compared women living in Scotland, Holland, the Gambia, the Philippines and Thailand. Leisure activities and the rate at which heavy work was done

**Fig. 12.3** *The cumulative energy costs of pregnancy. (Reproduced with permission from Hytten 1991.)*

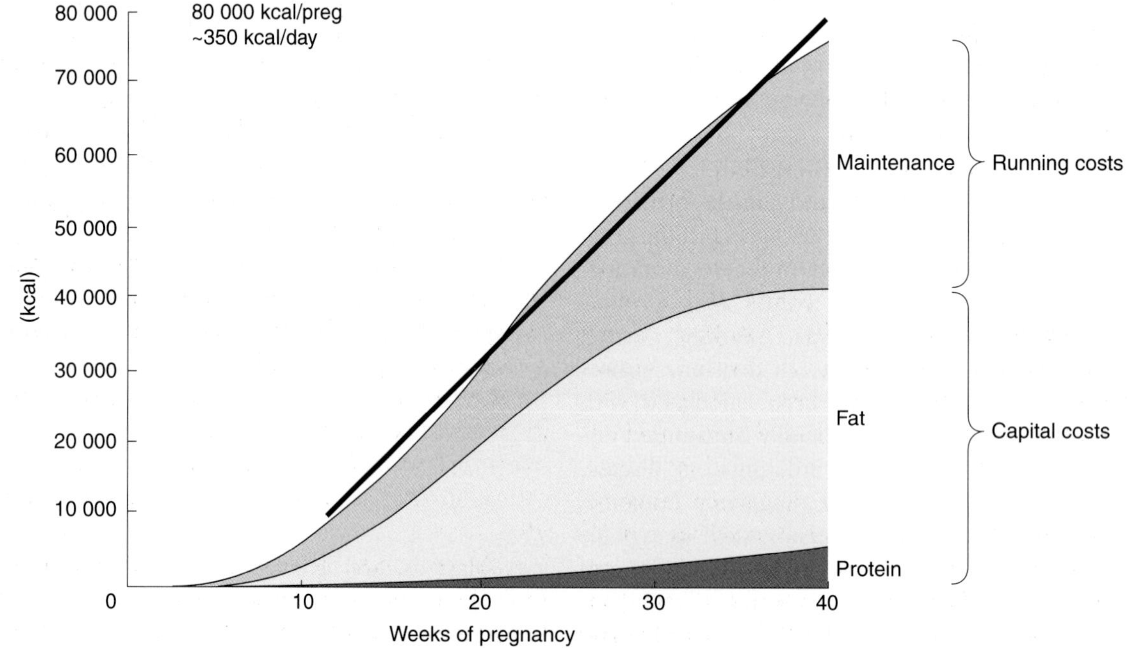

decreased. Women who have a long history of poor nutrition, for instance those in subsistence farming communities, seem to be able to adapt more to sparing nutrients and economizing to support the cost of the pregnancy. This may be because these women are more physically active and so can decrease their energy expenditure by a greater degree.

## Protein requirements

Protein requirements for the growth of maternal tissues and the growth of the conceptus can be calculated. The increased protein synthesis, and therefore increased dietary requirement, in late pregnancy is about 6 g per day. In Britain, where the NPU value is 0.7, this is equivalent to about 8–9 g additional dietary protein being required to maintain nitrogen balance, assuming that metabolism of protein is not affected by pregnancy. In pregnant rats, hepatic changes result in decreased urea production, which may spare protein for other roles (Naismith & Morgan 1976). Although such changes have not been observed in pregnant women, blood urea levels do fall (Campbell-Brown & Hytten 1998). The transfer of amino acids across the placenta is only just adequate for fetal protein synthesis so any factor adversely affecting amino acid transport mechanisms has the potential to limit growth.

During the pregnancy, there is a fall in blood protein levels from about 70 g/l to 60 g/l. Much of this fall is due to decreased plasma albumin concentration. Albumin functions as a non-specific carrier of lipophilic substances such as some drugs, hormones, free fatty acids, unconjugated bilirubin and some ions. It is has an important role in maintaining the plasma osmotic pressure. The fall in plasma colloid osmotic pressure increases movement of water out of the blood vessels (see Ch. 1), thus increasing lower limb oedema and affecting glomerular filtration rate. Plasma globulins increase in pregnancy.

Plasma levels of most amino acids fall in pregnancy. The most marked falls are observed in glucogenic amino acids, which can be used to form glucose, then those involved in the urea cycle and then the ketogenic branched-chain amino acids (Cox & Calarne 1978). Amino acids are actively transported across the placenta. Imbalances in maternal amino acid concentration will be reflected by placental uptake. For instance, women with phenylketonuria (PKU) are advised to resume a low-phenylalanine diet prior to conception as high levels of phenylalanine can harm the fetus, even if the fetus does not have PKU. High phenylalanine levels in pregnancy are associated with fetal IUGR, congenital heart disease, microcephaly and mental retardation.

The optimum birth weight in humans can be considered to be within the range of birth weights associated with the lowest incidence of perinatal mortality and morbidity, in the range 3500–4500 g (Wynn & Wynn 1991). Mothers of babies in the optimal birth-weight range tend to eat more protein than women who give birth to babies with lower birth weight. Maternal intakes of B vitamins and some minerals, particularly magnesium, have been found to correlate well with birth weight (Wynn & Wynn 1991). The main regulator of fetal growth seems to be availability of nutrients, which can affect growth directly, by changing the availability of substrates required for growth, or indirectly, by altering hormonal control of growth.

## Fat

In pregnancy, plasma lipids alter markedly. Free fatty acid levels fall early in pregnancy and then rise. The changes in handling of fatty acids are associated with changed sensitivity to insulin during the pregnancy (Robinson et al 1992). The low levels initially probably result from high rates of maternal fat storage. The rising level in the third trimester probably reflects mobilization of these stores. Lipids are transported as lipoprotein complexes, classified by their density (Fig. 12.4). Triglyceride levels increase throughout gestation. Placental uptake of triglycerides occurs in the form of very-low-density lipoproteins (VLDL). Placental lipase may hydrolyse VLDL, releasing the products for energy metabolism by the fetus (Robinson et al 1992).

Maternal fat stores, which are 3.5 kg on average, can subsidize a considerable part of the pregnancy. Oxidation of 3.5 kg of fat could theoretically produce 30 000 kcal. Fat accumulation is highest early in pregnancy when maternal maintenance costs of pregnancy and fetal growth are relatively low (Campbell-Brown & Hytten 1998). This appears to anticipate requirements later in pregnancy. In the later stages of pregnancy, when fetal requirements are maximal, maternal nutrient intake could be restricted by lack of availability of food or by effects of pregnancy on capacity for eating and gastrointestinal disturbances. Progesterone affects the control centres in the hypothalamus increasing maternal appetite, so food intake increases by about 200 kcal per day. However, this is augmented by decreased energy expenditure. Relaxation of

**Fig. 12.4** *Classification of lipoprotein complexes. (Reproduced with permission from Saffrey & Stewart 1997.)*

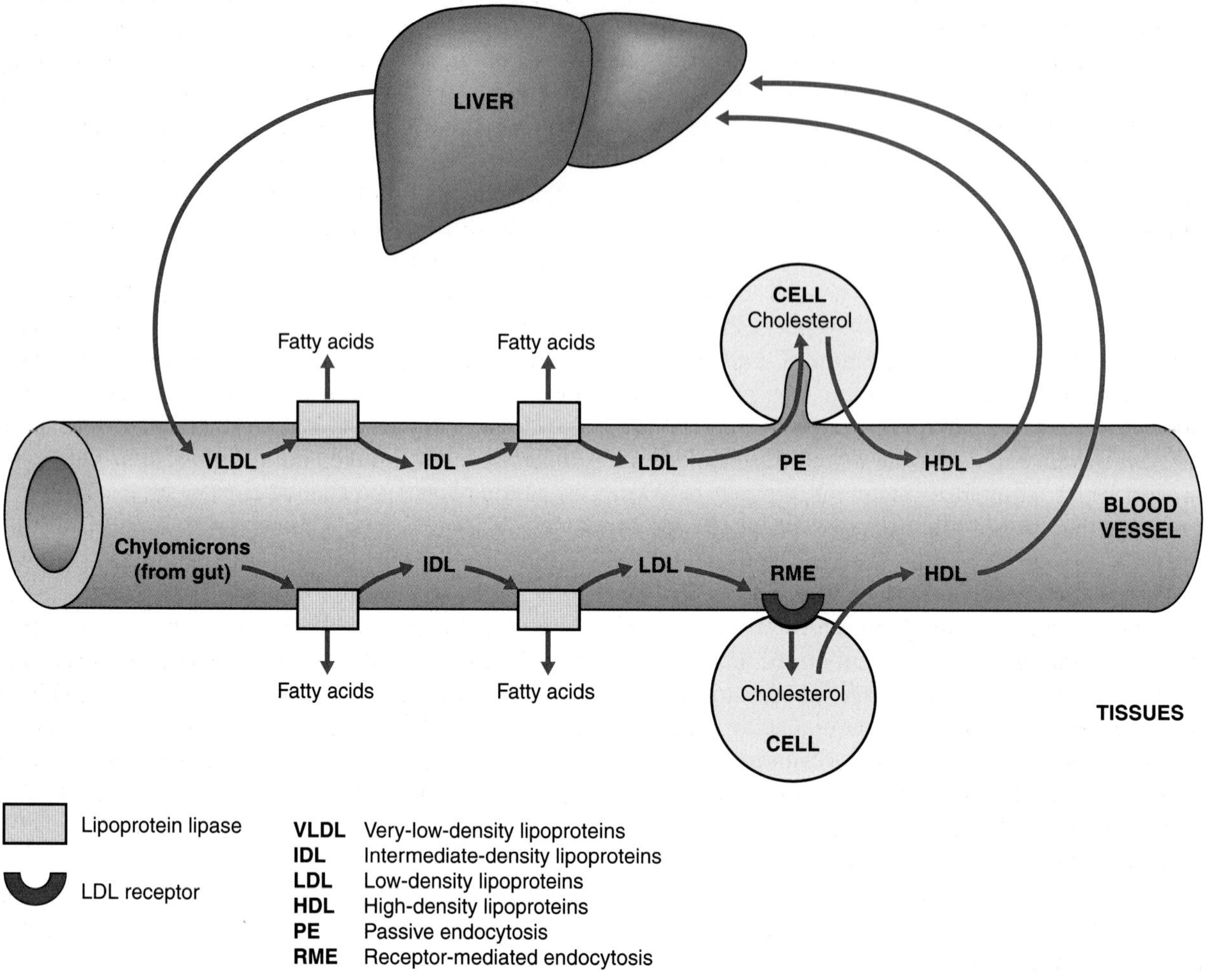

Lipoprotein lipase
LDL receptor

**VLDL** Very-low-density lipoproteins
**IDL** Intermediate-density lipoproteins
**LDL** Low-density lipoproteins
**HDL** High-density lipoproteins
**PE** Passive endocytosis
**RME** Receptor-mediated endocytosis

smooth muscle conserves energy and other metabolic activities such as thermogenic response to food may decrease (Illingworth et al 1987). Insulin sensitivity correlates well with postprandial thermogenesis (Robinson et al 1992).

The fall in fatty acid levels in early pregnancy and the later rise reflect high maternal uptake during the time of maternal fat deposition and decreased adipose storage and lipogenesis late in pregnancy. The change in lipid handling appears to be under control of the hormones of pregnancy.

## Vitamins and minerals

Specific increased requirements for vitamins in pregnancy have not been quantified. Both vitamin deficiency and excess are associated with adverse pregnancy outcome. The placenta can extract vitamins from maternal plasma and transfer them to the fetus, maintaining transport against a concentration gradient. Thus, fetal concentration of vitamins may be five to 10 times the level in maternal blood. The 'pump' mechanisms of the placenta appear to be specific for vitamins: most minerals are not transported by similar mechanisms. A good-quality maternal diet is probably able to provide the increased vitamin and mineral requirements of the pregnancy, particularly if energy intake is increased from a source of high-nutrient-density food. However, a poor-quality diet may adversely affect both fetal growth and the establishment of adequate stores for neonatal growth. Vitamin requirement is increased slightly in pregnancy but unless the woman is at the threshold of a deficiency, most women's diets should provide adequate reserve. Certain subgroups within the popula-

tion are at increased risk of vitamin deficiency, such as Asian women and vitamin D deficiency.

Levels of fat-soluble vitamins increase during pregnancy and levels of water-soluble vitamins fall. However, levels of vitamin A fall but levels of carotenoids rise. Fat-soluble vitamins cross the placenta more readily than water-soluble vitamins and their transport increases with gestational length. Urinary excretion of vitamins is increased in pregnancy and there are fetal demands. Excess vitamin A may present a teratogenic risk (Rosa, Wilk & Kelsey 1986) but toxic levels are probably impossible to achieve from usual dietary sources. Changes in animal husbandry, and increased use of growth-promoting agents and vitamin supplements given to animals, may make the livers of farmed animals considerably richer in vitamin A than they used to be. The B-vitamin requirements are related to energy intake and so increase in proportion in pregnancy.

Maternal plasma levels of most vitamins and minerals fall as the pregnancy progresses. This may be due to haemodilution rather than increased uptake by maternal and fetal tissue. Lower circulating levels of nutrients in pregnancy cannot be interpreted a deficiency. It is suggested that hormonal resetting of homeostatic mechanisms favours transfer of nutrients to the fetus (Campbell-Brown & Hytten 1998). The placenta can take up and store nutrients efficiently. Low levels of nutrients in maternal plasma may limit maternal cell uptake while optimizing placental uptake.

## Folic acid

Folic acid requirements in pregnancy have been studied in depth. Blood folate levels fall in pregnancy, probably reflecting the high rate of DNA synthesis and cell division. Any factor that reduces DNA, RNA and protein synthesis increases the risk of congenital malformations, which are usually associated with a reduced cell number rather than a reduced cell size. Folic acid supplements, of 400 μg per day, are offered to all pregnant women. Periconceptual consumption of folic acid at levels higher than could be achieved from the diet can markedly reduce the incidence of neural tube defects (NTD) (Smithells, Sheppard & Schoran 1981). It is possible that susceptible individuals have a genetically acquired block in folate metabolism, which can be overcome by high concentrations of folate (Scott et al 1994). It is recommended that women who have already had one conception affected by a NTD should consume 4 mg folic acid per day to reduce the risk of recurrence. Although pregnant women seem aware of campaigns recommending increased folic acid consumption, many seem reluctant to take it (Health Education Authority 1996). Possibly advice to supplement the diet with folic acid may appear to conflict with the health advice usually given to pregnant women about avoiding unnecessary drugs. Renaming folic acid as 'vitamin B9' as is done in some parts of Europe might alter the perception of folic acid as a drug.

The incidence of NTDs is 1.6 per 10 000 livebirths in England and 3.1 per 10 000 in Wales. It is difficult to increase levels of folate-rich food to the level recommended (Cuskelly, McNulty & Scott 1996). The argument for supplementing a staple food, such as bread or flour, with folic acid (Wald & Bower 1995) has been strengthened by the other advantages of increasing folate consumption. Increased folic acid consumption may protect against cardiovascular disease (Ward et al 1997), cancer (Jennings 1995) and depression and neuropsychiatric disorders (Bottiglieri 1996). However, folic acid supplementation can mask the symptoms of pernicious anaemia and may counter the activity of some anticonvulsant drugs used in the treatment of epilepsy. Animal studies have suggested that folate-resistant NTDs respond to another vitamin, myo-inositol (Greene & Copp 1997).

Case study 12.2 looks at the issue of folic acid supplementation.

**Case study 12.2**

Jane seeks preconceptual nutritional counselling. She has had a previous miscarriage and is keen to improve the quality of her diet. Jane expresses concern about taking drugs in pregnancy including folic acid and is adamant that the human race could not have evolved requiring nutrients that could not be provided by a healthy diet.

- How might a midwife summarize the characteristics of a balanced diet?
- What rich sources of folate could be identified and how might consumption be increased?
- Is the connection between a previous miscarriage and diet valid?
- How could Jane's fears about folic acid supplementation be addressed?

### Calcium

Calcium requirements increase, mostly in the third trimester when the fetal skeleton develops rapidly, incorporating a total of about 30 g calcium. However, this is a tiny proportion of the calcium deposited in the maternal skeleton, which can act as a reservoir if dietary calcium is low. However, if the mother's own skeleton is still growing, as in adolescent pregnancy, there may be competition between the maternal and fetal skeleton for calcium. Young girls who become pregnant within 2 years of starting to menstruate are most at risk.

### Iron

The requirements for additional iron in pregnancy remain controversial (see Ch. 11). It is estimated that about 600 mg of iron are required for the fetus and placenta and blood lost at parturition (Campbell-Brown & Hytten 1998). The expansion of maternal red blood cell mass accounts for about 290 mg iron (Letsky 1998) but this expansion probably accommodates for the blood lost at parturition. Amenorrhoea of pregnancy saves about 120 mg iron, which is not lost in menstruation (Hytten 1985) and iron absorption increases.

## Undernutrition in pregnancy

In experimental animals, maternal undernutrition in pregnancy usually leads to decreased birth weight. Maternal weight gain in human pregnancy is positively associated with birth weight and developmental outcome. However, in nutritional assessment it is important determine prepregnancy weight from objective data and to assess the level of oedema. Women who are underweight have an increased risk of pregnancy loss and small babies that have increased morbidity and mortality. It is difficult to dissociate the effects of a poor diet in pregnancy from other variables. Women who consume a poor diet in pregnancy are likely to have consumed a poor diet before pregnancy and probably in their developmental stages. Many of them are shorter than average and a poor diet is associated with an increased incidence of smoking. Maternal shortness is also associated with a poorer social background, young maternal age and less formal education.

### *Diet quality*

Although most nutritional studies have focused on energy requirements and consumption in pregnancy, the quality of the diet as well as the quantity may be important. In Britain, nutrient-deficiency diseases are rare but the quality of the diet varies markedly (see below). Mothers of low birth-weight babies have not only low energy intakes but also diets of low nutrient density. Even in affluent countries many women have daily intakes of B vitamins below the recommended level. Lifestyle changes, such as car ownership and less active work patterns, mean energy requirements fall. However, nutrient requirements may not fall in parallel; indeed pollution and smoking increase requirements of certain nutrients. This means that, although energy consumption needs to fall to match reduced energy expenditure, the density of nutrients within the diet may need to increase to ensure that requirements are met.

### *Supplementation*

Nutrient supplementation studies of the diet in pregnancy have produced inconsistent and inconclusive results. High-density protein supplementation depresses birth weight (Rush 1989). Lower concentrations of protein have disappointingly small effects. Some of the studies are probably methodologically flawed and supplements may be used as alternatives rather than increasing nutrient consumption, or the target group may not consume them. Supplementation in the second and third trimesters of pregnancy may be too late to have an effect on birth weight; however, it may benefit maternal health and work potential and improve breastfeeding efficiency. Earlier supplementation may have a greater effect because nutrient support of early follicular development and maternal nutrient stores prior to conception may programme the fetal growth trajectory.

### *Fetal adaptation to undernutrition*

Subjected to inadequate substrate levels, of either nutrients or oxygen, the fetus adapts by changing its metabolic activity in order to survive. Slowing of growth and reducing energy expenditure are part of this adaptation. Growth accounts for a large proportion of energy expenditure. Adapting to a lower growth trajectory means that nutrient requirement decreases and available nutrient levels may then be adequate. The

placenta, which has a high nutrient and oxygen requirement itself, may also adapt. Although a number of adult onset diseases are associated with impaired fetal nutrition (Fig. 12.5), they tend not to affect reproductive ability as they cause pathological problems late in life. Animal studies have demonstrated that marginal malnourishment for many generations requires optimal nutrition for several generations before normal size and behaviour are expressed (Stewart et al 1980). This intergenerational effect may be one of the reasons why dietary supplementation in pregnancy has such a small effect on outcome.

## *Malnutrition*

Interesting results come from studies looking at the effect of nutrient deprivation on previously well-nourished women. The Dutch Hunger Winter, from September 1944 to May 1945, was due to the Nazi blockade of food supplies exacerbated by very severe winter weather conditions. The severe nutritional deficiency affected fertility and birth weights and the birth rate fell dramatically, by about 50%, 9 months later (Lumley 1992, Stein & Susser 1975a). This was due to effects both on ovulation and an increased incidence of

**Fig. 12.5** *Association of adult onset diseases and impaired fetal nutrition. (Reproduced with permission from Barker 1995.)*

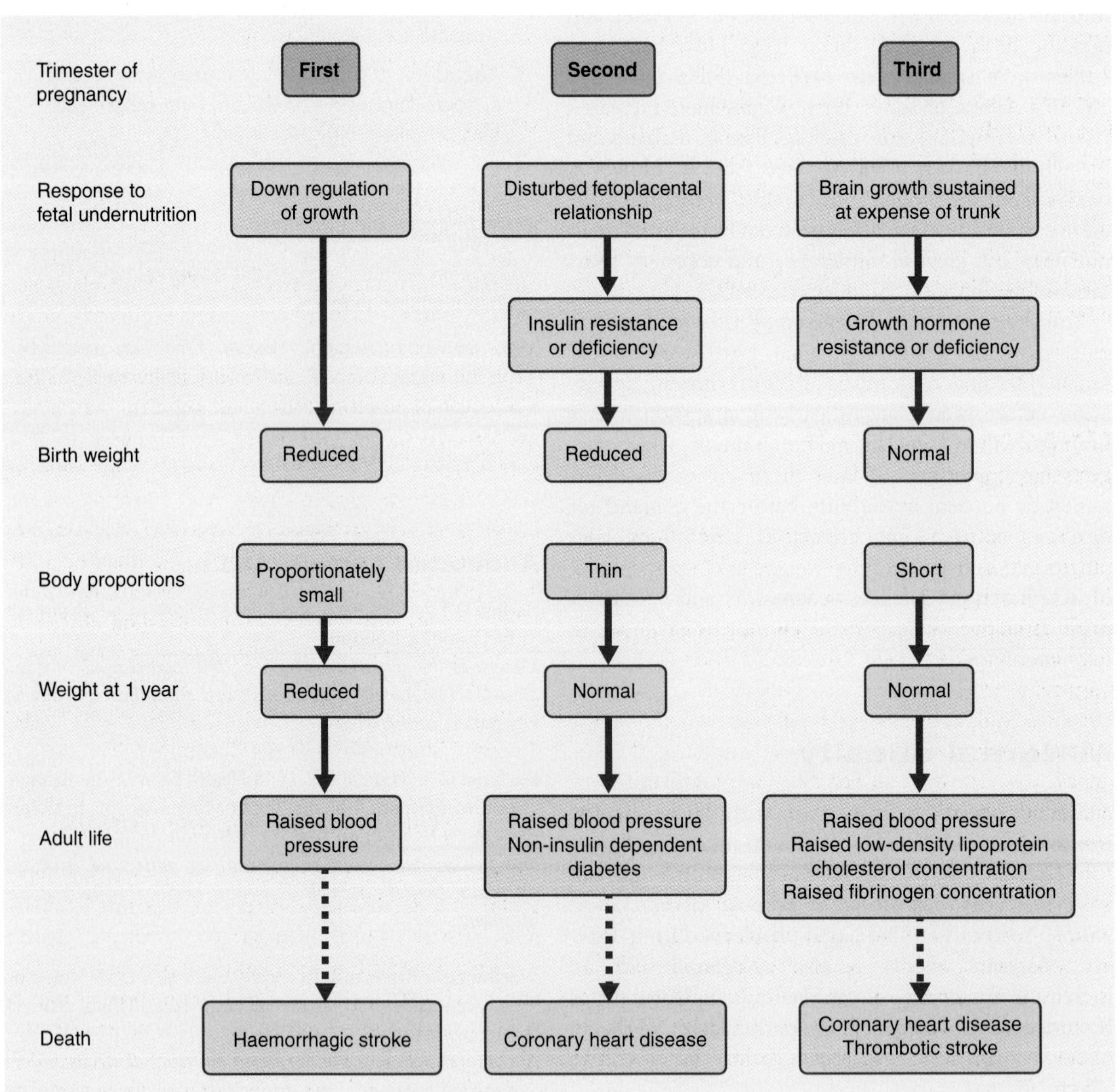

pregnancy failure. Congenital malformation rate increased among babies conceived during the famine or in the following 4 months.

However, many women were already pregnant at the time of the food shortage. If the women were deprived of energy in the second half of their pregnancy, the birth weight of their babies was reduced by 350 g on average. These babies were thin but of normal length. They appeared to develop and grow normally. However, in adulthood the male babies who had been exposed to deficiency late in development had lower rates of obesity compared with those who had experienced restricted nutrient levels early in development (Ravelli, Stein & Susser 1976). Young women who had been exposed to nutrient deficiency early in gestation, but not later, had normal birth weights themselves. However, their babies were smaller than expected (Stein & Susser 1975b). Adults of lower birth weight have increased risk of developing cardiovascular disease, diabetes and bronchitis (Barker 1998 and see Ch. 9). However, results from the longer, more severe, Leningrad siege do not show any association between intrauterine malnutrition and glucose intolerance and coronary heart disease in adulthood (Stanner et al 1997).

Transient nutrient deficiency may alter fetal growth patterns without affecting final birth weight very much (Harding & Johnson 1995). Nutrient deprivation before pregnancy or early in gestation affects brain growth and development in animals, which suggests 'programming' of later brain growth is determined by nutrient availability before the demand for nutrients occurs. Lung growth is affected by later nutritional deficiency; lung weight and composition, muscle function, defence mechanisms and surfactant production are all susceptible to nutritional insult in late pregnancy.

## Maternal obesity

Maternal obesity is associated with larger babies, macrosomia and increased perinatal mortality. Large-for-gestational-age babies are not longer on length but have increased deposition of adipose tissue. Obese women tend to have increased problems during delivery. Maternal obesity is also associated with an increased incidence of congenital malformations (Prentice & Goldberg 1996), particularly NTDs. In obese women, folic acid seems to lose its protective effect.

### Key points

- The diet before pregnancy, as well as that consumed during pregnancy, can affect the nutrient status of the woman.
- The increased energy requirements of pregnancy can be met by a combination of increasing intake, decreasing activity and changing metabolism.
- A good-quality, nutrient-dense diet can supply the additional protein, vitamin and minerals requirements of pregnancy.
- Energy restriction and obesity affect reproductive function: both fertility and fetal growth.
- Pregnancy-induced hormonal changes, including insulin resistance, affect transfer of nutrients to the placenta and fetus.
- Adaptation to poor nutrition in pregnancy results in changes in growth in utero and birth weight and may be linked to disease in adult life.

### Application to practice

Advice on nutrition is important during and for subsequent pregnancies.

Women who have a poor history of nutrition are at risk and the midwife needs to be aware of this to aid in the detection of problems associated with poor dietary intake.

## Annotated further reading

Barker D J P 1992 Fetal and infant origins of adult disease. BMJ Books, London

*Describes the research underlying the fetal origins of adult disease ('The Barker Hypothesis') in a compilation of the 31 key papers in this area.*

Edelman C L, Mandle C L 1998 Health promotion throughout the lifespan, 4th edn. Times Mirror-Mosby, St Louis

*Provides a focus upon health promotion including lifestyle and health choices in preconceptual, antenatal and the postnatal periods as well as health needs throughout the lifespan.*

Worthington-Roberts B, Rodwell-Williams S 1996 Nutrition in pregnancy and lactation, 6th edn. Times Mirror-Mosby, St Louis

*A comprehensive textbook about nutritional needs before and during pregnancy and during lactation. Includes practi-*

*cal information on assessing nutritional risk and counselling and supporting breastfeeding mothers.*

## References


Barker D J P 1995 Fetal origins of coronary heart disease. British Medical Journal 311:171–174

Barker D J P 1998 Mothers, babies and health in later life. Churchill Livingstone, New York

Bottigilieri T 1996 Folate, vitamin B12 and neuropsychiatric disorders. Nutrition Review 54:382–390

Campbell-Brown M, Hytten F E 1998 Nutrition. In: Chamberlain G, Broughton Pipkin F (eds) Clinical physiology in obstetrics, 3rd edn. Blackwell, Oxford, pp 165–191

Cox B D, Calame D P 1978 Changes in plasma amino acid levels during the human menstrual cycle and in early pregnancy: a preliminary report. Hormone and Metabolism Research 10(5):428–433

Cuskelly G J, McNulty H, Scott J M 1996 Effect of increasing dietary folate on red-cell folate: implications for the prevention of neural tube defects. Lancet 347:657–659

Durnin D V G A 1987 Energy requirements of pregnancy: an integration of the longitudinal data from the five country study. Lancet 2:1131

Franks S, Robinson S 1996 Nutrition, metabolism and reproduction. In: Hill SG, Kitchener HC, Neilson JP (eds) Scientific essentials of reproductive medicine. WB Saunders, Philadelphia, pp 242–249

Frisch R E 1990 The right weight, body fat, menarche and ovulation. Baillière's Clinics in Obstetrics and Gynaecology 4:3

Frisch R E, McArthur J W 1974 Menstrual cycles: fatness as a determinant of minimum weight necessary for their maintenance or onset. Science 185:949–951

Greene N D E, Copp A J 1997 Inositol prevents folate-resistant neural tube defects in the mouse. Nature Medicine 3:60–66

Harding J E, Johnson B M 1995 Nutrition and fetal growth. Reproduction, Fertility and Development 7:539–547

Health Education Authority 1996 Awareness, attitudes and behaviour towards folic acid amongst women: a report by the HEA. Feb. HEA, London

Hytten F 1985 Blood volume changes in normal pregnancy. Clinics in Haematology 14(3):601–612

Hytten F E 1991 Nutrition. In: Hytten F, Chamberlain G (eds) Clinical physiology in obstetrics, 2nd edn. Blackwell, Oxford, p 153

Hytten F E, Cheyne G A 1969 The size and composition of the human pregnant uterus. Journal of Obstetrics and Gynaecology of the British Commonwealth 76:400–340

Illingworth P J, Jung R T, Howie P J, Isles T E 1987 Reduction in postprandial energy expenditure in pregnancy. British Medical Journal 294:1573–1576

Jennings E 1995 Folic acid as a cancer-preventing agent. Medical Hypotheses 45:297–303

Lawrence M, Lawrence F, Coward W A, Cole T J, Whitehead R G 1987 The energy requirements of pregnancy in the Gambia. Lancet ii:1072

Letsky E 1998 The haematological system. In: Chamberlain G, Broughton Pipkin F (eds) Clinical physiology in obstetrics, 3rd edn. Blackwell, Oxford, pp 71–110

Lumley L H 1992 Decreased birthweights in infants after maternal in utero exposure to the Dutch famine of 1944–45. Paediatric & Perinal Epidemiology 6:240

McCrabb G J, Egan A R, Hosking B J 1992 Maternal undernutrition during mid-pregnancy in sheep; variable effects on placental growth. Journal of Agricultural Science 1189:127–132

Naismith D J, Morgan B L 1976 The biphasic nature of protein metabolism during pregnancy in the rat. British Journal of Nutrition 36(3):563–566

Pirke K M, Schweiger U, Lemmel W, Krieg J C, Berger M 1985 The influence of dieting on the menstrual cycle of healthy young women. Journal of Clinical Endocrinology and Metabolism 60:1174–1179

Prentice A, Goldberg G 1996 Maternal obesity increases congenital malformations. Nutrition Review 54:146–152

Ravelli G P, Stein Z A, Susser M W 1976 Obesity in young men after famine exposure in utero and early infancy. New England Journal of Medicine 295:349

Robinson S, Viita J, Learner J et al 1992 Insulin insensitivity is associated with a decrease in postprandial thermogenesis in normal pregnancy. Diabetic Medicine 10:139–145

Rosa F W, Wilk A L, Kelsey F O 1986 Teratogen update: vitamin A congeners. Teratology 33(3):355–364

Rush D 1989 Effects of changes in protein and calorie intake during pregnancy on the growth of the human fetus. In: Chalmers I, Enkin M, Kierse M J N C (eds) Effective care in pregnancy and childbirth, vol 1. OUP, Oxford, pp 255–280

Saffrey J, Stewart M (eds) 1997 Maintaining the whole. SK 220 Human biology and health, book 3. Open University Press, Milton Keynes

Scott J, Kirke P, Molloy A, Daly L, Weir D 1994 The role of folate in the prevention of neural tube defects. Proceedings of the Nutrition Society 53:631

Smithells R W, Sheppard S, Schorah C J 1981 Apparent prevention of neural tube defects by periconceptional vitamin supplementation. Archives of Disease in Childhood 51:911–918

Stanner S A, Bulmer K, Andres C et al 1997 Does malnutrition in utero determine diabetes and coronary heart disease in adulthood? Results from the Leningrad siege study, a cross sectional study. British Medical Journal 315:1342–1349

Stein Z, Susser M 1975a Fertility, fecundity, famine: food rations in the Dutch famine 1944/5 have a causal relation to fertility and probably to fecundity. Human Biology 47:131

Stein Z, Susser M 1975b The Dutch famine 1944–45 and the reproductive process. 1. Effects on six indices at birth. Paediatric Research 9:70

Stewart R J C, Sheppard H, Preece R, Waterlow J C 1980 The effect of rehabilitation at different stages of development in rats marginally malnourished for ten to twelve generations. British Journal of Nutrition 43:403–412

Wald N J, Bower C 1995 Folic acid and the prevention of neural tube defects. British Medical Journal 310:1019–1020

Ward M, McNulty H, McPartlin J, Strain J J, Weir D C, Scott J M 1997 Plasma homocysteine, a risk factor for cardiovascular disease, is lowered by physiological doses of folic acid. Quarterly Journal of Medicine 90(8):519–524

Wynn M, Wynn A 1991 The case for preconception care of men and women. AB Academic, Bicester

# 13 Physiology of parturition

**Learning objectives**

- To describe uterine changes in pregnancy and its preparation for labour.
- To discuss theories of the initiation and timing of parturition in humans.
- To relate factors thought to be involved with initiation of labour to methods for inducing labour, possible causes and treatment of preterm labour.
- To outline the physiology of pain in relation to childbirth and the rationale for choice of pain relief.
- To describe the effects of labour on maternal and fetal physiology.

## Introduction

The success of each pregnancy, and ultimately the survival of the species, depends on the baby being born healthy and mature enough to survive. In pregnancy and labour, the uterus has to fulfil two very different functions. It has to grow but remain quiescent during the pregnancy to allow fetal development and then, at the appropriate time, commence powerful and coordinated activity, which results in the delivery of the mature infant. The factors controlling the transition from one state to the other are poorly understood but are very important in understanding both the possible causes of preterm labour and how to induce labour successfully without eliciting fetal distress.

Most human infants are capable of surviving at delivery, and are born at term (defined as between the end of the 37th week and 42 weeks of pregnancy). Five per cent of preterm babies account for 85% of the early neonatal deaths that are not associated with a lethal deformity (Lopez Bernal et al 1993). The shorter the gestation the poorer is the prognosis. Even though very low birth-weight babies (i.e. those born below 1000 g) may now survive, it is generally at the expense of high morbidity rates and much distress for their parents, as well as a high financial burden on neonatal intensive care units. It could be argued that one of the principal objectives of obstetrics is to reduce preterm labour.

The control of the onset of human parturition is a mystery. There are marked differences between human and other mammalian species in the pathway of factors leading to parturition. It is not clear why the events leading to parturition should be so complex in the human or whether a variable length of gestation is advantageous. Humans have a very high rate of premature delivery (about 5–10%) compared with other species (less than 1% in sheep). Theoretically, the length of gestation does not matter to the mother. The crucial aspect is that the baby can survive at delivery. It seems likely, therefore, that the fetus controls the length of gestation. Certainly in animals there is proven fetal involvement in the timing of labour but it is difficult to obtain such evidence in humans.

Midwifery management of women in labour is often interventionist. This chapter covers the physiology of parturition; for information about clinical management, readers are referred to midwifery texts in the list of further reading.

## Definition of the stages of labour

From a clinical point of view, labour is often divided into three stages (Fig. 13.1). However, physiologically there is no abrupt transition between stages. The events leading to the onset of labour are gradually and inconspicuously initiated earlier in the pregnancy, and the three stages overlap. The first stage is the stage of progressive cervical dilatation timed from the onset of regular coordinated contractions accompanied by progressive effacement (thinning) and dilatation of the cervix. The end of this stage is marked by the full dilatation of the cervix as the uterine contractions pull the entire tissue of the cervix upwards, so it is incorporated into the lower uterine segment, continuous with the uterine walls. This stage lasts an average of 12–14 hours in primigravidae, but tends to be shorter in multigravidae. The second stage is the stage of fetal expulsion, from full cervical dilatation until the delivery of the baby. The contractions are strong and aided by the respiratory muscles. The second stage may take over an hour in primigravidae and as little as a few minutes in multigravidae. The third stage of labour involves separation and complete expulsion of the placenta and membranes, and control of bleeding from the uteroplacental circulation. The return to the prepregnant state is described as the puerperium (see Ch. 14).

## The uterus at term

### Uterine muscle

Towards term, the uterus stops being quiescent (having a low level of muscle activity) and is able to perform remarkable mechanical effort to expel its contents of baby and placenta, together with associated membranes and fluids, through the birth canal (Fig. 13.2). The anatomical structure of the uterus is predominantly bundles of 10–50 myometrial (smooth muscle) cells separated by connective tissue, formed of collagen and elastin. The distribution of the smooth muscle varies throughout the length of the uterus. The smooth muscle density is highest in the fundus of the uterus (approximately 90 : 10 smooth muscle fibres : connective tissue) and gradually declines until the cervix where the ratio is 20 : 80. The isthmus, which forms the lower segment of the uterus, has a lower smooth muscle content. The lower segment forms at about week 28 to 30 of pregnancy. Caesarean sections late in gestation are usually via the lower segment of the uterus (LSCS: lower-segment caesarean section), whereas the incision in a emergency 'classic' caesarean section earlier in pregnancy usually is on the midline of the uterus and is likely to dictate the method of delivery in future deliveries. Contractile strength is related to the proportion of smooth muscle (Petersen et al 1991). Therefore, the upper part of the uterus contracts strongly and the lower segment, which has a diminishing proportion of muscle, contracts weakly and passively (see Fig. 13.9, p. 279).

The uterine muscle forms three distinct anatomical layers, which are more evident with the hypertrophy of the uterus that occurs in pregnancy (Fig. 13.3). The innermost layer has muscle mostly in a longitudinal orientation. The outermost layer has longitudinal and circular fibres. The middle layer of uterine muscle has spiralling fibres and is particulary well vascularized. The blood vessels in the non-pregnant uterus are extremely tortuous and coiled (see Ch. 2); this allows them to adapt to the increased requirements of the expanding uterine tissue. Uterine blood flow increases in pregnancy as the blood vessel diameter increases and resistance to flow decreases.

### Uterine growth in pregnancy

The uterine muscle undergoes exceptional growth throughout pregnancy to accommodate the growing fetus. The prepregnant weight of the uterus is about 50 g in a nulliparous woman and about 60–70 g in a multiparous woman. During pregnancy, it increases 20-fold, to about a kilogram. Initially, the uterus grows by hyperplasia (increasing cell number). This is under the influence of oestrogen and, unlike later growth, occurs regardless of the site of implantation. By the 4th month, this growth has increased the uterine wall from 10 to 25 mm. Subsequent growth is due to hypertrophy (increasing cell size from 50 to 500 μm long) stimulated by uterine distension. The uterine wall thins and the smooth muscle cells increase markedly in length as they accumulate contractile proteins. The increased size is accompanied by a change in uterine shape from a sphere to a cylinder. By term, the organization of the myometrial cells allows coordinated, strong and effective contractions to develop. The uterine muscle is innervated by adrenergic, cholinergic and peptidergic fibres, which are more abundant in the cervix and uterine tubes. The uterus also has many sensory nerves.

**Fig. 13.1** ***Stages of labour***

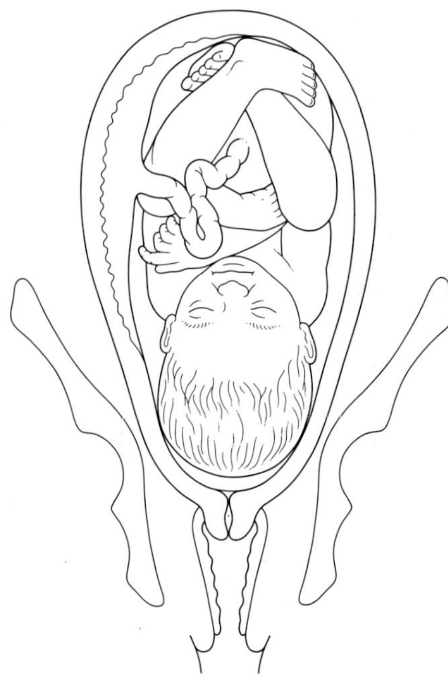

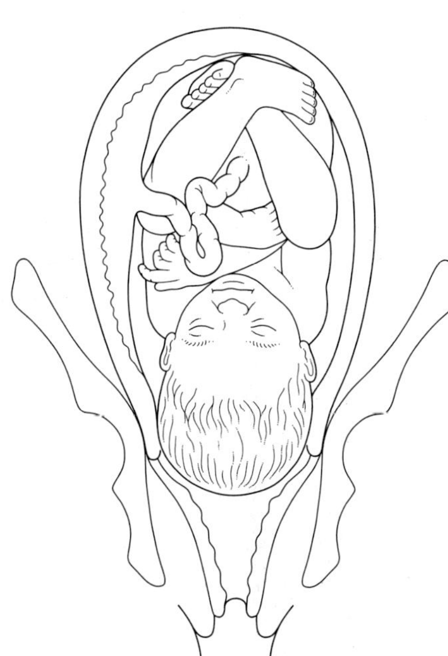

**First stage = DILATATION**
From onset of regular uterine contractions and effacement of cervix and dilatation of os ⟶ full dilatation of os uteri

**Second stage = FETAL EXPULSION**
From full dilatation ⟶ birth of baby

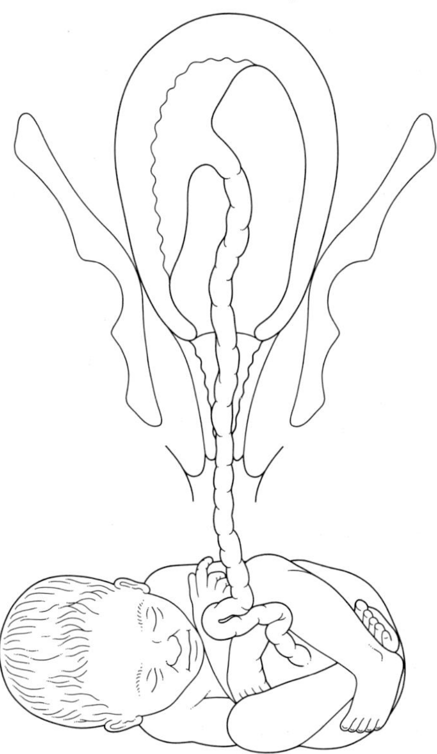

**Third stage**
From birth of baby ⟶ expulsion of placenta and membranes (and uterus retracted firmly)

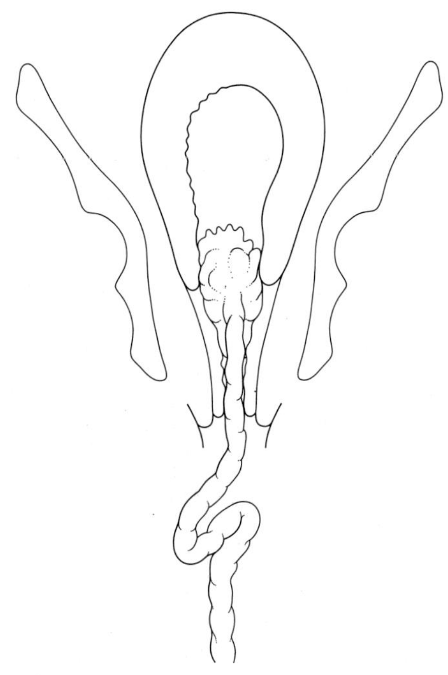

**Fig. 13.2** ***Expulsion through the birth canal.***

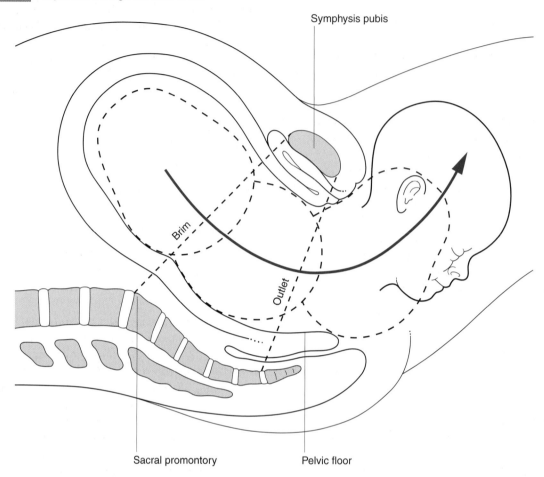



**Fig. 13.3** ***Uterine muscle layers: A the inner and outer muscle layers; B spiral organization of central smooth muscle fibres. (Reproduced with permission from Sweet & Titan 1996.)***

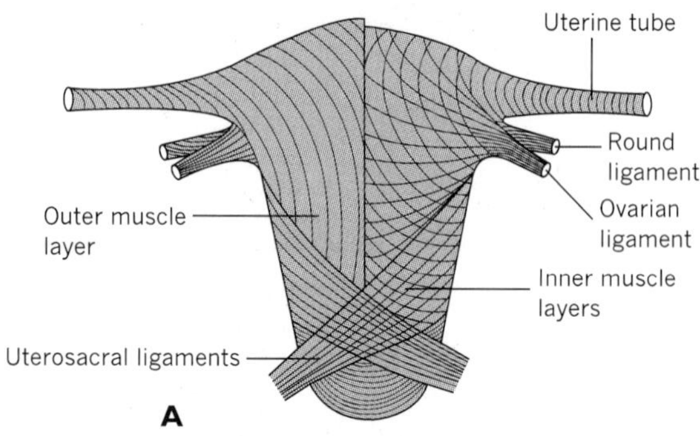


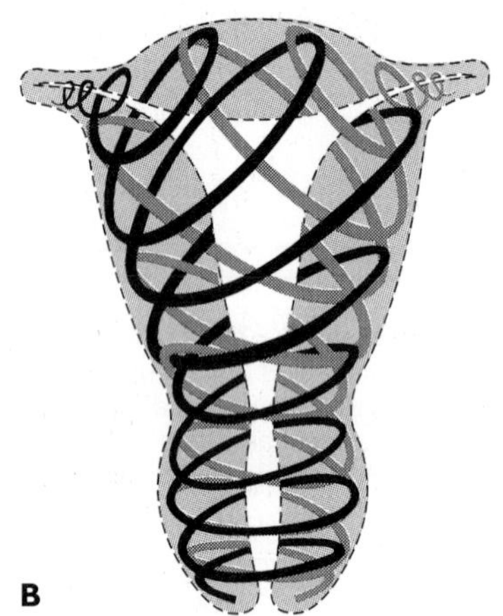

### Contractions

The uterus exhibits spontaneous contractility. A biopsy specimen of uterine tissue, placed in a physiological solution, will contract involuntarily every 2 to 5 minutes without stimulation. This rhythmic activity is inhibited by progesterone. However, the uterus is never completely quiescent. From about 7 weeks, the contractions, or 'contractures' are irregular, not synchronized and focal in origin; they have a very high frequency and a very low intensity (Wray 1993). From mid gestation, the contractions increase gradually in intensity and frequency until about 6 weeks before term when their intensity increases more markedly. The early Braxton–Hicks contractions can be perceived but, although strong, they are not normally painful as the cervix remains closed. In labour, the contractions become synchronized, regular and more intense with increased duration.

### The cervix

It is thought that the upright stance of human ancestors led to thickening and lengthening of the pelvic bones and the forward curvature of the sacrum (Stewart 1984); this stance imposes extra pressure on the pregnant cervix. Humans have a particularly high concentration of cervical collagen compared with other species. Unlike most other animals, where the cervix remains firmly closed until just before delivery, there is usually some degree of cervical softening relatively early in human pregnancy (Fig. 13.4); partial dilatation of the external os is evident by about 24 weeks (Anderson & Turnbull 1969). Because there is such a wide variation in the cervical changes among pregnant women, cervical assessment in isolation of other signs is an unreliable indicator of the imminence of labour. Towards the end of the first stage of labour, the changing shape of the cervix means that its tissue becomes integrated with the rest of the uterus (Fig. 13.5) (see below).

## The first stage of labour

### Cervical ripening

The consistency of the cervix changes in pregnancy to become softer in preparation for labour. Connective tissue changes affect the whole uterus but are more evident in the cervix. The uterine contractions imposed on the softened cervix result in it changing shape. During the pregnancy, the role of the cervix is to act as a closure for the uterus containing its contents and protecting them from ascending infection. Prior to the delivery of the baby, the cervix loses its structural rigidity and is pulled by the uterine contractions so it changes from being a tubular closure to becoming a wide-funnelled canal with very thin edges that is continuous with the rest of the uterine structure. In primigravida women, this shape change occurs in two distinct stages.

**Fig. 13.4** *A Prior to lightening: the fundus is in close proximity to the diaphragm and the lower uterine segment is still firm so the fetal head remains high. B After lightening (2–3 weeks before the onset of labour): the lower uterine segment has softened and dilated so the fetal head descends and the fundus sinks below the diaphragm, easing breathing. (Reproduced with permission from Bennett & Brown 1999.)*

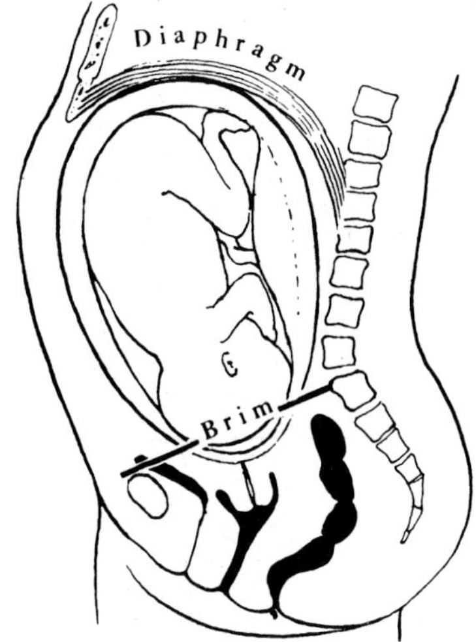


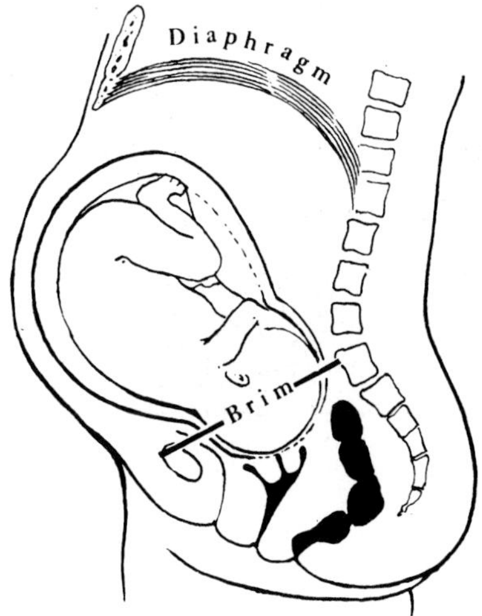

The first stage is effacement, where the cylindrical shape is transformed into a funnel, but the internal sphincter, or os, is still patent and closed. The longitudinal muscle fibres of the cervix shorten. The differential localization of the fibres means that the outer margins of the cervix develop more tension so maximum uptake of the cervix occurs at the lower end and the external os and softer cervical tissue moves upwards into the lower uterine segment (Gee & Olah 1993). During vaginal examination, a midwife might feel an 'effacement ridge' of the cervical tissue undergoing effacement (Fig. 13.5).

**Fig. 13.5** *A–C The differential movement of tissue planes at the time of cervical effacement and early dilatation. M direction of movement of collagen bundles; T, + differential tension across the myometrium. (Reproduced with permission from Sweet & Tiran 1996.)*

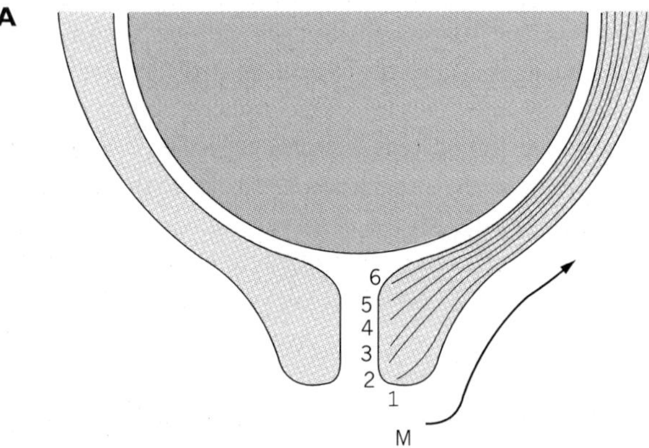


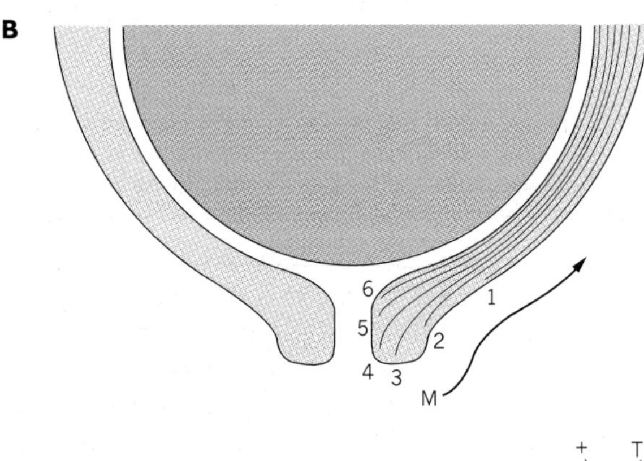


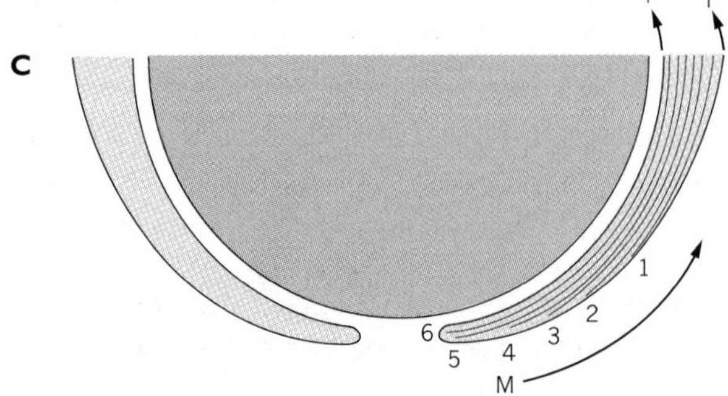


The second stage is dilatation (opening of the internal os); the uterus and vagina form one continuous 'sleeve' opening for the exit of the fetus. In multiparous women, the transition from one stage to the other is far less abrupt so effacement and dilatation occur simultaneously. Dilatation is due to the retraction or shortening of the upper part of the uterus, rather than pressure from the descending presenting fetal part. Therefore if there is no effective presenting part, as in a transverse lie, cervical dilatation still occurs. The dramatic changes in the cervix result from a combination of structural changes in the tissue and forces exerted by the uterine contractions.

The cervix is predominantly composed of fibrous connective tissue plus some smooth muscle and fibroblasts together with blood vessels, epithelium and mucus-secreting glands. There are two elements to cervical softening: increased vascularity and water content and structural changes in the connective tissue. At term, 90% of the weight of the cervix is water. Connective tissue is formed of collagen fibres and elastin held together by an extracellular matrix, or ground substance. The ground substance is predominantly composed of proteoglycans, which coat the collagen fibres and modify their physical properties, determining the water content of the tissue. Hormones that promote cervical softening affect the composition of the ground substance. Prior to the onset of labour, the composition of the proteoglycans changes so that dermatan sulphate decreases and hyaluronic acid increases. Dermatan sulphate binds collagen fibrils tightly, whereas hyaluronic acid has a lesser affinity for collagen and attracts water. Although the proteoglycans are a minor constituent of the cervix, they have an amazing ability to bind water; 1 g of hyaluronic acid can bind about a litre of water (Uldbjerg & Malstrom 1991). The increased level of hyaluronic acid may act as a signal to activate resident macrophages and neutrophils to secrete interleukins. Interleukins increase prostaglandin activity and neutrophil migration and degranulation (releasing collagenase and elastase).

The mechanical strength of the ground substance changes as the water content increases and the number of cross-links between elements of the connective tissue diminishes. The collagen increases in solubility and becomes disorganized and weakened (like a fraying rope) so it is more vulnerable to enzymatic digestion. Collagen is resistant to most proteases except collagenase from fibroblasts and neutrophil elastase. Amounts of neutrophil elastase in the cervix significantly increase at term. The association between intrauterine infection and premature labour may be linked to neutrophil infiltration and activation. The effects of oestrogen on cervical ripening are suggested to be mediated by IGF-I (Stjernholm et al 1996). Collagenolysis is a complex balance between availability of free collagenase and the inhibitory proteins. Connective tissue in the body of the uterus also changes at term altering uterine compliance. The level of elastin increases throughout the pregnancy. It provides the elastic recoil that coordinates the contraction–retraction cycle and is important in the return of the uterus to its normal shape after delivery.

Although the cervix has relatively little smooth muscle tissue, it may have an important functional role as a sphincter. The cervix constricts with uterine contractions in early labour (Olah 1994). It is suggested that this coordinated muscular activity is important in the maintenance of cervical integrity during Braxton–Hicks contractions before labour (Steer & Johnson 1998).

### Assessment of cervical effacement

In practice, the cervix can be assessed by using a simple scoring system, the Bishop's score (Table 13.1). This is particularly useful prior to induction of labour and for monitoring the changes in the cervix as the induction progresses.

If the cervix is soft, effaced and has started to dilate, induction may be implemented by artificial rupture of the membranes (ARM), which augments endogenous prostaglandin production. If the cervix is less favourable, prostaglandin $E_2$ ($PGE_2$) is administered into the posterior fornix of the vagina to facilitate effacement. However, $PGE_2$ should be used with caution in multiparous women, who have a greater sensitivity to it.

The cause of these structural changes in the cervix is not clear. It is thought to be hormonally controlled. Relaxin has been shown to be important in cervical ripening in rodents and has been used clinically to promote cervical ripening in humans. However, the levels of endogenous relaxin in pregnant women seem to be highest at the beginning of the second trimester. Oestrogen affects the synthesis of connective tissue components in vitro but has limited success when used pharmacologically as an induction method. $PGE_2$ causes cervical softening or 'ripening' and is produced naturally by both the cervix and the fetal membranes. $PGE_2$ appears to act by increasing collagenolytic activity rather than by changing the composition of the ground substance, which probably precedes prostaglandin use in successful induction of labour. Following delivery, glycoproteins that bind strongly to collagen are re-formed so the rigidity of the cervix is re-established; however, it never completely regains its original form (see Ch. 14). Damage to the cervix may have long-term consequences (Box 13.1).

**Table 13.1** *Bishop's score*

| Bishop's score | 0 | 1 | 2 |
|---|---|---|---|
| Station of presenting part | −3 | −2 | −1 |
| Position of cervix | Posterior | Mid | Anterior |
| Consistency | Firm | Soft | Very soft |
| Length | 3–4 cm | 1–2 cm | < 1 cm |
| Dilation of cervix | 0 | 1–2 cm | > 2 cm |
| Total = | (Bishop's score) | | |

## *Myometrial contractility*

The myometrium is formed of myometrial cells embedded in a collagen matrix. The cytoplasm of these myometrial cells is packed with long random bundles of actin and myosin. Compared with skeletal muscles, the concentration of actin is higher and the

**Box 13.1**

**Clinical issues relating to the cervix**

Longitudinal fibres allow full dilatation of the cervix to be achieved without the pressure of a presenting part, for instance in the case of a transverse lie. Artificial dilatation of an unprepared cervix may damage the collagen fibres. This can result in the cervix failing to remain intact during subsequent pregnancies, resulting in habitual spontaneous abortion, usually in mid trimester. Preoperative preparation to avoid this involves the administration of a prostaglandin derivative, which induces cervical softening and aids artificial dilatation of the cervix. This method is used prior to procedures involving exploration of the uterine cavity such as termination of pregnancy, evacuation of retained products of conception, surgical ablation of the endometrium and investigation of infertility.

Fig. 13.6 *Cell shortening and myosin contractile elements in myometrial muscle contraction: A relaxed; B contracted.*

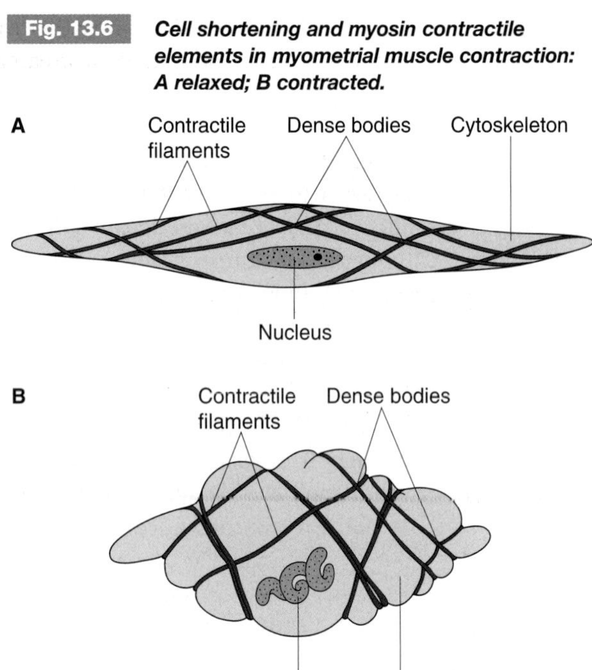


myosin has longer filaments, which increases the maximum shortening of the contractile cells. Myosin is both a structural protein and a Mg-ATPase, which can hydrolyse ATP and utilize the energy for movement. When ATP is hydrolysed (broken down), actin and myosin cross-bridges form so actin and myosin slide past each other, shortening the cell and the muscle contracts (Fig. 13.6). Myosin is made up of two heavy chains forming the ATPase and two light chains, which bind calcium and undergo phosphorylation. Phosphorylation is the binding of a phosphate group, which effectively activates the proteins.

## The role of calcium

Muscle contraction depends on intracellular calcium ions increasing; these bind to calmodulin, a protein that regulates the activity of many of the intracellular enzymes generating a cascade of reactions leading to binding of actin and myosin. Calcium binding to calmodulin activates myosin light-chain kinase (MLCK), which phosphorylates myosin so it can interact with actin, initiating contractions. Removal of calcium results in dephosphorylation of myosin by myosin dephosphorylase and causes muscle relaxation. Smooth muscle contraction can therefore be increased either by activating MLCK or by inhibiting myosin phosphatase.

Calcium enters from the extracellular fluid and is released from the sarcoplasmic reticulum of the myometrial cells. There is a good correlation between intracellular calcium concentration and the muscular force developed. Substances that stimulate myometrial contractility, such as prostaglandins and oxytocin, increase calcium influx and decrease calcium storage therefore increasing intracellular calcium concentrations and MLCK phosphorylation and increasing myometrial activity. Agents that relax the myometrium, such as progesterone, β-mimetics and prostacyclin, decrease intracellular calcium by promoting calcium uptake by the sarcoplasmic reticulum so free calcium levels decrease and the uterine muscle relaxes. Calcium channel blockers such as nifedipine prevent calcium entry into the cells promoting relaxation of the uterus.

## Hormonal control

Intracellular calcium levels (and myometrial activity) are hormonally controlled by various receptors on the myometrial cell surface. Most hormones that affect myometrial contractility bind to receptor sites that are coupled to one of two G-proteins (see Ch. 3) (Bernal et al 1995). The G-proteins act as transducers between the receptor and the effector regulating the cellular responses by generating an amplifying cascade of second messengers. The G-proteins allow the myometrial tissue to respond to a large number of agonists with a limited number of effects, either relaxation or contraction (Fig. 13.7). One of the G-protein pathways is linked to the inositol phosphate pathway. Binding of agonists that stimulate this G-protein activates phospholipase C generating inositol triphosphate and diacylglycerol. Inositol trisphosphate stimulates the release of calcium from the sarcoplasmic reticulum and other intracellular stores. Diacylglycerol is involved in calcium mobilization and activates protein kinase C, which in turn activates phospholipase A, which releases arachidonic acid, the precursor of prostaglandins. The result is a rise in intracellular calcium and therefore smooth muscle contraction. The other G-protein pathway activates adenylate cyclase, an enzyme that generates cyclic (cAMP) adenosine monophosphate causing a fall in intracellular calcium. Agonists that stimulate this pathway will cause dephosphorylation of myosin and uterine relaxation.

## Gap junctions

The onset of regular uterine contractions is gradual. As the pregnancy progresses, the resting potential of the myometrial cells falls so action potentials are gen-

Fig. 13.7 *The regulation of muscle contraction by G-proteins.*

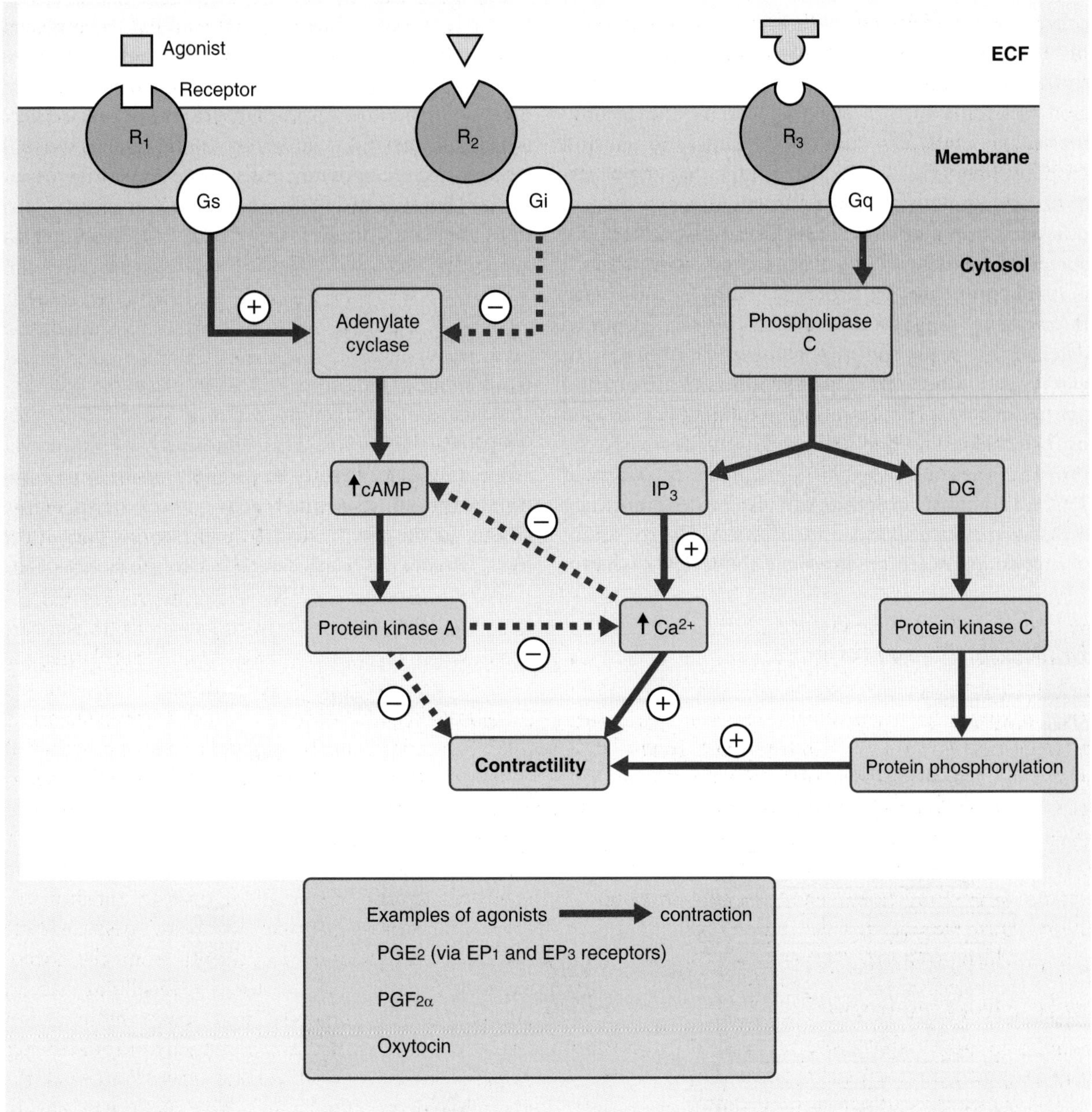


erated with greater ease. Initially spontaneous uterine contractility is inhibited but starts to reassert itself in mid gestation. At about 20–24 weeks, hardening of the uterus can be felt as muscle contractions start. Initially, uterine activity is mostly low amplitude and high frequency, with peak activity at night. This circadian rhythm stops about 3 weeks before delivery, and may be mediated by cortisol (Germain et al 1993). At first, small groups of myometrial cells contract together causing small fluctuations in intrauterine pressure. As pregnancy progresses, more cells are involved so the contractions become more coordinated. This increased coordination between the cells, allowing the muscular activity to become synchronized and propagated, is due to the formation of gap junctions between the cells. Factors that negatively affect myometrial contractility may be important in maintaining uterine quiescence through pregnancy; those that increase contractility may be important in facilitating the progression of labour.

Gap junctions are formed from bundles of proteins, called connexins, that align forming symmetrical channels protruding through adjacent cells, so allowing contact and communication. Gap junctions exist in other tissues that act together in a coordinated fashion, such as cardiac muscle and pancreatic islets. In the open state, gap junctions allow rapid transmission of signals such as electrical stimuli and second-messenger molecules such as calcium and inositol trisphosphate (Fig. 13.8). This means that depolarization and smooth muscle contraction in one cell are quickly communicated to an adjacent cell so there is a spread of excitement and synchrony of contractions.

As gap junctions are proteins, binding studies using fluorescently tagged antibodies can be carried out to determine the gap junction number. The number of gap junctions increases during gestation to about 1000 per myometrial cell. Gap junction number is increased by prostaglandins and oestrogen and decreased by progesterone and cAMP (MacKenzie & Garfield 1985). Gap junction density can also be determined by measuring electrical resistance of tissue. The resistance of human myometrium at term is about half of that in the non-pregnant uterus and much less than that in other smooth muscle, for instance bladder and stomach, which indicates that the cells of the pregnant myometrium are very well coupled. The increased numbers of gap junctions can be observed in the uterus of experimental animals prior to delivery. There is a higher density of gap junctions in human tissue if labour occurs spontaneously, whether at term or earlier (Beyer et al 1989). As the number of gap junctions increases, greater areas of the uterus contract generating increased intrauterine pressure levels.

## Uterine contractions

If softening of the cervix has taken place, the coordinated uterine contractions exert a steady pull thus stretching the cervix. This effacement of the cervix often takes place before the contractions become completely regular so it may occur a week or so before labour. As the cervix effaces, the presenting part of the fetus, usually the head, descends into the cavity of the

**Fig. 13.8** *The gap junction.*

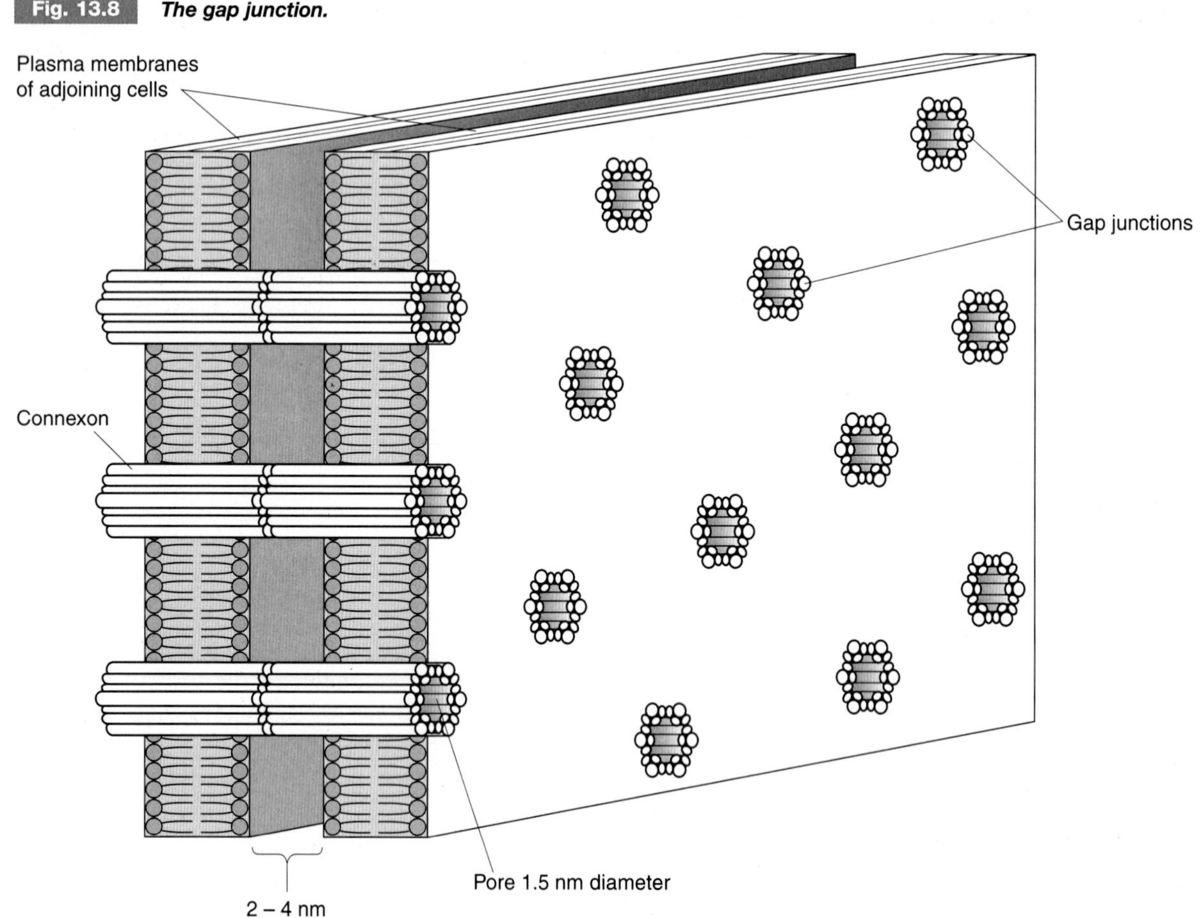

pelvis. The fetal position alters so that it fits well; this is described as engagement.

Contractions are involuntary and will therefore occur in an unconscious woman. However, they can be temporarily abolished by emotional disturbances (including moving from home to hospital and by a change in staff shifts). The frequency and strength of the contractions can be increased by enemas, prostaglandins and oxytocin preparations, and by stretching of the cervix or pelvic floor by the presenting part. Contractions are regular and intermittent. The intermittent nature is important as it allows recovery of both the uterus and the labouring woman and a resumed oxygen supply to the fetus.

Contractions begin to feel painful once the cervix starts to dilate. Backache often precedes cervical dilation. The pain is due to ischaemia in the muscle during the contraction because the uterine blood vessels are compressed. Similar pain occurs for the same reason in spasmodic dysmenorrhoea. Uterine pain is analogous to myocardial pain in angina when blood flow in the coronary arteries supplying the cardiac muscle is restricted. An increase in intrauterine pressure of about 20 mmHg can be felt by someone resting a hand on the woman's abdomen. Pain is often felt when the pressure rises above 25 mmHg. Pressures may rise to 50 mmHg in the first stage and to 75 mmHg in the second stage. Weak contractions have a shorter duration with longer intervals between each contraction. The sensation of pain is related not just to the strength of contraction and the interval between each contraction but also to the well-being of the mother. An

**Fig. 13.9** ***Contraction and retraction of uterine muscle cells. (Reproduced with permission from Sweet & Tiran 1996.)***

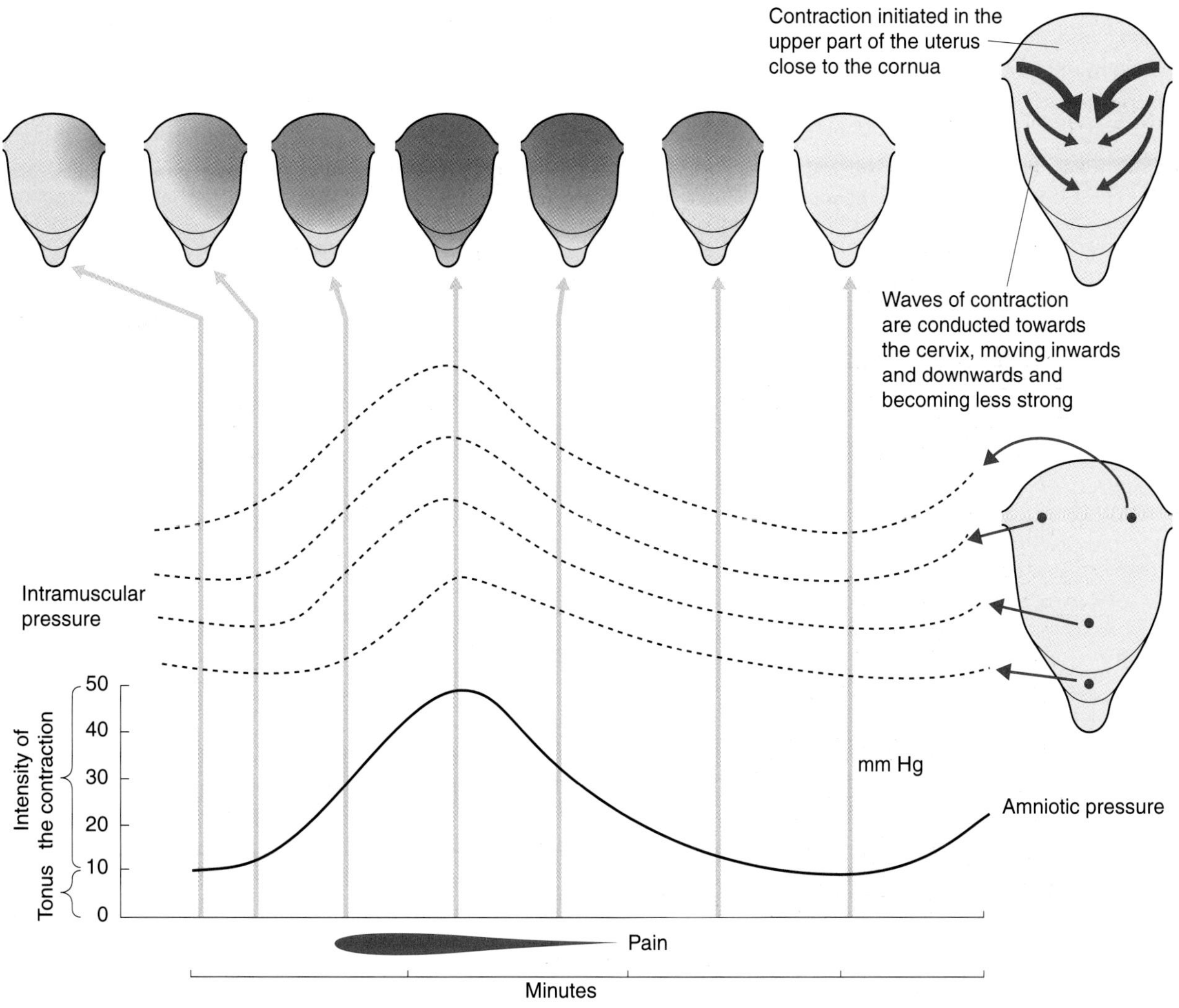

anxious or tired woman experiences pain at lower uterine pressure intensity (see below).

## Contraction waves

The uterus is also analogous to the heart in another respect in that it appears to exhibit pacemaker activity. Specific areas that depolarize more rapidly have not been identified, although it was believed that they were each side of the fundus, near the uterotubal junctions or cornuae. All myometrial cells have spontaneous pacemaker activity. The contractions tend to originate from cells near the fundus and spread as a wave, as the electrical activity moves through the gap junctions of the muscle fibres (Fig. 13.9). The waves are strongest at the fundus, which has the highest density of muscle fibres, and take about 30 seconds to travel down the length of the uterus. There is a polarity of wave contraction with rhythmic coordination between the upper segment (which contracts for longer and retracts) and the lower segment which contracts slightly and dilates. This is described as fundal dominance; it is similar to the peristaltic waves generated by smooth muscle in other viscera. If the wave pattern is abnormal, for instance if the lower part contracts first or more strongly, the waves become erratic and uncoordinated and labour does not progress efficiently. This is described as 'incoordinate uterine activity'.

The uterus relaxes between contractions, which is important for oxygenation of the fetus and myometrium. The upper part of the uterus does not relax fully between contractions but retracts instead. This means that the muscle fibres do not return fully to the original length but progressively and gradually get a little bit shorter and thicker with each contraction (Fig. 13.10). This means that the less active lower segment is pulled up towards the shortening upper part of the uterus. (If the uterine muscle relaxed completely following each contraction, the uterus would remain the same size and labour would not progress.) The weakest points are the os and cervix which are effaced and dilated, enlarging the opening of the uterus.

## Formation of hindwaters and forewaters

As the lower segment stretches and the cervix starts to efface and change its position, the chorion becomes

**Fig. 13.10** *Effacement and dilatation of the cervix: A in a primigravida; B occurring simultaneously in a multigravida. (Reproduced with permission from Sweet & Tiran 1996.)*

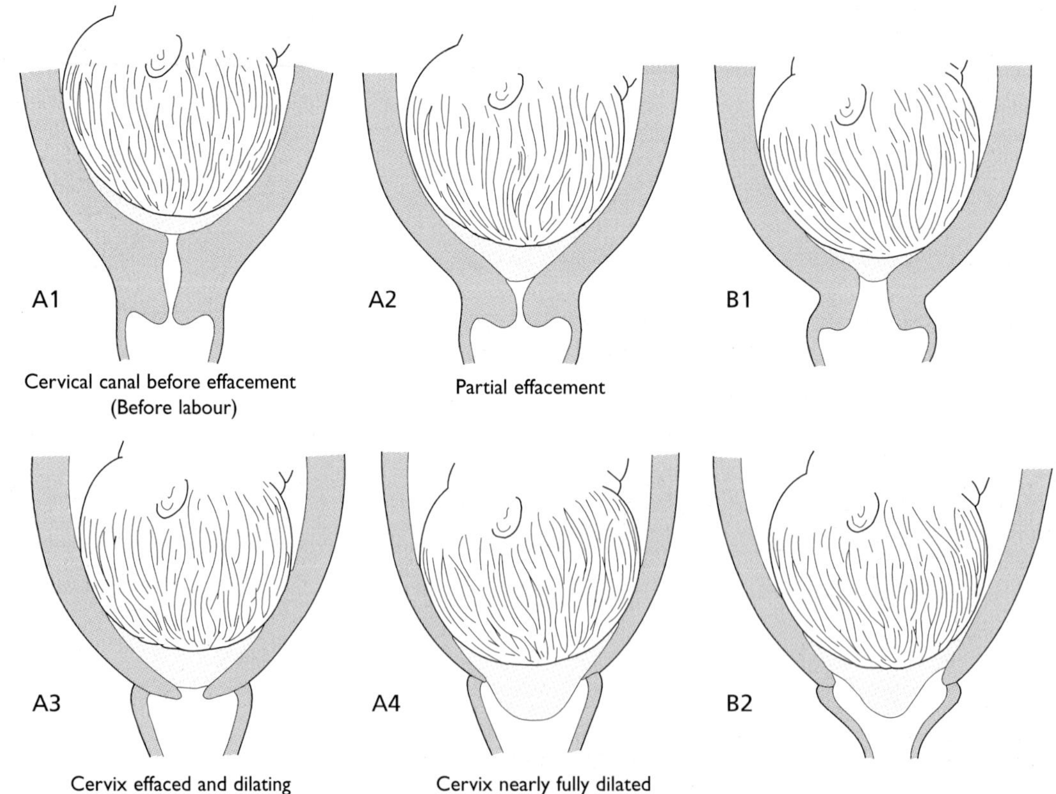

detached from the uterine wall. The operculum tends to become dislodged from the receding cervical canal. The loss of this mucus closure, which may be blood streaked, is described as 'the show' and indicates dilatation is progressing. The membranes are extruded through the opening cervix by the pressure of the amniotic fluid (Fig. 13.11). The head of the fetus tends to act as a ball-valve separating the amniotic fluid pushing through the cervix (forewaters) from the remainder of the fluid (hindwaters). The forewaters transmit the pressure generated from the waves of contraction, spreading the force evenly over the cervix, which aids its further effacement and dilatation. The hindwaters help to cushion the fetus from the contraction pressures. As the fundus presses on the upper aspect of the fetus (usually breech) during contractions, the pressure is transmitted through the fetal body to the lower segment and cervix (this is known as the fetal axis pressure). As uterine contractions progress, the pressure of the fluid in the forewaters rises and the membranes tend to rupture.

## Membrane rupture

In 5–10% of pregnancies, premature rupture of the membranes (PROM) occurs spontaneously as the earliest sign of labour (Duff 1996); about 60% of these are classified as term gestation. Spontaneous rupture of the membranes before 37 weeks' gestation often culminates in premature labour and delivery. Early rupture of the membranes as the first event in the course of labour is a cause for concern as it may indicate an ill-fitting presentation or high head at term in a primigravida, polyhydramnios or a local infection, such as chlamydia or streptococcal infection.

Rupture of the amniotic membrane is associated with collagen degradation in the membrane (Hampson et al 1997). Usually coordinated contractions and dilatation of the cervix follow rupture of the membranes but if there is a delay the fetus is at risk from ascending infections so clinical intervention may be necessary if labour has not followed within 24 hours. There is controversy about artificial rupture of membranes and the effect it has on speeding up labour; it is

**Fig. 13.11** *The forewaters: A in primigravida; B in multigravida. (Reproduced with permission from Sweet & Tiran 1996.)*

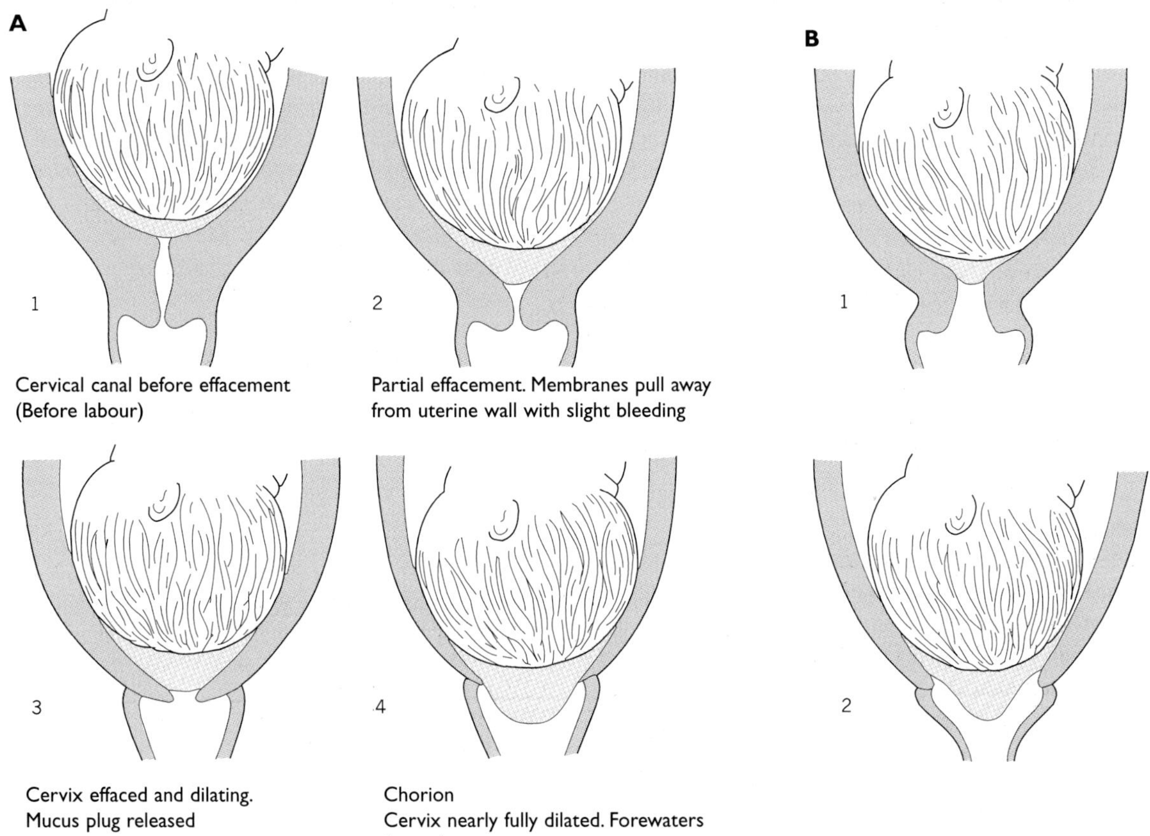

thought that labour may progress more abruptly and painfully (Barrett et al 1992).

### Size changes in the uterus and cervix

As the size of the upper segment of the uterus gradually diminishes because of the repeated cycles of contraction and retraction, the fetus is pushed into the lower segment so its presenting part (Box 13.2) exerts pressure on the obstructing maternal tissues. This results in increased oxytocin release from the posterior pituitary gland, which increases uterine activity by positive feedback (see Ch. 1). Later in labour, when the baby has been born and the placenta has been expelled, retraction aids the uterine walls to come together so the cavity is obliterated as the uterine walls lie in apposition. A physiological retraction ring forms at the junction between the thick retracted segment of the upper segment and the thin distended wall of the lower segment. Under normal conditions, this ring is not visibly evident or palpable by abdominal examination. A pathological visible 'Bandl's Ring' is the consequence of failure to recognize and manage obstructed labour appropriately and is a sign of imminent uterine rupture.

The rate of cervical dilatation is not constant; initially the cervix dilates slowly, but early changes are reinforced by positive feedback mechanisms and the rate accelerates. The latent phase of the first stage is slower and can take up to 12 hours (Box 13.3 and Fig. 13.12). It is during this stage, when dilatation to 3–4 cm is achieved, that the cervix positively contracts in response to oxytocin (Olah, Gee & Brown 1993). This probably facilitates effacement. After a transition stage of about 15 minutes when the cervix does not contract, the cervix then dilates in response to myometrial contractions during the faster active phase.

Case study 13.1 is an example of the first stage of labour.

**Box 13.2**
**Terms used for fetal presentation**

- Attitude—relationship between fetal head and limbs and fetal trunk
- Lie—relationship of fetus to long axis of uterus
- Presentation—part of fetus presenting in lower aspect of uterus
- Presenting part—part of presentation immediately inside internal os
- Position—relationship of presentation, or presenting part, to maternal pelvis
- Denominator—part of presenting part marking position

**Box 13.3**
**Progression of labour**

The medical model of care in labour has defined an acceptable rate of progress in labour. Failure of labour to progress at this rate is described as abnormal and used as the rationale for medical intervention. Progress in labour is assessed through the use of a partogram. Cervical dilatation at the rate of 1 cm/h is accepted as normal. Progression of cervical dilatation can be graphically plotted and compared with predefined lines of progress referred to as Studd curves (Studd & Duiagnan 1972). Intervention is usually recommended if the rate of progress falls below 2 cm of the expected progress.

**Case study 13.1**

Martha is a para 3; her previous pregnancies and labour were uneventful. She was admitted to the labour ward and confirmed to be in labour as her cervix was 6 cm dilated at 13:00 h. Four hours later on a repeat vaginal examination there was no further dilation, the membranes were intact, and cephalic presentation at the spines was judged to be in a direct OA position. Martha was coping well and there were no concerns raised over the fetal condition.

- Should the midwife refer Martha for an obstetric opinion?
- Is the fact that Martha has made no progress enough to justify intervention?
- How could the midwife justify her decision to leave Martha alone, if she felt that this were appropriate?
- What physiological processes/influences may be contributing to this situation?

## The second stage of labour

By the end of the first stage of labour, the lower uterine segment, the cervix, the pelvic floor and the vulval outlet form one continuous dilated birth canal. The forces required to expel the fetus are both from the uterine muscle activity and from the secondary muscles of the abdomen and diaphragm, which

**Fig. 13.12** *The partogram is a complete visual record of measurements made during labour and delivery. (Reproduced with permission from Symonds & Symonds 1997.)*

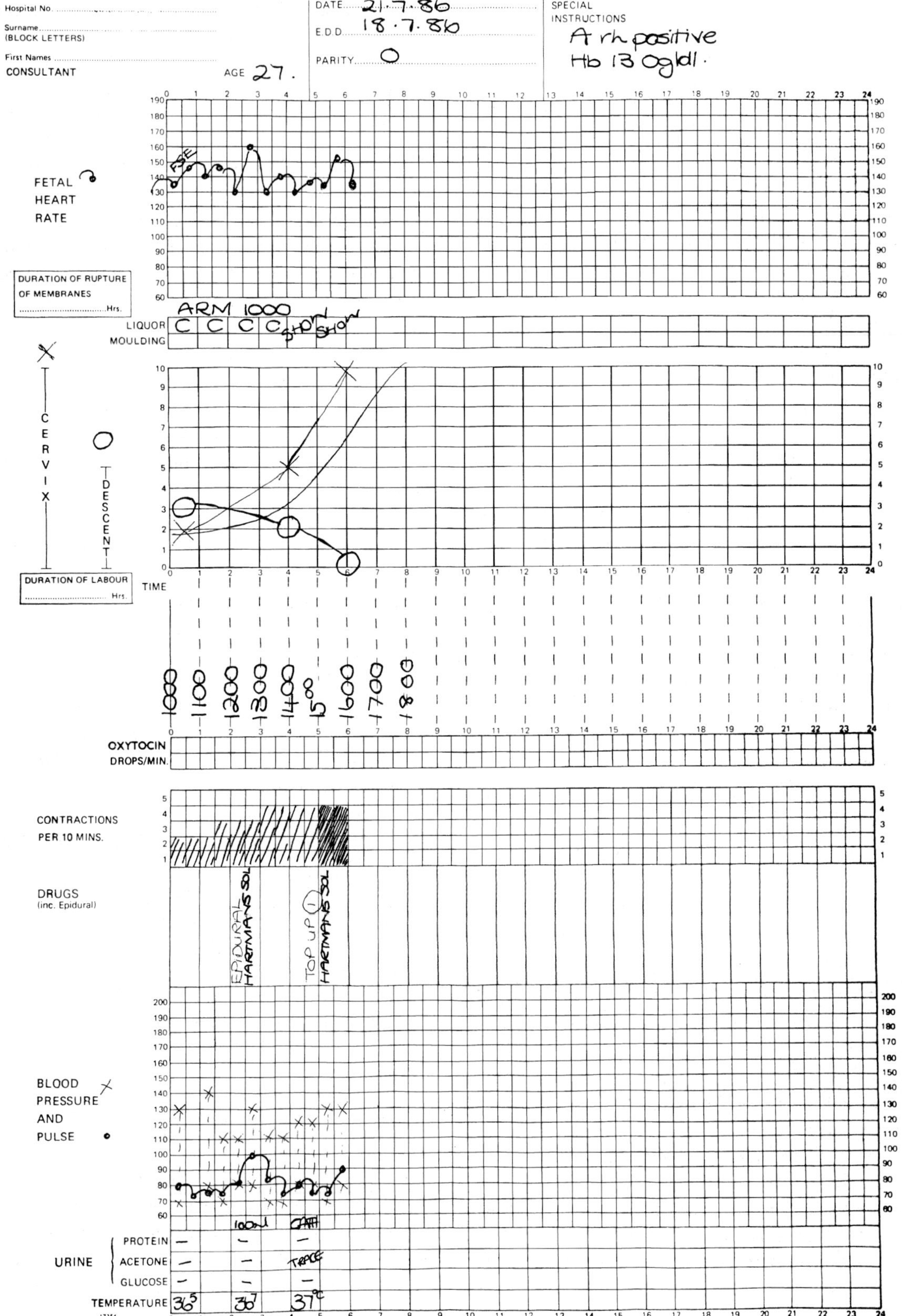

augment the contractions of the uterus. The forces generated by the uterus can be described as the primary power and the complementary force from the voluntary movement of the respiratory muscles as the secondary power. By this stage, the uterus is markedly retracted and undergoing a pattern of strong, regular and repetitive contractions. The mother is compelled involuntarily to bear down or push. As she inspires before pushing, the diaphragm is lowered and the abdominal muscles contract augmenting the contractile forces of the uterus. Bearing down by the mother helps to overcome the resistance of the soft tissues of the vagina and the pelvic floor. The fetal attitude (see Box 13.2) extends as it is directed through the birth canal, which aids the efficiency of the uterine contractions. The pain experienced in the second stage of labour is often less as cervical dilatation is complete and the woman is aware that progress is more rapid.

As the fetal head passes through the pelvis, the pressure on the sacral nerves may be associated with cramp in the legs and pain from the trauma to the tissue. The fetus distends the vagina and displaces the pelvic floor. The anterior part of the pelvic floor is drawn up causing the urethra to elongate and become compressed. The bladder is, therefore, repositioned within the protective environs of the abdomen. Posteriorly, the pelvic floor is stretched forward in relation to the presenting part and the rectum is compressed, which may lead to defaecation. The perineum is flattened and lengthened by the fetus.

During a contraction, the presenting part (usually the fetal head) advances forward. In the interval between contractions, the presenting part recedes slightly but, as the uterine muscle retracts with each contraction, progression in the forward direction is maintained. This progression has been likened to taking two steps forward and one step back. When the widest part of the fetal head (the biparietal diameter) distends the vulva, the stretching is at its maximum, hence pain may be severe if not managed effectively with analgesia. This is described as 'crowning' of the head. The severity of the pain may cause a labouring woman to gasp and inhale sharply. The momentary break in the bearing-down movement has an important role in protecting the perineum from too much trauma, which can cause tearing of the tissue. The birth is usually accomplished with the next contraction following 'crowning'. A gush of amniotic fluid escapes. The fetus undergoes a pattern of passive corkscrew movements as it follows the shape and curvature of the pelvis (curvature of Carus). The gutter shape of the pelvic floor facilitates the rotation of the presenting part enabling the widest diameters of the pelvis to accommodate the largest dimensions of the fetal head and shoulders (Fig. 13.13).

### *Influences of pelvic and pelvic floor morphology and parturition*

The passage of the fetus through the pelvis is described in practice as the mechanism of labour. Engagement describes the descent of the presenting part into the true pelvic cavity; the term relates to the widest transverse diameter of the fetal skull having negotiated the pelvic brim or inlet. If the baby has a cephalic (head-first) presentation, this is described in terms of number of fifths palpable (Fig. 13.14). Verification of the degree of engagement can be achieved through vaginal examination. With a cephalic presentation, the level of the biparietal prominences is judged in relation to the pelvic brim and the pelvic outlet at the level of the ischial spines. Engagement may occur long before the onset of labour, or may occur during, or even late on in labour (more common in multiparous women). In a primigravida, engagement usually occurs at about 36 weeks' gestation in response to effacement of the cervix. Engagement does not indicate cavity and outlet measurements.

## The third stage of labour

During the third stage, the placenta separates from the wall of the uterus and is expelled. The uterus retracts markedly and bleeding from the placental wound site is constrained. Following the safe delivery of a healthy baby, the third stage of labour still presents a number of potential hazards. Should part of the placenta be retained, control of bleeding is impaired and a life-threatening postpartum haemorrhage could ensue. Immediately after delivery, the uterus markedly decreases in size. The pattern of contractions is interrupted for a minute or so, until contractions resume. As the uterus retracts, the placental site is greatly diminished. The placenta is not elastic, thus it tends to wrinkle and be shorn off the elastic uterine wall (like a paper label coming away from a deflating balloon). It is at this stage that some fetal blood from the placental circulation can enter the maternal circulation, potentially causing problems if there is Rhesus incompatibility (see Ch. 10). The marked retraction of the uterus impedes the venous drainage of the maternal

**Fig. 13.13** *Rotation of the presenting part: A delivery of the head; B restitution; C external rotation. (Reproduced with permission from Bennett & Brown 1999.)*

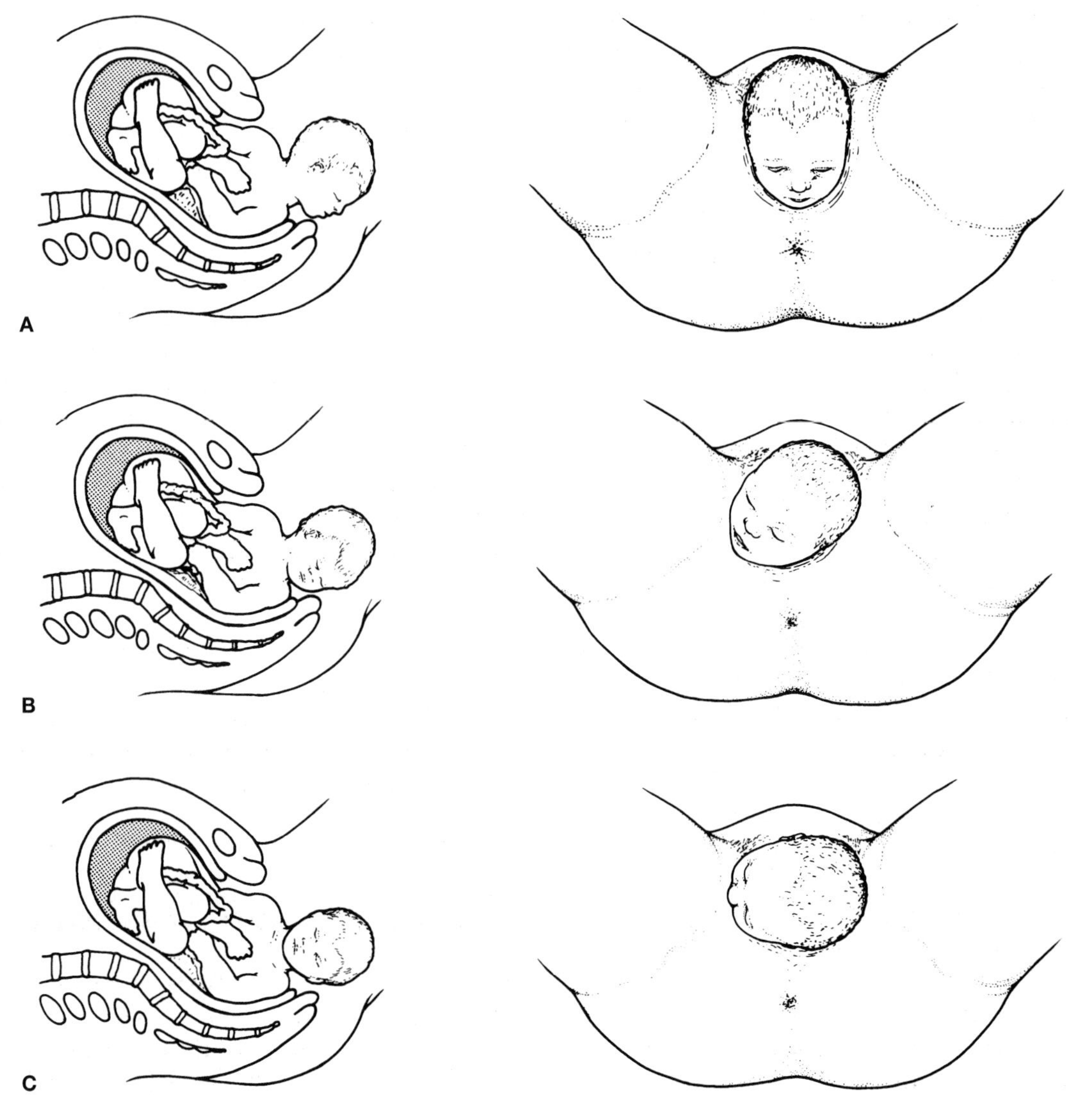


intervillous spaces. The extravasculated blood forms a clot under the shearing placenta, which aids its separation. As the uterus retracts, its progressively shortening muscle fibres tighten around the maternal vessels, forming 'living ligatures', which impede blood flow. This restricts the flow of maternal blood to the uterus and placental wound site, preventing excessive blood loss.

It is the commencement of spontaneous or stimulated uterine contractions following the completion of the second stage of labour that causes the placenta to separate from the uterine wall. The weight of the placenta completes the detachment of the membranes, which peel off and are expelled (Fig. 13.15). The site of placental implantation determines the speed of separation and the method of placental expulsion. The fetal membranes are expelled with the maternal or fetal surface prominent. The Schultze method of expulsion is more likely with a fundal site implantation and the Matthew–Duncan expulsion more likely with a lateral implantation.

## Active management

The third stage of labour can be physiologically managed, taking about 20–30 minutes to complete, but active management is widely practised by midwives, shortening the time of placental delivery to a

**Fig. 13.14** *A Flexion and descent of the presenting part into the pelvic cavity; B engagement of the head. (A reproduced with permission from Bennett & Brown 1999; B reproduced with permission from Sweet & Tiran 1996.)*

A

| $\frac{5}{5}$ | $\frac{4}{5}$ | $\frac{3}{5}$ |
|---|---|---|
| Occiput Sinciput above brim | Sinciput rises | Occiput below brim |

Brim

B

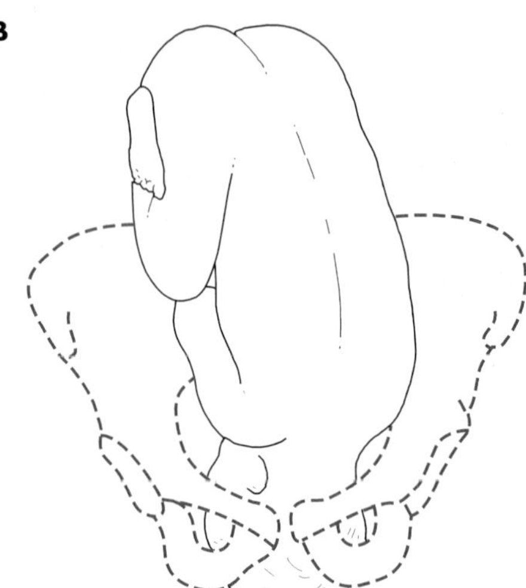

**Fig. 13.15** *The mechanism of placental separation and expulsion: A uterine wall partially retracted but not sufficiently to cause placental separation; B further contraction and retraction thicken uterine wall, reduce placental site and aid placental separation; C complete separation and formation of retroplacental clot (note: the thin lower segment has collapsed like a concertina following the birth of the baby); D Schultze method of expulsion; E Matthew–Duncan method of expulsion.*

*(Fig. 13.15D & E, see opposite)*

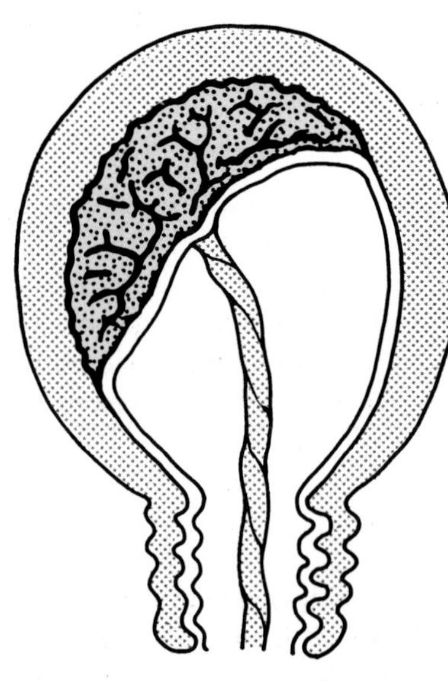

A

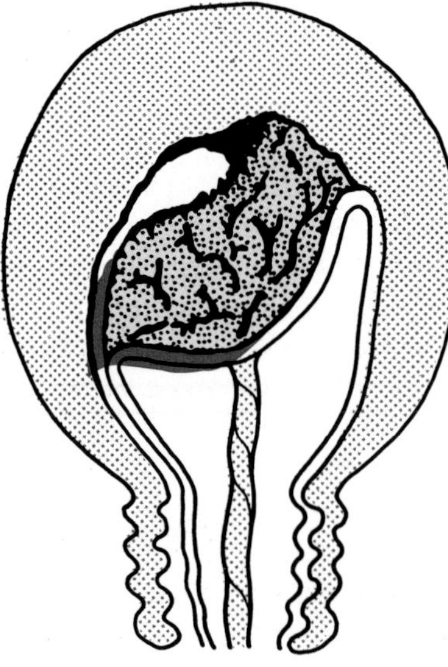

B

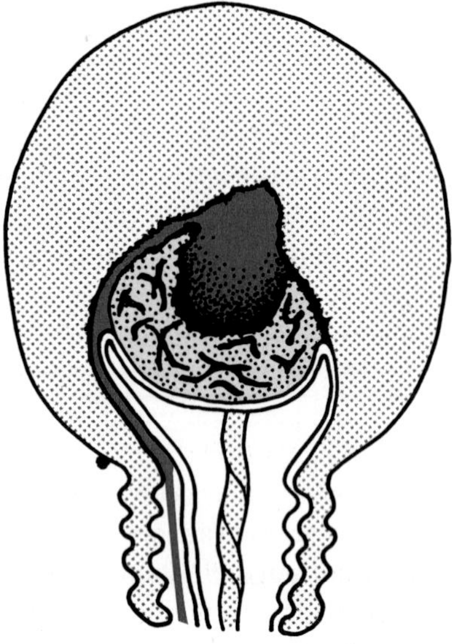

C

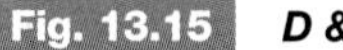
Fig. 13.15 D & E.

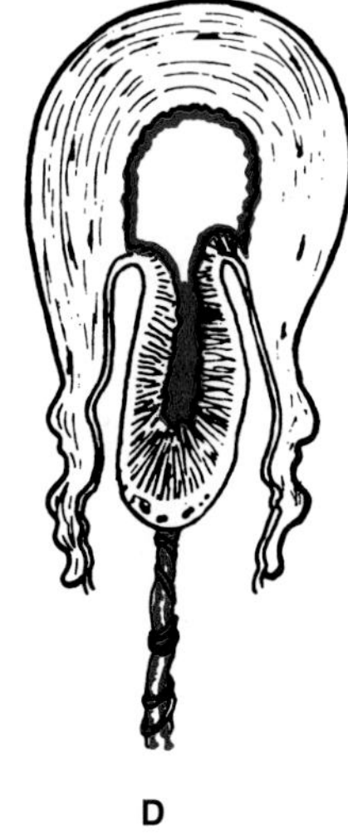


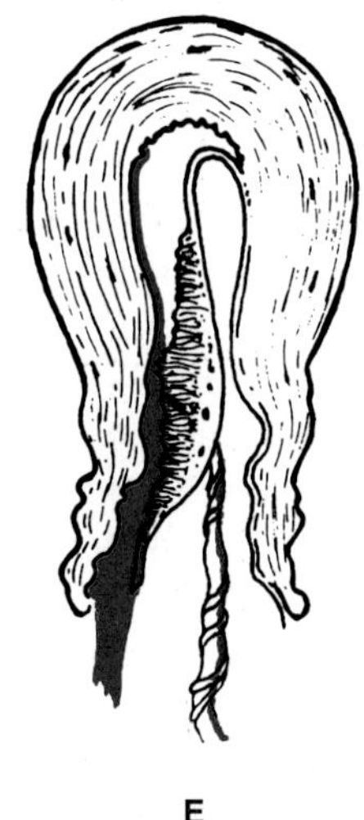


few minutes. Active management involves the injection of a tocolytic agent such as syntometrine at the birth of the anterior shoulder or shortly after the delivery of the baby and delivering the placenta and membranes by controlled cord traction (CCT). The placenta is extracted rather than expelled if active management of the third stage of labour is implemented.

Syntometrine is a combination of syntocinon and ergometrine. Syntocinon acts within 2 to 3 minutes following intramuscular injection, by causing intermittent contractions. These effectively continue the retraction process behind the placental site, thus encouraging separation and early expulsion. Ergometrine becomes effective about 5 to 7 minutes after administration. By this time, aided by CCT, the placenta has been expelled. The midwife applies cord traction by gripping the umbilical cord with one hand and applying a downward traction (Fig. 13.16). The other hand is placed on the lower abdomen, applying pressure to avoid inversion of the uterus. Ergometrine produces a sustained uterine contraction, which promotes the haemostatic action of the living ligatures. It is essential, therefore, to deliver the placenta before ergometrine stimulates closure of the cervix.

## Initiation of parturition in humans

The mean length of human gestation is 39.6 weeks and the majority of births occur between 38 and 42 weeks (Steer & Johnson 1998). Such a wide range of gestation times in normal pregnancy suggests the timing mechanism is not precise, possibly because it is affected by outside influences. The fetus seems to maintain the pregnancy actively. Labour invariably ensues after fetal death has occurred, although it might be delayed by a few weeks (and therefore be preempted by mechanical removal of the products of conception). Labour occurs sooner if placental damage has occurred. The critical events permitting extrauterine survival are adequate maturation of the fetal lung and nervous system. The fetal brain may monitor this maturation and control the timing mechanism.

Mothers of fetuses with brain abnormalities still progress into labour spontaneously but with a much wider range of gestation (see below). This suggests the fetal brain affects the precise timing of labour in humans, rather than controls the exact length of gestation.

Fig. 13.16 Controlled cord traction (Brandt–Andrews method). (Reproduced with permission from Bennett & Brown 1999.)

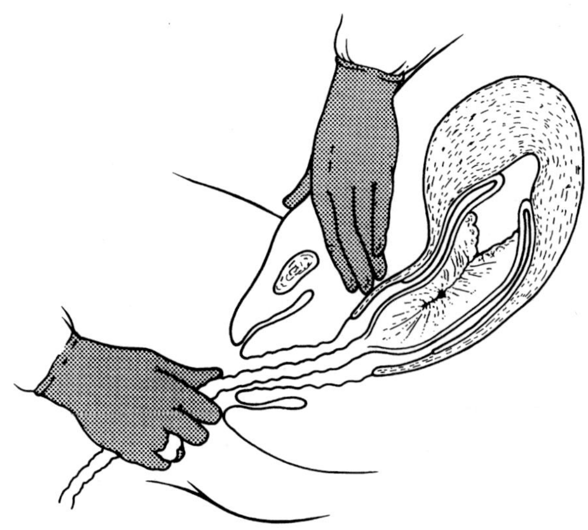

### Animal models of parturition

Parturition in the sheep has been studied in detail. Based on the assumption that mammals were likely to share similar physiological mechanisms for the onset of labour, a number of clinical procedures derived from labour in the sheep were developed, both for inducing labour and for inhibiting preterm labour in humans. About a week before delivery in ewes, there is a sharp rise in fetal cortisol levels due to mature secretion of ACTH from the pituitary gland and increased adrenal sensitivity to ACTH. This increase is the first indicator of impending labour. Removal or abnormal development of the fetal lamb pituitary gland prevents the onset of labour. Infusion of ACTH, cortisone or dexamethasone (a cortisol analogue, frequently used as an anti-inflammatory drug) into the sheep fetus induces labour. One suggestion is that hypothalamic release of NPY regulates cortisol levels and that stress (including hypoxia and hypoglycaemia) can increase NPY levels (Warnes et al 1998).

The effects of raised cortisol levels are to promote fetal organ maturity and to initiate labour. Cortisol induces 17α-hydroxylase activity in the placenta. This is enzyme converts progesterone to oestrogen so the progesterone : oestrogen ratio alters in favour of oestrogen. This increases prostaglandin ($PGF_{2\alpha}$) synthesis by the placenta and myometrium. The alteration in oestrogen and progesterone levels can be measured prior to the onset of labour. Exogenous oestrogen induces labour and infusion of progesterone inhibits labour in the sheep. Increasing oestrogen or decreasing progesterone levels stimulates the synthesis of $PGF_{2\alpha}$. Prostaglandins increase myometrial sensitivity to oxytocin. $PGF_{2\alpha}$ is important in cervical softening and increases uterine contractility. A positive feedback mechanism, known as the Ferguson reflex, amplifies the signals. The pressure of the fetal presenting part on the cervix activates a neurohumoral reflex whereby afferent nerves from the cervix impinge on the hypothalamus and increase oxytocin release from the posterior pituitary gland. Oxytocin stimulates uterine contractions and causes further release of $PGF_{2\alpha}$ from the uterus. However, initiation of labour in the human is markedly different, in a number of respects, from that in the sheep.

## Hormonal changes at parturition in humans

### The role of the fetal pituitary–adrenal axis

Human fetal malformations such as anencephaly (no cerebrum), malformed pituitary glands or hypoplasia of the adrenal glands are associated with an increased range of gestation length (both longer and shorter) but women still undergo spontaneous labour (Steer & Johnson 1998). This does not happen in sheep (Liggins, Kennedy & Holm 1967). This implies that fetal–adrenal axis acts as a fine tuner of gestational length in the human, rather than as the on–off switch of initiation of labour as in sheep.

#### *Cortisol*

It is evident that the human fetal anterior pituitary gland undergoes maturational changes in the last weeks of gestation as the profile of hormonal release changes. However, there are no defined changes measurable in the maternal circulation prior to the onset of labour. Some studies suggested that cortisol levels were higher in infants who had experienced a spontaneous delivery compared with those who had been induced or delivered by caesarean section. However, the cortisol seems to be maternally derived and levels are associated with maternal pain. Labour itself, whether spontaneous or induced, causes stress and therefore an increased production of cortisol, which can cross the placenta. It is possible to differentiate between cortisol of maternal origin and cortisol of fetal origin by comparing the levels in umbilical cord arterial blood with those in the cord vein. Blood in the vein flows from the placenta to the fetus so if cortisol levels are higher in the vein than the arteries this suggests the source of cortisol is maternal.

Exogenous corticosteroids (such as dexamethasone and betamethasone) given to a pregnant woman to promote fetal lung maturity (see Ch. 15) do not initiate parturition, although oestrogen and cortisol levels fall. Pharmacological doses of glucocorticoids introduced into the amniotic fluid increase uterine activity and induce labour; however, this effect is not observed with physiological doses. Most researchers have not been able to measure an increase in cortisol prior to the onset of labour, nor an effect on placental hormone production. Therefore, it now seems unlikely that cortisol is important in initiating labour in humans, although it has a vital role in fetal lung maturation. However, corticosterone, also produced by human fetal adrenal glands, has been reported to rise sharply late in gestation (Fencl et al 1980).

#### *Dehydroepiandrosterone sulphate*

DHEAS is the fetal precursor for placental oestradiol-17β and oestrone synthesis, which has been implicated as having a role in labour. It is the main product of the fetal zone of the adrenal glands, which is unique to humans and higher primates. This large zone disappears in the neonatal period and may be regulated by hCG levels. Production of DHEAS is controlled by ACTH from the anterior pituitary, which is itself regulated by hypothalamic corticotrophin-releasing hormone (CRH). Injection of ACTH to the fetus late in gestation results in increased DHEAS secretion by the fetal adrenal glands and a corresponding increase in maternal oestrogen levels. Injection of DHEAS in late gestation increases maternal oestradiol-17β levels and increases collagenolytic levels in the cervix causing cervical softening.

## Progesterone

Measurements of steroid hormone levels, prior to labour both in peripheral blood and in saliva, are inconsistent; however, most reports agree that absolute maternal progesterone levels do not measurably change before the onset of labour. In humans, the placenta does not express inducible 17α-hydroxylase activity and therefore cannot convert progesterone to oestrogen. However, increases in free oestriol levels have been observed in 70% of women before the onset of labour at term (Darne, McCarrigle & Lachelin 1987).

High progesterone levels inhibit myometrial activity during implantation and favour uterine quiescence throughout the pregnancy. This suppression of myometrial activity is essential to the maintenance of human pregnancy, although parturition begins without a measurable decrease in maternal peripheral progesterone levels. Large doses of progesterone are relatively unsuccessful in inhibiting preterm labour. Mifepristone, an antiprogestin also known as RU-486, blocks the effect of progesterone and can induce labour (Thong & Baird 1992).

However, it is possible that there could be local changes in progesterone concentration, not reflected in peripheral blood, that may affect myometrial activity. As the uterus enlarges during the pregnancy, the part of the uterine wall distal to the site of implantation, and therefore furthest away from the major source of progesterone production, may re-establish uterine contractions and trigger the onset of labour (Mitchell, Challis & Lukash 1987). Measurement of absolute progesterone levels may therefore be misleading as the biological effects will be altered by receptor density, levels of binding proteins or postreceptor changes. The fetal membranes have both progesterone-binding sites and enzymes that metabolize progesterone (Schwartz et al 1976). The fetal membranes also produce more cortisol as gestation progresses. Cortisol is antagonistic to progesterone and can increase the synthesis of CRH (Karalis, Goodwin & Majzoub 1996). Fetal membranes therefore offer a mechanism for local control of progesterone concentration.

## Oestrogen

Placental production of oestrogen increases throughout labour and the rate seems to increase in the latter part of gestation. However, spontaneous labour can occur in the absence of measurable changes in oestrogen concentration. Exogenous oestrogen causes transient increases in uterine activity and decreases the oxytocin threshold of the uterus but does not stimulate uterine contractions to a degree that would lead to delivery (Pinto et al 1964). Patients with low oestrogen levels tend to experience a prolonged gestation, particularly in the first pregnancy, and limited responses to induction techniques (Oakey, Cawood & MacDonald 1974). The changing ratio of oestrogen to progesterone may facilitate effective uterine contractions but is probably not critical for the induction of labour (Steer & Johnson 1998).

## Prostaglandins

Prostaglandins are known to be important in the progression of labour, and have been widely studied, but it is not clear whether they have a role in initiating labour and how their synthesis is regulated in the uterus. Prostaglandins are present in low concentrations and are cleared in the pulmonary circulation. They are difficult to measure as they have paracrine activity and a short half-life. Prostaglandins can be formed as a consequence of tissue trauma (including labour itself and any manipulative or tactile stimuli). In late pregnancy, prostaglandin synthesis is readily stimulated by minor local stimuli, such as coitus, vaginal examination, sweeping the membranes or amniotomy, which are associated with inducing labour. Exogenous prostaglandins can be used therapeutically to ripen the cervix and to induce uterine contractions and labour. Mid-trimester abortion can be induced by procedures, such as intra-amniotic injection of hypertonic saline, that result in the increased synthesis and release of prostaglandins. Increasing DHEAS or oestrogen concentration and decreasing progesterone concentration increase prostaglandin production (Gustavii 1975).

Prostaglandins are synthesized in the fetal membranes, decidua, myometrium and cervix; levels fall abruptly following placental separation. The rate-limiting step of prostaglandin production may be important in initiating labour. Activity of phospholipase $A_2$ ($PLA_2$) may regulate the level of arachidonic acid, which is the precursor of prostaglandins (see Ch. 3). Increased oestrogen (or decreased progesterone) simulates the release of $PLA_2$ from decidual lysozymes and therefore increases free arachidonic acid and subsequent prostaglandin synthesis (Gustavii 1975). Arachidonic acid can also be produced indirectly via phospholipase C activity. Alternatively, the activity of cyclo-oxygenase may be rate limiting (Aitken, Rice & Brennecke 1990).

The two most important prostaglandins appear to be $PGF_{2\alpha}$ and $PGE_2$. At term, concentration of $PGE_2$ and $PGF_{2\alpha}$ are higher in the decidua and myometrium (but these tissues are subject to tissue trauma so some authors believe raised prostaglandin levels are caused by increased uterine activity). Other authors have shown that, towards term, synthesis of prostaglandins, especially $PGE_2$, increases in the amnion, which may be the key event in the onset of labour (Okazaki et al 1981). $PGE_2$ is involved in cervical ripening and is metabolized by the myometrium to produce $PGF_{2\alpha}$. However, women with extrauterine pregnancies go into labour at term and experience painful uterine contractions even though there are no fetal membranes in contact with the uterus (Gustavii 1977).

Maintenance of human pregnancy may depend on the synthesis of $PGE_2$ being inhibited; inhibition of $PGE_2$ synthase is then attenuated at the onset of labour. Prostaglandin concentrations in the pregnant uterus are very low (about two hundred times lower than at any stage in the menstrual cycle), but increase sharply in the maternal circulation from 36 weeks' gestation (Dray & Frydman 1976). The human conceptus apparently interferes with the synthesis or metabolism of prostaglandins (it is not an effect of oestrogen or progesterone). Arachidonic acid, the precursor, is plentiful but synthesis of prostaglandins is inhibited, even if the pregnancy is extrauterine. Endogenous inhibitors of prostaglandin synthesis (EIPS) have been identified in maternal plasma; levels fall towards the end of gestation. Inhibitors of prostaglandin synthesis, such as aspirin and indomethacin, are used therapeutically to treat preterm labour. Proteins such as gravidin that inhibit endometrial cell $PLA_2$ have been found in amniotic fluid (Wilson, Liggins & Joe 1989).

Low doses of prostaglandins, particularly $PGF_{2\alpha}$, increase myometrial responsiveness to prostaglandins and oxytocin possibly by increasing the formation of gap junctions. In vitro, $PGE_2$ has a biphasic effect, stimulating at nanomolar concentrations and inhibiting at micromolar concentrations. It also has a dual action: when its effects are mediated by the $EP_1$ and $EP_3$ receptors, $PGE_2$ increases intracellular calcium concentration, but the $EP_2$ receptor is coupled to adenylate cyclase so $PGE_2$ acting at this receptor decreases intracellular calcium and favours relaxation. Variations in regional prostaglandin synthesis may occur (Wilmsatt et al 1995).

Prostacyclin ($PGI_2$) is synthesized in the myometrium and cervix. It has an important role in maintaining uterine blood flow; it causes vasodilation of smooth muscle and inhibits platelet aggregation. Placental thromboxane ($TxA_2$) has opposing effects and is important in the closure of the fetal ductus arteriosus and haemostasis after delivery. In pre-eclampsia, levels of prostacyclin are low and levels of thromboxane are high. This is the rationale for aspirin treatment of pre-eclampsia. Aspirin-like drugs are inhibitors of prostaglandin synthase and restore thromboxane levels in pre-eclampsia. Trials using aspirin caused a slight prolongation of gestation and diminution of uterine contractions, as well as increasing the risk of premature closure of the ductus arteriosus and postnatal bleeding problems in the mother.

Prostaglandins also have an important role in the establishment of a neonatal circulatory pattern (see Ch. 15). Respiratory distress syndrome is associated with high levels of $PGF_{2\alpha}$ in the infant's circulation and patent ductus arteriosus, with high $PGE_2$ levels. $PGE_2$ can prevent the ductus from closing and inhibitors of prostaglandin synthesis can promote closure of the ductus. There is indirect evidence (i.e. fetal breathing movements stop) that $PGE_2$ increases in the fetal circulation 48–72 hours before the onset of labour (Thorburn 1992). It is possible that this is mirrored by a local increase in $PGE_2$ concentration in uterine tissue, which initiates labour.

## Oxytocin

Oxytocin is used extensively for induction and augmentation of human labour and endogenous production can be stimulated, for instance by nipple stimulation, with a favourable outcome. However, it is not certain whether oxytocin is important in the normal physiological onset of labour. As oxytocin receptors are localized to the uterus, mammary glands and pituitary, oxytocin antagonists and agonists have few systemic effects. Maternal oxytocin levels are very low and do not change very much before labour. Maternal pituitary production of oxytocin dramatically increases in the first stage of labour. However, focusing on circulating levels of oxytoxin may be misleading. The concentration of oxytocin receptors in the myometrium and decidua dramatically rises (by 100–200 times) during late pregnancy so the sensitivity of the uterus increases (Fuchs et al 1984). This means the uterus can be stimulated by low concentrations of maternal oxytocin levels that previously had no effect. Therapeutic doses adequate to augment labour are very variable, which probably reflects individual differences in receptor number. The pattern of oxytocin release changes at the onset of labour, with an increased frequency of pulses (Fuchs et al 1991). It may be important that maternal oxytocin levels stay low during the pregnancy so the sensitivity of the uterus to oxytocin is maintained. Oxytocin antagonists are used to inhibit uterine contractility in preterm labour (see Table 13.2).

Exposing decidual cells to oxytocin increases the release of prostaglandins. Vaginal examination in late pregnancy stimulates the Ferguson reflex so oxytocin is released from the posterior pituitary, which stimulates uterine prostaglandin production. Earlier in pregnancy, this response does not occur, presumably because there are inadequate oxytocin receptors. Women who go into preterm labour seem to have an increased expression of oxytocin receptors and higher myometrial sensitivity to oxytocin. Failed induction of labour is associated with a reduced number of oxytocin receptors. Therefore the initiation of labour depends on mechanisms that induce the expression of oxytocin receptors in the myometrium rather affect the oxytocin level itself. Both oestrogen and prostaglandins increase uterine responsiveness to oxytocin.

Oxytocin is also synthesized by the decidua and may act locally (Miller, Chibbar & Mitchell 1993). The fetal posterior pituitary produces both oxytocin and ADH-vasopressin. Exogenous oxytocin can cause uterine contractions in sheep and anencephalic humans (Honnebier, Jobsis & Swaab 1974); however, the physiological relevance of this is not clear as maternal oxytocin secretion does not rise until labour has been initiated. In spontaneous labour, fetal secretion of oxytocin is high and transferred across the placenta at levels comparable to those used to induce uterine activity (Husslein 1985). The increment in oxytocin levels is greater in the umbilical arteries than in the umbilical vein and is much higher than maternal levels, suggesting it is synthesized by the fetus and transferred across the placenta. Initiation and maintenance of human labour may therefore be influenced by fetal oxytocin production. ADH-vasopressin is produced at even higher concentrations than oxytocin and may regulate prostaglandin production.

### Relaxin

Relaxin is a polypeptide hormone produced by the corpus luteum, and decidua and placenta in pregnancy, which promotes tissue remodelling during reproduction (Bani 1997). It has been found to inhibit myometrial contractility and promote vasodilation, via nitric oxide synthesis, until late pregnancy. It is also appears to promote cervical ripening at parturition. Concentrations of relaxin appear to be highest in the first trimester and then fall. A very early fall is associated with preterm labour. Histologically, the number of cells staining positively for relaxin are much less after spontaneous delivery compared with caesarean section. Relaxin may inhibit $PGE_2$ production during pregnancy but favours its production in labour. It may act synergistically with progesterone during the pregnancy, maintaining uterine quiescence and inhibiting oxytocin release.

### Corticotrophin-releasing hormone

Recent studies implicate placental CRH as having a possibly important role in the initiation of parturition. CRH is synthesized by the placenta and reaches the maternal circulation (Riley & Challis 1991). Levels steadily increase from mid term until about 35 weeks when levels sharply rise and are usually particularly high in pregnancies ending with premature labour (Wolfe et al 1990). CRH activity is modulated by CRH-binding protein (CRH-BP), which is synthesized by the liver, placenta and brain so most CRH is in the bound form during pregnancy. However, towards term, when levels of CRH increase, levels of CRH-PB simultaneously fall so circulating levels of physiologically active, free CRH markedly increase. CRH establishes positive feedback loops, increasing prostaglandin production (Petraglia et al 1995) and fetal glucocorticoid levels (Robinson et al 1988), both of which further increase placental synthesis of CRH.

### The maternal endocrine system

Ovaries are not necessary for the initiation of labour. Hypophysectomized women (who have no pituitary glands) and women with diabetes insipidus (a posterior pituitary defect) go into labour at term. However, the posterior pituitary stores oxytocin, which is synthesized in the hypothalamus. In the absence of a functional pituitary gland, oxytocin is probably secreted directly by the hypothalamus. Adrenalectomized women on corticosteroid maintenance therapy go into labour spontaneously but women with Addison's disease tend to have prolonged pregnancy.

## *The maternal nervous system*

There is a higher density of adrenergic and cholinergic innervation towards the cervix. The non-pregnant uterus contracts in response to both adrenaline and noradrenaline but, at term, noradrenaline increases uterine contractions and adrenaline causes relaxation. $\alpha$-receptor antagonists, such as phentolamine, decrease uterine activity and inhibit the response to noradrenaline so adrenergic drugs are used to suppress contractions in preterm labour; $\beta$-receptor antagonists, such as propranolol, increase uterine activity. Catecholamines both stimulate and inhibit uterine activity, acting via the $\alpha_2$-receptors and $\beta_2$-receptors respectively. The $\alpha_1$-receptors increase intracellular calcium concentrations and promote contractile activity. However, labour occurs normally in paraplegic women (who have no nervous input to the uterus), suggesting that the onset and progress of labour is under hormonal, rather than nervous, control. Neural control appears to modulate uterine activity but is subordinate to hormonal control.

### *Stretch*

In a normal pregnancy, growth of the uterus keeps pace with the growth of its contents and the limit of stretchability is probably not reached. However, overstretching, for instance with multiple pregnancy and polyhydramnios, is associated with a shorter gestation period. The probable mechanism is that stretching of the muscle fibres increases their excitability.

### *Other possible signals*

There are a number of other possible signals involved in the initiation of labour, including nitric oxide and cytokines. Nitric oxide has a role in maintaining maternal vasodilation and decreasing vascular responsiveness during the pregnancy. It also appears to cause myometrial relaxation. As its synthesis falls at term (Norman 1996), a possible role in the onset of labour has been investigated. Cytokines are a family of about 30 cellular-signalling molecules (see Box 4.3, p. 73), some of which are synergistic or interact with other hormones or cytokines. Activity of cytokines may affect prostaglandin synthesis. The role of interleukins, particularly interleukin 8, which may be involved with cervical softening, and interleukin 1, has been studied. They are of interest because their levels seem to increase in intrauterine infection associated with preterm labour. However, studies of interleukins in amniotic fluid suggest they are present as a consequence of normal term labour, rather than being the cause (Cox, Casey & MacDonald 1997).

## The timing of parturition

In some mammalian species there is a clear seasonal influence on ovulation and delivery. There are obvious advantages to ensuring the young are born at the optimal time of year when there is a plentiful food supply and less threat from predators. In these species, the length of the daylight period mediated by melatonin production appears to play an important role. The human fetus has the potential to survive birth as early as the 24th week of gestation. Most babies are delivered after the 37th week of gestation. However, there is a range of gestational periods producing healthy babies capable of survival. It is suggested that this variation in apparently normal gestation could allow changing environmental conditions to influence the precise timing. One suggestion is that the time of the lunar month could affect the timing after 37 weeks. Other suggestions are that gestational length may be linked to the length of the individual woman's ovarian cycle or may have a familial pattern. Women with longer menstrual cycles may have a lower level of oestrogen, which could affect the initiation of parturition (see above).

Mammals tend to labour most effectively during the period of the day in which they normally rest. This may be because the effect of the parasympathetic nervous system is then dominant; labour is inhibited by sympathetic stimulation. Both the start of labour and the actual time of delivery occur more frequently at night and in the early hours of the morning (Honnebier & Nathanielsz 1994). Circadian rhythms occur in several variables including pregnancy-associated hormones and prelabour myometrial activity. Uterine activity and oxytocin levels are higher at night until about 3 weeks before delivery. The maternal circadian system probably entrains fetal cooperation. Circadian rhythms do not occur in sheep (Apostolakis et al 1993).

## Intervention in labour

Humans have evolved to stand on two feet and to have a large brain. The development of bipedal locomotion has resulted in a changed pelvic structure and physiology. One suggestion is that eye contact in sexual intercourse has led to the vagina forming a right angle with the brim of the pelvis and uterus, presenting a laborious passageway in childbirth (Stewart 1984). The relatively straight cylindrical pelvis of our forebears has evolved into a tilted conical birth canal. Pelvic size has decreased to enhance adaptation to the upright posture and swift movement. The evolution of the human brain resulted in cephalization, the marked enlargement of head size in relation to overall body mass (Stewart 1984). This creates the potential problem of obstructed labour, which occurs at a much higher rate in humans than in other animals. The fetus has to negotiate rather than simply pass through the pelvic cavity. It seems that humans have adapted by the fetus completing in utero development at a relatively early stage, and being born at a much smaller proportion of the adult weight. As part of this evolutionary adaptation, two distinct signalling pathways seem to have evolved in humans (Fig. 13.17). The human fetus appears to undergo lung maturation 4 to

**Fig. 13.17** *The two distinct pathways controlling parturition and fetal development in the human.*

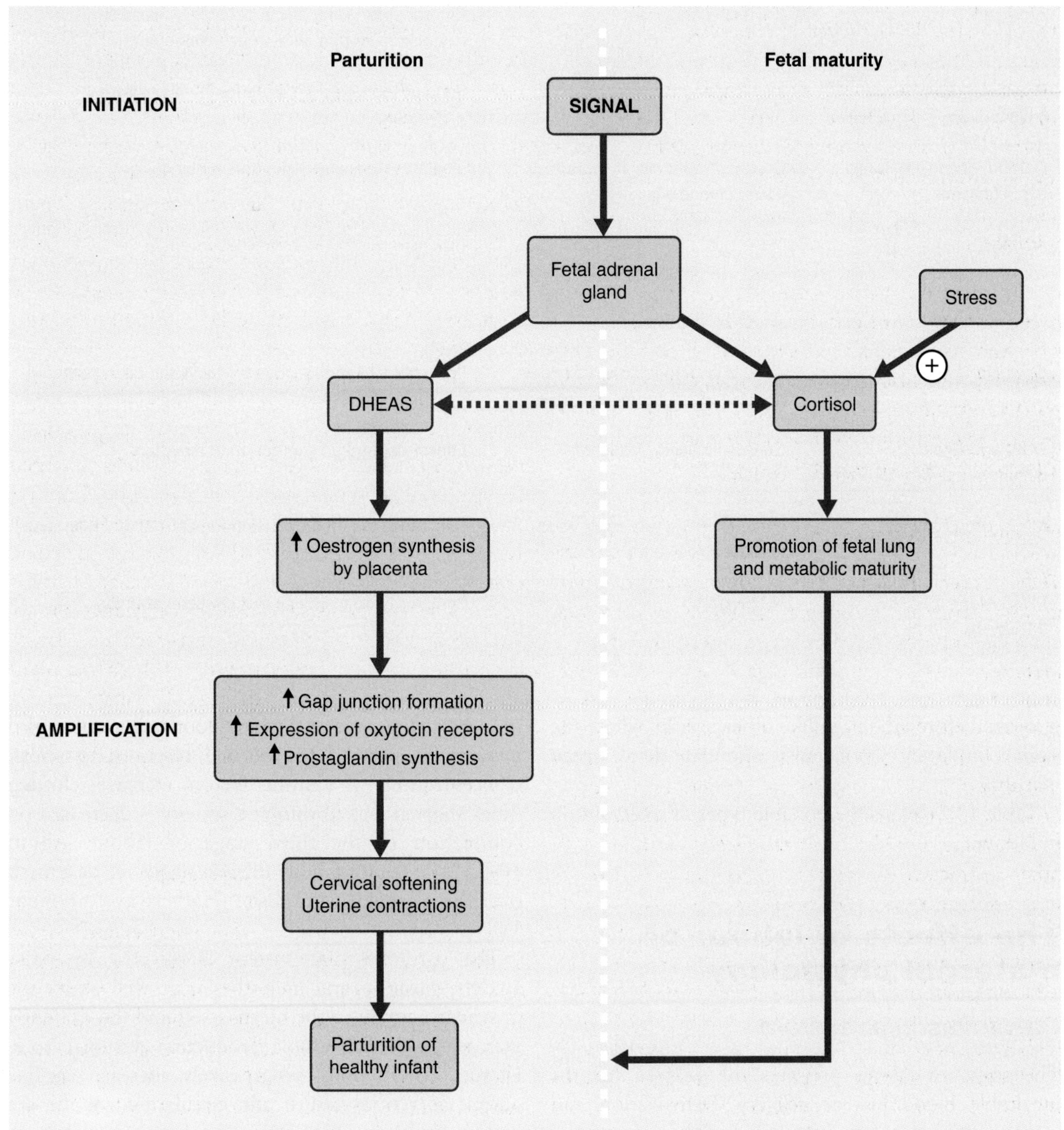

**Table 13.2** *Intervention in labour*

| Drug/treatment | Effect | Notes |
|---|---|---|
| *Treatment of preterm labour (tocolytic agents)* | | |
| Indomethacin | Inhibits prostaglandin synthesis | Adverse effects on fetal renal function, associated with oligohydramnios |
| β-adrenergic agonists e.g. ritodrine, terbutaline | Inhibit uterine contractions | Effects often short lived; unpleasant side-effects |
| Magnesium sulphate | Inhibits myometrial contractility | |
| Atosiban | Oxytocin antagonist | Clinical trials taking place; potentially useful as oxytocin receptors have limited distribution |
| Prostaglandin synthase inhibitors e.g. indomethacin | Inhibit preterm contractions | Serious neonatal complications in infants born < 30 weeks |
| Calcium channel blockers e.g. nifedipine | Decrease intracellular calcium, cause uterine relaxation | May affect placental and uterine blood flow |
| Alcohol | | Risk of aspiration and intoxication |
| *Treatment of post-term labour (methods of induction)* | | |
| Oxytocin | Used to augment labour; oxytocin has little effect on unripe cervix | Production of endogenous oxytocin can be increased by nipple stimulation |
| $PGF_2$ agonists e.g. dinoprostone, Cervidil, Prepidil | Cervical ripening, induction of labour | Effects depend on expression of receptors |
| Misoprostol (Cytotec) | Synthetic $PGE_1$ analogue; used to reduce acid in the stomach | Can cause the uterus to contract; nausea and diarrhoea |
| Mifepristone (RU-486) (Mifegyne) | Antiprogestin | Primarily used to induce first trimester abortion |

6 weeks before labour, unlike other species where the signals initiating labour also stimulate fetal organ maturity.

Table 13.2 details the possible types of intervention in labour.

## The effects of labour on maternal physiology

### *Cardiovascular system*

The stress of labour prepares the woman for the inevitable blood loss at delivery. Dehydration and muscle activity increase the haemoglobin concentration. Erythropoiesis and white blood cell number also increase as part of the normal response to stress. Concentrations of clotting factors increase, clotting times shorten and fibrinolytic activity is decreased on completion of the third stage of labour. About 10–15% of the total body fibrin is deposited as a mesh over the placental wound site (Hatherway & Bonnar 1987).

The cardiovascular system is affected by pain, anxiety, position and anaesthesia, as well as by the muscular activity of the uterus itself and the dramatic increase in catecholamine production during labour. Uterine contractions progressively increase cardiac output as venous return and circulating volume are increased. Each contraction can contribute 300 to

500 ml of blood to the circulation (Sullivan & Ramanathan 1985), which affects cardiac output and blood pressure. In the supine position, stroke volume and cardiac output tend to be lower and heart rate raised.

Catecholamines affect vascular tone and increase blood pressure; this effect is reduced with anaesthetics. Pain and anxiety result in tachycardia (increased heart rate) and affect blood pressure. During a contraction, systolic blood pressure increases by at least 35 mmHg and diastolic blood pressure may increase between 25 and 65 mmHg (Blackburn & Loper 1992). The increment in blood pressure precedes each contraction and falls to baseline between contractions. The greatest haemodynamic changes occur in women delivering their baby vaginally, which is an important consideration for women who have cardiac disease.

### Respiratory system

Labour affects the respiratory system as the muscular work increases metabolic rate and oxygen consumption. Respiratory rate and depth of respiration increase. Anxiety, drugs and use of a gas mask mouthpiece can all affect respiratory rate. There is a tendency for a labouring woman to hyperventilate. Hyperventilation is a natural response to pain. Contractions occurring at high frequency can affect oxygenation causing muscular hypoxia and acidosis. Hypoxia can increase the amount of pain experienced.

The increased ventilation causes a progressive and marked decrease in partial pressure of carbon dioxide (to about 25 mmHg) particularly if the contractions are painful. In early labour, hyperventilation can cause respiratory alkalosis and increased blood pH. This can result in the woman experiencing dizziness and tingling of her fingers and toes, and possibly developing muscle spasms. At extremely low $P_aCO_2$, blood flow can be affected and the oxygen–haemoglobin dissociation curve (see Ch. 1) shifts to the left so release of oxygen is impaired. The remedy of breath counting to slow respiratory rate, especially if the woman counts them with her partner or a midwife who deliberately slows down counting, can prevent or correct hyperventilatory effects.

By the end of the first stage, maternal acidosis due to isometric muscle contractions is likely and is compensated for, to a degree, by the respiratory alkalosis. The muscle contractions reduce blood flow to the uterine muscle, which becomes hypoxic and undergoes anaerobic metabolism. Flow to the intervillous space also decreases so fetal levels of carbon dioxide increase and the fetus tends to become acidotic. During bearing down, when the mother's accessory respiratory muscles are involved, mild respiratory acidosis is likely. In the second stage of labour lactate levels increase, thus pH falls. This metabolic acidosis is not compensated for.

### The renin–angiotensin system

Labour and delivery affect the renin–angiotensin system of both fetus and mother. Levels of renin and angiotensinogen increase, which is important in maintaining blood flow, but can also affect handling and excretion of drugs. Glomerular filtration rate, renal blood flow and sodium excretion are also affected by raised catecholamine levels or general anaesthetic. Oxytocin has structural similarities with ADH and has inherent antidiuretic properties, therefore fluid retention is increased in labour. Women in labour can be at risk of iatrogenic water intoxication due to loss of electrolytes, use of oxytocin, or intravenous fluid administration.

### Metabolic rate

Maternal glucose consumption markedly increases in labour to provide energy required by the uterus and skeletal muscles. Glucose and triacylglycerides are used as energy sources. Oxytocin has some insulin like properties. An increased body temperature during labour may indicate dehydration or infection. It is common for women to experience a transient postpartum chill about 15 minutes after the birth of the baby or delivery of the placenta. In the following 24 hours, postpartum women frequently have a slightly raised temperature secondary to dehydration.

## Nutrition in labour

Food and drink consumption in labour is controversial. There are two conflicting arguments. The first is that a woman in labour might possibly require a general anaesthetic and therefore should be treated as a preoperative patient (Douglas 1988). Pulmonary aspiration of gastric acid (Mendelson's syndrome) or particulate food matter, although rare, is a major cause of morbidity and mortality for women in labour. The risks of gastric aspiration are thought to be greatly reduced if oral intake is limited (Rowe 1997).

Pregnant women have a slower gastric emptying rate (see Ch. 11), which is further delayed by labour (Carp, Jayaram & Stoll 1992), and decreased tone of the lower oesophageal sphincter.

The opposing view is that a more liberal policy is more beneficial and that women are being needlessly deprived of food (Baker 1996, Ludka & Roberts 1993, Sharp 1997). It is argued that general anaesthesia is relatively rare now and that techniques have improved, which make aspiration of gastric contents unlikely. It is argued that prolonged fasting could have detrimental psychological and physiological effects, including increased anxiety and stress.

Pregnant women are predisposed to ketosis, particularly in labour. Starvation in pregnancy always causes ketonuria (Foulkes & Dumoulin 1983). It is estimated that a woman in labour has an energy requirement of 700–1100 kcal/h. When glycogen stores are exhausted, adipose tissue is mobilized. Fatty acid oxidation increases ketosis, an excess of ketone bodies in the plasma, which are excreted into the urine. Lipolysis provides fatty acid substrates for maternal energy needs and spares glucose for the fetus. The critical question is whether ketosis is detrimental to the progress of labour. Ketones can increase acidity, cause excessive renal excretion of sodium and cross the placenta to the fetus. A relationship between the length of labour and the degree of ketosis has been identified (Foulkes & Dumoulin 1983) but it is not clear whether longer labour results in increased ketosis or whether ketosis prolongs labour.

It is suggested that fasting in labour can increase the need for medical intervention. Allowing women to eat in labour reduces the plasma level of ketones, which may aid the progress of labour (Scutton, Lowy & O'Sullivan 1996). Ketonuria can be treated by administration of intravenous dextrose but this is associated with fluid and electrolyte imbalance. A number of women experience nausea and vomiting in labour. But, in practice, more maternity units are cautiously adopting a liberal policy offering a non-particulate diet while using antacids and $H_2$ antagonists to reduce gastric pH and decrease volume of gastric contents, thus minimizing the risk of aspiration and lung damage.

## The effects of labour on the fetus

Labour has profound effects on the fetus and is important in aiding the adaptation to extrauterine life (see Ch. 15). Understanding the effects of labour on the fetus is important in differentiating between normal healthy responses and diagnosing fetal distress.

### *Behaviour of the fetus during pregnancy*

After 36 weeks, the fetus exhibits a number of clearly definable behavioural states, which are analogous to the neonatal states (see Ch. 15). These states have characteristic patterns of fetal heart rate (FHR), fetal breathing movements (FBM), voiding and mouthing movements (Table 13.3) (Nijhuis et al 1982). The activity of the fetus changes with gestational age and is assumed to reflect the changes in its nervous development. The movements evidently demonstrate fetal ability to respond to external stimuli.

Fetal breathing movements are more regular in state 1F than 2F, occur more frequently in state 2F and are present but irregular in states 3F and 4F. It has been suggested that fetal breathing movements are more likely to be state dependent when maternal glucose levels are lower (Mulder et al 1994). Fetal voiding movements are inhibited in state 1F but occur at the transition to state 2F. Rhythmic mouthing movements are most often observed in state 1F, when they occur

**Table 13.3** *Fetal behavioural states*

| | |
|---|---|
| State 1F (1 fetal); quiet sleep | Fetal quiescence with brief gross startles; high-voltage electrocortical activity; no eye movement; FHR accelerations; minimal heart rate variability; isolated fetal heart rate |
| State 2F (2 fetal); active sleep | Paradoxical/irregular sleep; frequent and periodic stretches; retroflexion and movements of extremities; low-voltage electrocortical activity; continuous eye movements; increased FHR variability with frequent accelerations |
| State 3F (3 fetal); quiet awake | Absence of gross movements; continuous rapid eye movements; stable, but widely oscillating FHR, no accelerations |
| State 4F (4 fetal); active awake | Vigorous and continual movements; rapid eye movement; unstable heart rate—large, long accelerations and tachycardia |

in bursts of 10–20 minutes. States 1F and 2F account for about 90% of fetal life in late gestation. FHR patterns during these four behavioural states may mimic fetal distress. The fetal behavioural states and the transitions between them can be observed throughout labour. States 1F and 2F predominate as they do before labour. It is thought that diminished HR variability and absent accelerations in a healthy term fetus probably represent fetal sleep rather than fetal distress. In the deep sleep state 1F, FHR pattern is usually unaffected even by strong uterine contractions. A period of low fetal heart variability (FHV) or tachycardia may indicate that fetal oxygenation is being compromised. In the second stage of labour, the length of the behavioural cycles decreases; this is related to the gamut of sensory stimuli and head compression incurred during this stage of labour.

Fetal breathing movements increase in frequency and in length of episode as gestation progresses. By the third trimester, FBM occur for 30% of the time and are closely associated with behavioural state, especially active sleep (2F). A few days before the onset of labour, FBM are depressed, probably because increased levels of prostaglandin, especially $PGE_2$, inhibit the fetal respiratory centre. During the latent stage of labour, FBM occur for about 10% of the time but almost cease in the active stage. In preterm labour, the decrease in FBM is less acute. FBM may be affected by changes in oxygenation and pH. FBM require energy so the fetus decreases FBM in response to hypoxia as an adaptive response to conserve oxygen. The hypoxia-induced decrease in FBM is more marked near term possibly because the responses to hypoxia have become more sensitive as the respiratory centre becomes more mature. However, the respiratory centre remains inhibited until birth (Dawes 1984); possibly cord occlusion or changed oxygenation act to switch it on finally at delivery.

Although hypoxia normally decreases FBM, deeper, sustained inspiration or gasping is stimulated synergistically by raised carbon dioxide levels in the presence of hypoxia. In perinatal aspiration, this gasping can cause meconium inspiration. Paradoxically, maternal hyperventilation decreases FBM. Hypoglycaemia and CNS depressants, such as ethanol, barbiturates and diazepam, decrease FBM. Theophylline increases FBM and is used to treat postnatal apnoea in premature infants. Prostaglandin inhibitors, such as indomethacin, stimulate FBM but have to be used with caution because of their effects on fetal vascular function.

**Box 13.4**

**Changes in fetal behaviour during pregnancy**

**First trimester**

- Specific sequence of movements
- Continual activity
- Coordinated and graceful quality

**Second trimester**

- Body movements diminish
- Breathing movements increase
- Quiescence increases
- Rest–activity cycles develop

**Third trimester**

- Clear fetal behavioural states
- Specific combination of variables
- Stable with state transitions
- Breathing is state dependent

Changes in fetal behaviour over the course of pregnancy are summarized in Box 13.4.

## *Changes during labour*

The stress of labour causes a reflex increase in maternal catecholamine levels well above those seen in non-pregnant women or pregnant women before labour. The physiological stress and hypoxia associated with the pain and anxiety increase adrenaline secretion. The physiological work of labour, which is highest in the second stage of labour, increases noradrenaline release. Placental metabolism of maternal catecholamines reduces the transfer to the fetus. However, maternal catecholamines can affect placental blood flow and affect the fetus in labour. Animal studies show that adrenaline is associated with vasoconstriction and a reduction in uterine blood flow. As the rise in adrenaline level is associated with maternal stress in labour, there is a clear advantage to limiting maternal psychological distress and pain.

Normal labour and delivery are associated with an increase in cord levels of catecholamines in the neonate (Langercrantz & Slotkin 1986). The mechanism of the fetally derived catecholamines is not clear but may be a response to fetal compression, mild acidosis and other stimuli experienced during the birth. It is suggested that this is an adaptive response that facilitates extrauterine adaptation. The increased catecholamines stimulate breathing, increase fluid absorption from the lungs, stimulate surfactant release, enhance irritability, and play a role in metabolism by mobilizing glucose and fatty acids (Padbury et al 1987).

Fetal tissues are metabolically active; heat dissipation is via the placenta to the mother. Cord exclusion in animals results in an increase in fetal temperature. It seems likely that uterine contractions affecting uterine blood flow will impair heat transfer, particularly in active labour. At delivery, there is a transition from a heat-producing fetus to a neonate dependent on heat generation. In utero, $PGE_2$ and adenosine derived from the placenta may have a role in suppressing the activity of brown adipose tissue and therefore minimizing heat production by the fetus. Occlusion of the umbilical cord is the signal to increase heat generation. Non-shivering thermogenesis by brown adipose tissue is under the control of noradrenaline (see Ch. 1) released during labour.

A healthy term fetus has good energy stores and a normal base excess so it can tolerate temporary reductions in uterine perfusion in labour. There is a marked increase in fetal glycogen storage in the last month of gestation. The fetus also has the enzymes required for glycogenolysis. However, under normal uterine condition, placental transfer of maternal glucose means that the fetal glucose pool is of maternal origin. Until labour, the fetus still depends on maternal sources of glucose. The changes in catecholamine secretion boost neonatal metabolism.

The placenta also provides the route of oxygen transfer and carbon dioxide removal. Maternal hyperventilation in labour increases carbon dioxide diffusion across the placenta, therefore increasing respiratory alkalosis (increasing pH). However, respiratory depression caused by oversedation or magnesium sulphate could have the opposite effect. In the presence of a reduced oxygen supply, anaerobic metabolism will cause metabolic acidosis. Lactate diffusion across the placenta is slow and the fetal kidney is not efficient at clearing organic acids. It seems likely that the respiratory alkalosis related to maternal hyperventilation compensates for at least some of the metabolic acidosis, owing to anaerobic glycolysis, thus restoring fetal pH to a normal range. Normal labour nevertheless will cause a gradual decrease in fetal pH, oxygen and bicarbonate ions and a corresponding rise in partial pressure of carbon dioxide.

Uterine blood flow is largely determined by maternal blood pressure, cardiac output and uterine muscular tone. Labour compromises uterine blood flow. The maternal spiral arteries, which perfuse the intervillous spaces, are occluded and venous drainage of the spaces is obstructed during uterine contractions. Doppler measurements show that blood flow through the uterine arteries is gradually reduced during a contraction and gradually returns when the uterus relaxes. Most animal models demonstrate that the placenta has an anatomical redundancy; over 70% of the placental capillary bed must be occluded before impedance to gas exchange rises significantly. If placental reserve is reduced, uterine contractions may have a significant effect on fetal hypoxia and acidosis. Even with a healthy placenta and normal uterine blood flow, contractions with excessive strength of frequency can cause fetal hypoxia and bradycardia. Maternal conditions may exacerbate this by reducing uterine perfusion; supine posture can reduce venous return and therefore, cardiac output and regional anaesthesia can cause vasodilation so decreasing maternal cardiac output.

Labour promotes the clearance of fetal lung fluid. Transient tachypnoea, caused by residual lung fluid, is more common in babies born by elective caesarean section than in those experiencing a vaginal delivery. Chest compression mechanically expels a small volume of fluid. Late in gestation, the pulmonary epithelial cells actively secrete chloride ions, which creates a gradient maintaining adequate lung volume in utero. Before birth the lung epithelial cells change from being predominantly chloride secreting to being sodium absorbing, which draws fluid into the interstitial spaces. The sodium-pumping activity is increased in spontaneous labour; this may be related to the catecholamine surge.

A mature sucking pattern is evident from 36 weeks of gestation. Although fetal swallowing can be observed as early as 11 weeks' gestation, near term discrete episodes of swallowing occur, probably triggered by 'thirst', gastric emptying or changed composition of amniotic fluid (Boyle 1992). This swallowing may be important for gut development and maturation. In labour there is some evidence that swallowing increases. Meconium passage is rare until about 38 weeks when the control of intestinal peristalsis is more mature. Early meconium passage is associated with listeriosis. Meconium-stained amniotic fluid occurs in about a third of pregnancies beyond 42 weeks. Hypoxia induces vasoconstriction of the fetal gut, hyperperistalsis and anal sphincter relaxation so passage of meconium has been associated with fetal distress (Houlihan & Knuppel 1994). However, it has been argued that meconium-stained fluid could reflect normal maturity of the fetal gut function (Katz &

Bowes 1992). Less than 2% of babies born with meconium-stained fluid go on to develop severe meconium aspiration syndrome. It has been suggested that the primary cause of this syndrome is pulmonary epithelial damage or airway obstruction, which results in ineffectual clearance of meconium. The residual meconium can interfere with surfactant dispersal and increase the severity of the respiratory problems.

## The fetal skull and fetal presentation

The dimensions of the fetal head correlate well with those of the maternal pelvis. Examination of the shape of the baby's head soon after delivery shows how it passed through the pelvis (Fig. 13.18). The bones of the fetal skull are relatively mobile and mould under compression during labour. The sutures and fontanelles (Fig. 13.19) allow the skull bones to overlap partially so the dimensions of the presenting part can be reduced by about 0.5–1 cm. Diameters that are not compressed elongate to compensate for those that are reduced. If the pressure generated against the cervix impedes the circulation in the scalp then oedema may occur forming a caput or swelling. The area of the caput and the degree of moulding indicate the degree of head compression endured in labour. The caput is usually absorbed within a few days of delivery and requires no treatment. If the head is compressed in an abnormal diameter, or if the moulding is too excessive or rapid, the dura mater forming the falx cerebri may be pulled from the tentorium cerebellum resulting in rupture of the venous sinuses and intercranial haemorrhage (Fig. 13.20).

The position of the fetus (see Box 13.2, p. 282, for an explanation of terms) is determined on abdominal examination in later pregnancy and early labour (Fig. 13.21). The midwife can gently palpate the pregnant woman's abdomen to determine how the fetus is lying and how the presenting part of the fetus relates to the pelvis. The degree of engagement of the fetal head into the brim of the pelvis can also be ascertained. Auscultation of the fetal heart confirms the initial findings. The lie of the fetus describes the relative position of the long axis of the fetus to the long axis of the uterus. Usually the lie is longitudinal, rather than oblique or transverse, particularly in the last weeks of pregnancy. The attitude is the degree of flexion of the fetus. In the fully flexed attitude, the fit of the fetus in the uterus is comfortable. The presentation describes the presenting part of the fetus. Cephalic presentation occurs in most pregnancies. The fetal position is described by the relationship of the denominator (the presenting part) to areas of the maternal pelvis. The pelvic areas are: left and right, anterior, lateral or posterior areas. The occiput (the bone at the back of the fetal skull) is the denominator of a cephalic position so the fetus could, for instance, be described to be in a right occipito-anterior position (ROA). Anterior positions are more common because the fetal spine is against the mother's abdominal wall. Occipito-posterior positions tend to result in the fetus assuming a deflexed attitude, which can result in less effective contraction, prolonged labour, uneven cervical dilatation, increased risk of trauma to the perineum and unfavourable compression of the fetal head.

## Pain in labour

Many women experience severe pain in labour. Pain is a complex and personal phenomenon. Although it is easier to understand the neurophysiological aspects of tissue damage, the experience of pain is always subjective and is related to psychological state and past experience. Pain can be defined as a sensation evoked by tissue damage that stimulates the activity of specific receptors transmiting information to pain centres in the brain. Although pain can often be considered to be part of a protective mechanism against tissue damage there are some exceptions. For instance, pain associated with radiation (as in sunburn) or tumour growth tends to occur well after the tissue damage has occurred so it does not function as a warning. Chronic pain associated with degenerative diseases, such as arthritis, also cannot be regarded as a protective reflex. In labour, some aspects of pain experienced can be protective, such as the pain due to stretching of the soft tissue as the baby's head is crowned, which causes the woman to gasp.

The perception of pain depends on a number of physiological factors. The location and intensity of the stimuli affect the quality and severity of the perceived pain; generally, the higher the intensity of the stimuli, the greater is the pain experienced. However, psychological and cultural factors are important in the perception of pain (Box 13.5). Mood and personality type are important; generally, anxious or tired people are less able to tolerate pain but emotional arousal limits pain perception. In certain primitive cultures, the father has the 'labour pains' and the mother quietly gives birth.

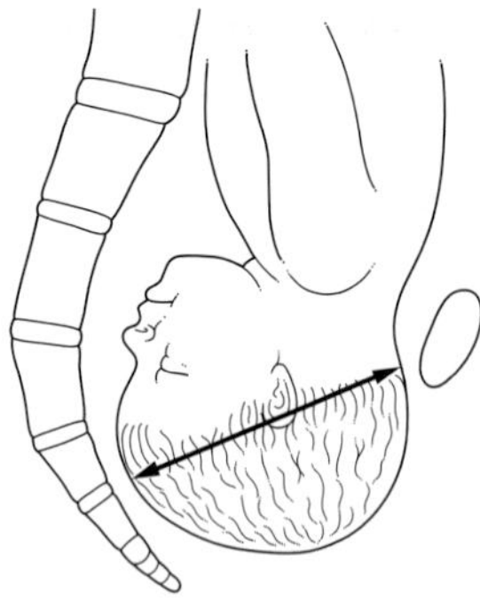

Suboccipitobregmatic 9.5 cm
vertex presentation

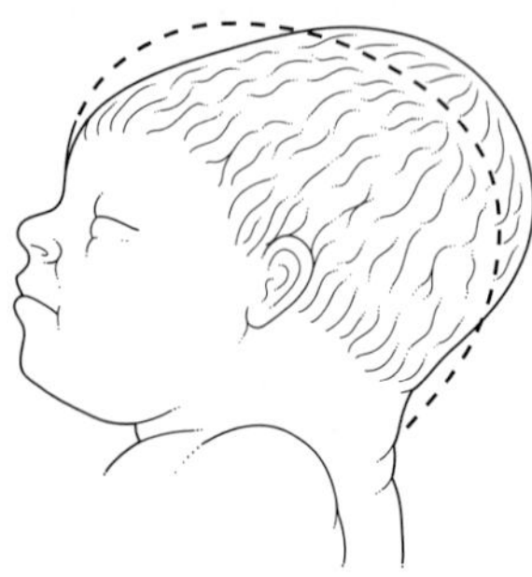

Occipito-anterior position

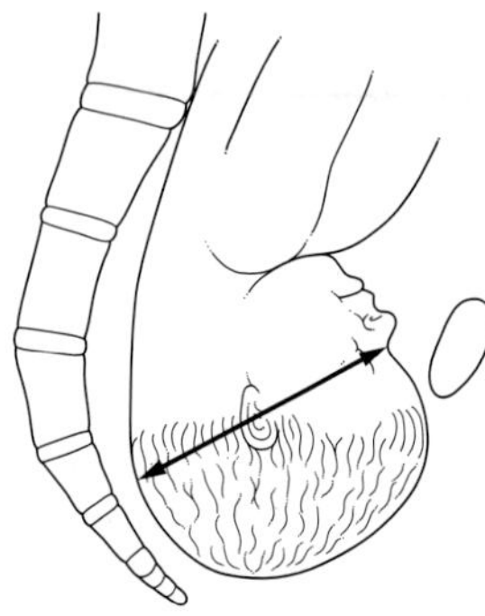

Occipitofrontal 11.5 cm persistent
occipitoposterior position

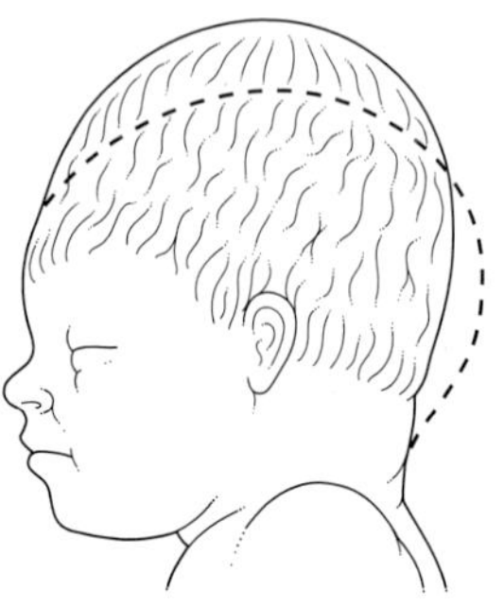

Persistent occipito-posterior position

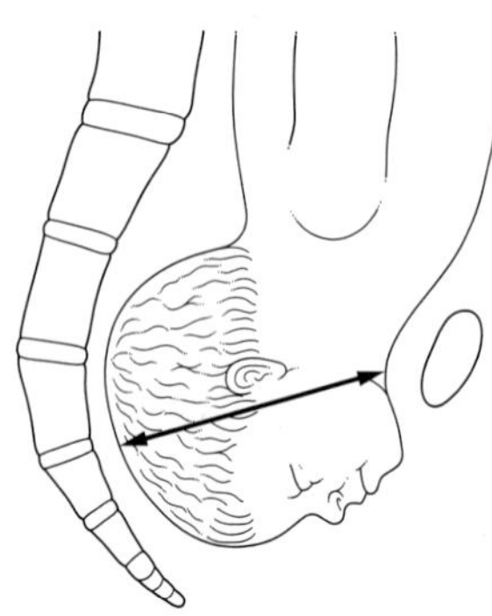

Submentobregmatic 9.5 cm
face presentation

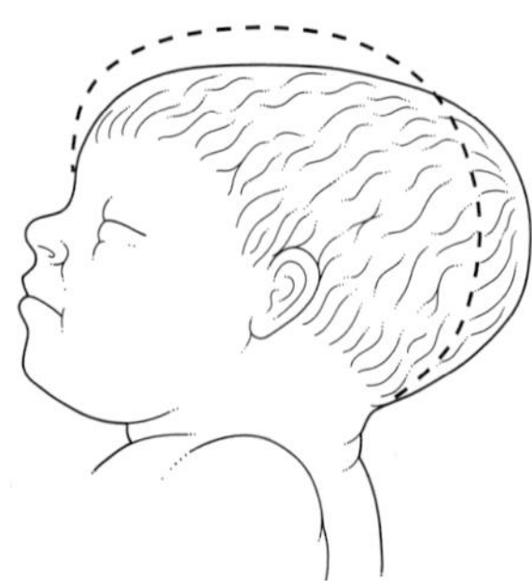

Face presentation

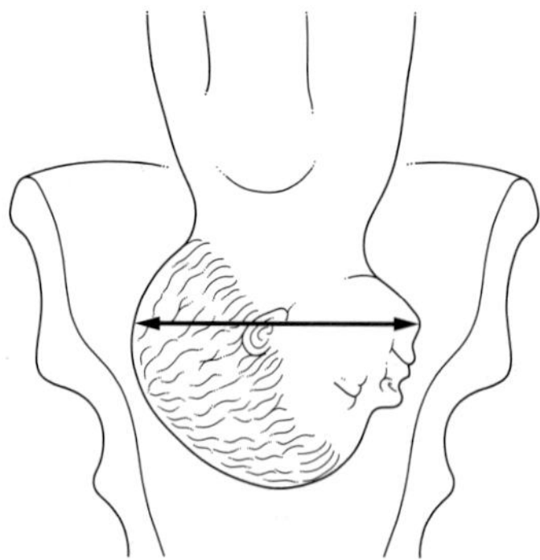

Mentovertical 13.5 cm
brow presentation

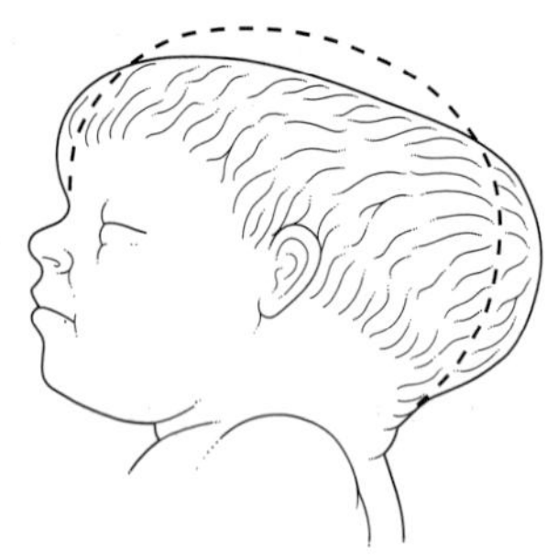

Brow presentation

**Fig. 13.18** *The relationship between the shape of the baby's head and the moulding of the fetal skull.*

**Fig. 13.19** *Sutures and fontanelles of the fetal skull.*

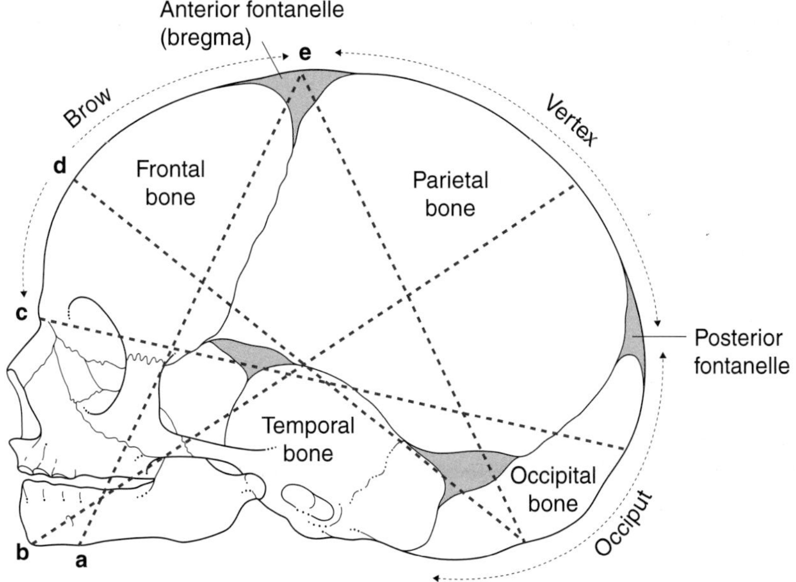


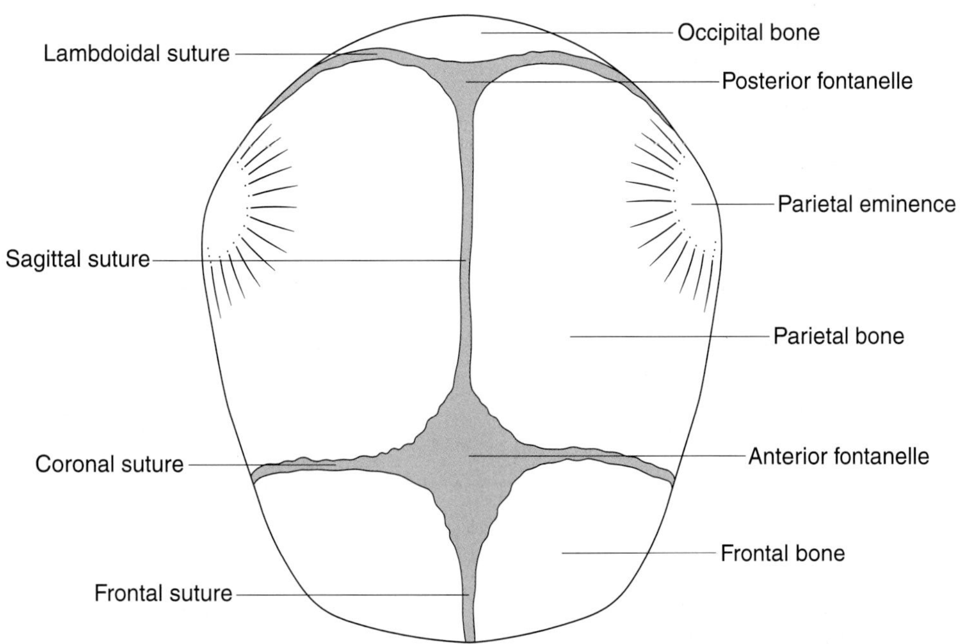

**Fig. 13.20** *Coronal section through the fetal head to show intracranial membranes and venous sinuses. (Reproduced with permission from Bennett & Brown 1999.)*

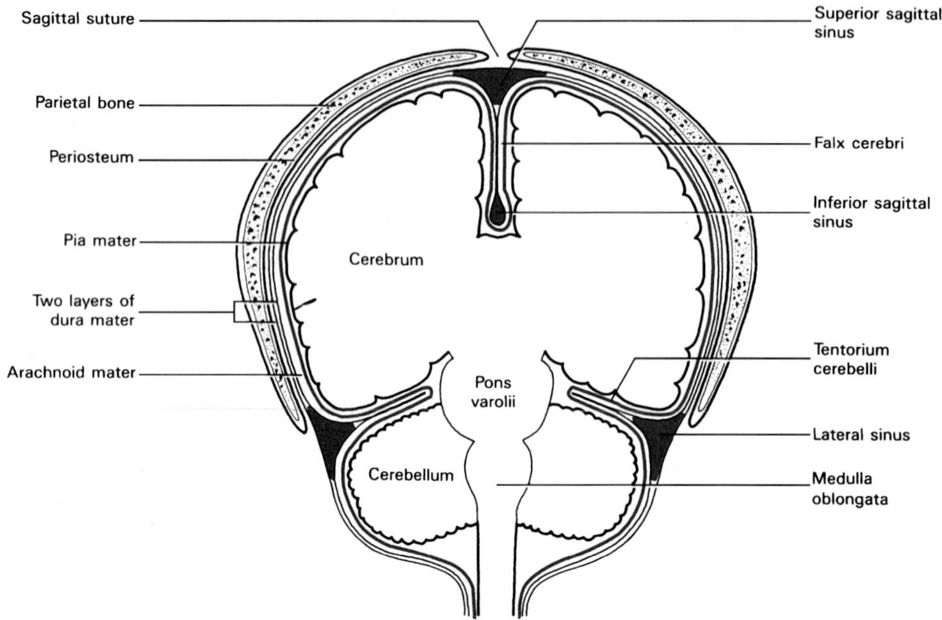


**Fig. 13.21** *A Attitude and B presentation of the fetus. (Reproduced with permission from Sweet & Tiran 1996.)*

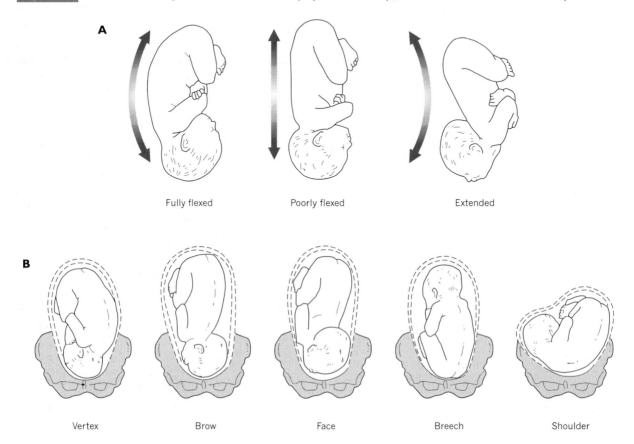

A

Fully flexed Poorly flexed Extended

B

Vertex Brow Face Breech Shoulder

**Box 13.5**

**Factors affecting pain perception**

- Anatomy
- Physiology
- Psychology
- Sociology
- Culture
- Cognition
- Learning

## Pain receptors

Pain or nociceptive receptors respond to stimuli that cause tissue damage. They are specific, responding to chemical mediators of tissue damage, such as plasmakinins, acetylcholine, histamine and substance P. Pain receptors are distributed unevenly with a higher density in skin, dental pulp, some internal organs, periosteum, meninges, arterial walls and joint surfaces. Pain receptors are free nerve endings that form part of small afferent myelinated Aδ fibres and larger (but unmyelinated) C fibres (Table 13.4). There is controversy over the pain being caused by overstimulation of other receptor types such as those that respond to temperature and pressure (Box 13.6).

**Box 13.6**

**Pain receptors**

*Large*

- Aα (Ia and b) (myelinated)—position proprioception, touch, pressure, vibration
- Aβ (II) (myelinated)—fine discriminative touch, pressure, vibration
- Aγ (myelinated)—burning sensation

*Small*

- Aδ (III) (myelinated)—well localizable sharp pain, temperature
- C (IV) (unmyelinated)—dull aching pain, temperature

## Pain transmission

Transmission of pain depends on the type of fibre in which the nerve ending triggers the impulse. In general the speed of transmission is faster in larger fibres and those that are myelinated (see Ch. 1). Sharp stabbing sensations are thought to be conducted by Aδ fibres and dull aching or burning pain by the slower unmyelinated C fibres. Myelinated fibres are more sensitive to ischaemia. Small unmyelinated fibres are more susceptible to local anaesthetics such as procaine, which is effective at blocking aching pain.

The nerve fibres enter the spinal cord and terminate in the grey matter of the dorsal horn (Fig. 13.22). Aδ fibres have a relatively direct route of transmission, synapsing with neurons in the dorsal horn to the brain-stem and via the spinothalamic tract to the thalamus and cerebral cortex. Therefore the pain is perceived as sharp and is easy to localize. The unmyelinated C fibres synapse in the grey matter of the spinal cord as well but are routed through the spinoreticular tract and reticular formation to the thalamus and cortex. Within the reticular formation, a number of physiological processes take place, stimulating the nervous system and affecting electrical activity in the brain, wakefulness and attention. The state of excitement that is generated means the pain is difficult to localize and produces unpleasant symptoms. The limbic system (which includes the hypothalamus and the amygdala) at the base of the brain is stimulated, which affects emotional responses such as fear, anger, pleasure and satisfaction. The thalamus integrates the sensation of pain and relays the information that tissue damage has occurred. The somatosensory cortex discriminates and identifies the precise position of the tissue damage and the parietal cortex is involved in interpreting the information and relating the learned meaningfulness to past experience.

**Table 13.4** *Fast and slow pain receptors*

| Fast pain | Slow pain |
|---|---|
| Bright, sharp, localized sensation | Dull, intense, diffuse unpleasant feeling |
| Aδ | C fibres |
| 2–5 μm diameter | 0.4–1.2 μm diameter |
| Myelinated | Non-myelinated |
| Conduct at 12–30 m/s | Conduct at 0.5–2 m/s |
| Terminate on neurons in laminars 1 and V | Terminate on neurons in laminars I and II |
| Spinothalamic tract | Spinorecticular tract |
| Somatic pain | Visceral pain |

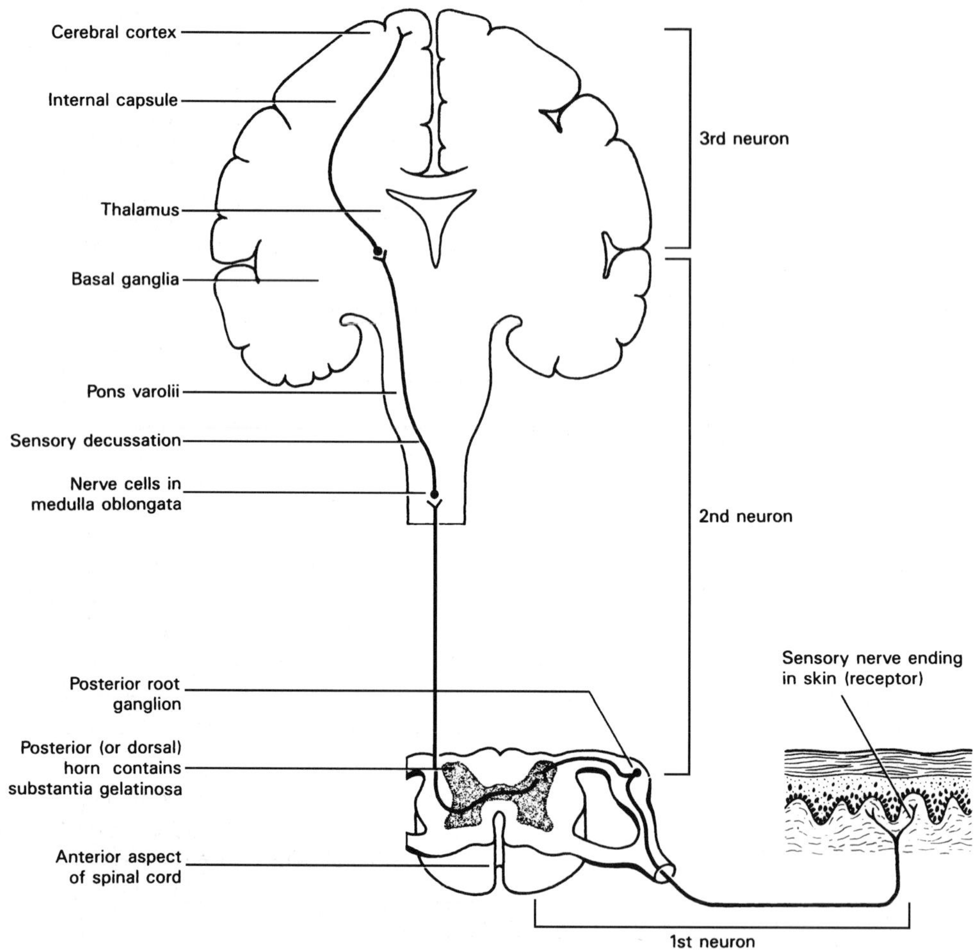


**Fig. 13.22** *Pathways of pain transmission. (Reproduced with permission from Bennett & Brown 1999.)*

## The gate control theory

There is a relationship between the pain receptors and the touch receptors at the level of the spinal cord. The pain gate control theory, proposed by Melzack & Wall in 1965, suggests interneurons in the substantia gelatinosa of the dorsal horn of the spinal cord can regulate the conduction of the ascending afferent nerve (Fig. 13.23). So input from the large-diameter myelinated fibres from the touch receptors can inhibit the impulses on the smaller-diameter fibres from the pain receptors, acting as a gate. This means that touch, like massage, can inhibit transmission from the pain receptor unless activity along the smaller fibres markedly increases. Descending fibres from the brain can also modify transmission of pain signals, thus 'opening' or 'closing' the gate. This explains the relationship between psychological factors and pain perception. If a labouring woman is feeling relaxed and confident, the descending inhibition is high so less pain is perceived. If she becomes tired or anxious, the descending inhibition is reduced. Transcutaneous electrical nerve stimulation (TENS) acts both to stimulate the large-diameter touch afferent nerves and possibly to stimulate powerful descending inhibitory pathways.

## Pain from muscle contractions

Both visceral pain from the uterus and somatic pain from trauma to the soft tissues of the birth canal are experienced in labour. Visceral pain tends to predominate in the first stage of labour when the uterus is contracting and the cervix is dilating. Rhythmic muscle contraction in the presence of an adequate blood flow does not usually cause pain. In labour, uterine contractions compress blood vessels and reduce flow; the ischaemic pain persists until the flow is restored. It is

**Fig. 13.23** *The gate control theory of pain.*

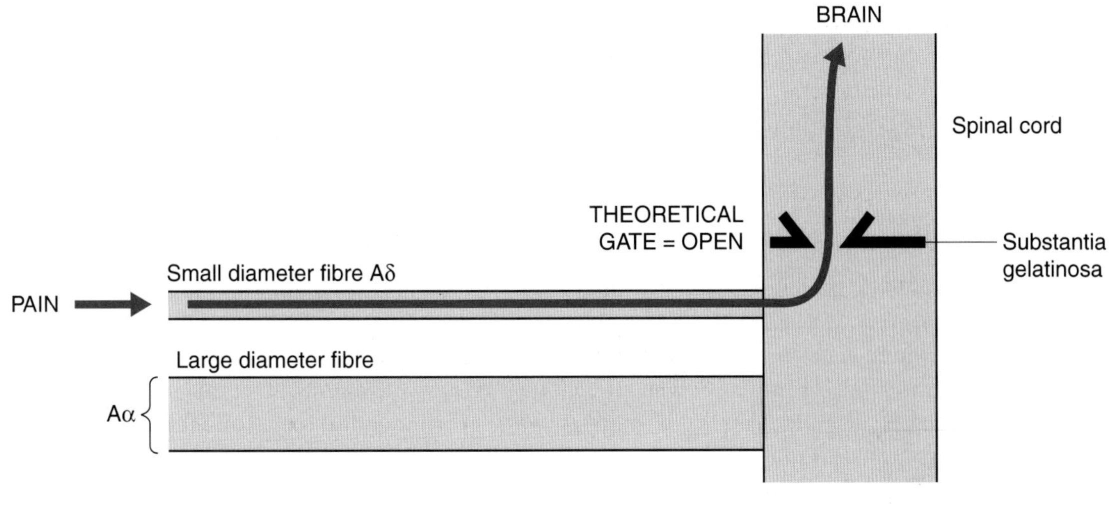


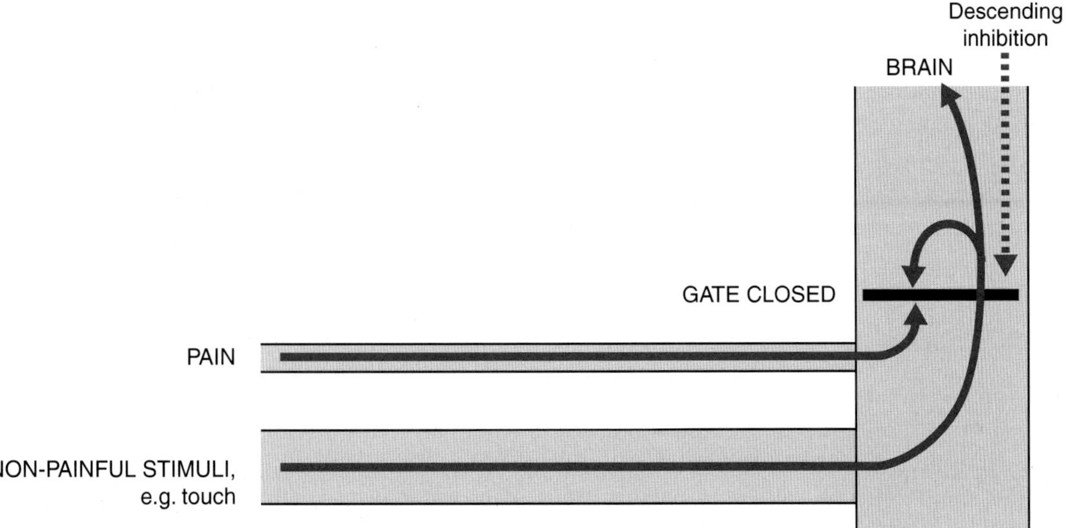


hypothesized that a chemical mediator reaches critical levels when flow is limited and stimulates the pain receptors. When flow is restored, the chemical mediator is diluted or metabolized. This is similar to exertion causing myocardial ischaemia and angina pain, which is relieved by rest and decreased myocardial oxygen requirements. Initially pain is transmitted by the afferent fibres entering the spinal cord at T11 and T12, spreading to T10 and L1.

## Referred pain

In referred pain, damage from one part of the body is experienced as though it had occurred in another part of the body. The pain fibres from the damaged area enter the spinal cord at the same level as the afferent nerves from the referred area. Usually the pain is referred to another tissue or structure that developed from the same embryonic structure or dermatome in which the pain originates. So, for instance, development of the diaphragm begins in the neck but, as the lungs develop, the diaphragm and the phrenic nerve migrate towards the abdomen. The afferent fibres in the phrenic nerve enter the spinal cord with the afferent fibres from the tip of the shoulder. Irritation of the diaphragm is therefore referred as a pain in the shoulder. However, previous experience is important in referred pain. Pain from the abdominal viscera includes the uterus is usually referred to the midline. But in patients who have experienced abdominal surgery, such as a caesarean section, the pain is referred to the scar site. Pain during this stage arising from the uterus and cervix may be referred. A labouring woman may experience pain over her abdominal wall, between the naval and pubic bone, radiating down her thighs and in the lumbar and sacral regions.

## Somatic pain

Somatic pain caused by the presenting part impinging on the birth canal, vulva and perineum tends to occur in the second stage of labour. Pain is transmitted by the pudendal nerves S2, S3 and S4. The conscious sensation of pain is accompanied by a number of physiological responses including increased ventilation and cardiac output, inhibition of gastrointestinal function, increased oxygen demand and metabolic rate and increased catecholamine release. The increased catecholamine release may detrimentally affect placental perfusion and uterine contractions. Non-pharmacological methods of pain relief, such as imagery, relaxation techniques and provision of information about the progress of labour, probably decrease anxiety and stress and responses mediated by the sympathetic nervous system.

## Endogenous opiates

The endogenous opiates are of particular interest in pain perceived in labour. These include β-endorphin, enkephalins and dynorphin, which are analgesic peptides. They bind to the presynaptic receptors on the neuron membrane and block pain transmission. Enkephalins comprise two short peptide chains (consisting of five amino acids) that are very unstable and have a half-life of less than a minute. Enkephalins are fragments of β-endorphin, which is more stable and also binds to opiate receptors; β-endorphin is a fragment of the pituitary hormone β-lipotrophin. Beta lipotrophin and ACTH are both derived from the same precursor.

Endogenous opiates inhibit prostaglandin synthesis. Prostaglandins are possible chemical mediators of pain. They also inhibit actions of a number of other pain transmitters. Beta endorphin levels increase throughout pregnancy, peaking at delivery, and may be further stimulated by the stress of labour. It is suggested that it is this high level of endogenous opiates that allows women to tolerate surprisingly high levels of pain during delivery; this phenomenon is known as 'pregnancy-induced analgesia'. Acupuncture may increase enkephalin activity. Placebo responses where pain relief occurs as a result of expectation of pain relief rather than because of being given an analgesic may be due to release of endogenous opiates and genuine analgesia.

## Pain relief

Pain relief in labour needs to work rapidly and effectively relieve the pain without slowing down the course of labour. It needs to be safe for the mother and fetus and not adversely affect the neonate. There is no ideal analgesic (Table 13.5); all have some side-effects but pain also can adversely affect the fetus. Maternal analgesia can alter the balance of factors promoting uterine contraction and can potentially result in increased effects of oxytocin, promoting tetanic uterine contractions, decreasing oxygen delivery and causing transient fetal bradycardia (Eberle & Norris 1996). There are three main mechanisms of pain relief blocking the pain receptors, the propagation of the action potential or the perception of pain within the CNS. Mild analgesics

**Table 13.5** ***Types of analgesics***

| Pain relief | Example | Mechanism | Disadvantages/advantages |
|---|---|---|---|
| Opioids | Pethidine | Depression of CNS | Nausea, vomiting, sedation; potentiate effect of epidural |
| Paracervical block | Spinal | Action potentials blocked from nerves | Risk of fetal injection; could provide surgical anaesthesia |
| Epidural | Bolus, intermittent or continuous infusion | Inhibition of neurotransmission across synapses | Maternal hypotension, motor blockade |

block at the pain receptor level. The sensitivity of the pain receptors is increased by prostaglandins. Drugs which inhibit prostaglandin synthesis, such as aspirin, decrease levels of prostaglandins both at the receptor and where prostaglandins are involved in pain transmission higher in the pathway.

### Local anaesthetics

Local anaesthetics prevent the propagation of action potentials by blocking the sodium channels. They are particularly effective in blocking pain carried by the C fibres, possibly because unmyelinated fibres allow easier penetration. For instance, lignocaine injected into the perineum is effective at blocking the pain of episiotomy.

### Centrally acting opiates

Centrally acting opiates or narcotics, such as morphine and pethidine, block nerve transmission in the brain and spinal cord and decrease pain perception. There are also opiate-binding sites in the substantia gelatinosa of the dorsal horn of the spinal cord, which affect the release of neurotransmitters. Opiates increase the activity of the descending inhibitory pathways from the brain-stem and act on the limbic system to elevate mood. Opiates have other physiological effects such as depressing the medullary respiratory centre, causing nausea and vomiting, sedating and affecting the heart rate.

## Position in labour

Certain positions have advantages in optimizing uterine efficiency or increasing maternal comfort (Blackburn & Loper 1992). The lithotomy position and lying supine are probably advantageous only to those assisting at the delivery, unless medical intervention/delivery is required. Fetal monitoring and a number of procedures can usually be adapted to a variety of maternal positions. There seems to be no physiological advantage in lying supine. Fetal alignment, pelvic diameter and efficiency of contractions are not optimal. Contractions are more frequent but less intense so labour is prolonged and drug use seems to be increased. Many women appear to choose a supine position because they are presented with a bed and have no alternative option.

A lateral recumbent position reduces obstructive pressure on maternal blood vessels so venous return and cardiac output are optimal for uterine perfusion and fetal oxygenation. Uterine contractions are more intense but less frequent and have increased efficiency. In an upright position, the abdominal wall relaxes and the effect of gravity will augment the effect of the fetal head pressing on the cervix and the subsequent feedback to the myometrial activity. Both frequency and intensity of contractions are increased so uterine activity is enhanced and labour tends to be shorter. Squatting increases maternal pelvic diameter, enhances engagement and the descent of the fetal head.

During bearing down, in the second stage of labour, directed pushing with a Valsalva manoeuvre against a closed glottis increases sympathetic discharge and catecholamine release. Minimal straining with an open glottis has lesser negative effects on maternal blood pressure, maternal and fetal oxygenation levels and is associated with reduced need for episiotomy.

## Key points

- Parturition in humans is poorly understood: animal studies offer limited insight into the process owing to the evolution of species-specific differences.
- Parturition is a continuous process: the defining of the various stages of labour enables clinical judgement of progress and thus intervention under the biomedical model of care.
- The fundal region of the uterus has the highest density of smooth muscle so it is responsible for the strong expelling contractions of the uterus during labour.
- Human cervical structure is complex owing to the upright stance causing an increased gravitational force as the contents of the uterus increase in mass. Structural changes within the cervix have to occur before dilatation can be achieved by uterine contractions.
- Coordinated effective contractions are facilitated by the development of gap junctions between the myometrial cells.
- The first stage of labour is measured from the onset of strong and regular effective contractions to full effacement and dilation of the cervix.
- The second stage of labour is characterized by strong expulsive contractions, aided by respiratory muscle involvement, until the fetus is delivered.
- The passage of the fetus through the pelvis is described as the mechanism of labour and is achieved through the contractions forcing the presenting part to rotate against the muscle tone, structural resistance and shape of the pelvic floor.
- The third stage of labour covers the delivery of the placenta and fetal membranes and staunching of maternal blood loss.
- Maternal blood loss immediately following separation of the placenta is limited by the myometrial fibres contracting, thus occluding the uterine vessels.
- The onset of labour is poorly understood; a fetal signal probably alters the ratio of progesterone and oestrogen and other factors, such as prostaglandin secretion and oxytocin receptor expression, are involved in the amplification of the signal.
- The evolution of bipedal locomotion and increasing cephalization have influenced parturition in humans so the presenting part has to negotiate, by rotational manoeuvres, rather than just pass through the pelvic girdle.
- The process of labour induces many changes within the fetus in preparation for extrauterine existence, which are mediated by increasing hypoxia and catecholamine production.
- Pain in labour has a complex aetiology; there are visceral and somatic components further complicated by psychological and social factors.

### Application to practice

Midwives need to understand the physiological interactions and external factors that can affect human parturition in order to underpin intrapartum care.

The development of observational skills allows the midwife not only to interpret how a woman may be coping with labour, but also to determine how the labour is progressing from observing behaviour and physical responses of the labouring woman. By ignoring, not noticing or misunderstanding certain physical cues, the midwife may inadvertently provide sub-optimal support.

Intervention in labour must be justified and decisions surrounding this must be underpinned to maximize maternal and fetal well-being. Knowledge of the effects of intervention upon fetal and maternal physiology is essential so that the midwife can judge the effectiveness and quickly identify possible adverse outcomes of such interventions.

## Annotated further reading

Blackburn S T, Loper D L 1992 Maternal, fetal and neonatal physiology: a clinical perspective. WB Saunders, Philadelphia
*An in-depth description of physiological adaptation to pregnancy and consequent development of the fetus and neonate that draws from physiological research studies. The chapters are clearly organized by physiological systems and link physiological concepts to clinical applications including the assessment and management of low- and high-risk pregnancies.*

Gee H, Glynn M 1997 The physiology and clinical management of labour. In: Henderson C, Jones K (eds) Essential midwifery. C V Mosby, St Louis, pp 171–202
*This chapter provides a useful overview to midwifery management of labour in relation to the physiological processes and their progression.*

Greer I A 1995 The physiology and biochemistry of labour. In: Chamberlain G (Ed) Turnbull's obstetrics, 2nd edn. Churchill Livingstone, New York, pp 551–567
*An in-depth exploration of the factors that may contribute to the onset and regulation of human parturition including interventions to inhibit preterm labour and induce labour at term.*

Liggins G C 1994 Mechanism of the onset of labour: the New Zealand perspective. Australian and New Zealand Journal of Obstetrics and Gynaecology 34:338–342
*A comprehensive and thoughtful review of the factors involved in the onset of parturition by one of the leaders in this field.*

Lopez Bernal A 1996 Parturition. In: Hillier S G, Kitchener H C, Neilson J P (eds) Scientific essentials of reproductive medicine. W B Saunders, Philadelphia, pp 364–375
*A good summary of factors which influence parturition in the human, their likely mechanisms and how these can be combined to create a model of physiological control of labour.*

Mander R 1997 The control of labour pain. In: Henderson C, Jones K (eds) Essential midwifery. CV Mosby, St Louis, pp 203–218
*Looks at pain pathways, management of pain and the interventions used at delivery to achieve pain relief.*

Morrison J 1996 Prediction and prevention of preterm labour. In: Studd J (ed) Progress in obstetrics and gynaecology, vol 12. Churchill Livingstone, New York, pp 67–85
*Examines the possible causes of preterm labour and the effectiveness and limitations of the obstetric interventions used in its management.*

Steer P J, Johnson M R 1998 The genital system. In: Chamberlain G, Broughton Pipkin F (eds) Clinical physiology in obstetrics, 3rd edn. Blackwell, Oxford, pp 308–355
*A comprehensive chapter describing the anatomy and physiology of the uterus and cervix. It includes changes in pregnancy and prior to labour, interaction of the placenta and uterus, factors influencing the onset of labour, and the involution of the uterus.*

Summers L 1997 Methods of inducing cervical ripening and labor induction. Journal of Nurse-Midwifery 42:71–85
*A succinct description of the rationale and practical aspects of the methods used for inducing labour.*

## References


Aitken M A, Rice G E, Brennecke S P 1990 Gestational tissue phospholipase $A_2$ messenger RNA content and the onset of spontaneous labour in the human. Reproduction Fertility and Development 2:575–580

Anderson A B M, Turnbull A C 1969 Relationship between length of gestation and cervical dilatation, uterine contractility and other factors during pregnancy. American Journal of Obstetrics and Gynecology 105:1207

Apostolakis E M, Rice K E, Longo L D, Seron-Ferre M, Yellon S M 1993 Time of day of birth and absence of endocrine and uterine contractile activity rhythms in sheep. American Journal of Physiology 264:E534–E540

Baker C 1996 Nutrition and hydration in labour. British Journal of Midwifery 4:568–572

Bani D 1997 Relaxin: a pleiotropic hormone. General Pharmacology 28:13–22

Barret J F R, Savage J, Phillips K, Liford R J 1992 Randomised trial of amniotomy in labour versus the intention to leave membranes intact until the second stage. British Journal of Obstetrics and Gynaecology 99:5

Bennett V R, Brown L K 1999 Myles' textbook for midwives, 13th edn. Churchill Livingstone, Edinburgh, pp 393, 396, 431, 451, 468, 473, 509, 993

Bernal A L, Europe-Finner G N, Phaneuf S, Watson S P 1995 Preterm labour—a pharmacological challenge. Trends in Pharmacological Science 16:129–133

Beyer E C, Kistler J, Paul D L, Goodenough D A 1989 Antisera directed against connexin 43 peptides react with a 43-kD protein localised to gap junctions in myocardium and other tissues. Journal of Cell Biology 108:595–605

Blackburn S T, Loper D L 1992 Maternal, fetal and neonatal physiology: a clinical perspective. W B Saunders, Philadelphia

Boyle J T 1992 Motility of the upper gastrointestinal tract in the fetus and neonate. In: Polin R A, Fox W W (eds) Fetal and neonatal physiology, vol 2. W B Saunders, Philadelphia, pp 1028–1032

Carp H, Jayaram A, Stoll M 1992 Ultrasound examination of the stomach contents of parturients. Anesthesia and Analgesia 74:683–687

Chamberlain G, Dewhurst J, Harvey D 1991 Ilustrated textbook of obstetrics. Gower Medical (Mosby), London, p 115

Cox S M, Casey M L, MacDonald P C 1997 Accumulation of interleukin-1 beta and interleukin-6 in amniotic fluid: a sequela of labour at term and preterm. Human Reproduction Update 3:517–527

Darne J, McGarrigle H H G, Lachelin G C L 1987 Saliva oestriol, oestradiol, oestrone and progesterone levels in pregnancy; spontaneous labour at term is preceded by a rise in saliva oestriol:progesterone ratio. British Journal of Obstetrics and Gynaecology 94:227–235

Dawes G S 1984 The control of fetal breathing and skeletal muscle movements. Journal of Physiology (London) 346:1–18

Douglas M J 1988 Commentary: the case against a more liberal food and fluid policy in labor. Birth 15:93

Dray F, Frydman R 1976 Primary prostaglandins in amniotic fluid in pregnancy and spontaneous labour. American Journal of Obstetrics and Gynecology 126:13

Duff P 1996 Premature rupture of the membranes in term patients. Seminars in Perinatology 20:401–408

Eberle R L, Norris M C 1996 Labor analgesia: a risk-benefit analysis. Drug Safety 14: 239–251

Fencl M D, Stillman R J, Cohen J, Tulchinsky D 1980 Direct evidence of sudden rise in fetal corticoids late in human gestation. Nature 287:225–226

Foulkes J, Dumoulin J G 1983 Ketosis in labour. British Journal of Hospital Medicine 6: 562–564

Fuchs A R, Fuchs F, Husslein P, Soloff M S 1984 Oxytocin receptors in the human uterus during pregnancy and parturition. American Journal of Obstetrics and Gynecology 150:734–741

Fuchs A R, Romero R, Keefe D, Parra M, Oyarzun E, Behnke E 1991 Oxytocin secretion and human parturition: pulse frequency and duration increase during spontaneous labour in women. American Journal of Obstetrics and Gynecology 165:1515–1522

Gee H, Olah K S 1993 Failure to progress in labour. Progress in Obstetrics and Gynaecology 10:159–181

Germain A M, Valenzuela G J, Ivankovic M, Ducsay C A, Gabella C, Seron-Ferre M 1993 Relationship of circadian rhythms of uterine activity with term and preterm delivery. American Journal of Obstetrics and Gynecology 168:1271–1277

Gustavii B 1975 The distribution within the placenta, myometrium, and decidua of $^{24}$Na-labelled hypertonic saline solution following intra-amniotic or extra-amniotic injection. British Journal of Obstetrics and Gynaecology 82(9):734–739

Gustavii B 1977 Human decidua and uterine contractility. Ciba Foundation Symposium (47):343–358

Hampson V, Lui D, Billett E, Kirk S 1997 Amniotic membrane collagen content and type distribution in women with preterm premature rupture of the membranes in pregnancy. British Journal of Obstetrics and Gynaecology 104:1087–1091

Hatherway W E, Bonnar J 1987 Haemostatic disorders of the pregnant woman and newborn infant. Elsevier, New York

Honnebier M B O M, Nathanielsz P W 1994 Primate parturition and the role of the maternal circadian system. European Journal of Obstetrics, Gynecology and Reproductive Biology 55:193–203

Honnebier W J, Jobsis A C, Swaab D F 1974 The effect of hypophysial hormones and human chorionic gonadotrophin (HCG) on the anencephalic fetal adrenal cortex and on parturition in the human. Journal of Obstetrics and Gynaecology of the British Commonwealth 81(6):423–438

Houlihan C M, Knuppel R A 1994 Meconium-stained amniotic fluid: current controversies. Journal of Reproductive Medicine 39(11):888–898

Husslein P 1985 Pregnancy and plasma oxytocin levels. Journal of Perinatal Medicine 13:314–315

Kanayama N, Terao T 1991 The relationship between granulocyte elastase-like activity of cervical mucus and cervical maturation. Acta Obstetrica et Gynecologia Scandinavica 70:29

Karalis K, Goodwin G, Majzoub J A 1996 Cortisol blockade of progesterone: a possible mechanism involved in the initiation of labour. Nature Medicine 2:556–560

Katz V, Bowes W A 1992 Meconium aspiration syndrome: reflections on a murky subject. American Journal of Obstetrics and Gynecology 166(1 pt 1):171–183

Langercrantz H, Slotkin T 1986 The stress of being born. Scientific American 254:100–107

Liggins G C, Kennedy P C, Holm L W 1967 Failure of initiation of parturition after electrocoagulation of the pituitary of the fetal lamb. American Journal of Obstetrics and Gynecology 98:1080–1086

Lopez Bernal A, Watson S P, Phaneuf S, Europe-Finner G N 1993 Biochemistry and physiology of preterm labour and delivery. Bailliere's Clinics in Obstetrics and Gynaecology 7:523–552

Ludka L M, Roberts C C 1993 Eating and drinking in labour. Journal of Nurse-Midwifery 38:199–207

MacKenzie L W, Garfield R E 1985 Hormonal control of gap junctions in the myometrium. American Journal of Physiology 248:C296–C308

Melzack R, Wall P D 1965 Pain mechanisms: a new theory. Science 150(699):971–979

Miller F D, Chibbar R, Mitchell B F 1993 Synthesis of oxytocin in amnion, chorion and decidua: a potential paracrine role for oxytocin in the onset of human parturition. Regulatory Peptides 45:247

Mitchell B F, Challis J R, Lukash L 1987 Progesterone synthesis by human amnion, chorion, and decidua at term. American Journal of Obstetrics and Gynecology 157(2):349–353

Mulder E J H, Boersma M, Meeuse M, Van der Wal M, Van De Weerd E, Visser G H A 1994 Patterns of breathing movements in the near-term fetus: relationship to behavioural states. Early Human Development 36:127–135

Nijhuis J G, Prechtl H F, Martin D B, Bots R S 1982 Are there behavioural states in the human fetus? Early Human Development 6:177–195

Norman J 1996 Nitric oxide and the myometrium. Pharmacology and Therapeutics 70:91–100

Oakey R E, Cawood M L, MacDonald M M 1974 Biochemical and clinical observations in a pregnancy with placental sulphatase and other enzyme deficiencies. Clinics in Endocrinology 3:131

Okazaki T, Casey M L, Okita J R, MacDonald P C, Johnston J M 1981 Initiation of human parturition XII: biosynthesis and metabolism of prostaglandins in human fetal membranes and uterine decidua. American Journal of Obstetrics and Gynecology 139:373–381

Olah K S 1994 Changes in cervical electromyographic activity and their correlation with cervical response to myometrial activity during labour. European Journal of Obstetrics, Gynecology and Reproductive Biology 3:157–150

Olah K S, Gee H, Brown J S 1993 Cervical contractions: the response of the cervix to oxytocic stimulation in the latent phase of labour. British Journal of Obstetrics and Gynaecology 100:635–640

Padbury J F, Agata Y, Ludlow J, Ikegami M 1987 Effect of fetal adrenalectomy on catecholamine release and physiologic adaptation at birth in sheep. Journal of Clinical Investigation 80:1096–1103

Petersen L K, Oxlund H, Uldberg N, Forman A 1991 In vitro analysis of muscular contractile ability and passive biomechanical properties of uterine cervical samples from non-pregnant women. Obstetrics and Gynaecology 77:772–776

Petraglia F, Benedetto C, Florio P et al 1995 Effect of corticotropin-releasing factor-binding protein on prostaglandin release from cultured maternal decidua and on contractile activity of human myometrium in-vitro. Journal of Clinical Endocrinology and Metabolism 80:3073–3076

Pinto R M, Fisch L, Schwarz R L, Montuori E 1964 Action of estriol 17β upon uterine contractility and the milk-ejecting effect in the pregnant woman. American Journal of Obstetrics and Gynecology 90:99

Riley S C, Challis J R G 1991 Corticotropin-releasing hormone production by the placenta and fetal membranes. Placenta 12:105–119

Robinson B G, Emanual R L, Frim D M, Majzoub J A 1988 Glucocorticoid stimulates expression of corticotropin-releasing hormone gene in human placenta. Proceedings of the National Academy of Sciences, USA 85:5244–5248

Rowe T F 1997 Acute gastric aspiration: prevention and treatment. Seminars in Perinatology 21:313–319

Schwarz B E, Milewich L, Johnston J M, Porter J M, MacDonald P C 1976 Initiation of human parturition V: progesterone binding substance in fetal membranes. Obstetrics and Gynecology 48:685–689

Scutton M, Lowy C, O'Sullivan G 1996 Eating in labour: an assessment of the risks and benefits. International Journal of Obstetric Anesthesia 5:214–215

Sharp D A 1997 Restriction of oral intake for women in labour. British Journal of Midwifery 5:408–412

Steer P J, Johnson M R 1998 The genital system. In: Chamberlain G, Broughton Pipkin F (eds) Clinical physiology in obstetrics, 3rd edn. Blackwell, Oxford, pp 308–355

Stewart D B 1984 The pelvis as a passageway I. evolution and adaptations. British Journal of Obstetrics and Gynaecology 91:611–617

Stjernholm Y, Sahlin L, Akerberg S et al 1996 Cervical ripening in humans: potential roles of estrogen, progesterone and insulin-like growth factor-I. American Journal of Obstetrics and Gynecology 174:1065–1071

Studd J, Duiagnan N 1972 Graphic records in labour. British Medical Journal 4(837):4

Sullivan J M, Ramanathan K B 1985 Management of medical problems in pregnancy: severe cardiac disease. New England Journal of Medicine 313:304–309

Sweet B, Tiran D 1996 Mayes' midwifery, 12th edn. Baillière Tindall, London p 31, 224, 225, 340, 358, 993

Symonds E M, Symonds I M 1997 Essential obstetrics and gynaecology, 3rd edn. Churchill Livingstone, Edinburgh, p 134

Thong K J, Baird D T 1992 Induction of abortion with mifepristone and misoprostol in early pregnancy. British Journal of Obstetrics and Gynaecology 99:1004–1007

Thorburn G D 1992 The placenta, PGE2 and parturition. Early Human Development 29:63–73

Uldbjerg N, Malstrom A 1991 The role of protcoglycans in cervical dilatation. Seminars in Perinatology 15:127–132

Warnes K E, Morris M J, Symonds M E et al 1998 Effects of increasing gestation, cortisol and maternal undernutrition on hypothalamic neuropeptide Y expression in the sheep fetus. Journal of Neuroendocrinology 10:51–57

Wilmsatt J, Myers D A, Myers T R, Nathanielsz P W 1995 Prostaglandin synthase activity of fetal sheep cotyledons at 122 days of gestation and term—expression of prostaglandin synthetic capacity in fetal cotyledonary tissue near labor is location-dependent. Biology of Reproduction 52:737–744

Wilson T, Liggins G C, Joe L 1989 Purification from cultured chorion of a phospholipase $A_2$ inhibitor active before but not after the onset of labour. American Journal of Obstetrics and Gynecology 160: 602–606

Wolfe C D A, Petruckevitch A, Quartero R et al 1990 The rate of rise of corticotropin releasing-factor and endogenous digoxin-like immunoreactivity in normal and abnormal pregnancy. British Journal of Obstetrics and Gynaecology 97:832–837

Wray S 1993 Uterine contraction and physiological mechanisms of modulation. American Journal of Physiology 264:C1–C18

# 14 The puerperium

**Learning objectives**

- To describe the physiological processes that achieve homeostasis in the early puerperium.
- To discuss the timing of the physiological changes in the puerperium.
- To understand the aetiology of the common problems experienced within the puerperium.
- To recognize signs of pathological conditions associated with the puerperium.

## Introduction

The puerperium has been traditionally defined as the 6-week period immediately following the birth of a baby and represents the period of time in which maternal physiology, particularly the reproductive system, returns to a near non-pregnant state. This probably stems from the tradition of 'churching', which was a religious ceremony where women were accepted back into the church after a period of 40 days during which they were considered unclean. With the rise of medical dominance, the end of the puerperium was marked by the postnatal examination of the woman by a doctor. This has structured the traditional descriptions of the puerperium as a period of maternal recovery, underpinned by the medicalization of pregnancy into a medical condition. It is the midwife's responsibility to maintain a careful watch on the physiological changes in the puerperium and to recognize signs of pathological conditions.

The puerperium is sometimes considered to be the 'Cinderella' of midwifery and obstetrics as the excitement of the birth is over and after delivery the effects of pregnancy on maternal physiology receive little emphasis. There is not very much research into the timing or mechanisms of the changes in the puerperium. However, the puerperal woman can be very vulnerable to physiological stress, which can become pathological. The midwife's role is to observe and monitor the early changes and to be able to differentiate between normal and abnormal changes.

During the puerperium, there is a marked decrease in the levels of oestrogen and progesterone within the maternal system. The fall in concentrations of steroid hormones facilitates the initiation of lactation (see Ch. 16) and allows the physiological systems to return to their prepregnant state. In reality, the puerperium should be described as a transitional phase. It begins at the birth of a child and it ends with the return of fertility. Women do not return to the same physiological and anatomical state, however. The puerperium also, within a social context, represents many transitions for the parents, child and other members of the family. Many of the physiological changes within the puerperium, such as the establishment of parenting skills, lactation and feeding, are modified by the past and present social interactions of the individuals within the new family situation.

# Physiological and structural changes

## Involution of the uterus

The puerperium begins as soon as the placenta and membranes are expelled from the uterus. Oxytocin released from the posterior pituitary gland induces strong intermittent myometrial contractions, and as the uterine cavity is empty the whole uterus contracts down fully and the uterine walls become realigned in apposition to each other. The myometrial spiral fibres that occlude the uterine blood vessels (see Ch. 13) restrict the blood supply to the placental site (Fig. 14.1). Uterine vascular resistance increases soon after delivery (Tekay & Jouppila 1993).

After about an hour after delivery, the myometrium relaxes slightly but further active bleeding is prevented by the activation of the blood-clotting mechanisms, which are altered greatly during pregnancy to facilitate a swift clotting response. Haemostasis is achieved in three ways:

- ischaemia
- pressure—apposition of the uterine walls forming the T-shaped cavity
- clotting mechanisms.

The midwife has the responsibility to inspect the placenta and membranes to assess that they are complete. If there is any doubt this may indicate that part of the placenta and membranes may have been left within the uterine cavity. Retained products may be the source of abnormal bleeding as they impede the contraction of the uterus. Retained products can also cause secondary postpartum haemorrhage (secondary PPH) as they become the focus of infection. Retained products are often spontaneously voided usually associated with the passing of a blood clot, which facilitates the cleansing of the uterine cavity.

Immediately after delivery the uterus weighs about 900–1000 g and the fundus is palpable about 11–12 cm above the symphysis pubis (Howie 1995). The placental site is raw and exposed. The uterus is continuous with the vagina with the cervix draping from the body of the uterus. Uterine involution is rapid so 50% of the total mass of the tissue is lost within a week (Howie 1995). There are rapid and

**Fig. 14.1** ***A Myometrial spiral fibres around uterine blood vessels; B occlusion of blood supply to the placental site. (Reproduced with permission from Sweet & Tiran 1996.)***

A

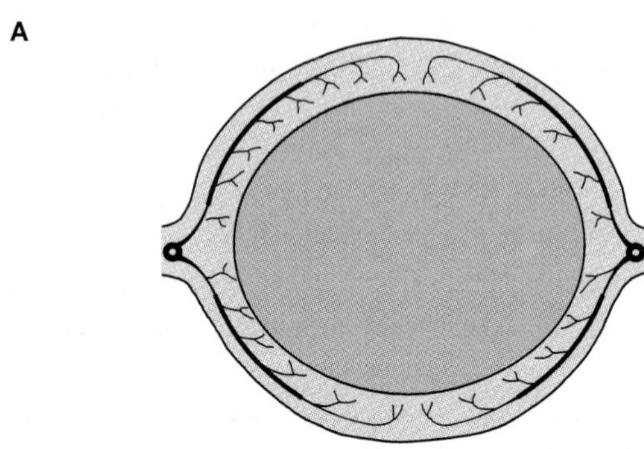

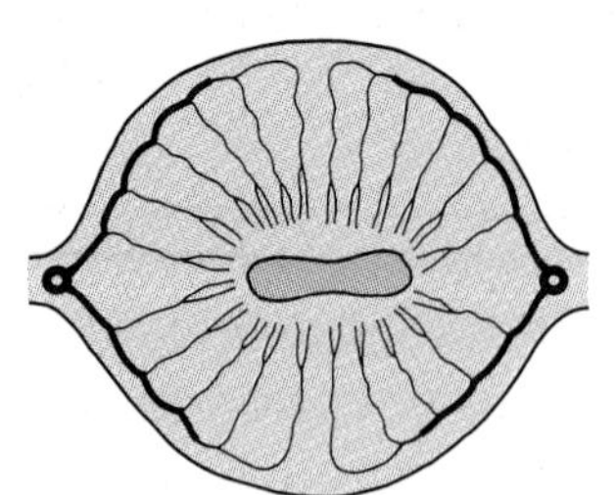

B

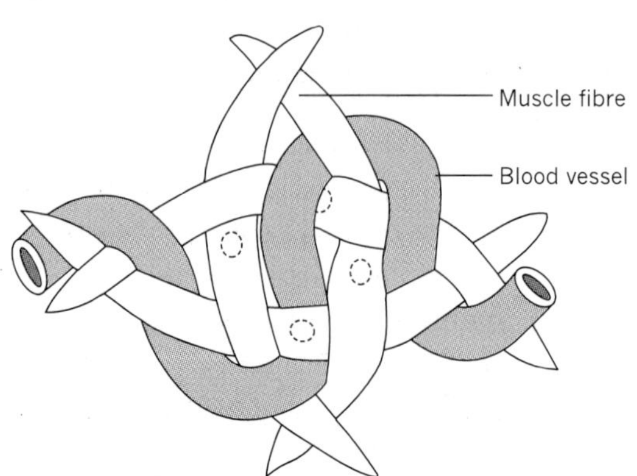


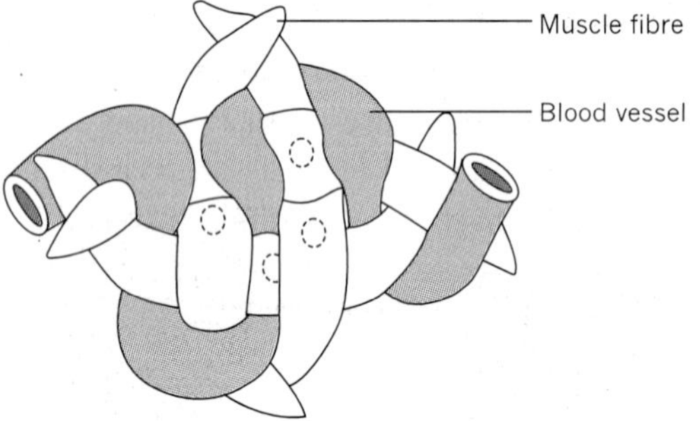

Fig. 14.2 *Reduction in size of myometrial cells. (Reproduced with permission from Miller & Hanretty 1998.)*

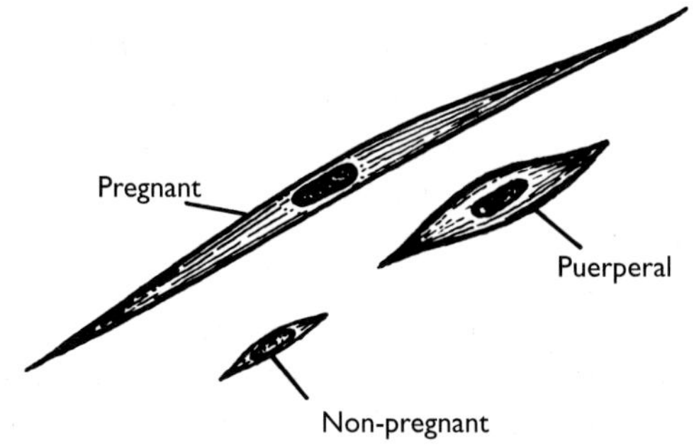


marked changes in collagen and elastin content (Stone & Franzblau 1995), and water and protein are lost. Involution results from a withdrawal of placental hormones and is thought to be mediated by hydrolytic and proteolytic enzymes released from myometrial cells, endothelial cells of blood vessels and macrophages. Cytoplasmic organelles are autodigested, and intracellular cytoplasm and extracellular collagen are reduced (Howie 1995). The breakdown of protein from the myometrial cells releases the amino acid components into the circulation and thence into the urine, thus a puerperal woman is in a state of negative nitrogen balance (see Ch. 12). The myometrial cells reduce in size (Fig. 14.2) and the uterus returns almost to its prepregnant size (Fig. 14.3) although the proportion of fibrous tissue present in the uterus is progressively increased with successive pregnancies.

Initially the cervix is soft, bruised and lacerated following a vaginal delivery. The cervix rapidly re-forms and closes; by the end of the first puerperal

Fig. 14.3 *Return of uterus to a size close to the prepregnant dimensions. A nulliparous uterus; B parous uterus. (Reproduced with permission from Miller & Hanretty 1998.)*

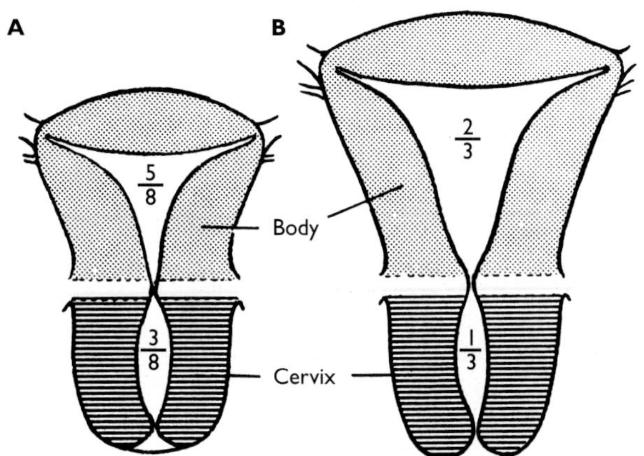


Fig. 14.4 *Re-formation of the external os. A nulliparous cervix; B parous cervix. (Reproduced with permission from Miller & Hanretty 1998.)*

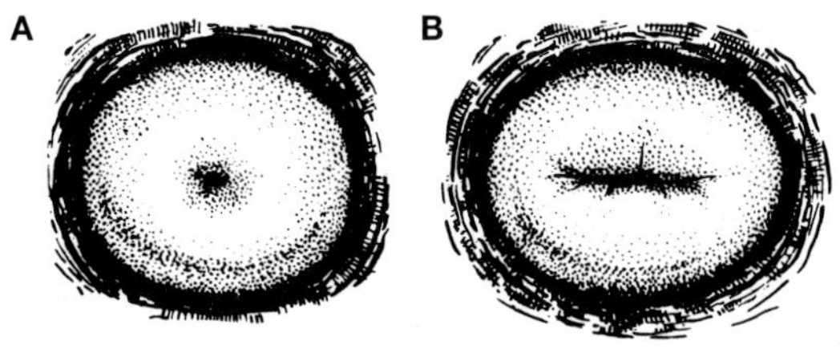


week, it will admit one finger. However, the cervix never returns to its original state and always shows evidence of parturition. The external os re-forms with a slit rather than the nulliparous dimple (Fig. 14.4).

The uterus involutes quite quickly, at about 1 cm a day; thus by the 10th day it can no longer be palpated above the symphysis pubis. Involution is slower in women who have undergone LSCS but it can be judged by a detectable decrease in fundal height. Subinvolution (a slow rate of uterine involution) may indicate retained products of conception and/or a secondary infection, which is usually found in conjunction with continued lochia rubra that may have an offensive odour. The uterus should be well contracted, hard and central; if it is higher than the umbilicus and soft on palpation (often described as 'boggy') then this may also indicate the presence of infection.

The initiation of breastfeeding and the infant suckling in the early puerperium augments stimulation of oxytocin release. The oxytocin stimulates further contraction of the myometrium and so aids the emptying of the uterine cavity. Involution of the uterus in breastfeeding mothers is more efficient. 'After-pains' associated with lactation are often experienced, particularly by multiparous women who often complain of increased vaginal loss while feeding. Initially oral analgesia such as paracetamol may be offered but the intensity of the pain usually subsides after about 24 hours when expression of myometrial oxytocin receptors is reduced as a result of oestrogen withdrawal.

The superficial layer of the decidua becomes necrotic and is shed in the lochia in the first few days of the puerperium. The epithelium rapidly regenerates, re-forming an intact layer over most of the surface within 7 to 10 days of delivery. The placental site takes up to 3 weeks to recover. The endometrium regenerates from the basal layers and grows in from the margins of the placental wound site and from glandular remnants within it (Howie 1995).

## Soft tissue damage and repair

It is not uncommon for soft tissue damage to occur during the delivery of a baby. Trauma to the female genital tract is described as follows.

- *Superficial*—this usually describes grazes to the skin where the epidermis has split owing to pressure of distension. These require no treatment; however, they often cause discomfort through stinging because of the disruption of the many nerve endings found within the superficial layer of the tissue. The voiding of urine can also be uncomfortable as the urine contacts with the grazes.
- *First degree*—this describes a tear in the skin and underlying superficial tissues (not including the muscle). Often the wound will heal on its own as the skin edges are usually in apposition. Ragged tears may result in the formation of excess scar tissue.
- *Second degree*—when a tear involves perineal muscle damage it is described as being second degree. Usually these wounds are sutured to aid healing.
- *Episiotomy*—this is a surgical incision to enlarge the introitus to facilitate the delivery of the baby. It falls into the same category as the second-degree tear.
- *Third degree*—here the muscle of the anal sphincter is involved. Obstetric repair is essential so that the sphincter activity of the muscle is restored thus avoiding complications of faecal incontinence at a later time.
- *Fourth degree*—when the tear is extensive the anal sphincter may become completely divided and the tear continues through the rectal mucosa. Specialist surgical repair is required to ensure the resumption of normal anal function.

Repair to the perineum involves the clinician suturing the perineum. There are a wide variety of suture materials and techniques for repair; however, suturing aims to achieve the following.

- *Haemostasis*—this is to ensure that any active bleeding points are ligated to minimize blood loss and the postnatal complication of a haematoma (formation of a blood clot within the wound) which can be extremely painful.
- *Alignment*—this is to bring the tissues back into alignment to optimize healing and to achieve a near pretear condition. If wounds are left gaping, alignment may not occur and as healing is by granulation this can result in the formation of scar tissue. This can result in a rigid misshapen perineum, which can cause dyspareunia (pain on intercourse).

The majority of perineal traumas can be described as being deep wounds as the tissue trauma involves layers below the epidermis and the dermis. Wound healing involves the following stages (see also Box 14.1).

1. First is the inflammatory response; inflammation is a normal reaction to tissue trauma. Perineal inflammation can initially cause great discomfort for women in the very early postnatal period. An analgesic such as Voltarol is useful as it acts as an anti-inflammatory agent. However, a degree of inflammation is vital to ensure tissue healing, so analgesics should be used only when the response is severe. The inflammation acts to isolate the damaged tissues, reducing the spread of infection. White blood cells, such as neutrophils and monocytes, invade the tissue owing to the increased vasodilatation in the surrounding blood vessels. These cells ingest any invading bacteria and break down any necrotic tissue within the wound.
2. The migratory phase involves the infiltration of the wound by mesenchymal cells that form fibroblasts, initially forming a scab over the open wound site. Following this, blood vessels grow into the wound and the wound is gradually filled from the bottom up by new tissue growth called granulation tissue.

**Box 14.1**

**The stages of wound healing**

*0–3 days*

- Blood clot forms, reinforced with fibrin fibres
- Acute inflammatory response occurs: polymorphs and macrophages migrate to site; high protein exudate leads to local oedema

*1 week later*

- Eschar dries out, hardens and eventually becomes detached
- Wound contracts
- Mitotic activity occurs in epidermal cells, which migrate over living tissue
- New blood capillary forms, formed from endothelial buds, bringing nutrients to healing tissue
- New connective tissue, formed by fibroblasts, supports capillary loops

*6 months later*

- Surface depression may still be visible at wound site; scar tissue becomes paler
- Epithelialization is complete
- Connective tissue is reorganized, less vascular and stronger

3. There then follows a proliferative phase where epithelial cells grow under the scab. It concludes with the maturation of the new cells and the shedding of the scab.

## Lochia

The initial vaginal loss is termed the lochia rubra and consists of blood that has collected within the reproductive tract and autolytic products of degenerated necrotic decidua from the placental site. The outward flow of blood lost at delivery and the subsequent discharge of lochia are important in removal of potential sources of ascending infection and protection of the placental wound site. The alkalinity of the lochia is also important in protecting the vulnerable site. Lochia is the normal discharge in the puerperium; it has a characteristic sweetish smell unless there is an infection.

Lochia may be described by its visual appearance (Box 14.2); normally, the lochia lightens progressively in both volume and colour. However, at about day 7 after delivery, the fibrinous mesh deposited over the placental site may be shed as part of the normal healing process so the vaginal loss may be transiently heavier and flushed with fresh blood. By day 10, the lochia is normally scant and pink in colour although discharge of lochia may persist for up to 6 weeks.

Heavy discharge of lochia with an offensive odour, maternal pyrexia and a feeling of general malaise can all indicate possible intrauterine infection. If the lochia remains abnormally heavy and further bleeding occurs, an obstetrician undertakes dilatation and curettage (D&C) to empty the uterine cavity. The procedure is also termed evacuation of retained products of conception (ERPC). The cervix is dilated and the retained products are scraped from the decidua. This procedure is not without complications, however. Excessive scraping can damage or remove the entire endometrium. If the basal layer of the endometrium is removed (see Ch. 2) then proliferation during the menstrual cycle fails to occur, affecting fertility; this is termed Asherman's syndrome.

**Box 14.2**

**Lochia**

- Lochia rubra (red)
  - decidua and blood from placental site
  - initially sterile then uterus begins to be colonized by vaginal flora
  - red colour persists for about 3 days
- Lochia serosa (pink/brown)
  - contains leukocytes, mucus, vaginal epithelial cells, necrotic decidua, non-pathological bacteria
  - may be blood stained for 3–4 weeks
  - characteristic sweetish odour
- Lochia alba (yellow-white)
  - mostly serious fluid and leukocytes
  - plus some cervical mucus and microorganisms

## Blood loss

Excessive blood loss—more than 500 ml or any amount that jeopardises the well-being of the mother—at and within 24 hours of delivery is termed a primary postpartum haemorrhage, or primary PPH. It is usually caused by failure of the myometrium to contract completely, or failure of the blood-clotting mechanisms, or both (see Ch. 1); PPH may be very serious (Box 14.3 and Case study 14.1).

The risk of primary PPH is lower 24 to 72 hours following delivery, but until involution of the uterus is complete there is a risk of a secondary PPH if there is an infection within the uterine cavity. The bleeding is usually due to the fibrinolytic action of bacteria such as

**Box 14.3**

**Disseminated intravascular coagulation**

Disseminated intravascular coagulation (DIC) is a condition caused by abnormal activation of the clotting mechanisms. The blood-clotting factors are induced on a wide basis resulting in fibrin deposits being produced that line the major part of the vascular bed. Once this has occurred bleeding continues owing to the absence of clotting factors, which were exhausted during the DIC phase and the activation of fibrinolysis. Liver dysfunction occurs in pre-eclampsia and may be associated with DIC and microangiopathic haemolysis (erythrocyte breakdown in small blood vessels). The acronym HELLP refers to *H*aemolysis, *E*levated *L*iver enzymes and *L*ow *P*latelet counts.

It is an extremely severe condition. Although such a life-threatening case would normally be managed by intensive care staff rather than by the midwifery unit, it is important that midwives are able to recognize the symptoms and implications of DIC.

**Case study 14.1**

Lucy is a 35-year-old primigravida who is delivered by emergency LSCS at 30 weeks' gestation owing to fulminating pre-eclampsia. Following delivery, the blood loss per vaginum is noted to be quite brisk and a syntocinon infusion is commenced in an attempt to control the bleeding. On investigation it is discovered that Lucy's platelet count is extremely low and that the clotting time for her blood is greatly prolonged. A provisional diagnosis of DIC secondary to HELLP syndrome is made.

haemolytic streptococcus. These bacteria are usually anaerobes (able to thrive in the absence of oxygen) and so specific antibiotic treatment with antibiotics such as metranidazole (Flagyl) may be required.

## Hormonal changes

In late pregnancy, most of the steroid hormones are derived from the placenta, although the corpus luteum and ovary continue to produce some. Levels of progesterone and oestrogen fall to non-pregnant levels within 72 hours of delivery. The placental protein hormones have a longer half-life so plasma levels fall more slowly. During pregnancy, production of the gonadotrophins is suppressed. FSH levels are restored to prepregnant concentrations within 3 weeks of delivery, but restoration of LH secretion takes longer, depending on the extent of lactation. Levels of oxytocin and prolactin also depend on lactational performance.

## The haematological system and cardiovascular changes

The blood lost at delivery, accepted to be about 300–500 ml normally, is adequately compensated for by the increase in blood volume acquired during pregnancy (see Ch. 11). Women can lose about 1000 ml of their predelivery blood volume before haemoglobin concentration is affected (Letsky 1998) (Case study 14.2). Erythropoiesis is stimulated before and after delivery (Ricther, Huch & Huch 1995). Diuresis further decreases plasma volume in the first days, although as interstitial fluid is mobilized subsequently the plasma volume tends to increase transiently causing haemodilution of both haemoglobin and plasma proteins, such as clotting factors. It is this variability in blood lost at delivery and restoration of normal water balance that may result in extremes of hypercoagulability due to raised concentrations of clotting factors. The tendency to coagulate is also affected by the loss of placental and fetal factors affecting clotting and water regulation (Blackburn & Loper 1992).

**Case study 14.2**

Prior to delivery Megan had a haemoglobin (Hb) concentration of 10.1 g/dl. At delivery, her blood loss is estimated at around 1000 ml. The midwife is quite concerned over this although Megan was asymptomatic. Prior to discharge on day 3 Megan's Hb concentration is rechecked and is estimated at being 9.8 g/dl.

- How can you account for the Megan's Hb concentration being relatively stable despite her suffering a postpartum haemorrhage?
- What advice/treatment would you give to Megan following her discharge?

Haemoglobin levels return to normal prepregnant levels within 4–6 weeks and white blood cell numbers fall to normal within a week of delivery (Blackburn & Loper 1992). Platelet number increases in the first few days following delivery, thereafter falling gradually to prepregnant levels. Fibrinolytic activity is maximal immediately after delivery for a few hours in response to the removal of the placenta, which produces fibrinolytic inhibitors (Hathaway & Bonnar 1987). The net result is that the hypercoaguable state of pregnancy is increased in the early puerperium and then slowly returns to a prepregnant state over a few weeks.

Mobilization is essential to optimize venous return to avoid stasis within the vascular bed, in order to minimize the risk of deep vein thrombosis (DVT) formation (see Complications of the puerperium, p. 322). Women who are unable to mobilize owing to obstetric complications, such as a LSCS, are given prophylactic treatment as the risks of DVT and complications are much increased. Women are advised to report any discomfort or swelling in the lower legs as this may indicate DVT formation; the risks of DVT progressively diminish.

The cardiovascular system is rendered transiently unstable by delivery owing to the blood loss and the ensuing compensatory mechanisms. During the period of transient instability of fluid balance in the 1st week after delivery, many women experience headaches.

Initially there is a marked increase in cardiac output as the uteroplacental flow is returned to the venous system and the gravid uterus no longer impedes the vena cava blood flow. This is augmented by the mobilization of extracellular fluid. Although pregnant women are normally able to tolerate normal blood lost at delivery, those women who had decreased vascular expansion during pregnancy, such as those with pre-eclampsia (see Ch. 11), may be less able to tolerate blood loss. Vaginal delivery is associated with a higher haemoglobin concentration than operative deliveries because vaginal delivery tends to have a lesser blood loss and to promote diuresis more markedly (Blackburn & Loper 1992).

Parameters of the cardiovascular system return towards prepregnant values but remain significantly different. Resolution of ventricular hypertrophy is slow. Vascular remodelling of pregnancy persists for at least a year after delivery and is enhanced by second and subsequent pregnancies (Clapp & Capeless 1997). Because circulating blood volume and cardiac output fall early in the puerperium and the hypertrophied ventricle is slowly remodelled, the stroke volume remains relatively high. This means that heart rate falls in the puerperium, as the stroke volume contributes proportionately more to the decreased cardiac output. Thus it is normal for puerperal women to exhibit bradycardia (a reduced pulse rate of about 60–70 beasts per minute). A raised pulse may indicate severe anaemia, venous thrombosis or infection (see below).

## Respiratory system

The decreased progesterone concentration following delivery of the placenta restores prepregnant sensitivity to carbon dioxide concentration so partial pressures of carbon dioxide return to prepregnant levels. The diaphragm can increase its excursion distance once the gravid uterus no longer impedes it so full ventilation of the basal lobes of the lung is possible. Chest wall compliance, tidal volume and respiratory rate return to normal within 1 to 3 weeks.

## Urinary system

It is important that bladder function is assessed in the early postnatal period. The trauma experienced by the bladder during delivery usually results in oedema and hyperaemia of the bladder, which has reduced muscle tone in pregnancy. Effects on the bladder are increased by prolonged labour, use of forceps, analgesia and anaesthetic procedures and pressure of the descending presenting part during delivery. The resulting transient loss of bladder sensation, which may cause overdistension and incomplete emptying, can last from days to weeks. Bladder changes are associated with increased risk of urinary tract infections in the puerperium. Trauma to the sphincter of the bladder increases the frequency of stress incontinence, which is marked by urine leakage occurring with coughing, laughing, sudden movement or exercise.

If bladder function is impaired, an indwelling catheter may be inserted to enable the damaged tissue to recover; however, catheterization increases the risk of an urinary tract infection (UTI). If the uterus can be palpated high up or is displaced over to one side following the woman voiding urine, this indicates that there is retention of urine as the full bladder displaces the uterus. This is compounded by the increased diuresis that occurs in the postnatal period due to the reduction of the increased plasma volume acquired during pregnancy. It is normal for women to have frequency of micturition as long as they are voiding large amounts of urine each time. Frequency involving just small amounts of urine being voided may indicate a degree of urinary retention.

Pain associated with micturition may indicate a UTI. Dilation of the ureters, overdistension of the bladder and instrumental or operative deliveries all increase the risk of infection. By day 10, full bladder function should be observed and assessed; there should be no evidence of unprovoked incontinence.

Parameters of the renal system, such as renal plasma flow, glomerular filtration rate and plasma creatinine, are back to normal non-pregnant levels by the 6-week check. Urinary excretion of mineral and vitamins is normal within the first week after delivery. Plasma renin and angiotensin levels adjust to the loss of fetal hormones affecting their control so levels fall and then increase before returning back to normal (Blackburn & Loper 1992). This fluctuation in hormone levels affecting water retention, together with the redistribution of body fluid, results in rapid and sustained natriuresis and diuresis, which is particularly marked between the 2nd and 5th day after delivery. Fluid and electrolyte balance is normal with 21 days after delivery. Oxytocin, which has ADH-like activity, falls after delivery, augmenting diuresis. The voiding volume increases and many women experience night sweats in the puerperium, which also increase fluid loss. Pregnancy-induced changes in the urinary system may persist for several months. Although the dilated smooth muscle of the urinary tract appears normal within a week of delivery, it remains potentially distensible. The kidneys return to their prepregnant size within 6 months of pregnancy.

## Gastrointestinal system and defaecation

During labour, gastric motility is reduced, particularly in association with pain, fear and narcotic drugs. The reduced tone of the lower oesophageal sphincter, reduced gastric motility and increased gastric acidity result in delayed gastric emptying. The tone and pressure of the lower oesophageal sphincter are normal by 6 weeks after delivery. However, in the early puerperium, the reduced gastrointestinal muscle tone and motility can relax the abdomen, increasing gas distension and constipation immediately after delivery.

The first bowel movement usually occurs within 2 or 3 days following delivery. This may become complicated by the presence of haemorrhoids, which are associated with evacuation problems. Due to the effects of progesterone on the venous system, the blood supply may become sluggish as the vessels become more torturous and so haemorrhoids are common during the latter half of pregnancy. Usually haemorrhoids resolve quickly after birth and cause only minor discomfort in the postnatal period. Sometimes, particularly if they are severe, owing to displacement by the passage of the presenting part through the birth canal they can become traumatized and localized thrombosis can occur. This can be further complicated if constipation develops and the woman, because of perineal trauma, is afraid to open her bowels. Problems with constipation are increased by intestinal atony, lax abdominal musculature, irregular food intake and dehydration in labour. By day 10, the woman should have achieved normal bowel function. Faecal incontinence may indicate anal sphincter damage or inadequate repair.

## Weight change

Although weight is lost at delivery of the products of conception, many women experience a weight gain in the first couple of days following delivery. This is due to a combination of increased ACTH, ADH and stress, all of which increase sodium and water retention. Weight usually starts to fall from the 4th day after delivery as diuresis increases. Weight is lost steadily, usually over a period of several months. Postpartum weight retention is affected by changes in lifestyle during and after pregnancy rather than by pregnancy itself (Ohlin & Rossner 1994). Weight loss tends to be greater with lower parity, maternal age and lower prepregnant weight.

## Other structural changes

Immediately after delivery, the vagina is smooth, soft and oedematous. The elasticity of the tissue returns within a few days. As the vagina is extremely well vascularized, episiotomies and tears usually heal well. The rugae of the vagina re-form but are less prominent than prior to pregnancy. The labia regress to a less prominent and fleshy state than in nulliparous women. The fall in oestrogen at delivery results in the vaginal epithelium becoming thinner and many women experience problems with vaginal lubrication immediately after delivery. Tags of the hymen remain and are renamed carunculae myrtiformes (Fig. 14.5).

Pelvic floor muscle strength and neuromuscular control are impaired to a greater extent in women who deliver vaginally and experience more mechanical trauma, particularly in the first week of the puerperium (Peschers et al 1997); however, for most women, muscular tone and strength are normal within 2 months. Weakened circumvaginal muscles are associated with perineal outcome, episiotomy, length of second stage of labour, the weight of the baby and pushing techniques (Cosner, Dougherty & Bishop 1991). Problems associated with a lax ineffective pelvic floor such as uterine prolapse, urinary incontinence and prolapse of the rectum are more likely as parity increases. Pelvic floor exercises help to restore the muscle tone and function of the pelvic floor;

**Fig. 14.5** *Carunculae myrtiformes. (Reproduced with permission from Miller & Hanretty 1998.)*

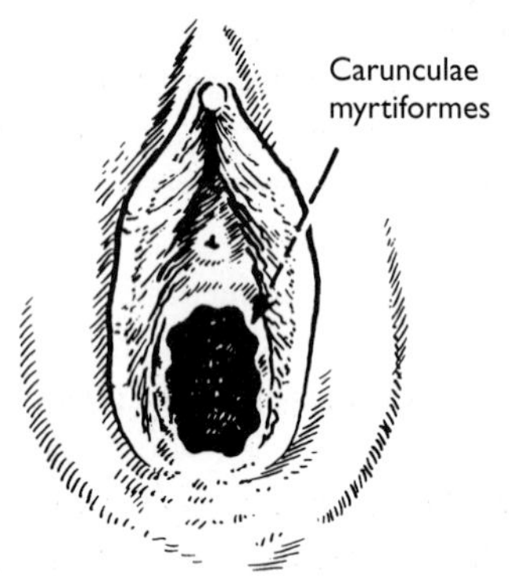

specialist advice from an obstetric physiotherapist may be required for persistent problems with incontinence.

The abdominal wall may remain soft and flabby for several weeks. Severe stretching, for instance in a multiple pregnancy or with polyhydramnios, can result in permanently lax muscles. The softened pelvic joints and ligaments slowly return to normal over a period of a few months. The striae gravidarum become paler over a period of several months but fade rather than completely disappear.

Pregnancy-induced changes in the skin spontaneously regress or fade. Hair loss may be marked following delivery and initial regrowth may be initially less abundant. Corneal sensitivity and pressure return to normal within 2 months of delivery. Nasal congestion and effects on the ear and larynx are restored to prepregnant status within a few days of delivery.

**Case study 14.3**

Sandra is a first-time mother who delivered a healthy male infant 3 days ago. She went home on the day of the birth as she appeared to be coping well with breastfeeding and caring for her infant. The community midwife visits at lunchtime on the 3rd day to find a very distressed mother, partner and infant. They have had no sleep and the baby has been very fractious and wakeful.

- What are the possible physiological causes that have contributed towards this situation?
- What would reassure the midwife that everything was normal and what support, help and advice could the midwife give to the family during this difficult period?

### *Body temperature*

In the first 24 hours following delivery, body temperature may increase slightly (to 38°C) in response to the stress of labour, particularly dehydration. This temperature fluctuation is normally transient; a persistent raised temperature may indicate infection (see below).

## Sleep

The puerperium is associated with disrupted sleep patterns, particularly immediately after delivery (Swain et al 1997). The first 3 days can be extremely difficult for the mother compounded by fatigue accumulated during labour and being unable to rest comfortably due to perineal pain (see Case study 14.3). Postpartum perineal pain correlates well with the duration of the 2nd stage of labour (Thranov et al 1990). Euphoria, urinary, breast and perineal discomfort and infant disturbances can all lead to reduced sleep, which may affect memory and psychomotor tasks. Theoretically, sleep patterns are close to normal within 2 or 3 weeks of delivery but breastfeeding mothers have a greater disruption of sleeping pattern (Quillin 1997).

## Psychological state

Usually by day 10 the mother and baby have established a feeding cycle. Although fatigue is common and normal, the mother should be developing strategies to cope with this, such as daytime sleeps. The mother should be independently caring for herself and the baby and interacting fully with members of her family and other people. Offspring provide their mothers with stimuli that elicit behavioural responses and emotional reactions; comparative studies suggest that these nurturing responses are evolutionarily conserved (Stern 1997).

Many women experience a lack of libido (sex drive) during the first few months following delivery. This may be complicated by trauma to the reproductive tract during delivery. Sexual desire, expression and satisfaction may be reduced after delivery. Sexual activity may be affected by fatigue, altered body image, marital adjustment, dyspareunia, lactation, traditional taboos, vaginal bleeding or discharge, insufficient lubrication or fear of waking the baby.

## Return to fertility

Women who do not breastfeed begin to menstruate, on average, about 55 to 60 days after delivery and to ovulate at about 40 to 50 days after delivery (Wang & Fraser 1994), whereas lactation delays ovulation to 30 to 40 weeks after delivery and menstruation to 8–15 months, depending on the duration and extent of breastfeeding. A proportion of women become pregnant during lactational amenorrhoea but the degree of suppression of fertility depends on infant-feeding patterns and perhaps on maternal nutrition. Lactational effects on fertility are reduced as the spaces between the feeds increase and as the baby receives supplementary feeding. However, lactational amenorrhoea appears to provide relatively good contraception for about 6 months (Lewis et al 1991), although it is probably more successful in achieving birth spacing.

Many women purposely choose to limit the number of children they wish to have. There are many economical and social issues that impinge on this; however, it is important to recognize that there are some women for whom certain (or all) methods of contraception are not acceptable on cultural and religious grounds. The return of fertility is very difficult to assess as factors such as breastfeeding, cultural and religious practice, genetic variation and disease may all compound the identification of return of the fertility cycle. It is important to emphasize that ovulation precedes menstruation so amenorrhoea does not guarantee the absence of fertility.

## The role of the midwife

Usually most women are discharged from midwifery care by day 10; however, the midwife may visit up to day 28 in the postnatal period if required. Once the midwife is satisfied that the physiological transition is progressing normally then the discharge can be completed. The health visitor and general practitioner (GP) continue care of the mother and baby. The responsibilities of the midwife in the puerperium and at discharge include giving advice to women on a number of issues including infant feeding, parentcraft, pelvic floor exercises, contraception and sources of psychological support.

## Complications of the puerperium

### *Thromboembolic disorders*

The increase in potential clot formation can have a physiological disadvantage both in pregnancy and following delivery in that thrombi (blood clots) can form within the venous system. Thromboembolic disorders are relatively common in pregnancy. During the third trimester the pregnant woman develops a state of hypercoagulation, thus that her blood is more likely to clot than it would in the non-pregnant state and the effects of progesterone on venous muscle tone increase stasis of flow. The risk of thromboembolic disorders in pregnancy is about six times higher than previously, and increases further in the puerperium. This is enhanced by a decrease in fibrinolytic activity (the breakdown of fibrin forming a blood clot) and raised concentration of clotting factors. This tendency of the blood to clot more readily imparts a physiological advantage to the woman to prevent excess blood loss during and immediately after delivery of the placenta and membranes. Haemoconcentration of the blood from physiological diuresis following delivery augments the increase in clotting factors.

#### Thrombophlebitis

Thrombophlebitis is a thrombus (clot) in a superficial vein. The commonest site of thrombus formation is in the saphenous vein supplying the calf of the leg. Symptoms include a tender reddened area over the thrombosed vein and possibly a small increase in pulse and temperature. Motility and elevating the legs at rest reduce the risk of thrombus formation; compression stockings may be helpful. Thrombophlebitis is unlikely to progress to pulmonary embolism.

#### Deep vein thrombosis

DVT is less common but carries the risk of a clot dislodging, which can cause pulmonary embolism. Hypercoagulability is increased with increased maternal age, parity, dehydration following delivery, and delivery by caesarean section. Women are at increased risk if they have a previous history of thromboembolic problems, pregnancy-induced hypertension (and associated lack of vascular expansion), anaemia, or if they have artificial heart valves or have had an operative delivery (Weiner 1985). It has been observed clinically that there is an increased risk of DVT in the left leg, especially after a caesarean section, because blood flow velocity is reduced to a greater extent (Macklon & Greer 1997). DVT may cause no symptoms or the woman may experience pain and swelling over the affected area and occasionally pyrexia. There may be marked differences in calf size or, in extreme cases, circulation to the leg below the thrombosis may be affected so the leg appears cold and white and possibly oedematous. DVT is confirmed by Doppler ultrasound or impedance plesthysmography.

#### Pulmonary embolism

Pulmonary embolism (PE) is an obstetric emergency that may follow DVT or occur without warning. PE is a condition that contributes towards maternal mortality associated with pregnancy. If a thrombosis (fragment of the blood clot) breaks away and enters the venous system, it is then carried in the venous system to the right side of the heart and the pulmonary circulation. As the pulmonary arteries reduce in size, the thrombus may occlude arterial vessels within the lungs, causing major damage. Symptoms are sudden collapse, acute severe chest pain, dyspnoea, cyanosis, haemoptysis and shock. A woman with a PE will require intensive treatment and care.

Women assessed to be at increased risk of thrombus formation are treated with prophylactic anticoagulants, such as heparin and synthetic analogues such as enoxaparin. DVT is usually treated with heparin, and if required long-term anticoagulation therapy with drugs such as warfarin is commenced.

## *Risk of infection*

In the puerperium, the woman is at increased risk of infection particularly that associated with the genital tract, urinary system, breast and any site of thrombophlebitis. The placental wound site, lacerations and incisions of the perineum and the lax urinary system are especially vulnerable. The lochia provides ideal culture conditions for microorganisms. Other predisposing factors include anaemia, fatigue, malnutrition, traumatic delivery and the presence of retained tissue in the uterus. Both maternal and neonatal infection (see Ch. 15) may be caused by endogenous or exogenous organisms (Box 14.4).

Symptoms of infection include pyrexia (up to 40°C), tachycardia (up to 140 beats per minute), subinvolution of the uterus, headache, malaise, lower abdominal pain and offensive heavy lochia. Infection in the acute phase can inhibit lactation. When choosing antibiotics to treat infection in the puerperium one needs to take into consideration whether the woman is breastfeeding and the potential effect of the transfer of the drug into milk.

**Box 14.4**

**Examples of microorganisms causing puerperal infection**

- Endogenous:
  - *Escherichia coli*
  - *Clostridium perfringens*
  - *Streptococcus faecalis*
  - *Pseudomonas aeruginosa*
- Exogenous:
  - β-haemolytic streptococci
  - *Staphylococcus aureus*

## *Breast discomfort and after-pains*

The establishment of lactation is covered in detail in Chapter 16; however, it is worth mentioning here two common problems that can occur during this period in relation to breastfeeding.

- If the baby has been incorrectly positioned, often because it is fractious or hungry and wanting to feed constantly, the nipple may become sore, cracked and bleed as a consequence. A break in the integrity of the nipple skin increases the risk of mastitis—localized and ascending infection usually caused by *Staphylococcus aureus*. Women experiencing early feeding problems need a lot of help and support. The baby needs to 'fix' or 'latch on' properly in order to provide adequate nipple stimulation to establish the feeding cycle.
- Sometimes the breasts become engorged or extended. Initially this may be a venous cause due to the increased vascularization of the breast. However, when milk production increases (described as the milk 'coming in'), the breast may initially be overproductive. The breasts may overfill with milk causing them to become distended and hardened, which may be uncomfortable or painful. The baby may need help achieving an appropriate position; however, once the feeding cycle is established the demand/supply balance is achieved and the breast engorgement problems will resolve.

## *Pharmacological effects*

The majority of deliveries within the UK have the third stage actively managed as opposed to passive or physiological management where the women delivers the placenta naturally (see Ch. 13). However, the administration of a tocolytic drug such as syntometrine, which contains ergotamine, may cause side-effects following completion of the third stage such as:

- nausea and vomiting
- transient rise in blood pressure
- palpitations and tachycardia
- chest pain
- headache.

Also during the early puerperium women may suffer side-effects from pharmacological methods of pain relief administered during labour. Pethidine may induce drowsiness, fatigue and nausea within the mother and reduce the suckling instinct of the infant, thus interfering with feeding. The effects of an epidural anaesthetic may take several hours to wear off, which affects maternal mobility and the ability to void urine.

## *Psychological problems*

Women in the postpartum period have increased vulnerability to affective disorders, such as postpartum 'blues', depression and psychosis. It is estimated that over half of all puerperal women experience transient emotional disorders at about day 3 described as 'the blues' (Kumar 1985). A further 10% develop true depressive illness, which may have a later onset (or referral) and delayed recovery. A few women (0.2%) develop severe prolonged psychotic illness following childbirth. Although many of these cases may be recognized in the early postnatal period, some become evident much later. Certain symptoms are recognized to be important in the diagnosis of postnatal depression (Box 14.5).

The aetiology of these depressive disorders is not fully understood. Immediately after delivery, the infant may feed often and this may be increased at night adding to maternal fatigue. Initially the mother's fatigue is overcome by intense feelings of relief and excitement at the birth of her baby. By day 3, however, the woman may become emotional, tearful and tired and need a lot of support and comfort during this period. This low ebb of hormonal withdrawal is physiologically marked by the commencement of full lactogenesis following the initial production of small volumes of colostrum (see Ch. 16). The 'blues' coincide with lactation, breast engorgement, perineal pain and wound discomfort.

It has been controversially proposed that progesterone withdrawal results in depression (Dalton 1980); progesterone suppositories (e.g. Cyclogest) have been used prophylactically to treat women with a history of postnatal depression, but the studies have been criticized for lack of scientific rigour and appropriate controls. Oestrogen has also been associated with psychological well-being (Brace & McCauley 1997); sudden changes in oestrogen levels such as those experienced in the puerperium may result in effects on neurotransmitter release.

Other authors suggest that levels of cortisol or β-endorphin have a stronger association with postnatal depression (Harris et al 1996). The hypothalamic–pituitary–adrenal axis is very active in the third trimester as placental CRH production increases and CRH-binding protein levels fall. Suppression of hypothalamic CRH secretion is implicated in the aetiology of postnatal depression (Magiakou et al 1996). The relationship between breastfeeding and postnatal depression is controversial. However, hormones involved in lactation affect cortisol levels (Amico, Johnston & Vagnucci 1994). Lactation may also predispose the breastfeeding mother to depression by isolating her and increasing levels of fatigue. Women who develop postnatal depression make a good recovery with the right treatment and support. Exercise programmes have been found to decrease anxiety and depression in the puerperium significantly (Koltyn & Schultes 1997). The recurrence of postnatal depression is high, which allows identification of women at increased risk.

Case study 14.4 is an example of a hormonal complication of the puerperium.

**Box 14.5**

**Classic signs of postnatal depression**

- Depressed mood
- Sleep disturbance not related to discomfort and infant wakening
- Unable to cope—guilt
- Thoughts of harming self or baby
- Rejection of baby
- Altered libido
- Anxiety

**Case study 14.4**

At delivery Lucy suffered from a large haemorrhage that was difficult to control and finally underwent a hysterectomy following a total blood loss of over 4 litres. Her recovery was uneventful but within 6 months she was diagnosed as suffering from Sheehan's syndrome—necrosis of the pituitary gland.

- What would her symptoms be?
- What endocrine function would be disrupted as a result of this condition?

## Key points

- Maternal physiology and anatomy adapt rapidly to the withdrawal of steroid hormones, following the delivery of the placenta. These dramatic physiological changes increase the risk of infection, haemorrhage and psychological and emotional changes.
- The uterus rapidly involutes after delivery; normal involution can be monitored by assessment of fundal height and characteristics of the lochia.
- After delivery, there is a dramatic and rapid decrease in circulating volume followed by a return to normal cardiovascular parameters. As stroke volume initially remains high, bradycardia is common, particularly in the first 2 weeks.
- The postpartum physiological changes allow the woman to tolerate considerable blood loss at delivery but alteration in clotting factor concentration and venous stasis predispose the woman to thromboembolic disorders; the risk is enhanced by immobility and sepsis.
- Marked diuresis is normal in the puerperium but overdistension, or decreased sensitivity, of the bladder can predispose the woman to urinary problems.
- Ovulation occurs before menstruation and is delayed by breastfeeding; lactational amenorrhoea is useful in birth spacing rather than being a reliable method of contraception.

### Application to practice

In comparison to pregnancy, when the changes induced by endocrine effects are at a relatively slow pace, the reversal of this in the puerperium is much more rapid. These rapid changes occur at the same time as another endocrine-induced change resulting in lactation.

Fatigue from labour, perineal pain from trauma and the demands of a newborn infant can also complicate the situation.

The midwife needs to use her knowledge of the puerperium to support women through this often difficult period of adaptation.

## Annotated further reading

Abbott H, Bick D, McArthur C 1997 Health after birth. In: Henderson C, Jones K (eds) Essential midwifery. C V Mosby, St Louis

*Describes the postnatal period and the care required for the mother and baby from a health perspective.*

Bonnar J 1995 Venous thrombosis and pulmonary embolism. In: Chamberlain G (ed) Turnbull's obstetrics, 2nd edn. Churchill Livingstone, New York

*A detailed description of these pathological problems associated with the vascular system during and after pregnancy and how they may be recognized and treated.*

Geary M 1997 The HELLP syndrome. British Journal of Obstetrics and Gynaecology 104:887–891

*A review of the HELLP (haemolysis, elevated liver enzymes, and low platelets) syndrome covering aetiology, diagnosis and care in pregnancy.*

Montgomery E, Alexander J 1994 Assessing postnatal uterine involution: a review and a challenge. Midwifery 10:73–76

*Structured review of literature relating to the assessment of postnatal uterine involution which found no evidence that any form of anthropometric assessment of uterine involution in the early postnatal period had preventative or predictive value.*

Pugh L C, Milligan R M 1993 A framework for the study of childbearing fatigue. Advanced Nursing Science 15:60–70

*This article identifies factors that may predispose a woman to fatigue in childbearing and looks at the effects of maternal fatigue upon childbirth, providing a framework of intervention designed to prevent or reduce fatigue.*

Smith R, Thomson M 1991 Neuroendocrinology of the hypothalamic–pituitary–adrenal axis in pregnancy and the puerperium. Baillière's Clinics in Endocrinology and Metabolism 5:167–186

*Describes alterations in hormones during and after pregnancy and examines the role of placental hormones on maternal physiology. Includes a description of hormones affecting diurnal rhythm and possible links between hormonal changes and the development of postnatal mood changes.*

Van Gelderen C J 1995 Puerperal sepsis. In: Chamberlain G (ed) Turnbull's obstetrics, 2nd edn. Churchill Livingstone, New York, pp 285–318

*A thorough examination of the factors associated with puerperal sepsis and how to treat it.*

Varner M W 1998 Medical conditions of the puerperium. Clinics in Perinatology 25:403–416

*This article reviews the physiological and emotional changes that occur during the puerperium and the clinical management of common problems such as infection and haemorrhage.*

Vekemans M 1997 Postpartum contraception: the lactational amenorrhea method. European Journal of Contraception and Reproductive Health Care 2:105–111

*Describes the lactational amenorrhoea method (LAM) as a way of physiologically spacing births and supporting breast-feeding. Includes the underlying hormonal control of suppressed fertility and considers natural family planning and cultural issues.*

## References


Amico J A, Johnston J M, Vagnucci A H 1994 Suckling-induced attenuation of plasma cortisol concentrations in postpartum lactating women. Endocrinology Research 20:79–87

Blackburn S T, Loper D L 1992 Maternal, fetal, and neonatal physiology: a clinical perspective. W B Saunders, Philadelphia

Brace M, McCauley E 1997 Oestrogens and psychological well-being. Annals of Medicine 29:283–290

Clapp J F, Capeless E 1997 Cardiovascular function before, during, and after the first and subsequent pregnancies. American Journal of Cardiology 80:1469–1473

Cosner K R, Dougherty M C, Bishop K R 1991 Dynamic characteristics of the circumvaginal muscles during pregnancy and the postpartum. Journal of Nurse-Midwifery 36:221–225

Cox J L 1986 Postnatal depression. Churchill Livingstone, New York

Dalton K 1980 Depression after childbirth. OUP, Oxford

Harris B, Lovettt L, Smith J, Read G, Walker R, Newcombe R 1996 Cardiff puerperal mood and hormone study III: postnatal depression at 5 to 6 weeks postpartum, and its hormonal correlates across the peripartum period. British Journal of Psychology 168:739–744

Hathaway W E, Bonnar J 1987 Hemostatic disorders of the pregnant woman and newborn infant. Elsevier, New York

Howie P W 1995 The physiology of the puerperium and lactation. In: Chamberlain G (ed) Turnbull's obstetrics, 2nd edn. Churchill Livingstone, New York

Koltyn K F, Schultes S S 1997 Psychological effects of an aerobic exercise session and rest session following pregnancy. Journal of Sports Medicine and Physical Fitness 37:287–291

Kumar R 1985 Pregnancy, childbirth and mental illness. Progress in Obstetrics and Gynaecology 5:146–159

Letsky E 1998 The haematological system. In: Chamberlain G, Broughton Pipkin F (eds) Clinical physiology in obstetrics, 3rd edn. Blackwell, Oxford

Lewis P R, Brown J B, Renfree M B, Short R V 1991 The resumption of ovulation and menstruation in a well-nourished population of women breastfeeding for an extended period of time. Fertility and Sterility 55:529–536

Macklon N S, Greer I A 1997 The deep venous system in the puerperium: an ultrasound study. British Journal of Obstetrics and Gynaecology 104:198–200

Magiakou M A, Mastorakos G, Rabin D, Dubbert B, Gold P W, Chrousos G P 1996 Hypothalamic corticotrophin-releasing hormone suppression during the postpartum period: implications for the increase in psychiatric manifestations at this time. Journal of Clinical Endocrinology and Metabolism 81(5):1912–1917

Miller A W F, Hanretty K P 1998 Obstetrics illustrated, 5th edn. Churchill Livingstone, New York, p 336

Ohlin A, Rossner S 1994 Trends in eating patterns, physical activity and socio-demographic factors in relation to postpartum body weight development. British Journal of Nutrition 71:457–470

Peschers U M, Schaer G N, DeLancey J O, Schuessler B 1997 Levator ani function before and after childbirth. British Journal of Obstetrics and Gynaecology 104:1004–1008

Richter C, Huch A, Huch R 1995 Erythropoiesis in the postpartum period. Journal of Perinatal Medicine 23:51–59

Quillin S L 1997 Infant and mother sleep patterns during the 4th postpartum week. Issues in Comparable Pediatric Nursing 20:115–123

Stern J M 1997 Offspring-induced nuturance: animal-human parallels. Developmental Psychobiology 31:19–37

Stone P J, Franzblau C 1995 Increase in urinary desmoline and pyridoline during postpartum involution of the uterus in humans. Proceedings of the Society of Experimental Biology and Medicine 210:39–42

Swain A M, O'Hara M W, Starr K R, Gorman L L 1997 A prospective study of sleep, mood, and cognitive function in postpartum and nonpostpartum women. Obstetrics and Gynecology 90:381–386

Sweet B, Tiran D 1996 Mayes' midwifery, 12th edn. Bailliere Tindall, London, pp 405, 406

Tekay A, Jouppila P 1993 A longitudinal Doppler ultrasonographic assessment of the alterations in peripheral vascular resistance of uterine arteries and ultrasonographic findings of the involuting uterus during the puerperium. American Journal of Obstetrics and Gynecology 168:190–198

Thranov I, Kringelbachh A M, Melchior E, Olsen O, Damsgaard M T 1990 Postpartum symptoms: episiotomy or tear at vaginal delivery. Acta Obstetrica et Gynecologia Scandinavica 69:11–15

Wang I Y, Fraser I S 1994 Reproductive function and contraception in the postpartum period. Obstetrics and Gynecological Survey 49:56–63

Weiner C 1985 Diagnosis and management of thromboembolic disorders of pregnancy. Clinics in Obstetrics and Gynecology 28:107

# 15 The transition to neonatal life

## Learning objectives

- To identify the key steps in the transition to successful neonatal life.
- To describe the vulnerability of the neonate, with particular reference to the potential risk of respiratory problems, jaundice and hypoglycaemia.
- To outline thermoregulation in the newborn.
- To compare the fetal and neonatal circulatory and respiratory systems, describing the transition stages.
- To describe factors, relating to the neonatal gastrointestinal, renal and nervous systems, that make breast milk the ideal food.

## Introduction

During fetal life, the placenta carries out the crucial physiological roles of gas exchange, nutrition, elimination of waste products and additional aspects of circulation. Within minutes of birth, the placental support ceases so the baby's own cardiovascular, respiratory, gastrointestinal, renal and metabolic systems must function independently. The transition from fetal to neonatal life needs to be smooth, swift and successful: the majority of infant deaths occur within the neonatal period (first 28 days) (Bernal et al 1993) and these are linked to inadequate progression to neonatal physiological functions.

One of the most important transitional stages in the adaptation to extrauterine life is the establishment of the neonatal circulation. In fetal life, the source of oxygen is the placenta so most of the blood flow bypasses the fetal lungs. At birth, circulation perfuses the lungs and flow through the fetal vascular structures ceases.

The process of birth is stressful with fluctuations in placental blood flow resulting in a degree of hypoxia and respiratory acidosis. Increased secretion of adrenal catecholamines, stimulation of the sympathetic nervous system and the subsequent mobilization of glycogen and lipid stores are fundamental in the activation of essential physiological mechanisms that result in an alert and active baby at birth. However, a prolonged or difficult delivery and marked hypoxia/anoxia and acidosis can result in an overstressed or seriously asphyxiated baby.

Both the fetus and the neonate can tolerate degrees of hypoxia and anoxia that would result in serious morbidity or mortality in an adult. The neonate retains the capability to divert a considerate proportion of its cardiac output to the brain thus protecting it. Although the brain is vulnerable to hypoxia, the compensatory mechanisms can increase tolerance to hypoxic states (Parer 1998). However, severe asphyxia can cause cerebral microhaemorrhages resulting in a spectrum of damage from impaired intellectual development to spasticity and irreversible brain damage.

# The cardiovascular system

## *Blood*

### Before birth

Fetal blood (Table 15.1) contains larger and more numerous erythrocytes (red blood cells) with a higher haemoglobin content which maximizes their uptake of oxygen (Oh 1986). Fetal haemoglobin with its two $\alpha$- and two $\gamma$-chains has a higher affinity for oxygen in the slightly more acid fetal environment. Less effective binding of 2,3-BDP (or 2,3-DPG) means that the oxygen–haemoglobin dissociation curve of the fetus and neonate is shifted to the left (Fig. 15.1). Shifts of pH in the placenta further increase both dissociation of oxygen from maternal haemoglobin and its uptake by fetal haemoglobin. This means that, although fetal haemoglobin has an increased oxygen take-up, it is less efficient at releasing oxygen to the tissues.

At term, the ratio of HbF: HbA (fetal haemoglobin: adult haemoglobin) is 80:20; by 6 months production of the $\beta$-chain replaces the $\gamma$-chain so the ratio is 1 : 99 (Fig. 15.2). Preterm infants tend to have an even higher HbF level and a decreased 2,3-BDP concentration therefore oxygen unloading at the tissue level is even less efficient. The raised levels of HbF in the neonate mean that haemoglobinopathies caused by altered synthesis of $\beta$-chains (such as $\beta$-thalassemia) or altered structure of $\beta$-chains (such as sickle cell anaemia) are not evident immediately at birth but manifest themselves when the infant is at least 2 months old. It is possible to detect fetal blood cells in the maternal circulation, an observation that is utilized in the management of Rhesus incompatibility (see Ch. 10) (Lamvu & Kuller 1997).

### After birth

At birth, fetal blood has an increased population of nucleated erythrocytes (even more so if the baby has been subjected to increased stress, is immature or has Down's syndrome). For the first 3 months of life, the erythrocytes are more fragile, have an increased metabolism and a shorter half-life and erythropoietin production is suppressed (Box 15.1).

## *Haemostasis*

Neonates, particularly those born prematurely, have an increased risk of haemostatic problems (Andrew 1997). The most common example (Kuehl 1997) is DIC due to accelerated inappropriate coagulation, which exhausts the supply of plasma clotting factors. Susceptibility is increased because, first, the immature neonatal reticuloendothelial system has a decreased capacity to remove intermediary products of coagulation so they can further stimulate coagulation and consumption of clotting factors and, secondly, synthesis of

**Table 15.1** *Fetal and adult blood*

| | Fetal/neonatal | Adult |
|---|---|---|
| Blood volume | 80–100 ml/kg<br>90–105 ml/kg (preterm) | 75 ml/kg |
| Red blood cell number | 6–7 × $10^6$/ml | female: 4.8 × $10^6$/ml<br>male: 5.4 × $10^6$/ml |
| Haemoglobin content | 20.7 g/dl | female: 14 g/dl<br>male: 16 g/dl |
| Oxygen content of 100 ml saturated blood | 21 ml (theory)<br>13 ml (practice) | 16 ml (theory)<br>15.7 ml (practice) |
| Red blood cell lifespan | 80–100 days<br>60–80 days (preterm) | 120 days |
| Haemoglobin type | HbF: $\alpha_2\gamma_2$ | HbA: $\alpha_2\beta_2$ |

**Note**: the theoretical value is the amount of oxygen the blood can be saturated with whereas, in practice, the blood is saturated to a lesser degree because the transfer of oxygen across the placenta is less efficient than the transfer of oxygen across the alveoli.

**Fig. 15.1** *The maternal and fetal oxyhaemoglobin dissociation curves.*

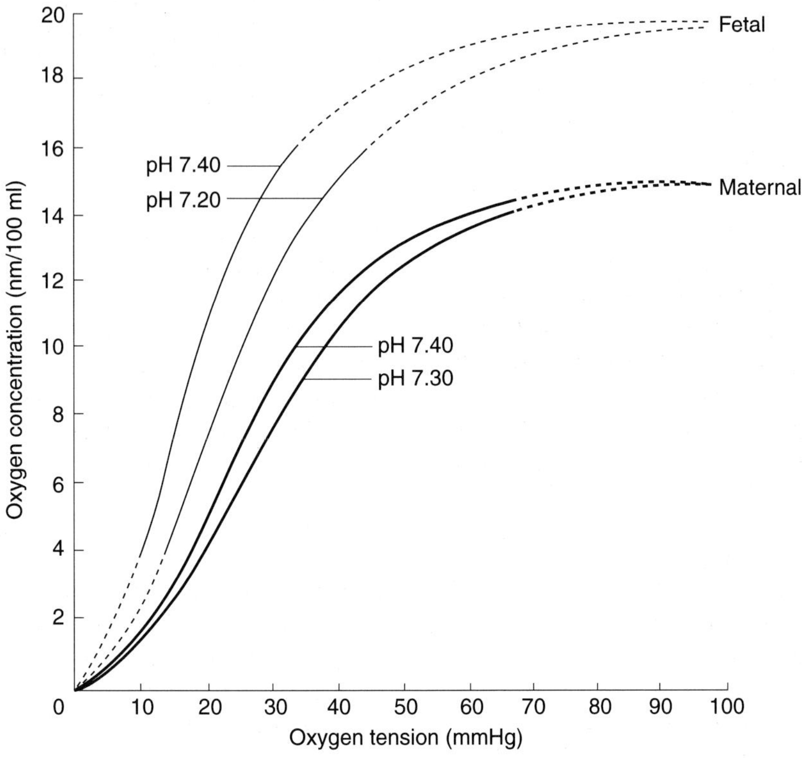


**Fig. 15.2** *Changes in fetal:adult haemoglobin (HbF:HbA) ratios in fetal and infant blood. (Reproduced with permission from Begley et al 1978.)*

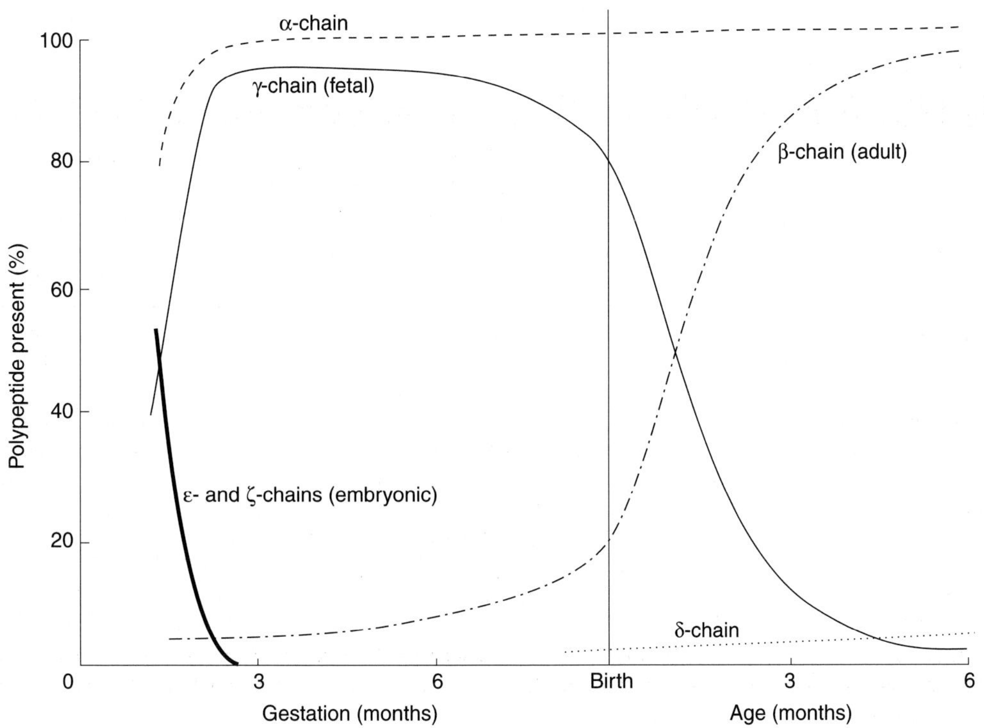

**Box 15.1**

**Physiological anaemia of infancy**

Haemopoiesis (red blood cell production) is controlled by the hormone erythropoietin, which increases when oxygen delivery to the kidney is reduced; it stimulates red blood cell production by the bone marrow. The increased oxygen levels inhibit erythropoietin levels in the neonate postnatally (Strauss 1994). Levels remain low for 2 to 3 months (longer in preterm infants) and then increase resulting in increased bone marrow activity and red blood cell production. As the neonate appears to tolerate the fall in haemoglobin concentration without ill effects, it is deemed to be physiological. The haemodilution effects are increased by rapid growth being matched by total blood volume, which precedes any change in red blood cell number.

**Box 15.2**

**Haemorrhagic disease of the newborn (HDNB)**

- Bleeding from the gut, umbilicus, circumcision wounds and oozing from puncture sites
- Evident 2 to 3 days after birth
- Associated with antibiotics, which affect colonization of the gut with vitamin K-synthesizing bacteria
- Associated with anticonvulsant drugs (e.g. phenobarbitol, diphenyl hydantoin), which concentrate in the fetal liver and antagonize the effect of vitamin K
- Associated with maternal warfarin treatment, which decreases levels of vitamin K-dependent clotting factors and prolongs prolonged clotting times
- Prophylactic vitamin K is routinely administered to all babies born in the UK (Hilgartner 1993) but studies have implicated intramuscular vitamin K administration in childhood cancer (Golding et al 1992)
- Term babies respond well to vitamin K therapy but synthesis of clotting factors is further limited in preterm babies by inadequate hepatic synthesis of precursor proteins

clotting factors by the immature liver is inefficient. Vitamin K levels in the neonate are about 50% of adult values, which affects the efficiency of the clotting cascade. Vitamin K levels are low because placental transport of the vitamin is poor and there is a lack of gut colonization by bacteria that synthesize vitamin K. The consequent reduced level of all vitamin K-dependent clotting factors is associated with an increased bleeding tendency, which can predispose to haemorrhagic disease of the newborn (HDNB) (Box 15.2). Neonatal platelets exhibit decreased aggregation and adhesiveness because their production of thromboxane $A_2$ is impaired. This appears to protect the term neonate against thrombosis but to increase the vulnerability to bleeding of the preterm or sick baby. Placental transfer of maternal drugs such as aspirin can affect coagulation in the neonate.

## *The circulation*

### Before birth

As the fetal oxygen source is the placenta rather than the lungs, blood in the fetal circulation flows in a circuit that perfuses the placenta and largely bypasses the lungs (Fig. 15.3). In order to do this, the fetal circulation has several additional structures: the umbilical vein, which carries blood rich in oxygen and nutrients to the underside of the liver to the ductus venosus (a venosus is a shunt that connects a vein to a vein), which inserts into the inferior umbilical vein en route to the right side of the heart. The hypogastric arteries, which branch off the internal iliac arteries, become the umbilical arteries of the umbilical cord, returning blood to the placenta. The lungs are bypassed by two structures: the foramen ovale, which allows blood to move directly from the right atrium to the left, and the ductus arteriosus, which connects the pulmonary arterial trunk to the descending aorta.

The oxygenated and nutrient-enriched blood is taken from the placenta in the umbilical vein that goes through the abdominal wall to the underside of the liver. This is the only unmixed blood and is about 80% saturated with oxygen; the blood goes through the ductus venosus to the inferior vena cava where it mixes with oxygen-depleted blood returning to the heart from the lower body (Fig. 15.4A). The inflows of blood from the inferior and superior venae cavae do not mix thoroughly because of their angle of entry and the shape of the right atrium. Because the entry of the inferior vena cava is aligned with the foramen ovale, most of the blood from the inferior vena cava travels from the right atrium through the foramen ovale into the left atrium and thence to the left ventricle and the ascending aorta.

Most blood entering the right atrium from the superior vena cava passes through the tricuspid valve into the right ventricle and to the pulmonary arterial trunk. The ductus arteriosus is inserted into the vessel

**Fig. 15.3** *The fetal circulation. (Reproduced with permission from Goodwin 1997.)*

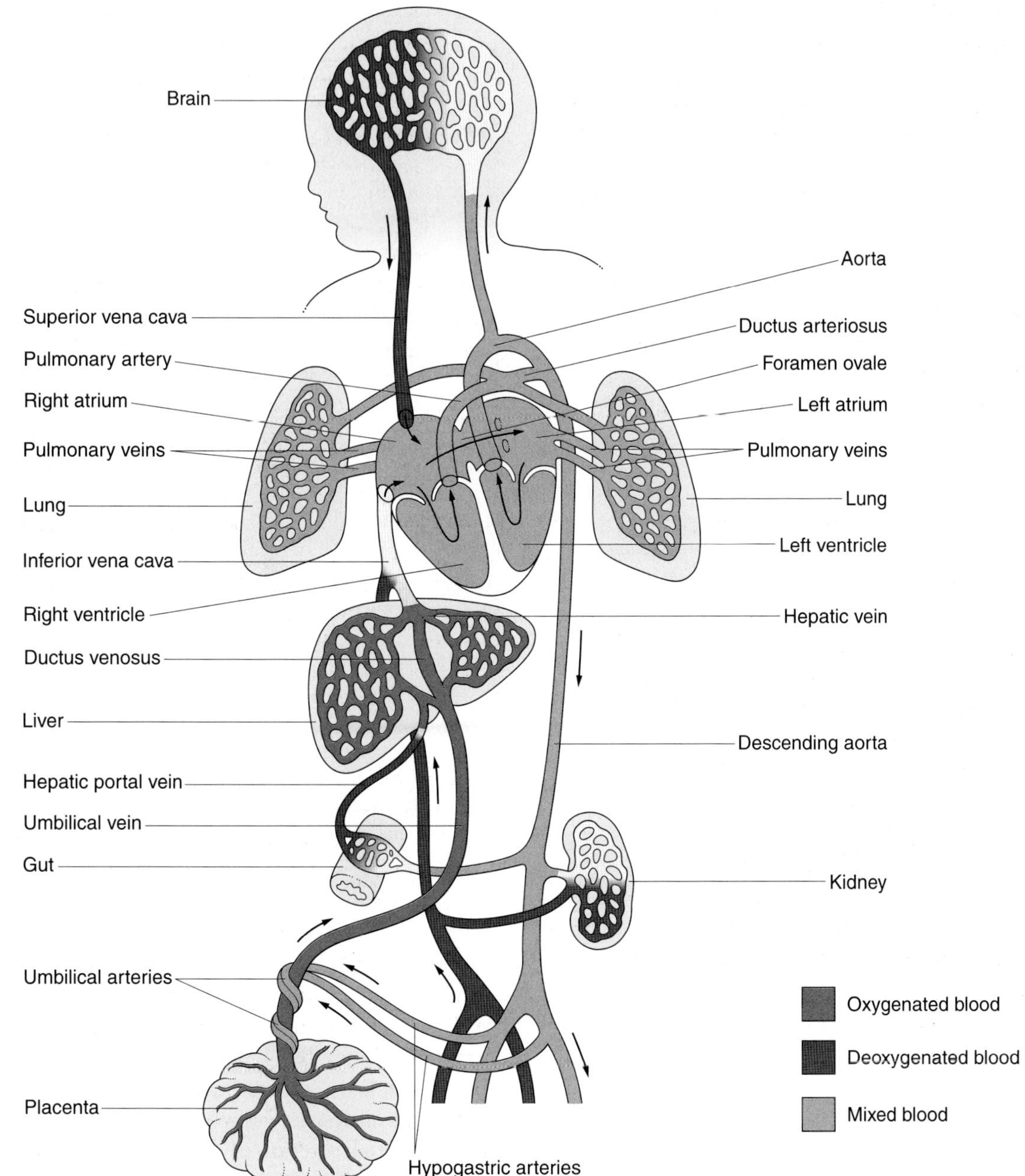


at the bifurcation of the right and left pulmonary artery (taking blood to the right and left lung respectively); it shunts blood from the pulmonary arterial route into the descending aorta. The pulmonary circulation is vasoconstricted and has a high vascular resistance. Only about 10% of the output of the right ventricle continues into the pulmonary circulation; the rest is diverted through the ductus arteriosus. From the descending aorta, the blood supplies the remaining organs and the lower body. The hypogastric arteries branch off the internal iliac arteries and return to the placenta via the umbilical arteries.

The upper body and head are fed from arteries which branch off from the aortic arch before the insertion of the ductus arteriosus and the subsequent mixing of slightly less well-oxygenated blood. The early branching of the coronary and carotid arteries means the heart and brain receive slightly better oxygenated blood. The advantages conferred by the early branching of the subclavian arteries which supply the

Fig. 15.4 *Changes in circulation at birth: A fetal circulation showing oxygen saturation of blood; B neonatal circulation. (Reproduced with permission from Chamberlain et al 1991.)*

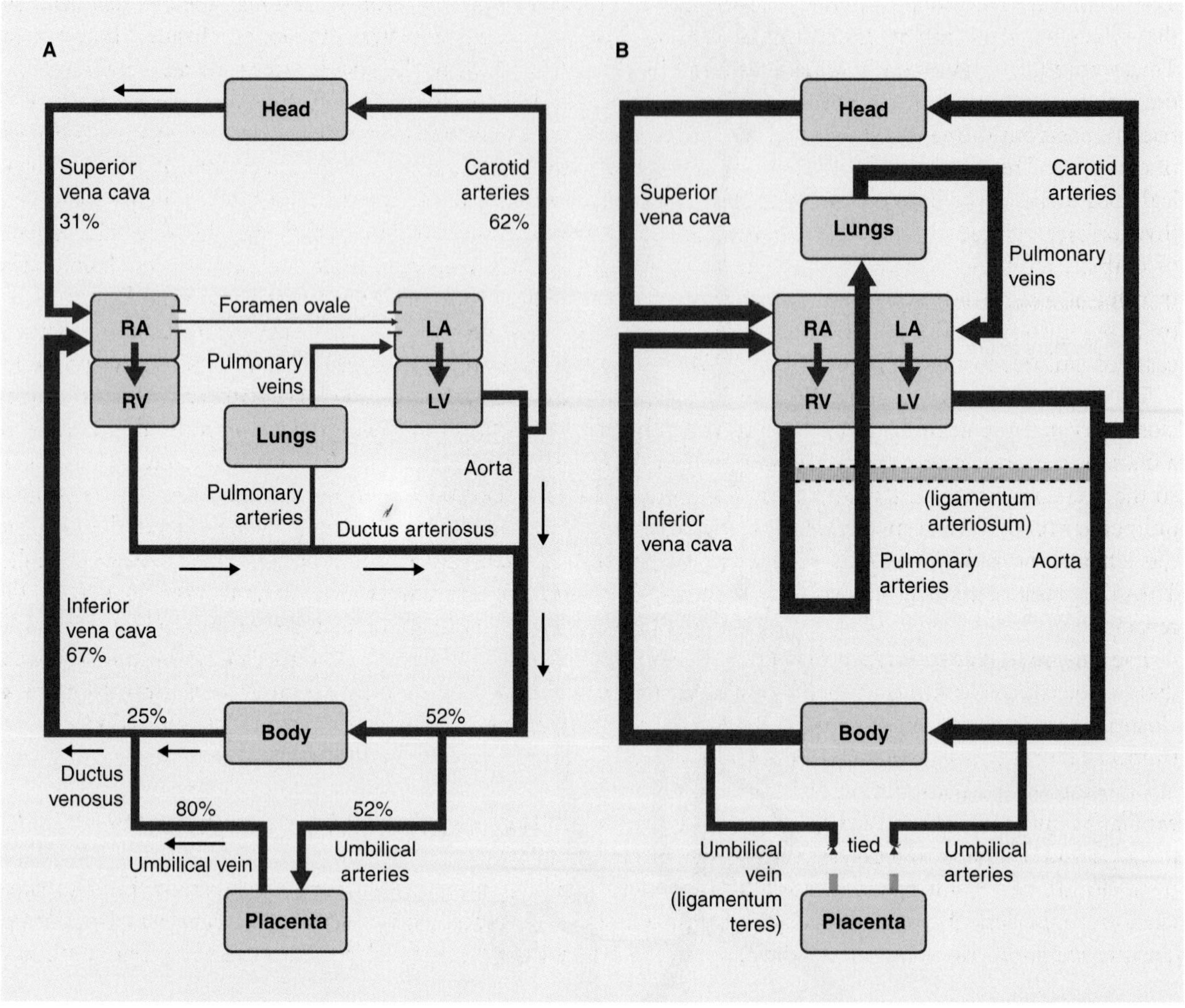


upper limbs can be illustrated by the enhanced development of arms compared to the legs.

## After birth

At birth, the changes that mark the transfer of the fetal into adult-type circulation (see Fig. 15.4B) are not rapid or immediate. They are initiated within 60 seconds of delivery but may not be fully completed for a few weeks. The two determining events that initiate the closure of the fetal shunts are the arrest of the umbilical circulation, and therefore placental perfusion, and the lung inflation and expansion, which results in increased pulmonary blood flow. The first breath results in lung expansion and vasodilatation of the pulmonary vessels in response to increased partial pressure of oxygen. The tortuosity of the capillaries is reduced and the pulmonary circulation changes from a high- to a low-resistance pathway so 90% of the blood flows through the pulmonary vascular bed. There is a brief reversal of flow through the ductus arteriosus, which vasoconstricts in response to the change in oxygen level, mediated by prostaglandins, especially decreased $PGE_2$ (Thorburn 1992).

The smooth muscle of the umbilical artery walls is not innervated but is irritable. Vasoconstriction is stimulated by stretching and handling the cord, by cooling, and in response to stress-related catecholamine release. The thicker walls of the umbilical arteries are able to generate high intraluminal pressure, which arrests the placental circulation, preventing flow from the infant to the placenta. This is augmented by the increased synthesis of prostaglandins and thromboxanes in response to the raised oxygen level due to breathing, which increases vessel irritability and vasoconstriction. The umbilical vein remains dilated; blood flow from the placenta to the infant can continue via gravity. Thus initial neonatal blood volume is affected by the timing of clamping of the umbilical cord and by the relative positions of the infant and placenta at the time of clamping. The usual practice is to clamp the umbilical cord earlier if the baby is subject to fluid overload (hydropic), or if the baby is polycythaemic (e.g. infants of diabetic mothers or growth retarded), to limit the transfer of maternal analgesia agents or antibodies or to avoid possible baby-to-baby transfusions in the cases of multiple births (Kinmond et al 1993).

The flap of the foramen ovale (Fig. 15.5) is pushed closed because the decreased umbilical flow results in a decreased venous return from the inferior vena cava so the pressure in the right atrium falls. The increased pulmonary blood flow results in an increased return to the left atrium and consequent increase in pressure. Thus the pressure gradient across the foramen ovale is reversed.

The closure of the fetal structures may not be immediate or permanent and may never be completed. The closure of the foramen ovale is reversible at first; interruption of ventilation or a drop in alveolar oxygenation results in constriction of the pulmonary capillaries and consequent reversal of pressure across the atria and reversion to fetal circulation. The incomplete closure can result in intermittent and reversible cyanotic episodes. After a few days of functional closure, the tissue associated with the foramen ovale fuses and closure becomes permanent. In many adults, a patent foramen ovale can be demonstrated (a probe can be passed through) although the pressure gradient maintains effective functional closure. Intermittent flow through the ductus arteriosus may initially occur during each cardiac cycle when aortic pressure is maximal following ventricular contraction. Fibrolysis and obliteration of the lumen are usually complete within 8 days; continued patency is very serious and can result in left ventricular failure. The ductus venosus constricts when umbilical flow is halted. The obliterated vessels remain as anatomical ligaments.

The nervous control of the cardiovascular system is well developed in the neonate with mature physiological control of blood pressure and cardiac output demonstrable. The systemic arterial blood pressure is relatively low in the first few weeks as vascular tone develops which increases vascular resistance. Pulmonary arterial blood pressure is initially high but falls to mature values as pulmonary resistance falls. The neonate's heart rate is fast like the fetus. As in the fetus, control of cardiac output is largely achieved by changing heart rate. At birth, the wall of the right ventricle is thicker than the left, which hypertrophies in response to the changed postnatal circulation.

## The respiratory system

The primitive air sacs are developed by the 20th week of gestation, and by 26 weeks, respiratory bronchioles with a rich capillary supply are evident. Although

**Fig. 15.5** *Initiation of neonatal circulation and closure of the foramen ovale between the right atrium (RA) and left atrium (LA).*

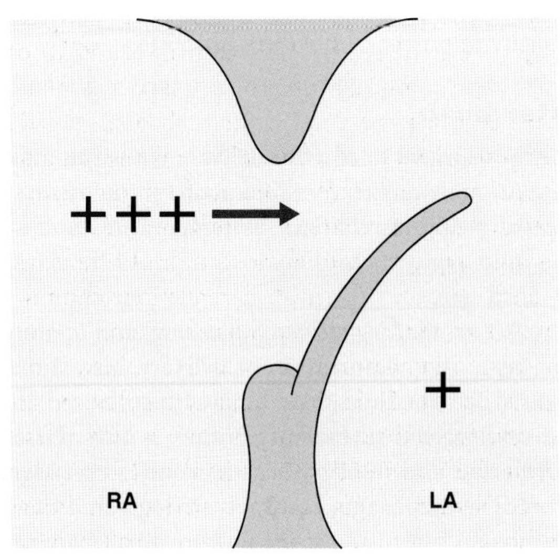


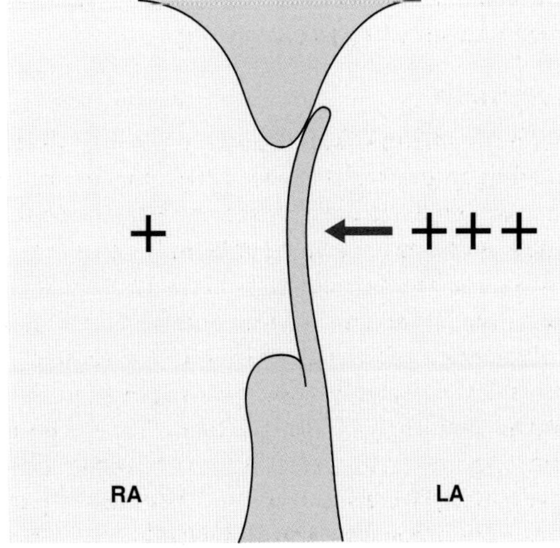

the enzymes for synthesis of phospholipid– lipoprotein components of surfactant are present from week 18, the type II pneumocytes secrete surfactant only from week 26 with a surge in production after week 30. Surfactant, a detergent-like wetting agent, allows increased compliance so the force required to inflate the alveoli is reduced thus increasing compliance. A lack of surfactant causes respiratory distress syndrome (RDS) (see below). The lecithin:sphingomyelin (L:S) ratio of the surfactant can be determined by amniocentesis indicating the maturity of the respiratory system (Fig. 15.6). By week 35 the L:S ratio in a healthily developing fetus is 2:1. This ratio is decreased in pre-eclampsia, prematurity, narcotic addiction, maternal diabetes and other problems in pregnancy. Administration of cortisol (dexamethasone) to the mother prior to delivery of a baby born from 24 to 34 weeks' gestation increases fetal surfactant production within 24 hours and can be used to decrease the risk of RDS (Hutchison 1994). Premature infants may require instillation of exogenous surfactant down endotracheal tubes to alleviate respiratory distress.

**Fig. 15.6** ***Lecithin:sphingomyelin (L:S) concentration in the amniotic fluid—the concentration rises very sharply after 30 weeks' gestation. (Reproduced with permission from Chamberlain et al 1991.)***

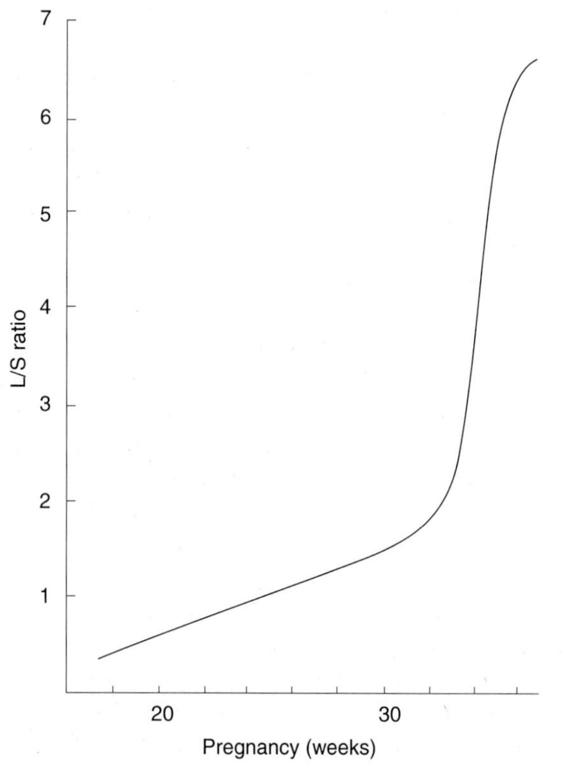


## *The lungs*

### Before birth

In fetal life, the lungs are filled by fluid secreted by the lungs, which exchanges with amniotic fluid. At birth, 10–25 ml/kg fluid will be expelled or resorbed. Fetal breathing movements (FBM) are observed on ultrasound from the first trimester. Initially, they are intermittent, rapid and irregular. As gestation progresses, FBM increase in strength and frequency, occurring up to 80% of the time in an organized pattern (Nijhuis 1986). The lung fluid is 'breathed' out by the fetus into the amniotic fluid; it is thought to promote growth and to allow rehearsal of the respiratory muscles. Patterns of FBM dominate during the daytime and are correlated with fetal behavioural states. Fetal wakefulness and arousal are associated with sustained vigorous respiratory patterns. Quiet sleep is associated with less FBM. Adrenergic and cholinergic compounds, prostaglandin synthesis inhibitors and raised maternal carbon dioxide levels stimulate FBM. They are inhibited by hypoglycaemia, cigarette smoking, alcohol consumption and accelerated labour. Despite the relatively low partial pressure of oxygen and high partial pressure of carbon dioxide, the fetus makes only shallow respiratory movements although severe hypoxia and acidosis may stimulate gasping. Mild hypoxia leads to quiet sleep and reduced energy expenditure and oxygen consumption, which may be protective. The movement of the diaphragm generates about 25 mmHg pressure for between 1 and 4 hours per day in a pattern that coincides with rapid eye movement sleep. FBM are important in lung development (Harding & Hooper 1996), allowing rehearsal of the respiratory actions. The fluid volume in the fetal airways correlates with the functional residual capacity in postnatal life (Strang 1991).

### After birth

The most urgent need after delivery is the initiation of ventilation. Many factors interact to stimulate the first breath, including changes in temperature and state. The mild asphyxia and acidosis induced by clamping the cord sensitizes the medullary chemoreceptors that increase ventilatory drive. Squeezing and manipulation, as in the compression of delivery, also stimulate respiration. The fluid-filled lung with collapsed alveoli and undispersed surfactant proffers a high resistance to inflation and the first breath requires considerable effort. The diaphragm contracts strongly and the flexible ribs and sternum of the newborn baby are pulled concave in the effort of the first breath. Once the lungs are inflated, the lung fluid is rapidly resorbed into the pulmonary lymphatic vessels. Subsequent breaths require less changes in pressure and less mechanical work. The thoracic compression of a vaginal delivery aids fluid loss from the upper respiratory tract. Most babies gasp within 6 seconds and have patterns of normal breathing and gas exchange within 15 minutes. The risk of transient tachypnoea is increased in babies who are delivered by caesarean section or those who experience perinatal hypoxia.

The rate of ventilation of the newborn is high compared with an adult but is similar when relative size is taken into account. Ventilation is often irregular with the baby exhibiting periods of fetal-like shallow breathing. The reflexes associated with lung inflation also appear to be different. As well as the Hering–Breuer reflex (where filling of the lungs increases expiratory centre activity), the newborn infant demonstrates the paradoxical reflex of Head (where filling the lungs excites the inspiratory centre thus stimulating further inspiration) (Petersen 1987). For the first few weeks, babies breathe via the nose and suck via the mouth. Control of ventilation by chemoreceptors is functional but qualitatively different in that hypoxia tends to increase depth of respiration (rather than respiratory rate) and that the response is temperature dependent and is abolished in cold temperatures. The chemoreceptors seem to be more sensitive to raised $CO_2$ levels.

Babies have relatively large oxygen consumption, which reflects their heat generation, and their more metabolically active tissues (for instance, liver and brain) are of proportionally larger size. The high airway resistance means the energy cost of respiration is higher. Pulmonary vascular resistance drops 6–8 weeks after birth when the diameter of the small arterioles increases. The relatively high requirement for oxygen means that neonates are more susceptible to asphyxia than other age groups. Neonatal resuscitation aims to prevent mortality and morbidity. The aims of neonatal resuscitation are to promote and maintain adequate ventilation and oxygenation, to initiate and maintain adequate cardiac output and perfusion and to maintain body temperature and adequate blood glucose levels.

### *Respiratory distress syndrome*

RDS is caused by a deficiency in surfactant, which results in alveolar collapse and increased airway resistance. Surfactant deficiency is usually inversely related to gestational age and lung maturity. Abnormal pH, stress and inadequate pulmonary perfusion also inhibit surfactant synthesis and recycling. RDS is worsened by asphyxia and is the most common cause of respiratory failure in the preterm infant. The reduced surface tension affects alveoli expansion. Small alveoli tend to collapse and normal alveoli are overdistended. Segments of the lung close and hypoxaemia and carbon dioxide retention progressively increase. The resulting metabolic and respiratory acidosis further limits the production of surfactant from the type II pneumocytes. Hypoxaemia causes vasoconstriction of the pulmonary arteries thus compromising pulmonary perfusion and increasing the likelihood of right-to-left shunting through the foramen ovale and ductus arteriosus. Local ischaemic damage affects the alveolar tissue and capillary endothelium. Changes in pulmonary pressure brought about by the infant attempting to maintain adequate air flow, together with the low plasma protein level common in preterm infants, tends to cause displacement of fluid into the alveoli. Fibrinogen in the exudate is converted into fibrin and lines the alveoli thickening the membrane. The thickened membrane and excess fluid increase the diffusion distance and impair gas transfer.

The infant responds to the respiratory difficulties by increasing respiratory rate and effort. The clinical signs appear early and increase in severity over 2 or 3 days. The infant may grunt, and exhibit oedema and cyanosis. Cyanosis tends to be progressive and is due to high levels of deoxygenated haemoglobin in the capillaries. It is enhanced by right-to-left shunting, alveolar hypoventilation and impaired gas diffusion across the alveolar membranes. The baby grunts because expiration is against a partially closed glottis, which increases pressure and retards expiratory flow so increasing gas exchange. RDS risk is increased in prematurity, babies of diabetic mothers (because insulin is antagonistic to cortisol), antepartum haemorrhage and second-born twins. Male babies are twice as susceptible to RDS. Chronic hypertension, maternal heroin addiction, pre-eclampsia and growth retardation appear to protect against RDS.

## Temperature regulation

### *Before birth*

In utero, the fetus depends on its mother for temperature regulation. The fetus is a net heat producer although raised maternal temperature may compromise it (Edwards, Walsh & Li 1997). Research has focused on raised maternal temperature due to fever, exercise and external raised temperature (such as hot baths and saunas). The results are inconclusive. However, maternal fever has effects not only on temperature gradients but also on oxygen consumption and haemodynamics and may be associated with teratogenesis and preterm labour.

### After birth

As environmental temperature is usually less than maternal temperature, the baby will experience a temperature loss at birth. Heat transfer is affected by two gradients: the internal gradient involving transfer from the core to the surface of the baby and the external gradient involving heat transfer from the body surface to the environment. Transfer of heat through the internal gradient depends on insulation and blood flow. Neonates have less subcutaneous fat than adults do (about 16% body fat compared with 30%) and a higher surface area: mass ratio (about three times the relative surface area of an adult). Should the baby be born small, it will not only have an even larger surface area to mass ratio but the insulation provided by its subcutaneous fat will also be further compromised and skin permeability will be increased. Small-for-dates babies have proportionately bigger heads and higher metabolism and are disadvantaged in that their heat losses are higher. Changes in peripheral circulation affect heat loss via conduction.

Heat loss across the external gradient depends on the temperature difference between the body and the environment. Conduction, convection, evaporation and radiation transfer heat from the baby. Warming objects that will come into contact with the neonate, and increasing insulation by wrapping, limit heat loss by conduction. Evaporation offers the greatest route for heat loss immediately after delivery but drying the baby, especially the head, immediately after delivery is effective at reducing the loss. Skin keratinization is inadequate in immature infants so evaporative heat losses are higher. Evaporative insensible heat loss increases with respiratory problems, activity, the use of radiant heaters or phototherapy and low relative humidity. Convective losses are related to draughts and are affected by ambient temperature and humidity. Higher air temperatures, minimal air circulation, swaddling and baby hats reduce heat loss by convection. Radiation is the major form of heat loss from babies in incubators. It involves the transfer of radiant energy to surrounding objects not directly in contact with the baby. Consideration, therefore, has to be given to the temperature of objects in the local environment including the incubator, walls and windows.

The mechanisms of heat conservation and generation mediated by the peripheral nervous system are insufficient in the neonate (Okken 1991). Infants can produce heat from metabolic processes and by increasing activity. Postural changes are also important in conserving heat. Shivering is not so important in infants but heat generation by non-shivering thermogenesis is important. Non-shivering thermogenesis (NST) is carried out in brown adipose tissue (BAT), a specialized type of adipose tissue that is well vascularized and has cells densely packed with mitochondria (Fig. 15.7). Adults have little brown adipose tissue, around the kidneys and great blood vessels, which generates minimal heat. However, 2–7% of the term infant's body weight is BAT, which has a major role in heat production in the neonate. BAT is formed from about 30 weeks gestation until about 4 weeks' post-birth. Stores of BAT are lower in preterm infants. BAT is located in the interscapular and perirenal regions (Fig. 15.8). It generates heat by uncoupling electron transport from oxidative phosphorylation in the mitochondria so the energy released by electron transport will not be used to synthesize ATP but will be liberated as heat instead (Fig. 15.9). Heat production per unit mass of the neonate is higher than an adult; thermogenesis begins when a critical temperature difference of 12°C between the environment and the skin is exceeded. The drop in temperature stimulates release of noradrenaline from sympathetic nerve endings that stimulate the brown adipose cells (Gunn et al 1991). Catecholamines from the adrenal medulla and thyroxine ($T_4$) from the thyroid gland augment the effect of noradrenaline. Oxygen consumption and metabolic rate increase markedly in response to a drop in temperature. Heat generation involves lipolysis of BAT, which depends on the availability of oxygen, ATP and glucose. There is a strong interrelationship between ventilation, feeding and temperature regulation, which means that hypoglycaemia, hypoxia or acidosis can affect the ability of the neonate to produce heat (Fig. 15.10).

Mechanisms for losing heat are not well developed in the neonate (Power 1992). The neonate can lose some heat by sweating (which increases evaporation) but peripheral vasodilatation is the main source of heat loss. Although the density of neonatal sweat glands is high in some areas, they are less responsive and less efficient at sweat production. Phototherapy

**Fig. 15.7** ***Structures and development of white and brown adipose tissue. (Reproduced with permission from Robinson 1994.)***

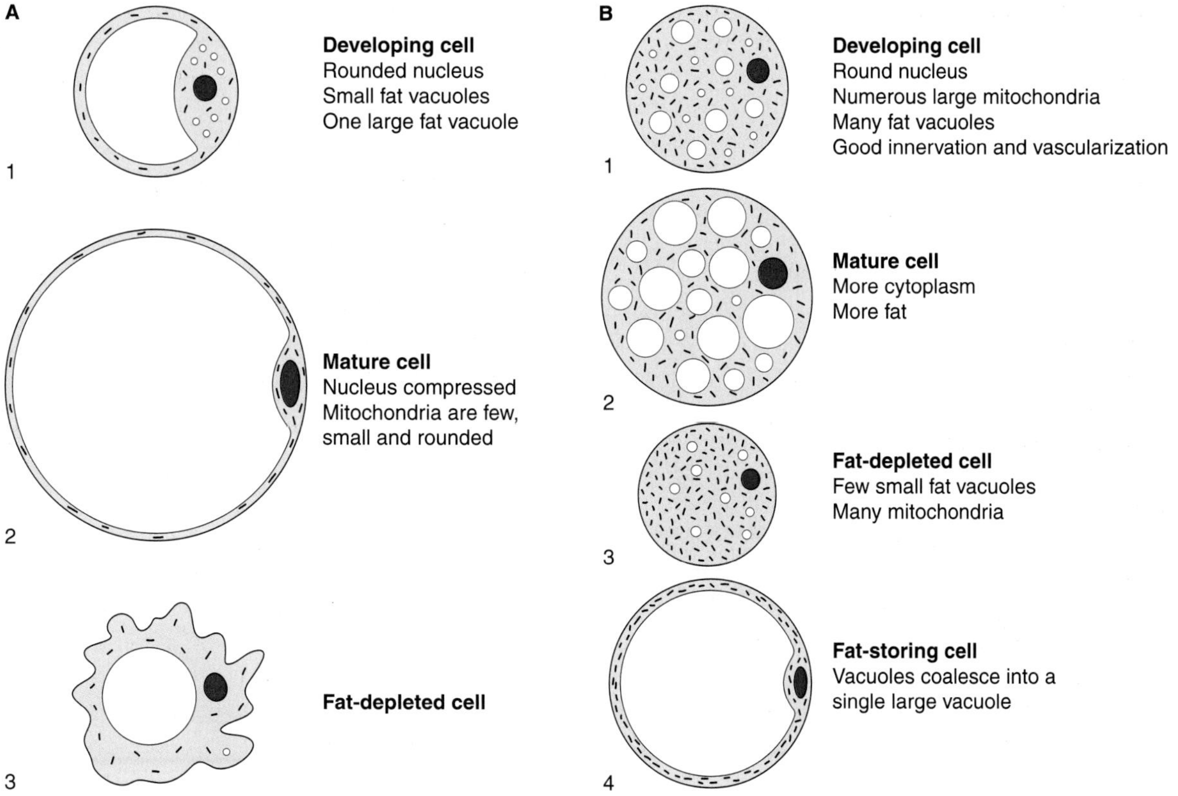

**A**

1

**Developing cell**
Rounded nucleus
Small fat vacuoles
One large fat vacuole

2

**Mature cell**
Nucleus compressed
Mitochondria are few, small and rounded

3

**Fat-depleted cell**

**B**

1

**Developing cell**
Round nucleus
Numerous large mitochondria
Many fat vacuoles
Good innervation and vascularization

2

**Mature cell**
More cytoplasm
More fat

3

**Fat-depleted cell**
Few small fat vacuoles
Many mitochondria

4

**Fat-storing cell**
Vacuoles coalesce into a single large vacuole

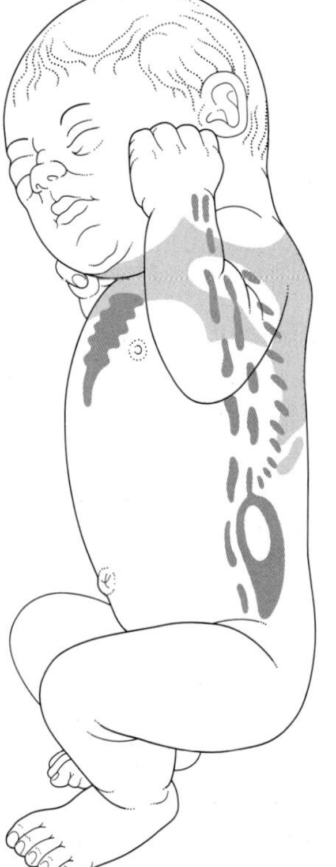

**Fig. 15.8** ***Location of brown adipose tissue in the human infant.***

**Fig. 15.9** *Metabolic pathways in brown adipose tissue: triglycerides break down to yield useful heat (about 160 kcal/mol are produced during each turn of the cycle). (Reproduced with permission from Begley et al 1978.)*

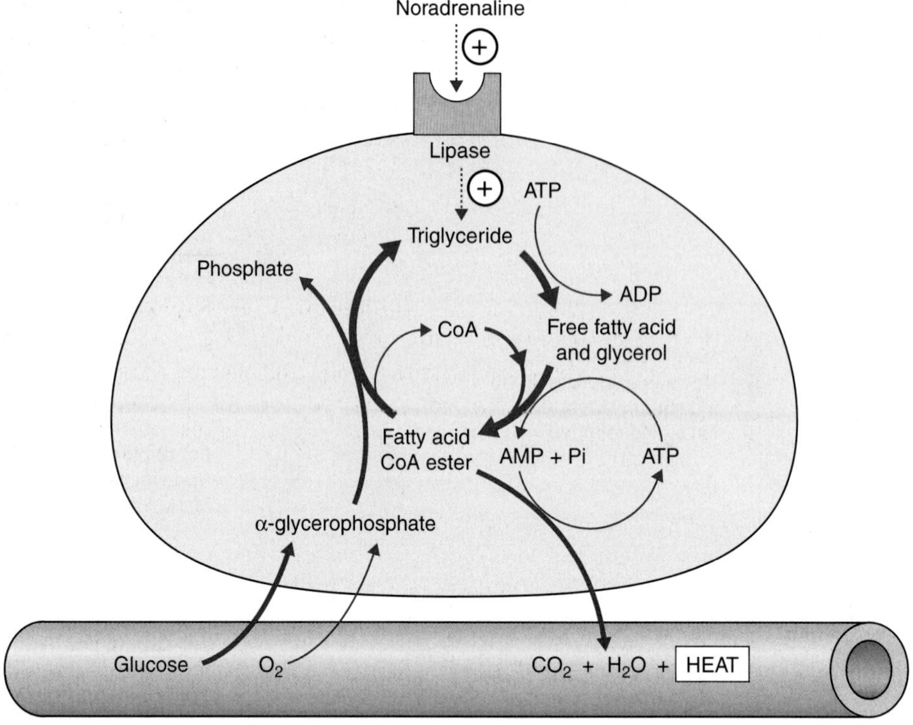


**Fig. 15.10** *Interrelationship between temperature regulation, glucose concentration and respiration.*

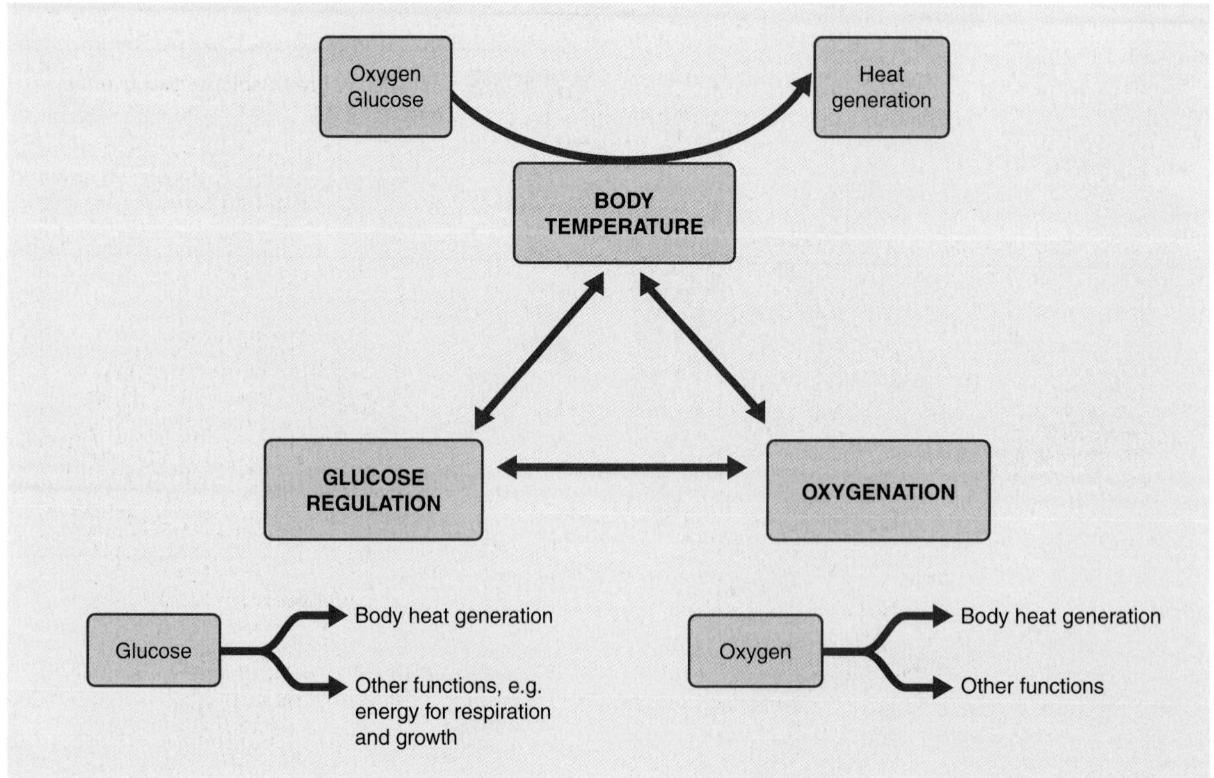

increases water loss. Sweating is more inefficient in preterm babies and those with CNS dysfunction. As the baby gets older and can rely on physical methods of generating heat, NST becomes less important. Brown adipose tissue gradually diminishes in the 1st year.

## The neonatal liver

### Bilirubin

The functions of the neonatal liver are similar to those of an adult but are relatively immature. The abilities to synthesize plasma proteins and to metabolize foreign substances are inefficient. This, together with immature intestinal processes, means the neonate is at increased risk of developing hyperbilirubinaemia (Blackburn 1995). Before birth, bilirubin is cleared by the placenta and then handled by maternal metabolism. If bilirubin accumulates in the neonate, jaundice can occur. As the blood–brain barrier of the neonate is more permeable, free bilirubin can cross easily and in sufficient concentrations can cause kernicterus, resulting in a range of symptoms from convulsions and abnormal behaviour to cerebral palsy, deafness or death.

Bilirubin is a breakdown product of haemoglobin from red blood cells (Fig. 15.11). Iron from red blood cells is recycled. Haeme, the pigment, is degraded by macrophages of the reticuloendothelial system to biliverdin and then bilirubin. Unconjugated (indirect)

**Fig. 15.11** *Breakdown of haemoglobin to form bilirubin.*

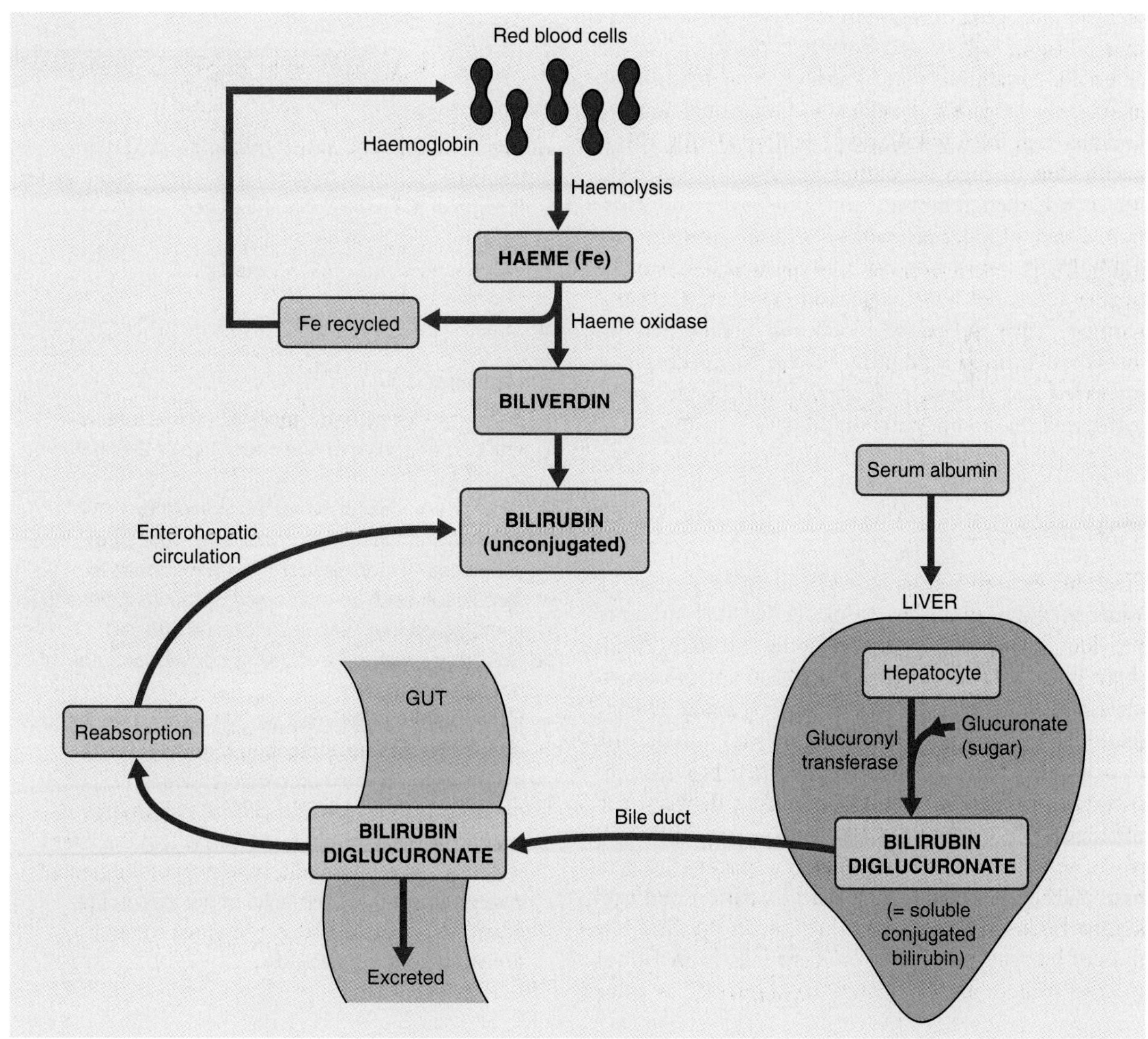

bilirubin is insoluble and cannot be excreted. It is transported bound to plasma albumin to the liver to be metabolized into conjugated (direct) bilirubin, which is soluble. Conjugation involves binding of glucuronide sugars to bilirubin forming bilirubin diglucuronate. Conjugated bilirubin is excreted into bile and so into the intestines. It is a major component of bile and faeces. In the intestine, conjugated bilirubin is further metabolized by bacterial flora to produce urobilin and stercobilin (which give the characteristic colour of faeces). Some of the breakdown products of bacterial metabolism of bilirubin are deconjugated and absorbed across the gut wall to be recirculated. Small amounts of bilirubin are also excreted via the kidneys.

Decreased production of plasma proteins can result in raised unconjugated bilirubin levels. The pathways in the liver that deconjugate bilirubin to its water-soluble, and therefore excretable, metabolite may also be compromised. As meconium is rich in bilirubin, delayed passage of meconium increases the possibility that bilirubin will be deconjugated, absorbed and re-enter the circulating pool. Production of bilirubin in neonates is inversely correlated to gestational age and remains high for a few weeks (Lockitch 1994). This is partly due to high circulating levels of blood cells, which are then removed, and also to having more fragile red blood cells with a shorter lifespan (see Table 15.1 earlier). The risk of hyperbilirubinaemia is further increased by other conditions that stress this pathway such as excess blood cell breakdown (as in excessive trauma at birth or due to infection) or increased red blood cell breakdown (as in polycythaemia due to maternal diabetes).

## Fuel storage

Fetal metabolism is dominated by anabolic pathways, whereas the neonate has to catabolize fuel stores to provide nutrients between periodic neonatal feeds (Hay 1994). The last weeks of gestation are an important time for laying down lipids and glycogen. During fetal life, glycogen is stored in the skeletal muscle and, to a lesser extent, in the liver. Glycogen provides the substrate for energy metabolism during delivery and the first few hours of postnatal life (Nelson 1994). Fat stores serve as an alternative energy source; the neonate markedly increases fatty acid oxidation and uses ketone bodies for energy production. In the first few days of life, the respiratory quotient falls from 1.0 (as glucose sources are exhausted) to about 0.7 (a value similar to that seen in adult diabetics) as fat and protein are mobilized until adequate milk is consumed.

## Glucose regulation

Blood glucose levels in the neonate tend to fall after delivery because the immature liver is better at promoting glycogen synthesis than glycogenolysis, and because the baby has increased activity and metabolism at birth. The large brain and large red blood cell number have a high requirement for glucose. The stress of delivery and cooling at birth stimulate the release of catecholamines, which stimulate glucagon release and suppress insulin release and are important in activating the metabolic pathways in the liver. The neonate is unable to regulate blood glucose efficiently (Smith 1995) and is usually hypoglycaemic (glucose levels are about 2 mmol/l) (Box 15.3). The enzymes

**Box 15.3**

**Risk factors and symptoms of hypoglycaemia**

**Risk factors**

- Hypothermia, evaporation, draughts, cold room
- Babies who do not feed or have a poor response to feeding in the early postnatal period
- Intrauterine growth retardation
- Prematurity
- Maternal diabetes
- Stress

**Symptoms**

- Lethargy: 'floppy baby' (normal muscle tone is reduced to conserve glucose usage of skeletal muscle)
- Drowsiness, difficult to rouse, indicating neurological function is impaired by lack of glucose
- Jitteriness—an adverse tremor in response to stimulation such as loud noise or touch, indicating neurological inhibition of reflexes is affected
- Coldness—may be a cause or consequence of hypoglycaemia
- **Note:** many babies may be hypoglycaemic without clinical symptoms, indicating that they are maintaining normal neurological function by other metabolic pathways. The clinical symptoms indicate these pathways are failing and the infant is at risk. Hypoglycaemic screening of the neonate involves measuring the level of glucose in the infant's blood by analysis of a small amount obtained from a heel prick.

involving glucose metabolism do not reach optimal levels in the liver for 2–3 weeks so glycogenolysis and gluconeogenesis are relatively slow in correcting falls in blood glucose. If the delivery is protracted, the neonate may deplete its glycogen stores. Also the response to raised levels of glucose is slow; although adequate concentrations of insulin are present in the pancreas, the β-cells initially lack sensitivity to glucose, responding better to amino acids. Thus neonatal blood glucose levels fluctuate. Values as low as 1.0 mmol/l have been recorded. In an adult, such a level of hypoglycaemia would cause convulsions, hypoglycaemic coma and probable neurological damage, whereas in the newborn they might cause an apnoeic attack. The central nervous system of the neonate exhibits a degree of plasticity and is partially protected as it can utilize fatty acids and ketones efficiently.

## The gastrointestinal system at birth

The gut completes anatomical development by week 24 and the term neonate is able to digest and absorb milk from birth. Species-specific growth factors in milk are important in promoting postnatal development of the gut. The neonatal gut has immature digestive and absorptive capacities but there are a number of compensatory mechanisms, particularly for babies who are breastfed (Lebenthal & Leung 1988).

### *Feeding reflexes*

From birth, a normal infant can suck from the breast, convey milk to the back of the mouth and swallow it for a period of 5–10 minutes while breathing normally. There is an innate programme of reflexes and behaviour, which become evident within an hour or so following delivery, including the ability to move from the mother's abdomen to her breast, coordinated hand–mouth activity, rooting for the nipple, attaching to the breast and feeding vigorously before falling asleep. Touching the palate triggers the sucking reflex. The neonate exhibits rhythmic jaw action, which creates a negative pressure, and the peristaltic action of the tongue and jaw strips milk from the breast and moves it to the throat thus triggering the swallowing reflex. These breastfeeding reflexes are strong at birth in the normal neonate and are evident in preterm babies from about 32 weeks (about 1200 g). Extremely preterm babies and those that are sick or have a very low birth weight have markedly decreased or absent reflexes. Other babies who experience feeding problems include, for instance, those with physical problems such as cleft lip or palate and those subjected to obstetric sedation, analgesia or extreme stress at birth.

The sucking and swallowing reflexes are aided by the particular morphological configuration of the neonate's mouth, which has a proportionately longer soft palate. The neonate also has an extrusion reflex in response to the presence of solid or semisolid material in the mouth. This reflex is lost at 4–6 months and is replaced by a pattern of rhythmic biting movements coinciding with the development of the first teeth at 7–9 months.

### *Hormone and enzyme production*

Gastric secretion is developed but low; responses to gut regulatory hormones appear also to be low. The effect is that the gastric juice has a pH close to neutral (compared with a pH of 2 in an adult's stomach). The high gastric pH means that salivary amylase is not inactivated in the stomach so starch digestion can continue. Reflux of gastric contents is common, as the lower oesophageal sphincter is immature in both musculature and neurological control. Less acidic gastric juice does not cause painful tissue damage to the oesophageal mucosa but also is less effective at denaturing proteins including microorganisms. It has been suggested that a reflux of human milk is advantageous as very small amounts of milk may reach the upper part of the respiratory tract conferring an immunological benefit there. Breastfed babies have a lower incidence of respiratory problems. Decreased acid production in the stomach means that the activation of pepsinogen to pepsin is restricted, limiting protein digestion in the stomach. The decreased acidity and protein digestion may enhance the defence mechanism promoting the activity of immunoglobulins and antigen recognition in the gastrointestinal tract as these proteins survive the gentler gastric environment.

Pancreatic amylase levels are low in the newborn but breast milk contains mammary amylase, which can augment starch digestion. Colostrum is particularly rich in mammary amylase. Lactase activity is relatively late in developing, reaching adequate levels after 36 weeks' gestation. However, many preterm babies can digest lactose satisfactorily as unabsorbed lactose can be metabolized by colonic bacteria to short-chain fatty acids, which can then be absorbed thus salvaging the energy. The low pancreatic lipase levels are compensated for by lingual and gastric lipase produced by the neonate (stimulated by suckling) and by bile salt-stimulated lipase in human milk. Bile acid formation is low but human milk is rich in taurine, which is used for neonatal conjugation of bile salts.

### *Bowel movements*

Passage of meconium, a mix of mucus, epithelial cells, fatty acids and bile pigments (which gives it the characteristic greenish-black colour), confirms that the lower bowel is patent. Passage of a changing stool (meconium and food residue), usually within 24 hours, indicates the whole gut is patent. At birth, the stomach capacity is 10–20 ml, which rapidly increases to 200 ml by 1 year.

## The kidneys

### *Before birth*

In utero, from 9 to 10 weeks' gestation, the fetus produces large volumes of dilute urine, which is an important source of amniotic fluid (Box 15.4). However, the regulatory and excretory functions of the kidneys are minimal before birth (Guillery 1997). The placenta corrects any osmotic imbalance. Mature kidney function is not developed until about 1 month; until then the urine is fetal-like. The neonatal kidneys, weighing about 12.5 g each, have a low glomerular filtration rate and relatively low surface area. The ability to reabsorb or excrete sodium ($Na^+$) is poor so the urine produced is of low specific gravity and hypotonic reaching 1.5 times plasma concentration (700–800 mOsm) compared to adult values of 3–5 times plasma concentration (1200–1400 mOsm).

**Box 15.4**
**Clinical symptoms of Potter's syndrome**

- Bilateral renal agenesis (absence of kidneys)
- Urine is not excreted into amniotic fluid
- Results in oligohydramnios (defined less than 500 ml of amniotic fluid at term)
- Incidence: about one in 3000 livebirths
- Incompatible with postnatal life; most affected babies die within a few hours of birth
- Causes: pulmonary hypoplasia because of restricted space for thoracic expansion and an imbalance of fluid for filling the lungs; musculoskeletal abnormalities because fetal movement is constrained; abnormal facies because face is moulded by compression; cord compression in labour and fetal distress (Scott & Goodburn 1995)

### *After birth*

At birth, the normal obligatory water loss means the baby loses 5–10% of its birth weight in the first 4 days as a result of the loss of water and $Na^+$ ions. Neonatal renal function can efficiently prevent dehydration and eliminate the lower level of metabolic waste products of the breastfed infant. Changing fluid intake (or increasing the solute load) can result in osmotic imbalance, acidosis or dehydration. The risks are lower if the baby is feeding on demand, however, the very immature renal function of preterm babies requires careful calculation of fluid and electrolyte balance as $Na^+$-rich urine may be produced despite low plasma $Na^+$ levels. This can be crucial if there is high extrarenal water loss, for instance in the presence of fever or high ambient temperature.

The ability to excrete protons or hydrogen ions ($H^+$) is also limited thus increasing the neonate's susceptibility to acidosis. Elimination of drugs such as antibiotics cleared by the renal system is decreased so the half-life of the drug in the circulation is increased necessitating a requirement for decreased frequency of dose. The neonate should urinate within 24 hours of delivery. Initially, 15–30 ml/kg of urine is produced per day increasing to 100–200 ml/kg by day 7 as the fluid intake increases. Mature renal function is not achieved until 12 months to 2 years.

## The nervous system

### *Before birth*

The fetus responds to noises, intense light, noxious stimulation of the skin and decreased temperature by changing autonomic responses such as heart rate and by moving. Fetal movements can be felt from about week 14; the 'exercise' is thought to aid muscle growth and limb development. By term, the nervous system is prepared to process and receive information. Human cortical function is relatively immature compared with that of some other mammalian species. Complete myelination of the long motor pathways occurs after birth, therefore fine movements of the fingers, for instance, are not evident until several months after birth.

### After birth

After birth, the nervous system undergoes accelerated development in response to increased sensory input. Reflexes may be slightly depressed for the first 24 hours, particularly if there has been transplacental transfer of narcotic analgesia, after which several reflexes can be elicited. In cases of severe asphyxia, low Apgar scores (see Examination of the newborn p. 344) or neurological damage, reflexes are depressed and may take longer to appear. The grasping reflex and the Moro embrace are used to assess the reflex ability of the newborn. Babies also demonstrate a strong palmar grasp and a rhythmic stepping movement. Many reflexes common to the neonate disappear unless there is pathological interference, in which case they may be exhibited in the adult. The baby exhibits general awareness to its surroundings and reacts to sound and light.

Babies are born with active sensory pathways (Haith 1986). Studies have demonstrated that neonates can recognize the smell of their mother's milk. They can differentiate between tastes and appear to have a preference for sweet tastes. Although babies can see at birth, there are big postnatal developments in visual capability, particularly in the first 6 months. The neonate has limited visual acuity but appears to focus at a distance of 20 cm. From birth, babies can discriminate between contrast and contours and can follow movement. The neonate is able to hear and discriminate between sounds particularly those of low to middle range frequency. Studies have demonstrated neonates' ability to recognize their mother's voice and to demonstrate a preference for rhythmic sing-song intonation (DeCasper & Fifer 1980). Neonates are reassured by the rhythmic sounds of breathing, heartbeat and gut peristalsis, which they hear, for instance, while being held.

## Sleep and behavioural states

The fetus exhibits slow wave and REM sleep between patterns of wakefulness. The neonate sleeps about 16 hours per day, 40% in REM sleep, compared with a total of 12 hours asleep at 2 years old (20% in REM sleep). Sleep patterns are not diurnal and do not follow a light–dark cycle. Six sleep–wake states are recognized: quiet (deep) sleep, active (light) sleep, drowsy state, awake (quiet) alert, active alert and crying (Wolff 1966). The proportion of time in each state varies with postconceptual age. Quiet deep sleep is restful and the baby is in an anabolic state when growth hormone secretion is high, mitotic rate is high, oxygen consumption is low and there is little movement. In active sleep, the eyes are closed but the baby moves its face and extremities. Respiration and heart rate are irregular. The baby exhibits 'paradoxical' REM sleep, in which the brain activity is similar to awake states. This state is associated with learning and synapse development. The drowsy state is transitional between being awake and asleep. The eyes are open and the baby is alert but has little movement. The baby appears to focus on visual stimuli and appears to be processing sensory information. In the active alert state, respiration rate is increased and is irregular. There are skin colour changes, much activity and the baby has increased sensitivity to stimuli. Crying is the method of communication usually in response to unpleasant stimuli. Characteristically, neonates close their eyes, grimace and make sounds. However, preterm infants may not be capable of making a noise.

At one time, it was believed that the immature degree of myelination and lack of experience meant that neonates were unable to perceive pain. The anatomical and functional requirements for pain perception are developed early and the neonate demonstrates similar physiological responses to the adult (Porter 1989). Catecholamine and cortisol release increases, heart rate and respiration rates change, metabolic rate and oxygen consumption increase and blood glucose levels rise. The rate of transmission may be slower but a probable shorter distance between the pain receptor and brain compensates for this. Assessment of pain can be difficult as pain may be expressed differently; facial expressions may be used but some babies tend to withdraw and increase passivity and sleep patterns in response to pain.

## The skin and immune system

The skin of a neonate appears relatively transparent and soft and velvety. It is important in temperature regulation, as a barrier and as a sensory organ. Part of the appearance is due to the lack of large skin folds and localized oedema. Melanin production and pigmentation are low in the newborn so the skin is vulnerable to damage by ultraviolet rays. However, residual levels of maternal and placental hormones can produce transient pigmentation of certain skin areas. During delivery, the skin is subject to changes in blood flow and mechanical stress from the pressure of contractions and from maternal structures that can result in abrasions and ischaemia. Obstetric interventions, for example fetal monitoring, scalp sampling, and use of amnio-hooks, forceps and vacuum extraction also compromise the integrity of the skin. Immediately after birth, most fair-skinned babies have a characteristic pink coloration with blue but warm extremities.

Vernix caseosa is a superficial fatty substance that coats the fetal skin from the middle of gestation and decreases in amount in direct relation to gestational maturity. Lanugo is the first generation of downy body hair that is fine and unpigmented; it appears from the 12th week and is mostly shed before birth. Vernix caseosa tends to accumulate at the sites of dense lanugo growth and is evident on the preterm baby on the face, ears and shoulders and in folds. At term, traces of vernix are present on the brow, ears and in the skin creases. Vernix caseosa is composed of sebaceous gland secretion and skin cells and is rich in triacylglycerides, cholesterol and fats. Its role is to protect the fetus from the amniotic fluid and to prevent loss of water and electrolytes. It provides insulation for the skin and helps to reduce friction at delivery.

The barrier properties of the stratum corneum of the skin increase with increased gestational age, especially after 24 weeks (Rutter 1996). The epidermis of a preterm baby might be only five layers thick compared with about 15 layers in a term infant. A thinner epidermal layer results in increased transepidermal water loss, decreased ability to cope with friction, thermal instability because of the increased blood supply to the surface and increased permeability to microorganisms and chemicals (such as topically applied substances and reagents on clothes). Premature babies have translucent shiny red skin that becomes pinker through to the white thick skin of term infants. Drying out of the skin is a normal maturation process. Substances that interfere with the keratinization process, such as emollients, can delay the development of the skin becoming effective as a barrier. The transepidermal water loss can be limited by use of a thermal blanket, altering the air flow and maintaining an insulating layer of saturated air in contact with the skin.

The neonate is a compromised host, vulnerable to nocosomial (cross) infection. Host defence mechanisms are immature, partly because of lack of previous exposure to common organisms and partly because the neonate has limited cellular responses (see Ch. 10). Breaks in the delicate mucosa and skin from delivery and invasive obstetric procedures provide opportunities for the entry of pathogenic bacteria. In relation to artificial feeding, neonates are at increased risk of developing gastrointestinal infections, which may be associated with later development of allergies. Preterm infants, especially those of less than 34 weeks' gestation, are very vulnerable as they have less maternal IsG transfer. At birth, the neonate leaves the sterile fetal environment for one loaded with microorganisms (Jarvis 1996). Ingestion and inhalation provide routes for bacterial colonization after birth, initially with organisms derived from the maternal genital tract. The neonate's skin, umbilical cord and genitalia are colonized first, followed by the face, respiratory system and gut. Skin flora is increased in infants with little vernix caseosa and is limited by antiseptic agents and alkaline soaps. Initially gut colonization is with organisms that the infant comes into contact with at and immediately after delivery. The profile of organisms is affected by the diet; breastfed babies have optimal conditions for the growth of the protective lactobacilli and bifidobacterium. Different patterns are seen in babies of very low birth weight and those who require feeding or ventilatory assistance. Meconium in vivo is usually sterile but when excreted provides rich culture conditions for microorganisms. The use of antibiotics changes the pattern of bacterial colonization of the neonate and can encourage the growth of resistant bacteria.

Case study 15.1 is an example of neonatal infection.

## Examination of the newborn

After delivery, the baby is always examined by a midwife who in accordance with professional legislative requirement must refer any deviation from the normal to a medical practitioner. There is a statutory requirement to document findings.

### *The Apgar score*

The baby's condition, including mental and physical development and level of awareness, is assessed using the Apgar score (Table 15.2).

**Case study 15.1**

During a routine visit, the midwife examines Tracy, a 3-day-old baby, who was delivered in hospital and discharged the day before. Her umbilicus appears moist and sticky so the midwife takes a swab for culture and sensitivity. Two days later it is revealed that Tracy's umbilicus has been colonized with methicillin-resistant *Staphylococcus aureus* (MRSA). The infant appears well, has been exclusively breastfed and has regained her birth weight.

- What treatment, if any, would Tracy require and what reasons could be applied to argue against the use of antibiotic therapy?
- Do you think it is necessary to try and identify the source of the infection?
- What should the midwife do to ensure that further cross-infections do not occur?
- What factors may put other individuals at risk?

Although the interpretative value of the Apgar score has been questioned, it is a means of assessing a baby for the absence or presence and degree of birth asphyxia. It is quick and simple and no other test has been routinely adopted. The Apgar test scores the baby's heart rate, respiratory effort, colour, muscle tone and reflex responses at 1 and 5 minutes following birth. It is repeated at 5-minute intervals when active resuscitation measures are undertaken. The 1-minute score may be low as the baby has been subjected to physical stress including a drop in temperature. Dark-skinned babies are assessed out of a total score of 8 omitting evaluation of skin colour.

Measurement of heart rate can be done by palpating the heart via the anterior chest wall or listening to the heart with a stethoscope. A heart rate of 110–150 beats per minute is considered normal. A baby who is crying is obviously breathing in order to produce sound. Breathing can be seen easily even on quiet babies. The respiratory rate of a healthy newborn baby is about 40–60 breaths per minute and should not be punctuated by grunting. A high-pitched or irritable cry may indicate brain damage or cerebral irritation due to oedema or haemorrhage.

The colour of the mucous membranes inside the mouth and the eye lids is assessed. If the blood flow is good, as in a healthy baby, these areas will be pink. If the tissues are being deprived of oxygen, they appear purplish or navy blue if the deprivation is severe. Healthy babies often appear bluish at the extremities but this is may be due to cold rather than poor circulation. The face may appear congested if the cord was around the neck or if pressure from the delivery was prolonged. Pale babies may be anaemic and polycythaemic babies (with an excess of red blood cells) tend to look very red.

The rooting reflex, turning of the head towards a touch on the cheek, is noted. Alternative reflexes include the baby curling the toes if the sole of the foot is stroked or responding with a grabbing movement if the palm of the hand is stroked (palmar grasp reflex). Abnormal responses such as the toes curling upwards are often associated with abnormalities. The Moro reflex is looked for by startling the baby. If the head is allowed to drop back a few centimetres, the baby responds by flinging the arms outwards, usually accompanied by crying.

Muscle tone is more difficult to assess. All newborn babies have poorly developed musculature and seem fairly floppy but babies who are especially floppy because they have immature coordination do not resist limb movement. Healthy babies have flexed limbs and respond to handling; the normal procedure is to lie the

**Table 15.2** *Apgar score*

| | 0 | 1 | 2 |
|---|---|---|---|
| Heart rate | Absent | Slow (<100 b.p.m.) | Fast (>100 b.p.m.) |
| Respiratory effort | Absent | Irregular, slow | Regular, cry |
| Muscle tone | Limp | Some flexion in limbs | Well-flexed limbs |
| Reflex irritability | Nil | Grimace | Cough, cry |
| Colour | White, blue | Body pink, extremities blue | Completely pink |

baby on the midwife's hand resting on its stomach and to observe position of the limbs.

A baby that needs urgent resuscitation is pale and floppy, has a sluggish pulse and makes no respiratory effort. This is apparent and needs immediate response without having to calculate the Apgar score first. The Apgar score indicates the baby's capability to survive without intervention. If the Apgar score is above 7, little intervention is required but a baby with an Apgar score of 5–7 will often need suction and oxygen via a face mask. A score of 3–5 usually requires administration of oxygen via an 'Ambu' bag and a lower score requires immediate active treatment.

Case study 15.2 is an example of a baby possibly in need of resuscitation.

**Case study 15.2**

Paul is only 10 seconds old. He appears blue, not moving, limp and does not respond to touch. The midwife summons help and a paediatrician is called. The paediatrician arrives 4 minutes later to find a healthy, well-perfused infant, crying whilst being held by his mother.

- Was the midwife justified in being cautious by summoning a paediatrician early?
- How many midwives in practice wait a full minute before their initial assessment of the newborn?

## Body measurements and inspection

Once these tests are completed, further examination of the newborn can take place. An initial development check is followed by a paediatric check 24 hours later. The baby's weight, length and head circumference are measured and recorded. Babies with birth weights above the 90th centile or below the 10th centile have an increased risk of becoming hypoglycaemic. Examination of the genitalia allows assignation of the sex of the baby. In male infants, the scrotum is felt for the presence of both testes and the position of the urethral exit on the penis is checked. In female babies, the vaginal and urethral orifices are inspected. Presence of meconium demonstrates patency of the anus; this may become evident on rectal temperature measurement.

Moulding of the head and oedema of the scalp are common at birth because of the pressure imposed by the birth canal (see Ch. 13). The normal term infant is well endowed with subcutaneous fat and usually has vernix caseosa in the skin folds. Postmature babies may have dry and peeling skin. The fontanelles and suture lines are observed. Bulging fontanelles may indicate an increased pressure and sunken fontanelles that the baby is dehydrated. An abnormal-shaped head indicates abnormal moulding (see Ch. 13). Eyes and ears are checked for abnormalities; the eyes should be clear and free from discharge. Low-set, absent or deformed ears may be associated with chromosomal abnormalities. The baby's mouth is inspected for the presence of teeth, which can be removed, or other extraneous material. Both the soft and hard palate are checked; the baby should demonstrate a sucking reflex. Minor skin blemishes are common. Hypertrophic sebaceous glands or milia present as white spots on about 40% babies. Both these spots and 'stork marks'—minor capillary haemangiomas—usually on the nose or eye lids, disappear within a few months of delivery.

The overall morphology of the baby should be symmetrical. The insertion of the umbilicus should be central, and is checked for swellings. The nipples, of either male or female babies, may be swollen and producing milk in response to maternal hormones circulating. Respiratory movement of the chest of a healthy baby is symmetrical and the abdomen is rounded. The limbs are checked for equal length and free movement; short limbs can indicate achondroplasia. The digits are counted; extra digits and webbing between the digits are relatively common. The feet and ankles are examined for talipes and other abnormalities.

Visible signs of congenital dislocation of the hips (CDH) are asymmetry of the pelvis, asymmetrical creases in the groin and apparent differences in leg length. Midwives may be discouraged from undertaking manipulative tests of the hips as there is a danger of malpositioning the head of the femur into the acetabular cup, which can trap the femoral blood flow resulting in necrosis of the head of the femur. Midwifery units usually have local policies and protocols for the screening of hips for congenital dislocation.

The neck is observed for shortness, webbing or folds of skin on the back of the neck; these characteristics are associated with chromosomal abnormalities, such as Turner's syndrome. The spine is checked for swellings or defects and for pilonidal dimples or hairy patches, which may indicate occult spina bifida. Before the baby is discharged from the postnatal ward, there should be confirmation that the baby is feeding normally; excretion of urine and meconium normally occurs within 24 and 48 hours of delivery respectively. Early screening is important both to reassure the parents and to detect any abnormality or problem requiring further investigation.

## Key points

- Many changes must occur at birth for successful transition to neonatal life including initiation of breathing, conversion from fetal to neonatal circulation and physiological homeostatic control of thermoregulation and metabolism.
- The transition to neonatal circulation requires closure of the fetal shunts and vasodilatation of the pulmonary circulation; oxygen is a major stimulant.
- Successful breathing requires adequate maturation of the lungs, particularly the presence of adequate surfactant and neuromuscular control, and clearance of lung fluid.
- The relatively large surface area of neonates means they are vulnerable to excessive heat loss; body temperature is maintained by non-shivering thermogenesis. Efforts to reduce heat loss at birth are essential.
- Normal newborn infants are able to maintain adequate blood sugar levels; this can be compromised by a stressful labour, a shortened third trimester and abnormal maternal metabolism.
- Human milk and early physiological conditions compensate for the immature development of the neonatal gut.

## Application to practice

An understanding of the transition to neonatal life is important for the following reasons. Many infants require some degree of intervention to enable establishment of respiration after birth. An infant who does not appear to adapt fully at birth (i.e. is cyanotic) may have an underlying cardiac defect.

The midwife should use her assessment of adaptation as part of the neonatal check and not solely check for visible abnormalities.

Many parents are distressed at the appearance of a baby that has just been born and need reassurance that the transition is not always completely spontaneous and that this is quite normal.

## Annotated further reading

Blackburn S T, Loper D L 1992 Maternal, fetal, and neonatal physiology: a clinical perspective. W B Saunders, Philadelphia

*An in-depth description of physiological adaptation to pregnancy and consequent development of the fetus and neonate that draws from physiological research studies. The chapters are clearly organized by physiological systems and link physiological concepts to clinical applications including the assessment and management of low- and high-risk pregnancies.*

Henderson C, Jones K (eds) 1997 Essential midwifery. C V Mosby, London

*A research-based midwifery textbook covering biological, social and psychological aspects of midwifery care applied to conception, pregnancy, infancy and development of the family. It has a holistic approach, integrates theory and practice well and includes factors influencing midwifery such as politics.*

Lowe N K, Reiss R 1996 Parturition and fetal adaptation. Journal of Gynaecology and Neonatal Nursing 25:339–349

*This article focuses on how the process of labour facilitates the fetus in the transition to extrauterine existence.*

Polin R A, Fox W W (eds) 1992 Fetal and neonatal physiology. W B Saunders, Philadelphia

*This text provides a comprehensive description of normal and abnormal physiology of the fetus and neonate, stressing developmental aspects and the clinical significance of abnormal physiology including pathophysiology of neonatal disease.*

Rennie J M, Robertson N R C (eds) 1999 Textbook of neonatology, 3rd edn. Churchill Livingstone, New York

*This is a comprehensive reference book covering care of the normal neonate and the pathophysiology, diagnosis and management of disorders in the newborn.*

Silver R A, Soll R F 1976 Physiological adaptation at birth. In: Hillier S G, Kitchener H C, Neilson J P (eds) Scientific essentials of reproductive medicine. W B Saunders, Philadelphia

*This chapter, from a textbook focusing on molecular and cellular fundamentals of reproductive biology, provides a comprehensive guide to the physiological basis of neonatal transition to extrauterine life.*

Sinclair J C, Bracken M B (eds) 1992 Effective care of the newborn infant. OUP, Oxford

*This book provides an invaluable review of the research evidence on the effects of the various care practices carried out during pregnancy, childbirth and the early days after birth.*

## References


Andrew M 1997 The relevance of developmental hemostasis to hemorrhagic disorders of newborns. Seminars in Perinatology 21:70–85

Begley D J, Firth J A, Hoult J R S 1978 Human reproduction and developmental biology. Macmillan, New York, pp 160, 199

Blackburn S 1995 Hyperbilirubinaemia and neonatal jaundice. Neonatal Network 14:15–25

Bernal A L, Watson S P, Phaneuf S, Europe-Finner G N 1993 Biochemistry and physiology of preterm labour and delivery. Bailliere's Clinics in Obstetrics and Gynaecology 7:523–552

Chamberlain G, Dewhurst J, Harvey D 1991 Illustrated textbook of obstetrics. Gower Medical (Mosby), London, pp 14, 15, 16

DeCasper A J, Fifer W P 1980 Of human bonding: newborns prefer their mother's voices. Science 208:1174

Edwards M J, Walsh D A, Li Z 1997 Hyperthermia, teratogenesis and the heat shock response in mammalian embryos in culture. International Journal of Developmental Biology 41:345–358

Golding J, Greenwood R, Birmingham K, Mott M 1992 Childhood cancer, intramuscular vitamin K and pethidine given during labour. British Medical Journal 305:341–346

Goodwin B 1997 Health and development: conceptions to birth. Open University, Milton Keynes, p 259

Guillery E N 1997 Fetal and neonatal nephrology. Current Opinion in Pediatrics 9:148–153

Gunn T R, Ball K T, Power G G, Gluckmann P 1991 Factors influencing the initiation of nonshivering thermogenesis. American Journal of Obstetrics and Gynecology 164(1 pt 1):210–217

Haith M M 1986 Sensory and perceptual processes in early infancy. Journal of Pediatrics 109:158

Harding R, Hooper S B 1996 Regulation of lung expansion and lung growth before birth. Journal of Applied Physiology 81:209–224

Hay W Jr 1994 Placental supply of energy and protein substrates to the fetus. Acta Paediatrica (Suppl) 405:13–19

Hilgartner M 1993 Vitamin K and the newborn. New England Journal of Medicine 329:957

Hutchison A A 1994 Respiratory disorders of the neonate. Current Opinion in Pediatrics 6:142–153

Jarvis W R 1996 The epidemiology of colonisation. Infection Control and Hospital Epidemiology 17:47–52

Kinmond S, Aitchison T C, Holland B M, Jones J G, Turner T L, Wardrop C A 1993 Umbilical cord clamping and preterm infants: a randomised trial. British Medical Journal 306:172–175

Kuehl J 1997 Neonatal disseminated intravascular coagulation. Journal of Perinatal and Neonatal Nursing 11:69–77

Lamvu G, Kuller J A 1997 Prenatal diagnosis using fetal cells from the maternal circulation. Obstetrics and Gynecology Survey 52:433–437

Lebenthal E, Leung Y K 1988 Feeding the premature and compromised infant: gastrointestinal considerations. Pediatric Clinics of North America 35:215

Lockitch G 1994 Beyond the umbilical cord: interpreting laboratory tests in the neonate. Clinical Biochemistry 27:1–6

Nelson N 1994 Physiology of transition. In: Avery G B, Fletcher M A, MacDonald M G (eds) Neonatology, pathophysiology and management of the newborn, 4th edn. Lippincott, Philadelphia, pp 223–247

Nijhuis J G 1986 Behavioural states: concomitants, clinical implications and the assessment of the condition of the nervous system. European Journal of Obstetrics, Gynecology and Reproductive Biology 21:301–308

Oh W 1986 Neonatal polycythemia and hyperviscosity. Pediatric Clinics of North America 33:528

Okken A 1991 Postnatal adaptation in thermoregulation. Journal of Perinatal Medicine 19 (suppl 1):67–73

Parer J T 1998 Effects of fetal asphyxia on brain cell structure and function: limits of tolerance. Comparative Biochemistry and Physiology A. Molecular Integrated Physiology 119:711–716

Petersen E S 1987 The control of breathing pattern. In: Whipp B J (ed) The control of breathing in man. Manchester University Press, Manchester, pp 1–28

Porter F 1989 Pain in the newborn. Clinics in Perinatology 16:549

Power G G 1992 Fetal thermoregulation: animal and human. In: Polin R A, Fox W W (eds) Fetal and neonatal physiology. W B Saunders, Philadelphia, p 447

Robinson D (ed) 1994 Temperature and exercise. (Book 2 of S324 Animal physiology). Open University, Milton Keynes, p 96

Rutter N 1996 The immature skin. European Journal of Pediatrics 155 (suppl 2):s18–20

Scott R J, Goodburn S F 1995 Potter's syndrome in the second trimester: prenatal screening and pathological findings in 60 cases of oligohydramnios sequence. Prenatal Diagnosis 15:519–525

Smith S L 1995 Hypoglycaemia in the neonate. In: Alexander J, Levy V, Roch S (eds) Aspects of midwifery practice: a research-based approach. Macmillan, Basingstoke, pp 154–176

Strang L B 1991 Fetal lung liquid: secretion and reabsorption. Physiological Review 71:991–1016

Strauss R G 1994 Erythropoietin and neonatal anemia. New England Journal of Medicine 330:1227–1228

Strickberger M W 1968 Genetics. Macmillan, New York

Thorburn G D 1992 The placenta, $PGE_2$ and parturition. Early Human Development 29:63–73

Wolff P H 1966 The causes, controls and organization of behaviour in the neonate. Psychological Issues 5 (monogram 1):1

# 16 Lactation and infant nutrition

## Learning objectives

- To describe the anatomical structure of the breast.
- To outline the hormonal control of lactation.
- To describe how the physiology of lactation can be applied clinically.
- To describe the mechanisms of milk secretion.
- To discuss maternal adaptations during lactation: the effects on fertility, maternal behaviour and nutritional requirements.
- To explain why breastfeeding provides optimal nutrition of the neonate.
- To describe the non-nutritional advantages of breast milk.

## Introduction

Infant feeding is the result of a complex interaction between infant nutritional demand and maternal physiology. The physiological basis of lactation is important in understanding and facilitating successful breastfeeding. Despite increased awareness of the health benefits of human milk, many women discontinue breastfeeding because they perceive that they have insufficient milk supply. Most breastfeeding problems have an identifiable physiological, rather than a pathological, cause and are best addressed by considering the interaction between the mother and baby. Successful breastfeeding has nutritional, emotional, developmental and economic benefits. It can be argued that the nutrient requirement of the infant is one of the best understood areas of nutrition. Human milk, however, does not just provide the optimal balance of nutrients in a form appropriate to the developmental needs of the infant, it also compensates for the immature digestive capability and vulnerable immune status of the neonate.

## Anatomy of the breast

The tissue of the breast extends from about the second to the sixth rib (depending on posture). The extension of the tail of the tissue into the axilla (Fig. 16.1) can result in discomfort in the early puerperium when it may become swollen. The main constituents of the breast are glandular cells with associated ducts and a variable amount of adipose tissue and connective tissue. The breast is divided into sections or lobes by fibrous septae, which run from behind the nipple towards the pectoralis muscle. These septae are important in localizing infections, which are often visually evident as a wedge of red inflamed skin on the surface of the breast. Each of the 15 to 20 lobes, separated by connective tissue, contains glandular tissue arranged

**Fig. 16.1** *The position of the breast.*

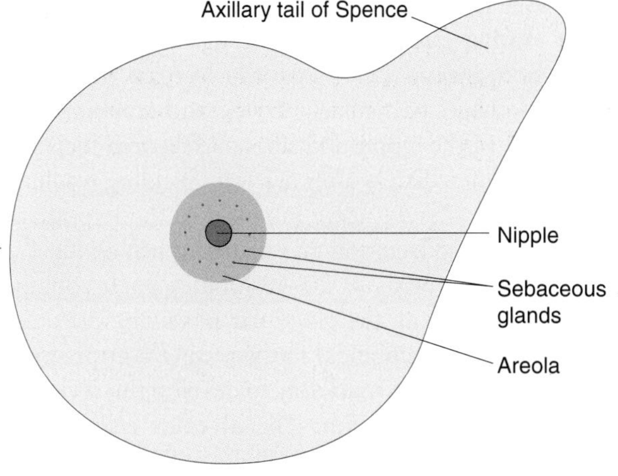

**Fig. 16.2** *The ductal–alveolar system of the breast arranged in lobes. (Reproduced with permission from Pond 1992.)*

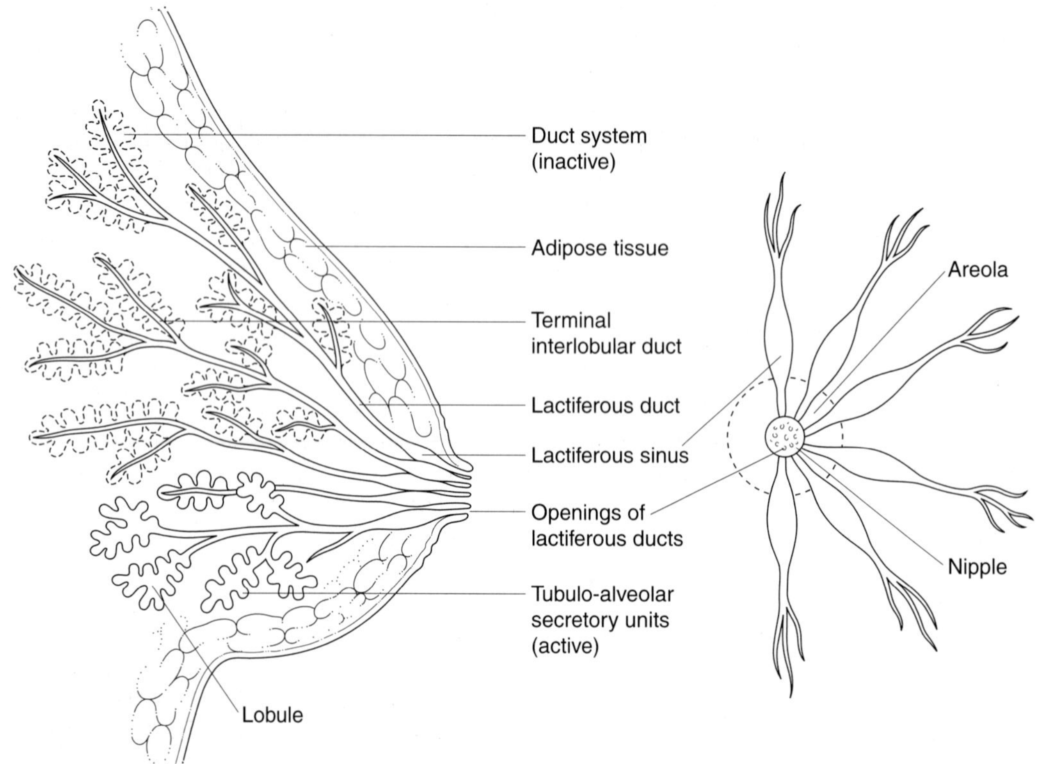


as a ductal–alveolar system (Fig. 16.2). The alveolar secretory cells are grouped in grape-like lobules around an extensive branching system of ducts, which join to form the main lactiferous ducts leading to the nipple. The lactiferous ducts dilate into the ampulla, or sinus, immediately at the base of the nipple and open to the exterior via the ejectory ducts.

The nipple is surrounded by the areola, a pigmented area of varying size, which darkens during pregnancy and has rich vascular supply and sensory nerve inputs. Surrounding the nipple are Montgomery's tubercles—sebaceous glands that hypertrophy and become prominent during pregnancy, providing lubrication and protection. Heavy use of soap can increase the risk of nipple damage, particularly drying and cracking. The sensitivity of the nipple and surrounding area increases markedly immediately after delivery. Suckling results in an influx of afferent nerve impulses to the hypothalamus controlling lactation and maternal behaviour.

Each lobe consists of 20–40 lobules, each containing 10–100 alveoli, the glandular physiological units. Alveolar cells are cuboidal in the resting non-pregnant breast and change remarkably to develop full secretory features during lactation. The alveolar cells secrete milk into the lumen of the small ducts. These secretory cells are surrounded by oxytocin-sensitive myoepithelial (contractile) cells, which are important in milk ejection. The ducts are also lined by contractile cells that open the ducts widely during the milk ejection reflex to assist flow.

## Breast growth and development

Mammary growth and development can be divided into four phases: resting, development (pregnancy), milk secreting (lactation) and involution. At birth, the structure is simply the nipple and a few rudimentary ducts, with few or no alveoli reflecting their evolutionary origin of modified apocrine sweat glands. Until puberty, the only degree of development may be a little branching of the ducts. There is a decreased incidence of breast cancer in populations with a high consumption of phyto-oestrogens (oestrogen-like compounds derived from plants). It is suggested that the phyto-oestrogens stimulate development of the mammary cells in childhood and puberty before pregnancy; these well-differentiated cells may be more resistant to tumour formation (Adlercreutz 1995).

The human is unusual, even when compared with other primates, in the major degree of development at puberty, rather than at pregnancy, resulting in an erotic significance. During puberty the proliferation of the milk ducts, which sprout and branch, is primarily dependent on secretion of oestrogen with further contributions from growth hormone and adrenal hormones. The modest alveolar development at this stage is stimulated by progesterone, providing the tissue has been primed by oestrogen. Prolactin may also play a role although the interaction between the adrenal and pituitary glands and the ovaries is not fully understood. The hormonal fluctuations of the menstrual cycle give repeated exposure of the tissue to oestrogen and progesterone, which allow additional but limited growth. Many non-pregnant women experience cyclical changes, especially premenstrually, in breast volume, which is associated with water retention. However, some secretory activity may occur within the alveoli and a mammary secretion may be expressed premenstrually.

Once an adult woman has developed breasts, minimal stimulation is required to begin milk secretion (Box 16.1). The hormones required for breast development during pregnancy are less than those required for other species. In humans, neither hPL nor GH is essential.

In early pregnancy, breast size and areolar pigmentation increases. The tubercles of Montgomery enlarge and the nipples become more erect. Blood flow to the breast doubles so blood vessels become more prominent and the skin may appear to have a translucent marbled appearance. There is a sharp increase in ductal and glandular elements so the breasts tend to feel slightly lumpy in early pregnancy. This initial hyperplasia is followed by alveolar cell hypertrophy and initiation of secretory activity in later pregnancy.

Oestrogen plays the dominant role in development of the ducts and progesterone in the development in glandular tissue, although insulin and other growth factors (such as EGF and TGFα) have a role in regulation. Changes in pregnancy depend on the lactogenic hormones, prolactin and human placental lactogen with placental oestrogen and progesterone playing important modulatory roles. Under these hormonal influences, prominent lobules form in the breast so the alveolar lumen becomes dilated by mid pregnancy and the secretory cells fully differentiated (Box 16.2). The areola becomes pigmented and a secondary patchily pigmented areola may develop. By the 4th month of pregnancy, the epithelial cells accumulate substantial amounts of secretory material and the mammary glands are fully developed. Prolactin levels progressively increase throughout the pregnancy and are maximal at term. Full milk production is inhibited by high steroid levels so copious milk production is not established until after parturition.

**Box 16.1**
**Relactation**

Relactation, or induced lactation, is the process whereby lactation is initiated at a time not associated with delivery. For instance, an adoptive mother who has not borne a child may wish to breastfeed her adopted baby or a mother may want to resume feeding her own child. Relactation is easier if the woman has previously lactated or been pregnant and if the infant is young. Hormonal support such as oxytocin nasal sprays may be used. The woman is advised to eat well and rest, and to stimulate the nipple and breast often, either by hand or with a breast pump. Supplementary formula milk is given to the baby by spoon or dropper; bottle teats and dummies are avoided. Use of a 'Lact-Aid' supplementer is often found helpful. This device allows the baby to feed on formula milk from a tube attached to the mother's nipple. As the baby feeds, it stimulates the nipple and increases endogenous prolactin secretion. The formula milk is in a bag maintained at body temperature because it is in contact with the mother's body. As breast milk production increases the amount of formula milk can be reduced.

**Box 16.2**
**Changes to the breasts in pregnancy**

- Increased vascularization—may cause tingling
- Dilatation of superficial veins—fair skin appears 'marbled'
- Hypertrophy—full development of lobules
- Dilatation of alveoli and ducts—may feel nodular
- Thickening of nipple skin
- Pigmentation of nipple and areolar—persists after pregnancy
- Secondary areola may appear in dark-skinned women
- Montgomery's tubercles become prominent
- Small quantity of clear colostrum can be expressed in latter half of pregnancy

# Physiology of lactation

Lactation can be considered as two phases: lactogenesis, the initiation of lactation, and galactopoiesis, the maintenance of milk secretion. The initiation of lactation is related to the drop in oestrogen, progesterone and possibly hPL from the maternal circulation at delivery. The two most important hormones involved in lactation are prolactin, which stimulates production of milk, and oxytocin, which is involved in milk ejection (Table 16.1, Fig. 16.4).

## *Prolactin*

Suckling results in the firing of afferent impulses via the anterolateral columns of the spinal cord to the brain-stem and hypothalamus. The hypothalamus subsequently decreases release of dopamine (formerly described as prolactin inhibitory factor) into the portal circulation to the pituitary gland. It was postulated that a dopamine-stimulating factor existed but, although several hormones positively modulate prolactin secretion, control is largely by the lifting of the tonic inhibition from dopamine. The abrogation of the dopamine inhibition stimulates the release of prolactin from the cells of the anterior pituitary. Secretion of prolactin is modified by oestrogen and TSH. Studies in rats have demonstrated that VIP, released from the pituitary gland, is an extremely potent prolactin-releasing factor and affects mammary blood flow. The number of signals affecting prolactin release indicates a complex neuroendocrine axis (Ben-Jonathan, Laudon & Garris 1991). Beta endorphin and MSH, which are coreleased from the intermediate lobe of the pituitary gland, also seem to have a role. Beta endorphin blocks dopamine inhibition of prolactin and MSH stimulates the release of prolactin by lowering the threshold of the lactotrophs (Porter et al 1994).

Levels of prolactin begin to rise within 10 minutes of suckling, peak about 30 minutes after initial stimulation and then progressively fall back to basal levels within a further 3 hours. This delay in prolactin secretion following suckling led to the concept that the rise in prolactin was the 'order for the next meal'. Areolar stimulation is essential for prolactin release; negative pressure alone is not adequate and denervation of the nipple prevents prolactin release in response to nipple stimulation.

Prolactin levels fall abruptly about 2 hours before delivery then dramatically rebound. These fluctuations in prolactin level probably relate to changing oestrogen concentrations. The level of prolactin seems to be important in establishing lactation but levels are much diminished after 6 weeks at a rate dependent on suckling frequency and duration (Johnston & Amico 1986). The peak prolactin levels in response to suckling also fall progressively.

Prolactin has a pulsatile release. A diurnal rhythm of prolactin secretion is apparent, with higher circulating levels during sleep. The exact quantitative relationship between prolactin levels and milk production is not clear. In the early puerperium bromocriptine, a dopamine $D_2$ receptor agonist, causes a fall in prolactin levels and abolishes milk secretion. Dopamine-receptor blockers (such as metoclopramide, haloperidol, domperidone and sulpiride) increase prolactin levels and milk production. Dopamine binds to receptors on the pituitary and is internalized resulting in the increased breakdown of prolactin within the secretory granules. However, women who have had pituitary surgery and

**Table 16.1** *Prolactin and oxytocin*

| | Prolactin | Oxytocin |
|---|---|---|
| Source | Anterior pituitary gland | Posterior pituitary gland (but synthesized in hypothalamus) |
| Primary control | Lifting of dopamine inhibition | Neural pathway |
| Modulating factors | Positively stimulated by oestrogen, TSH, VIP | Neurotransmitters |
| Peak response | 30 minutes | 30 seconds |
| Stimulus | Suckling | Suckling, sound, sight and thought of baby |
| Target cell | Alveolar cell | Myoepithelial cell |
| Effect | Milk synthesis | Milk ejection |

have prolactin levels just above non-pregnant level can breastfeed. The evidence seems to suggest that a threshold prolactin level is required but then there is no correlation between prolactin level and milk production (Howie et al 1980).

Prolactin binds to receptors on the secretory alveolar cells, acting at several sites to increase synthesis of several components of the milk including casein, lactalbumin and fatty acids. During pregnancy the mitochondria proliferate and the biosynthetic apparatus of the cell, the endoplasmic reticulum and the Golgi apparatus undergo development.

## *Biosynthesis of milk*

The secretory cells of the alveoli (Fig. 16.3) synthesize or extract the components of milk, which are secreted into the alveolar lumen. The cells are joined near their apical surface by tight junctions. The apical plasma membrane has a smooth surface with few microvilli in contrast to the tightly folded basal membrane, which facilitates uptake of substrates such as amino acids, glucose, acetate and fats from the extracellular space. Proteins, fats and lactose are synthesized in the cell and packaged into vesicles. The vesicles move to the apex of the cell where exocytosis takes place.

The composition of the maternal diet can influence the components of breast milk, especially those passing from blood to milk with little modification by the alveolar cell, such as lipids. Fat droplets are secreted by an apocrine mechanism whereby they are enclosed by cell membrane. Water, electrolytes and water-soluble constituents diffuse across the alveolar membrane via pores, thus reflecting maternal diet, or

**Fig. 16.3** ***The alveolar secretory cells of the breast. (Reproduced with permission from Pond 1992.)***

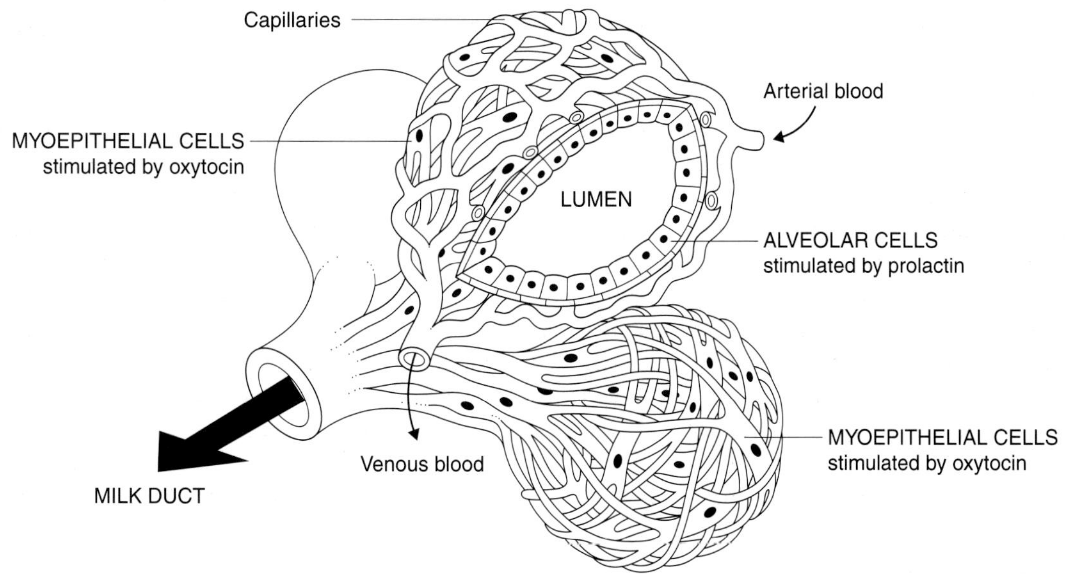


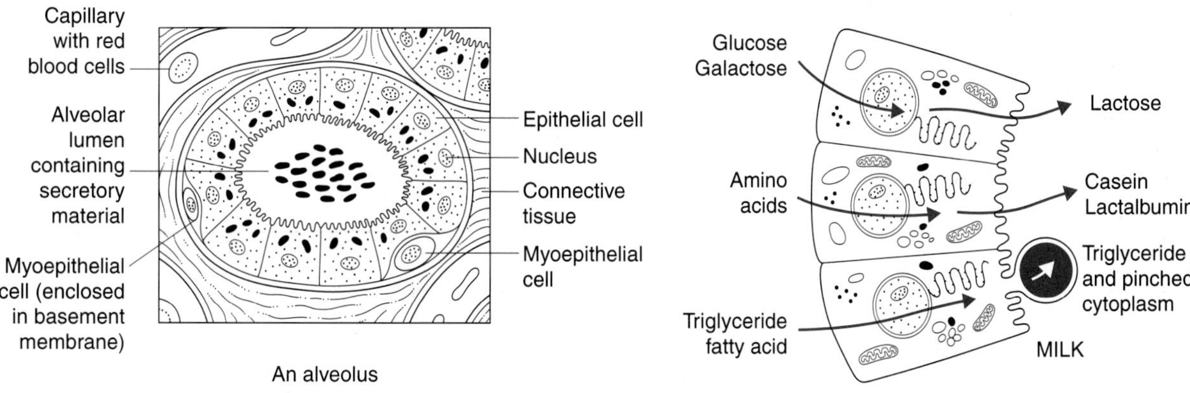

are transported by active transport. Active transport of calcium, amino acids, glucose, magnesium and sodium takes place. Large blood cells follow a paracellular route, squeezing between the alveolar cells.

### *Oxytocin*

The milk ejection reflex, which is responsible for the transfer of the milk from the breast to the baby, is controlled by oxytocin levels. Oxytocin stimulates the myoepithelial cells so the alveolar sacs are compressed, increasing the pressure, and the ducts shorten and widen. Although secretion of oxytocin is under a similar neuroendocrine reflex to prolactin, it is physiologically independent. Oxytocin synthesis in the hypothalamus, and its release from the posterior lobe of the pituitary gland, is increased in response to handling the baby, hearing cries or thinking about feeding as well as by tactile stimulation at the nipple. Oxytocin is released in short-lived bursts of less than a minute immediately in response to stimuli. Frequently, the largest response is to the baby crying before feeding so maximum release of oxytocin may occur before suckling starts. Between feeds, isolated pulses of oxytocin are released (McNeilly et al 1983) possibly in response to other babies' cries or fleeting images of the baby. Unlike prolactin secretion, the milk ejection reflex can be conditioned—as demonstrated by dairy farmers who clanged their buckets to stimulate oxytocin and a good milk yield. Similarly, a baby's cry can often trigger oxytocin secretion which is why the practice of babies 'rooming-in' with their mothers (sleeping close to their mother's bed) is often associated with successful breastfeeding.

The milk ejection reflex is very sensitive to inhibition by physical and psychological stresses such as emotions, tiredness, embarrassment and worry. The limbic system, which coordinates the body's responses to emotions, is involved in oxytocin release. The likely mechanism is catecholamine inhibition of oxytocin release and adrenergic vasoconstriction of mammary blood vessels limiting access of the oxytocin to the myoepithelial cells. Women experiencing problems in establishing milk flow are often helped by covering their breasts with warm flannels which appears to aid blood flow and oxytocin access.

Surprisingly, denervation of mammary glands in experimental animals appears to have little effect on milk production (Williams, McVey & Hunter 1993). This suggests that the afferent nerve pathway may not be so important as the interactions of neurotransmitters. Transmitters that have been implicated in the control of the milk ejection reflex include noradrenaline, β-endorphin, serotonin and dopamine. As with control of prolactin secretion, the number of factors influencing oxytocin secretion suggests that the pathway is much more complicated than originally thought. Stimulation of the female reproductive tract, especially the vagina and cervix, increases oxytocin release so milk may be ejected from the breasts during coitus.

Oxytocin binds to specific receptors on the myoepithelial cells around the milk-secreting cells and to longitudinal cells in the duct walls. Contraction of the myoepithelial cells results in milk being expelled into the ducts, which shorten as the longitudinal cells contract. Oxytocin-induced contraction generates pressure waves within the breasts and is responsible for prickly sensations associated with breastfeeding. When the milk ejection reflex is well established, milk may be spontaneously ejected from both breasts.

Oxytocin pulses increase in amplitude during labour and are involved in the positive feedback amplification in labour (see Ch. 1). Oxytocin is associated with changes in maternal behaviour and increased alertness at delivery. The pulses of oxytocin induced by feeding have an effect on the uterus, stimulating uterine contractions and involution. These contractions or 'afterpains' are felt with increased intensity by multiparous women. Women who do not want to breastfeed may find the physiological changes in the breasts at delivery uncomfortable; various techniques are recommended to inhibit lactation (Box 16.3).

## Suckling and milk transfer

In feeding from the breast, the baby takes the whole nipple into its mouth and places its tongue under the adjacent areola. The baby milks the ampullae of the breast, which lie deep in the nipple, with a stripping

**Box 16.3**
**Suppression of lactation—methods**

- Bromocriptine (dopamine agonist) (used with great caution)
- Treatment with sex steroids to antagonize prolactin effects
- Breast binding
- Application of ice-packs

action. In contrast, milk is removed from the bottle by negative pressure.

Babies exhibit two distinct patterns of suckling (Turgeon-O'Brien et al 1996). Nutritive suckling is a continuous stream of strong slow sucks, which efficiently allows milk transfer. This occurs predominantly in the early part of the feed. Non-nutritive suckling increasingly replaces nutritive suckling during the progression of the feed. It is characterized by alternation of rapid shallow bursts of suckling and rests. It is thought that patterns of thumb sucking may reflect these two conducts. Breastfed babies have two distinct rhythms of thumb suckling and tend to put more of the root of the thumb into their mouths. Although non-nutritive suckling is associated with a decreased transfer of milk, it is still very effective in stimulating prolactin release and so may be important in successful lactation.

The amount of milk produced is extremely variable; that mothers can feed multiple babies and produce additional milk for banking or storage suggests that the mammary synthetic capacity exceeds the normal requirement of single infants. A demand-fed baby consumes irregular quantities of milk at irregular times. The suggestion that the baby determines milk yield by local control is supported by the strong correlation between degree of breast emptying and rate of milk synthesis. Some women feed exclusively from one breast (and not at all from the other). The autocrine factor capable of overriding the central hormone control was first identified in goats (Wilde, Prentice & Peaker 1995) and has been named factor inhibiting lactation (FIL). This protein inhibitory factor has also been found in the whey fraction of human milk. It is secreted from the alveolar cells and accumulates in milk. The factor inhibits secretion of lactose, probably by blocking the action of prolactin, and therefore provides the mechanism to adjust supply to demand. When milk is not removed from the breast, the concentration of the factor increases and blocks the action of prolactin thus reducing the rate of milk synthesis. It helps to explain why maternal dietary intake has relatively little influence on the amount of milk produced.

## Involution

After ceasing lactation, involution takes about 3 months. Milk accumulates in the alveoli and small lactiferous ducts, which causes distension and mechanical atrophy of the epithelial cells and rupture of the alveolar walls, creating large spaces. Milk secretion is therefore suppressed by local mechanical factors rather than by diminishing prolactin levels. Phagocytosis of the cells and glandular debris results in fewer and smaller lobular–acinar structures. The alveolar lumens decrease in size and may disappear. The alveolar lining changes from a single secretory layer to a non-secretory double layer. If breastfeeding is stopped suddenly, the process is more intense and painful. The breasts remain larger after lactation as the deposits of fat and connective tissue are increased. Involution after lactation is different to the structural atrophy and loss of adipose tissue occurring in postmenopausal mammary cells deprived of oestrogen.

## Problems associated with lactation

### *Milk insufficiency*

Most problems have an identifiable physiological basis; breast milk insufficiency is frequently overdiagnosed and is usually simply resolved (Woolridge 1996). The majority of women with apparently insufficient milk supply have unsubstantiated worries and require confidence, improved technique, especially positioning, encouragement or advice. This can be supported by physiological strategies such as electric breast pumps and pharmacological (antidopamine) agents. Iatrogenic low milk supply may be attributed to excessive down-regulation of supply probably during the calibration period. It is possible that baby milk manufacturers inadvertly exploit the importance of the calibration period by offering free milk samples early in lactation. If the initial calibrated volume cannot be increased, the mother will then be unable to increase her milk supply later and will be forced to provide alternative inferior sources of milk, which are expensive and can be harmful if water supplies are contaminated, as happens in a number of developing countries.

Behavioural problems that are acquired by the baby as coping strategies to avoid aversive events may also induce a low milk supply. These problems include discomfort during positioning at the breast and problems with breathing. Self-limitation of intake and lack of persistence may account for the condition described as 'contented underfed babies' (Woolridge 1996). Pathophysiological failure is rare and probably affects less than 2% of women with apparent milk insufficiency. Rare causes include mammary hypoplasia, or absence of normal breast development at puberty or in pregnancy. Retained placental products affect lactation reversibly but Sheehan's syndrome, necrosis of the anterior pituitary due to acute hypovolaemic shock, as in antepartum haemorrhage (for instance due to placental abruption) or postpartum haemorrhage, is more serious.

## Drugs

Many drugs are secreted into breast milk, but the data on the effects of specific drugs on the breastfed infant is often not available. Of particular concern are those drugs with CNS activity as the postnatal development of the infant's nervous system is vulnerable. The benefits of maternal treatment and the advantages of breastfeeding have to be balanced against the risk of exposure of the neonate to the medication. Passive diffusion of the unbound, unionized form of the drug into the breast milk is the major mechanism of transfer. Therefore, it is affected by maternal compartmentalization and molecular properties and the composition of the breast milk.

Drug elimination by the neonate is often limited so exposure to apparently low doses of the drug in milk can have an accumulative effect, particularly in premature babies and those who have prolonged exposure. Drugs tend not to accumulate in the milk but have a bidirectional transfer. Therefore, the amount of drug received by the infant will be reduced if the mother takes the drug immediately after a feed so the baby does not feed when the drug is at peak concentration in the maternal plasma and milk. Assessment of adverse drug reactions in infants is difficult. Drugs that are minimally excreted into the breast milk, are metabolized quickly by the neonate and are not associated with adverse effects are obviously the preferred choice.

Socially used drugs such as alcohol (Menella & Beauchamp 1991) and nicotine (Woodward et al 1986) also cross into the milk. How much these affect the baby is not clear. Production of breast milk is also a method of excretion and contains drugs, viruses, food additives, chemical contamination, pesticides and radioactivity. Chemical residues of pollutants are detected in most human milk throughout the world. Heavy metals are of concern because of the susceptibility of the infant's nervous system. Mammals do not have a mechanism to excrete pesticide residues such as 1,1,1-trichloro-2,2,bis(p-chlorophenyl)ethane (DDT). However, the residues do cross the blood–breast barrier so lactation is the only way to reduce the body load. The burden is then transferred to the breastfed infant (Rogan et al 1987). The health risks are not clear. Usually breastfeeding is not contraindicated.

## Viruses

Maternal viruses may enter the milk. Transfer of HIV and TB has been confirmed. It is probably inadvisable for mothers with TB to breastfeed as the infection tends to be reactivated by maternal tiredness and stress (Box 16.4). However, advice about HIV-positive mothers is unclear. The immunological properties of breast milk are probably important in protecting against illnesses that accelerate the development of AIDS, particularly in areas of the world where it is endemic (Van de Perre 1995).

Case study 16.1 is an example of concerns about breastfeeding.

**Box 16.4**
**Contraindications to breastfeeding**

- Maternal illness
- Maternal drug consumption
- Congenital abnormalities, e.g. cleft palate
- HIV-positive—controversial
- TB infection (depending on strain and treatment)

**Case study 16.1**

Elma expressed concerns about breastfeeding throughout her pregnancy. She complained that the midwives running the antenatal classes were biased towards breastfeeding and that bottlefeeding was just as good. Elma described her own family as an example; she is the oldest of five children all of whom were bottlefeed by her mother and were well and healthy. Two days after delivery, Elma experienced breast discomfort and tentatively asked a midwife whether it was too late to try breastfeeding.

- How would you as the midwife explain and encourage Elma to breastfeed throughout the antenatal period?
- What factors would increase her chances of being successful in breastfeeding?
- What support would she require from the midwives?
- Would breastfeeding or anything else help to relieve the breast discomfort?

## Inhibition of fertility

Breast milk is also important to the infant because suppression of fertility is an advantage. An adequate birth interval is important for both maternal and child health. Lactational amenorrhoea may last from 2 months to 4 years. It is particularly important in developing countries where breastfeeding prevents more pregnancies than all the other methods of contraception put together. The variability in duration of suppressed fertility seems to be related to a number of factors; the most important seems to be frequency of suckling. At the end of pregnancy, levels of gonadotrophins are very low because high levels of oestrogen continue to impose negative feedback. At delivery, the placental hormones begin to disappear, at different rates depending on their half-life. hPL disappears from the plasma within hours. Oestrogen and progesterone levels fall to prepregnant levels within a week (Martin et al 1980). Levels of hCG are negligible about 3 weeks after delivery. There is a gradual recovery in the ovarian–pituitary axis over the first 4 months after delivery; this recovery is delayed by regular suckling.

In non-lactating women, body temperature measurements and the first menstrual bleeding suggest that the earliest ovulation may occur at 4 weeks after delivery but is usually delayed until 8–10 weeks (Gray et al 1987); most women have resumed normal menstrual patterns by 15 weeks. The first menstrual cycle is often anovulatory or associated with an inadequate luteal phase. Most cycles are ovulatory by the third cycle. Fifty per cent of non-lactating women who do not use contraception conceive within 6–7 months.

Menstruation and ovulation return more slowly in a lactating woman. Ovarian activity usually returns before the end of lactational amenorrhoea. Therefore, menstruation is a poor indicator of fertility; conception can occur without menstruation. Neither ovulation nor menstruation normally occurs within 6 weeks, but about half of all contraceptive-unprotected breastfeeding mothers conceive within 9 months of lactation, 1–10% during lactational amenorrhoea. Between 30 and 70% of first cycles are ovulatory; the longer is the period of lactational amenorrhoea, the more likelihood there is of an ovulatory cycle prior to the first menstruation.

The precise mechanisms involved in lactational amenorrhoea are not clear. High prolactin levels abolish the pulsatile LH secretion and decrease the pituitary response to gonadotrophin-releasing hormone. The mid-cycle positive feedback in response to oestrogen is absent. The sensitivity to negative feedback is enhanced and that to positive feedback is decreased. So, even if enough LH and FSH are present to stimulate follicular development, the inhibitory effect of oestrogen results in an inadequate luteal phase. Prolactin is inhibitory at the level of the ovary, blocking the effects of LH and FSH. It also has a direct effect on the brain, possibly affecting libido.

As prolactin secretion has a pulsatile rhythm with larger amounts being released at night, the night-time feeds are particularly important in maintaining prolactin levels high enough to suppress fertility (Howie & McNeilly 1982). The duration and number of feeds are important because the prolactin levels are augmented before they return completely to the basal secretory level (Anderson & Schioler 1982). Prolonged amenorrhoea is associated with maternal malnutrition (Rogers 1997). Poor nutrition is associated with suppression of fertility in non-lactating women. The extra nutrient requirement for milk production can increase the degree of maternal malnutrition. Also, although women receiving less than optimal nutrition can breastfeed their babies adequately, they secrete milk more slowly so the infants feed more often and for longer. This will raise their circulating prolactin levels.

## Maternal behaviour

The demands of the parent and offspring during lactation may conflict. It is suggested that parents will tend to maximize the survival of their young but not to the extent that would limit investment in other offspring, including those as yet unborn (Peaker 1989). This theory means that, although mothers will try to recoup the investment of pregnancy by favouring the offspring's survival, should this cost compromise their future reproductive ability there are genetic advantages in discontinuing this investment in favour of a more favourable future offspring. There may be genetic components affecting the time-course of lactation or the upper limit of milk production. The rate of milk secretion and duration of lactation vary with nutritional state. Some mammals respond to decreased food supply in ways that favour the succeeding pregnancies, such as killing some or all of the litter. Species with long gestation and long-term commitment to the offspring, such as humans, tend to favour the well-being of live offspring.

Behavioural changes include preparatory behaviour such as nest building and increased aggression. Care and protection are associated with lactation. These behavioural patterns are associated with the progressive independence of the young. In humans, this behaviour is more difficult to observe than in other species.

The nutritional status of the mother may affect feeding and interaction with her infant (Britton 1993). The effect of maternal malnutrition can affect infant development, depending on its duration and the timing. Infants malnourished in utero may have decreased capacity to respond to appropriate cues and therefore an increased likelihood of social and further nutritional deprivation. Malnourished infants have poorer muscle tone, increased lethargy, irritability and frequency of illness, decreased attention and responsiveness and altered sleep–wake states. Malnourished mothers experience more fatigue, which can affect their own sensitivity to cues from the baby, such as responses to stress and attention–behavioural patterns.

## Nutrition of the lactating mother

Human growth rate is much slower than that of other animals. Neurological development is relatively late and the duration of human lactation is longer. During lactation, daily nutrient input and reserves laid down in pregnancy are juggled. Milk output is largely independent of the mother's ethnic origin and nutritional status. A balanced diet in lactation appears to favour the health of the mother.

### *Energy requirements for milk production*

The energy output of milk is a significant proportion of the total energy output of the lactating woman; it is estimated to be about 25% of the energy expenditure for women who are exclusively breastfeeding. In dairy animals, the level of food intake strongly correlates with milk yield. However, it may not be valid to apply knowledge of nutrition and physiology of dairy animals, which are completely milked twice a day, to mammals who suckle their young according to natural patterns of behaviour. Anthropological studies on human hunter–gatherer communities suggest that babies feed every half hour at 2 weeks and every 4 hours at 4 months. The characteristics of mammalian milk relate directly to the interaction between the mother and child. Marsupials and animals that bear their young during hibernation and are always present produce milk that is dilute and has a low fat content. In contrast, in animals where the mother nurses her young at widely spaced intervals, for instance a hunting lioness, the milk is very concentrated and high in fat. Human milk has most resemblance to the former; it is dilute with a low fat content suggesting that humans have evolved as a species where the young have unlimited access to milk and there is high attentiveness shown by a constantly present mother (Prentice & Prentice 1995). The stress of human lactation is relatively low compared with species with faster growing or multiple young, but this is countered by the high cost of maintaining a dependent infant for a prolonged period. The high level of maternal investment in pregnancy and slow reproductive cycle mean that humans are committed to sustain a conception.

There is a discrepancy between the theoretical calculated energy requirement for milk production and the actual intake of lactating women, even taking into account the fat reserves laid down in pregnancy. Current recommendations are that an exclusively breastfeeding woman requires an additional 650 kcal/day and an increase of 20 g protein per day (Dewey 1997). However, it is thought that 150 kcal/day will be provided by the maternal fat stores for the first 6 months so the net increment needed is 500 kcal/day. In practice, these requirements are much higher than the observed intakes in successfully lactating women even when offered unlimited access to food. Lactational performance is particularly resilient in humans as demonstrated by the efficiency of lactation in undernourished and impoverished communities.

In animals, a decrease in non-shivering thermogenesis (inhibition of brown-fat heat generation) and therefore the provision of extra energy for milk production is suggested to account for this difference. The mechanism in humans is not thought to be mediated by changes in non-shivering thermogenesis but the lactating woman has increased sensitivity to insulin (Illingworth et al 1986). This energy-sparing effect and efficient energy utilization of lactating women has a particularly big implication in developing countries.

Increased incidence of obesity in Western societies is of concern with about a third of women having a BMI over 25 kg/m$^2$. Pregnancy is a risk factor for the development of obesity and it is suggested that postpartum weight loss may not be inevitable (Ohlin & Rossner 1996). Possibly the changes in energy metabolism associated with pregnancy and lactation may remain after weaning. If so, lactation could contribute to the problem. Different species of mammal lay down body fat during pregnancy to different degrees. In lactation, mammals rely on the deposited fat to different extents. Whales and seals, for instance, rely entirely on body fat and protein reserves to sustain lactation whereas dairy cows and laboratory rats are very dependent on increased intake to provide energy for milk yield. Pregnant women deposit fat and have a changed hormonal environment. The reported studies tend to conflict and do not show significant differences in weight loss with different patterns of infant feeding. However, interpretation of the studies is confused by confounding factors such as different duration and extent of feeding and the increased tendency of women who are not breastfeeding to reduce their weight deliberately. There is also a large variation in the energy content of the milk produced (see below).

### *Calcium and iron*

Both pregnancy and lactation present a drain on the calcium status of the woman. The fetal skeleton requires 5 mmol calcium per day. The average daily production of 800 ml of milk contains 6.25 mmol calcium. Demand for calcium can be met by one or more of the following: increased dietary calcium, increased absorption, decreased excretion, or increased bone demineralization (net loss of bone). In the third trimester, absorption of calcium increases. Increased renal losses are measured but calcium balance remains positive possibly because the increased oestrogen protects bone mass. In lactation, increased reabsorption of calcium in the renal tubule occurs but absorption of calcium is no longer high. The oestrogen level is relatively low so the bone mass is not protected to the same extent.

Lactation is associated with a net drain of calcium from the body, with a selective decrease in trabecular bone. This reduction is independent of parathyroid and vitamin D levels. So lactation may appear to increase future risk of osteoporosis, but risk factors shown to be associated with fractures do not necessarily include breastfeeding (Sowers 1996). During weaning, an imbalance between bone resorption and bone formation results in the recovery of bone mass. The implications for birth spacing and prolonged breastfeeding are not clear. Modern practices of delaying childbearing resulting in decreased time for recovery before menopause are probably countered by the cumulative effect of having fewer children. Prolonged lactational amenorrhoea may help to restore maternal iron status.

## Infant nutrition and the composition of human milk

Human milk optimally fulfils the nutritional requirements of the human neonate. It has a unique composition that is particularly suitable for the rapid growth and development of the infant born with immature digestive, renal and hepatic systems. Unique features of human milk are able to compensate for the underdeveloped neonatal capabilities. Human milk contains not only the macronutrients, vitamins and minerals but also non-nutrient growth factors, hormones and protective factors.

There are at least 100 components of human milk, including substances yet to be identified and their roles elucidated. In the *Koran* breast milk is described as 'white blood'. This is a particularly apt description because the early milk has more white blood cells than blood itself. Milk is a solution in which other substances are dissolved, emulsified or colloidally dispersed. The value of breast milk is undisputed; rarely should breastfeeding be discouraged.

The unique characteristic of humans is the large complex brain, which undergoes much development in the first 2 years of life. Human milk provides levels of lactose, cysteine, cholesterol and thromboplastin, which are required for CNS tissue synthesis. However, as breast milk appears to be perfect nutrition, analysis of its composition has allowed good substitutes to be produced as formula feeds. Infant formula milk will never completely mimic human milk, however. A number of the factors that make breast milk qualitatively superior are heat-labile.

Although breast milk may be considered perfect nutrition, its composition is variable. It varies from person to person, from one period of lactation to another, and hourly through the day. Its composition is related to the timing of the feed, how much is produced and parameters relating to the last feed (Emmett & Rogers 1997); it has also been suggested that maternal age, parity, health and social class affect the composition of the milk. Mothers of premature infants produce milk that has a higher concentration of some nutrients, but this probably reflects the small volumes produced for small infants. Except for vitamin and fat content, the composition is largely independent of maternal nutrition unless the mother experiences severe malnutrition. There are a lot of difficulties encountered in the estimation of the volume of milk produced. Weighing either the mother or baby before and after the feed is fraught with problems. Although double-labelled water measurements have allowed more accurate estimations (Lucas et al 1987), the variability within a fed and from feed to feed make it very difficult to ascertain precisely the nutrient consumption of a healthy growing baby. These estimates of about 60 kcal/100 ml are lower than UK food composition tables (69 kcal/100 ml).

The low levels of gastric secretion and other immature digestive characteristics of the neonatal gut confer a number of immunological advantages which were described in Chapter 15 (p. 341).

## Colostrum

In the first 3 days postdelivery, the mother produces about 2 to 10 ml of colostrum per day. More colostrum is produced sooner if the woman has had previous pregnancies, particularly if she has lactated before. In some cultures, colostrum is thought to be old milk or 'pus' and is not fed to infants.

Colostrum is transparent and is yellow from the high β-carotene content. Mature milk in contrast looks less viscous and slightly blue. Colostrum has more protein and vitamins A and K and less sugar and fat than the later milk. It is easily digested and well absorbed. It has a lower energy content of 58 kcal/100 ml compared with 70 kcal/100 ml in mature milk. Levels of sodium, potassium, chloride and zinc are high in colostrum but probably reflect the low volume produced rather than the infant's requirements for a bolus dose of certain nutrients. The composition is extremely variable, which reflects its unstable secretory pattern.

Colostrum is believed to facilitate the colonization of the gut with *Lactobacillus bifidus* (Wharton, Balmer & Scott 1994). Meconium also contains growth factors for *Lactobacillus bifidus*. Colostrum seems to have a laxative effect, stimulating the passage of meconium. The high protein content is largely due to the abundant antibodies, which protect against gastrointestinal tract infection. IgA forms 50% of the protein content of colostrum, falling to 10% by 6 months.

During the first 30 hours or so, the secretion (colostrum) has a high protein to lactose ratio. In the following days, as the baby suckles more and stimulates the nerve endings, the resulting increase in prolactin secretion stimulates production of the major whey protein, α-lactalbumin, which is a specific component of the lactose synthetase enzyme and so regulates lactose production. The effect of increasing lactose production is that water is drawn into the secretion to maintain ionic equilibrium so the volume increases thus diluting the protein content. The absolute amounts of protein secreted into the milk are maintained or increased even though the concentration falls.

The composition of the milk becomes relatively stable from about day 5 but is variable in volume. The amount of breast milk produced is related to the weight and requirement of the infant; there is a steady increase in volume in the first few weeks. Milk production appears to get under way without any reference to the size and requirements of the baby, although hPL levels may play a role in the increased production of milk in mothers of twins. The early weeks of lactation can be considered to be a time of calibration between maternal production and infants' demand. The volume of milk produced is usually increased to match demand. Downregulation may be irreversible. It is suggested that mothers of small or preterm babies who initially express milk should therefore express as much as they can (i.e. peak yield rather than only enough for the baby's transiently limited requirement).

Milk secretion in women who do not suckle their baby may persist scantily for 3 or 4 weeks while prolactin levels are still high. The effect of suckling is to stimulate the release of prolactin and oxytocin, which are essential for the maintenance of lactation (Fig. 16.4). Provided breastfeeding is regular, lactation can last for several years. Most studies suggest that the average daily volume of milk produced is about 800 ml. Measurement of the milk produced is notoriously difficult but it is clear that there is much variation depending on demand: mothers of twins produce about twice as much milk.

## Protein

Protein is the limiting nutrient for growth and development. It also provides nitrogen and amino acids required for membrane and transport proteins, hormones, enzymes, growth factors, neurotransmitters and immunoglobulins. Human neonates have a very slow growth rate compared with other species therefore human milk has low protein concentrations (0.7–0.9 g protein/100 ml compared with 3.5 g/100 ml in cow's milk). Excess protein intake can present an excessive solute load to the immature kidneys, which results in acid–base imbalance and metabolic acidosis.

Fig. 16.4 *Suckling stimulates the release of prolactin and oxytocin.*

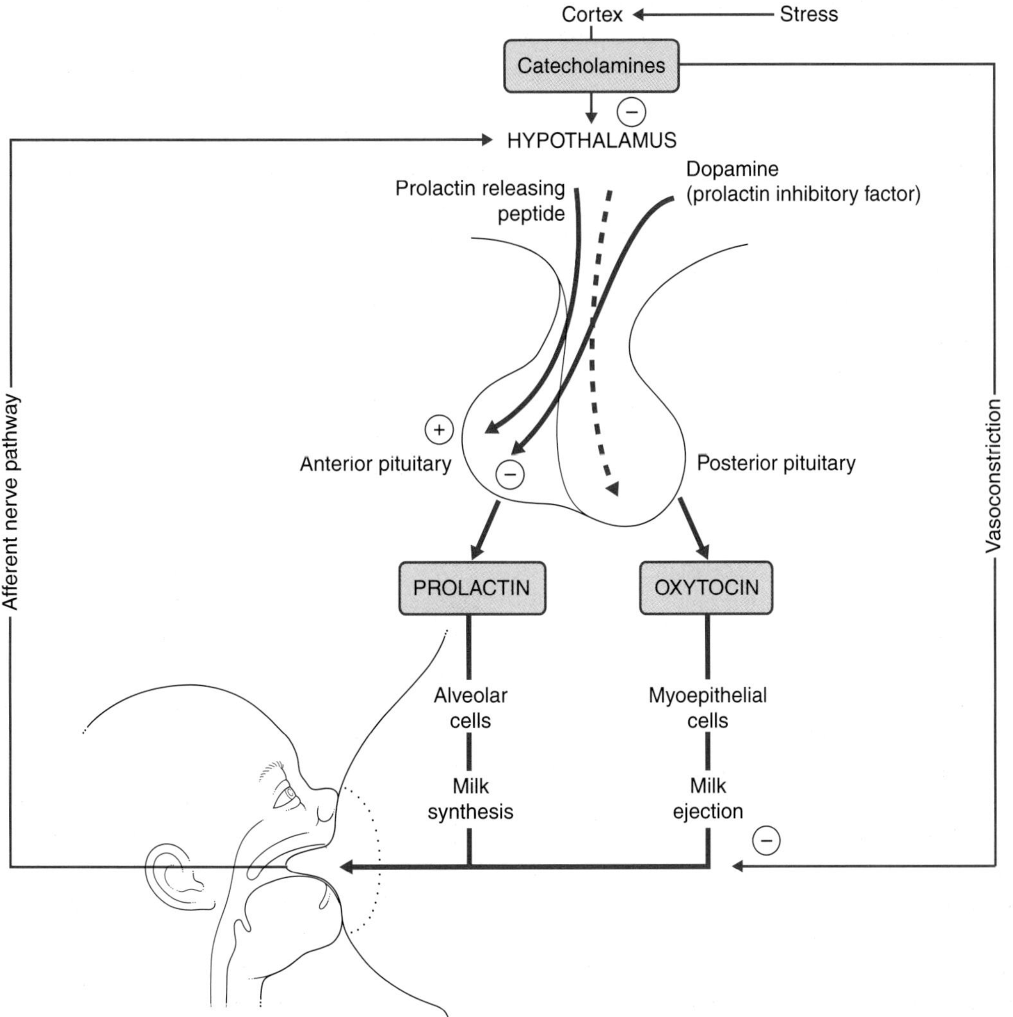


Chronic protein undernutrition or prolonged lactation may result in changes in the protein composition of milk. Protein supplementation of the mother's diet tends to increase milk volume rather than affecting protein concentration but has an important role in supplementing maternal health.

When milk proteins are exposed to the relatively acidic environment of the neonatal stomach they separate into casein, proteins that precipitate the formation of curds, and whey, those proteins that are still soluble. This means that there is a continuous flow of nutrients, initially as soluble lactose and whey proteins, and later from digested curd. Whey proteins include α-lactalbumin, lactoferrin and secretory IgA. They are easy to digest by a human neonatal gut, which has particularly low levels of trypsin and pepsin. The whey-dominant content of milk reduces the risk of lactobezoars (obstructive milk curd balls) forming in the stomach (Schreiner et al 1979). Human α-lactalbumin is easier to digest than bovine β-lactalbumin.

The ratio of whey to casein in human milk is 60:40 (1.5). The β-casein in human milk forms curds that are soft and flocculent with a low curd tension, which are easily digested. Peptides formed from hydrolysis of human milk casein may be important in stimulating the neonatal immune system (Ebrahim 1990). In contrast, cow's milk has a whey:casein ratio of 20:80 (0.25). Bovine casein is predominantly α-casein, which forms a tough rubbery precipitate unless heat-treated, which is more difficult for human infants to digest and decreases the bioavailability of calcium and other cations. Human β-casein tends to form smaller micelles incorporating minerals that are easier for the neonate to digest. κ-casein in cow's milk has a marked effect on the development of the bovine gastrointestinal physiology, stimulating the secretion of chymosin, which is the dominant protease of the fourth stomach.

## The immune response to cow's milk

A high proportion of dietary casein of bovine origin is associated with an increased incidence of intestinal allergy and inflammation and is implicated as one of the possible triggers of necrotizing enterocolitis. As the neonatal gut is permeable, large proteins can be absorbed intact across the gut. Some of these proteins stimulate maturation of the gut and immune system. However, others may present an immunological challenge that produces a response which can cause problems later in life. It has been controversially hypothesized that proteins in cow's milk formula are associated with an increased incidence of diabetes (Karjalainen et al 1992). The hypothesis suggests that a large bovine protein crosses the infant's gut and stimulates the immune system (Monte, Johnston & Roll 1994). Because of similarities between this protein and proteins of the endocrine pancreas, the immune system may direct an autoimmune response against the cells of the pancreas destroying the insulin-producing β-cells. For whatever reason, the incidence of insulin-dependent diabetes mellitus is lower in children who have breastfed.

## Essential amino acids

Proteins are formed of 20 amino acids. Some of the amino acids cannot be made in the body; these are essential amino acids (see Table 12.1, p. 254). The other amino acids, which can be formed within the body from the essential amino acids, are described as non-essential. The neonate has limited capabilities of converting some essential amino acids into non-essential amino acids so some amino acids are conditionally essential for the neonate. The biological value of a protein can be assessed by the proportions of amino acids in a food compared with how efficiently the amino acids can be assembled into proteins. A food with a deficiency of an amino acid has a low net protein utilization (NPU) value. A normal Western omnivorous diet has an NPU of about 0.7, meaning that 70% of the amino acids are utilized from the diet. Human milk has an NPU of 1.0 because it is fully utilized by the neonate as its amino acids are exactly in proportion to requirement. Few other foods have such a high value. By the end of the second week of life, 90% of the ingested nitrogen-containing substances in milk are absorbed, suggesting that milk contains the optimal pattern of amino acids.

Aspartame is a sweetener composed of aspartic acid and phenylalanine. If maternal consumption of foods containing aspartame is increased, there is an increase in plasma levels of phenylalanine but levels in milk only increase marginally suggesting that the mammary gland regulates the transfer of amino acids into the milk.

## Non-protein nitrogen (NPN)

More than 25% of the nitrogen found in human milk comes from sources other than protein. This is the non-protein nitrogen (NPN) fraction (Box 16.5). Methods for protein determination rely on measuring

**Box 16.5**
**Non-protein nitrogen (NPN)**

The protein content of human milk was initially overestimated because it was based on the assumption that the nitrogen fractions within the milk would all be components of protein. In fact, about 25% of the nitrogen-containing components in the milk are not within proteins. This is high compared with other species; for instance cow's milk contains only 5% of the total nitrogen as non-protein nitrogen.

The non-protein nitrogen includes:

| | |
|---|---|
| Amino sugars | which promote the growth of *Lactobacillus bifidus* and are also incorporated into neural tissue and gut epithelial membrane |
| Taurine | a free amino acid that is a component of bile salts and, therefore, contributes to fat digestion |
| Peptides | these have roles as growth factors and hormones |
| Cysteine | a free amino acid that is conditionally essential in the infant because the conversion of methionine to cysteine is limited |
| Binding factors | these facilitate absorption of other nutrients |
| Urea<br>Creatine<br>Creatinine<br>Uric acid | the role of these factors is not clear |

the total nitrogen in a foodstuff and calculating the average amount of protein that would contain that much nitrogen. Therefore, the protein content of human milk was overestimated before it was clear how large the proportion of NPN was. Each mammalian species has a characteristic amount and profile of NPN, which is probably of nutritional significance. The NPN of human milk is derived from maternal blood and includes a variety of compounds such as peptides and free amino acids, traces of inorganic compounds, urea, creatinine and glycosylated amines. Some of the NPN compounds are of developmental importance but the biological significance of others is uncertain.

The amino acid content of human milk, especially whey proteins, is ideal for the growth requirements of the human infant. Neonatal metabolism of certain amino acids (for example, phenylalanine, tyrosine and methionine) is initially limited because the enzymes involved in their metabolism are expressed late in development. If these amino acids reach high concentrations, they can cause damaging effects. Human milk is relatively low in tyrosine, phenylalanine and methionine but high in amino acids that the infant cannot synthesize in adequate amounts. The inability to synthesis adequate quantities of histidine, cysteine and taurine means that these become conditionally essential for infants and need to be provided in the diet. The enzyme that converts methionine to cysteine, cystathionase, is low or undetectable in the neonate. Cysteine is required for growth and development. Infants, especially preterm infants, fed unmodified cow's milk may develop hyperphenylalaninaemia and hypertyrosinaemia, which can increase the net acid load and adversely affect development of the CNS.

Humans cannot synthesize taurine well. Infants use taurine for bile acid conjugation (in contrast to adult conjugation by glycine) so this amino acid is important in the digestion and metabolism of cholesterol and fats. There are high levels of taurine in fetal brain tissue; it may act as a neurotransmitter or neuromodulator in the brain, and be involved in myelinization of nerves and the optimal maintenance of retinal integrity (Carlson 1985). The absolute requirement for taurine is unknown but it is added to formula milk at the levels found in human milk.

## Fat

Fat is the main source of energy in the milk. The nutritional status of the mother affects the fat concentration of the milk and therefore the energy content, fatty acid composition and immunological properties. The total fat content of milk has a considerable variation; it is influenced by the maternal diet, parity and the season of the year. The sampling method used to measure fat is important as hindmilk has 3 to 5 times the fat content of foremilk. Fat content of milk also falls during the day. This diurnal rhythm of milk composition is related to GH secretion. The fatty acid pattern is variable reflecting maternal energy intake and dietary fat consumption. It is possible to discriminate between the milk of vegetarian and non-vegetarian mothers (Sanders, Ellis & Dickerson 1978). If maternal energy intake falls, the fat composition of the milk resembles maternal adipose fat composition as fat stores are mobilized. If maternal carbohydrate consumption is increased, the content of lauric and myristic acids is increased. As fat concentration affects the energy content of the milk, these variations in fat content make it particularly difficult to arrive at the average energy content of human milk. Overestimation of energy consumption may have led to the overfeeding and potential obesity problems of previous generations.

Ninety per cent of fat is present as triacylglycerides. The remaining 10% is made up of free fatty acids, phospholipids, cholesterol, diglycerides and monoglycerides, glycolipids and sterol esters. Fat provides the vehicle for fat-soluble vitamins and essential fatty acids required for brain development. Phospholipids are critical components of cell membranes and are a component of surfactant. The fatty acid composition of human milk is very different to that of cow's milk. Human milk has more essential fatty acids (linoleic, α-linoleic and oleic), has a higher proportion of unsaturated fatty acids and is rich in long-chain fatty acids. Cow's milk has more short-chain fatty acids ($C_4$–$C_8$) and a higher content of saturated fatty acids. The products of lipase digestion are predominantly 2-monoglycerides and free fatty acids, which can be absorbed. Most of the triacylglycerides in human milk have palmitic acid (16:0) or oleic acid (18:0) at position two of the molecule. Bovine triacylglycerides usually have palmitic acid at position one or three so digestion of cow's milk fat can release free palmitic acid, which is precipitated by calcium as a soap. This can result in the loss of absorption of both fat and calcium.

Human milk and vegetable oil fats are better absorbed than is the saturated fat of cow's milk. Long-chain fatty acids require bile salt micelle formation and lipase activity. Short- and medium-chain fatty acids can be absorbed intact.

## Cholesterol

Human milk has a high content of cholesterol, which is required for myelin synthesis (important for the CNS development). The amount of cholesterol in the milk falls as the infant gets older. There may be a connection between cholesterol exposure early in life and the development of enzymes for cholesterol degradation and amounts of endogenous cholesterol synthesized (Bayley et al 1998). The cholesterol content of breast milk is not affected by maternal diet.

As lactation progresses, triacylglyceride levels increase and cholesterol levels fall but phospholipid content remains stable. Usually, 20% of the milk in a feed remains in the breast; this contains about half of the fat. This effect may be due to absorption of fat globules on the surface of the alveolar cells. It has been observed that babies suck in longer bursts and decrease the rest intervals when they are feeding on hindmilk (Woolridge & Fisher 1988).

## Essential fatty acids

Essential fatty acids (see Ch. 12, Table 16.2) are required for cell proliferation, retinal development and myelinization of the CNS. The neonate has a limited ability to desaturate and elongate fatty acid chains thus limiting the conversion of linoleic acid into arachidonic acid so arachidonic acid becomes conditionally essential in the diet. Human milk is particularly rich in arachidonic acid (AA) and docosahexaenoic acid (DHA). Proportions of AA and DHA are high in membrane phospholipids of brain grey matter, retinal photoreceptor cells and vascular tissue. Research has implicated long-chain fatty acids, particularly DHA, in breast milk with both raised IQ levels and better visual perception (Lucas et al 1992).

The variation in milk probably reflects the variation in maternal diet (Sanders, Ellis & Dickerson 1978). A low-fat maternal diet may maximize de novo synthesis of fatty acids for milk triacylglycerols but should contain adequate quantities of long-chain polyunsaturated fatty acids. As a species, human have a uniquely large brain, which is composed of about 60% lipid. The essential dietary requirement for long-chain polyunsaturated fatty acids required for the development of the human cerebral cortex has some interesting evolutionary aspects. It has been proposed that the freshwater lakes of the Rift Valley in East Africa provided the optimal environment to promote development of *Homo sapiens* (Broadhurst, Cunnane & Crawford 1998). Freshwater fish and shellfish are particularly rich in long-chain polyunsaturated fatty acids and have a ratio of arachidonic acid to docosahexaenoic acid similar to that of the human brain (Table 16.2).

**Table 16.2** *Long-chain polyunsaturated fatty acids*

| | Omega 6 (n-6) family | Omega 3 (n-3) family |
|---|---|---|
| Predominant source | Vegetable oils | Marine oils |
| Essential fatty acid | Linoleic | α-linolenic |
| Converted to | Arachidonic acid | Docosahexaenoic acid |

The importance of the long-chain fatty acid ratios may explain some of the observed benefits of breast milk such as the decreased incidence of multiple sclerosis (Pisacane 1994). Animal fats, including human milk, tend to have more omega 6 fatty acids (Crawford 1993). Formula milks are supplemented with fat derived from vegetable sources so tend to be far richer in linoleic acid than the omega 3 family of long-chain polyunsaturated fats. Several manufacturers of milk intended for preterm babies now supplement their formula milk with AA and DHA because premature babies have limited capability in elongating and desaturating fatty acids.

## Lipases

Human milk contains lipases, which are supplemented by unique production of neonatal lipases; these together compensate for limited pancreatic lipase activity. Lipoprotein lipase (serum-stimulated lipase) may appear in milk because of leakage from mammary tissue. Refrigerated and frozen milk undergo lipolysis; the enzyme responsible for this appears to have activity similar to that of pancreatic lipase; it is present in the fat fraction of the milk and is inhibited by bile salts. The most important lipase is the bile salt-stimulated lipase, which occurs in milk of humans and other primates. This enzyme is stable and active in the gut. It has a significant effect on the hydrolysis of milk triacylglycerides and is activated by concentrations of bile salts even lower than those required for micelle formation.

Lipase activity occurs in the saliva (and there may be additional gastric lipase activity). This lingual lipase is stimulated by the presence of milk in the mouth and by suckling, even non-nutritive suckling. Human milk fat digestion is 85–90% efficient compared with less than 70% efficiency of the fat digestion in cow's milk-derived formulas. Human milk fat globules are enclosed in maternal alveolar cell membranes, which aid in maintaining optimal surface area for emulsification and absorption and also protect the fat from lipolysis and oxidation. These factors mean that human milk stores well.

### Carnitine

Human milk contains carnitine, which has an important role in facilitating the entry of long-chain fatty acids into mitochondria where they are oxidized. Carnitine is synthesized from the essential amino acids lysine and methionine, but neonates may have limited synthetic capacity. Carnitine also is involved in the initiation of ketogenesis and in the regulation of heat generation from brown adipose tissue. As infants use fat as a major source of energy and have limited ability to synthesize carnitine, they have an increased need for carnitine.

## *Carbohydrate*

Lactose, which is unique to mammalian milk (and probably therefore important in the development of the mammalian order), is the major carbohydrate of milk. Levels of lactose do not vary and appear to control the volume of milk produced. As well as lactose, there are also trace amounts (about 10%) of 130 other sugars, the most prevalent of which are glucose, galactose, glucosamine and other oligosaccharides. Some of the non-lactose sugars may contribute to favourable gut colonization. Nitrogen-containing oligosaccharides, including the complex sugar 1-fucose, promote the growth of *Lactobacillus bifidus* resulting in increased gut acidity, which is unfavourable to pathogenic bacteria.

### Clinical application: nutritional problems of preterm infants

Human milk is nutritionally inadequate for preterm infants, leading to poor growth rates and osteopenia. However, it does have clear advantages. It has valuable immunological properties, protecting against necrotizing enterocolitis. It is associated with improved cognition and it stimulates gut maturity. The ideal food for a preterm infant able to tolerate lactose is the baby's own mother's milk fortified with additional calories, protein and minerals. Babies requiring parenteral feeding benefit from receiving some milk in the gut. One of the problems of tube feeding is the loss of energy as the fat tends to stick to the tubes. If the mother has a good supply of milk, the energy content can be increased by fractionating the milk and feeding the baby the fat-rich hindmilk. Skin-to-skin contact has also been found to be important for premature babies and it helps to stimulate the mother's lactational capabilities. It also increases the maternal IgA in the milk, which is specific to the nocosomial flora of the hospital environs.

Lactose is a disaccharide that is digested by the enzyme lactase into its component monosaccharides, glucose and galactose. Lactase activity develops rapidly in late gestation and is adequate from 36 weeks; its activity cannot be prematurely induced by exposure. Lactase is not produced by most mammals and many humans after infancy. The ability to produce lactase throughout life seems to be related to continual exposure to lactose in communities that have a strong economic dependence on dairy farming.

Lactose is relatively insoluble and is slowly digested and absorbed in the small intestine. It promotes the growth of microorganisms that produce organic acids and synthesize many B vitamins. The acidic environment is inhospitable to many pathogenic bacteria. Lactose forms soluble salts so the absorption of calcium, phosphorus, magnesium and other metals is increased in the presence of lactose.

In preterm babies, with low lactase activity, a large proportion of lactose reaches the large intestine in an undigested form. Here it is metabolized by colonic bacteria to produce organic acids, hydrogen and carbon dioxide. The organic acids are absorbed across the mucosa and a proportion of the energy is recovered. This means that preterm babies are able to utilize a large proportion of the energy contributed from lactose. The extent of colonic salvage can be determined by measuring the amount of hydrogen in the baby's breath and can be severely compromised by antibiotics or surgery disrupting the colonic flora. It is suggested that over-accumulation of organic acids in the lower gut may be a factor in the initiation of necrotizing enterocolitis (Lucas & Cole 1990) (Box 16.6).

Although the evolution of mammalian species has obviously depended on the unique properties of lactose, intolerance to lactose may occur. Although galactose is directly involved in the synthesis of glycoproteins and glycolipids of the CNS, it is not essential in the diet. Galactose can be synthesized from glucose in the liver so glucose can substitute for lactose in a

**Box 16.6**
**Necrotizing enterocolitis**

- Seen predominantly in premature infants
- Associated with infection, hypertonic feeds, hypovolaemia and perinatal asphyxia
- Most prominent in jejunum, ileum and colon
- Clinical signs usually appear at 3–10 days old
- Symptoms may include abdominal distension, blood in stools, vomiting, lethargy, respiratory distress and poor thermoregulation
- Human milk fed enterally is protective—possibly by stimulating gut maturity and integrity, providing substrates for enzymes and increasing perfusion

lactose-free diet. Alternatively, lactase can be added directly to bottles or milk or milk can be fermented prior to ingestion.

Table 16.3 compares the composition of human colostrum, mature human milk and cow's milk.

### Starch

Starch digestion in young babies is possible. Infant saliva contains some amylase activity but levels rapidly increase from 3 to 6 months. Pancreatic amylase activity is minimal in the first 3 months and remains low until about 6 months. Mammary amylase in human milk has a high activity in colostrum, which is retained for about 6 weeks. Intestinal mucosa has both disaccharidases and glucoamylase, which hydrolyses oligosaccharides and disaccharides. Glucoamylase is a brush-border enzyme that can hydrolyse glucose polymers in formula milk. Formula feeds derived from cow's milk often contain maltodextrin, a polymer of maltose and glucose. This has the advantages of being easily digested and increasing the viscosity and mineral content of the formula. Babies are born with relatively high levels of glucoamylase activity, which further increases after birth. Glucoamylase is less susceptible to being affected by intestinal mucosal damage and is distributed along the length of the small intestine, which increases the efficiency of hydrolysis and uptake of its products.

There is evidence that the ability to digest starch can be induced if starch is present in the diet. Adaptation is not quick and may take days to weeks. Undigested starch causes gastrointestinal disturbances, such as diarrhoea, which interfere with the absorption of other nutrients so affected infants may exhibit symptoms of failure to thrive. Hypoxia and ischaemia result in decreased intestinal perfusion, which alters the structure of the epithelial cells affecting uptake of monosaccharides.

### Oligosaccharides

Milk contains about 130 different oligosaccharides. Human milk seems to have a particular diverse profile of oligosaccharides, which vary genetically and with the duration of lactation and the time of day. The role of oligosaccharides in milk is protective. They are not absorbed and appear to act as substrates for beneficial bacteria and to bind pathogens competitively thus mopping them up (McVeagh & Miller 1997). Oligosaccharides thus promote a particular bacterial flora in the gut of breastfed babies, which results in a characteristic pH and may protect against urinary infections. The oligosaccharide sialic acid occurs in high concentrations in breast milk. It is found in high concentrations in the brain and is associated with brain development and increased learning behaviour in animals (Tram et al 1997).

## *Vitamins*

A plentiful breast milk supply from a well-nourished woman contains all the vitamins required by a term neonate, with the possible exceptions of vitamins D and K. As fat is the most variable constituent of the milk, the level of fat-soluble vitamins is relatively unstable. There is a seasonal variation in the vitamin A content of cow's milk. Human milk may have a seasonal variation in vitamin C content. Dietary taboos practised during lactation in some cultures may affect breast milk vitamin content. Vitamin $B_{12}$ deficiency is associated with maternal diet.

### Vitamin D

Breastfed babies rarely develop rickets although the level of vitamin D in breast milk is low. The vitamin D content of foods is measured by assessing the vitamin D content of the fat fraction. However, breast milk may contain an aqueous vitamin D sulphate, which is not included in the fat fraction, so the vitamin D content of breast milk may be underestimated. Neonates have stores of all fat-soluble vitamins, including vitamin D, and they are able to synthesize vitamin D on exposure to sunlight from an early age. Vitamin D-deficient milk is associated with low exposure to sun, long winters, Northern climes, dark skins and cultural practices. Increased levels of pollution may also affect vitamin D synthesis in the skin. Certain ethnic groups, such as Rastafarians in the UK, have an increased risk of vitamin D deficiency.

**Table 16.3** *Comparison of human colostrum, human milk and cow's milk*

| | Colostrum | Mature human milk (100 ml) | Cow's milk (100 ml) | Comments |
|---|---|---|---|---|
| Energy<br><br>Water | | 70 (kcal) | 66 (kcal) | Colostrum is produced in small but easier to digest amounts—produced during first 3 days of life—neonate may feed frequently as metabolic process adapts from the constant feed environment of the uterus to an extrauterine fast/feed cycle |
| Protein | Immunoglobulins account for increased protein content | 1.3 g (mostly whey); lactoalbumin; immunoglobulins; lactoferrin lysozyme; enzymes; hormones | 3.5 g (high casein content | Colostrum rich in passive immunity factors to provide initial protection to infant; cow's milk harder to digest owing to increased casein, also contains lactoglobulin not found in breast milk (may be responsible for cow's milk allergy); protein ratios differ owing to the calf having a faster growth trajectory than the human infant |
| Lactose | Less lactose | 7.0 g provides 37% of energy requirement | 4.9 g | Breast milk tastes sweeter than cow's milk |
| Fat | Less fat | 4.2 g (98% triglycerides) provides approx. 50% of energy requirements | 3.7 g | All mammalian milks are rich in fats owing to the high-yielding energy from fat metabolism |
| Sodium<br>Potassium<br>Chloride<br>Calcium<br>Phosphorus | | 15 mg<br>60 mg<br>43 mg<br>35 mg<br>15 mg | 22 mg<br>35 mg<br>29mg<br>117 mg<br>92 mg | Higher concentrations of organic ions in cow's milk; the neonatal kidney may be unable to regulate higher ion concentrations owing to immaturity |
| Magnesium | | 2.8 mg | | |
| Vit A | Increased level | 60 μm | less | |
| Vit D | | 0.01 μm | | |
| Vit E | Increased level | 0.35 μm | | |
| Vit K | Increased level | 0.21 μm | 6 μm | |
| Thiamin | | 16 μm | 44 | |
| Riboflavin | | 30 μm | 175 μm | |
| Nicotinic acid | | 230 μm | | |
| $B_{12}$ | | 0.01 μm | 0.4 μm | |
| $B_6$ | | 6 μm | | |
| Folates | | 5.2 μm | 5.5 μm | |
| Pantothenic acid | | 260 μm | | |
| Biotin | | 3.8 μm | | |
| Vit C | | 3.8 mg | 1.1 mg | |
| Iron | | 76 μm | 5 mg | Breast milk has low levels of iron; however, it is absorbed approx. 20 times more efficiently than iron supplements |
| Copper | | 76 μm | | |
| Zinc | | 295 μm | | |
| Iodine | | 7 μm | | |

### Vitamin E

Vitamin E, mostly in the form of α-tocopherol, is an antioxidant. Deficiency compromises the integrity of the red blood cell membrane and can lead to microhaemorrhages if severe. In formula feeds, the α-tocopherol to polyunsaturated fat ratio is held constant (1 IU vitamin E per gram of linoleic acid).

### Vitamin K

Vitamin K deficiency is associated with haemorrhagic disease of the newborn (see Ch. 15) and is usually due to low stores of vitamin K rather than low levels in the milk. The major source of vitamin K is a by-product of bacterial metabolism but the baby is born with a sterile gut, and gut colonization capable of producing vitamin K is not adequate until the baby is at least 6 weeks old. Concentrations of vitamin K are higher in colostrum and early milk, particularly the hindmilk as the vitamin is fat soluble. Breast milk stimulates colonization of the gut by vitamin K-producing bacteria. A prophylactic dose of vitamin K is routinely given at birth to protect against haemorrhagic disease of the newborn.

### Vitamin A

Vitamin A requirement is increased if stores are inadequate or there are problems with fat absorption. A deficiency of vitamin A in infancy is associated with bronchopulmonary dysplasia. This may result from a low intake or increased requirement for the vitamin in healing the damaged lung epithelium.

## *Minerals*

The mineral content of milk is slightly affected by maternal diet but milk provides all the major minerals and trace elements required by the normal term infant. Usually the mother's dietary deficiency or excess intake of mineral does not affect the composition of her milk very much as maternal homeostasis protects the infant against fluctuations of most minerals in the maternal diet. Parenteral feeding of infants, rather than frank deficiencies, has elicited most information about mineral requirements. Deficiencies are usually associated with short gestation or severe placental insufficiency.

The concentration of most minerals remains generally low but the bioavailability is high. Human milk has a number of binding proteins, notably for iron, calcium and zinc. The absorption of iron from human milk is particularly efficient, aided by the lactoferrin and transferrin content of milk and its low pH. The binding of iron is bacteriostatic.

The sodium content of human milk is inversely related to the volume of milk produced so it is higher initially and at weaning. Cow's milk has four times the sodium content of human milk. Hypernatraemia, caused for instance by hot weather, mild infection or overconcentrated formula reconstitution, can result in dehydration.

Calcium absorption is affected by vitamin D, calcium and phosphorus concentrations, fatty acids and lactose. It is particularly enhanced by the acid environment and low phosphorus content of human milk. The calcium:phosphorus ratio of human milk is 2:4 (compared with 1:3 in cow's milk). If phosphorus levels are high, there is increased phosphorus absorption at the expense of calcium absorption as they compete for the same mechanism of transfer across the gut wall. The resulting fall in plasma calcium concentration can cause hypocalcaemia with symptoms of jitteriness, tetany and convulsions.

## *Milk-borne trophic factors*

As well as nutritive and immunological factors, human milk contains a group of biologically active factors that affect growth. These factors can be classified into three groups: hormones and peptide growth factors, nucleotides and nucleosides, and polyamines. The hormone group includes insulin, GH, IGF-I, somatostatin, EGF, prolactin and GH-releasing factor. Some of these hormones and growth factors are absorbed across the permeable neonatal gut into the body where they affect metabolism and promote growth and differentiation of organs and tissues. Other hormones, such as somatostatin, appear not to be absorbed but resist proteolysis having an effect directly on the wall of the gut. They may protect gastrointestinal cells and therefore reduce the risk of necrotizing enterocolitis.

Both human and bovine colostrum are rich in nucleotides, which are precursors of nucleic acids. Nucleotides appear to have a role in enhancing growth and differentiation. They are particularly involved in liver cell function, lipid metabolism and lipoprotein synthesis. They also affect the development of the gut-associated lymphoid tissue (GALT). Unlike cow's milk, mature human milk maintains high levels of nucleotides. Up to a fifth of the breastfed neonate's

**Case study 16.2**

Isla is 11 days old and has just regained her birth weight. She has been breastfed since birth and appears to be very healthy and alert. Julia, her mother, contacts the midwife because she is concerned about Isla who is sleeping 12 hours at night and feeds only four times a day. Julia's elder sister also gave birth recently and her 21-day-old baby feeds every 2 hours, day and night, and has been progressively gaining weight. Julia's sister reported that her midwife told her that this is how a newborn baby normally behaves and advises Julia to stop breastfeeding because her baby is not growing properly.

- How can the midwife reassure Julia that Isla is well, feeding normally and gaining adequate nutrition?
- What concerns, if any, would you have for Julia's niece or how would you reassure Julia that all was normal?
- Why do some babies have different patterns of feeding and weight gain?

requirement for nucleotides is derived from milk. Dietary nucleotides may facilitate iron absorption and promote development of the immune response.

The polyamines, spermine and spermidine, are present in all cells but human milk has about 10 times as much polyamine content as cow's milk. Levels of polyamines are particularly high in the first days of lactation. They may have mitogenic, metabolic and immunological effects promoting gut development of the newborn.

Case study 16.2 is an example of concerns about newborn nutrition.

## Immunological properties of human milk

Milk has an important non-nutritive protective role. Human milk discourages bacterial growth whereas cow's milk promotes bacterial growth in the upper small bowel, which is optimal for ruminants (Jackson & Golden 1978). Breastfed infants have fewer infections (Box 16.7), but some of this effect may be due to a decreased exposure to other foods bearing microorganisms (Golding, Emmett & Rogers 1997). The protective properties of milk are also important in protecting the breasts themselves from infection. Many cultures use breast milk topically—for instance using it

**Box 16.7**

**Advantages of breastfeeding**

- Optimal infant nutrition
- Convenience, cost and lack of contamination
- Reduced risk of mortality—from necrotizing enterocolitis and sudden infant death syndrome
- Reduced infection—gastrointestinal, respiratory, urinary tract, ear, meningitis, intractable diarrhoea
- Reduced risk of maternal cancer—breast, ovarian
- Reduced atopic disease—eczema, asthma
- Increased intelligence
- Reduced risk of autoimmune disease
- Enhanced immunity

to treat eye infections. Immunological properties of human milk are increased with better maternal nutrition (Chang 1990).

### *Immunoglobulins*

The immunoglobulins (antibodies) in milk are distinct from those found in maternal serum. The major immunoglobulin is secretory IgA but milk also contains minor amounts of monomeric IgA, IgG and IgM. Secretory IgA is at very high concentrations in the colostrum but declines to lower levels by day 14 as milk volume increases. The mother will produce specific immunoglobulins to every pathogen she encounters. The transfer of IgA into the milk is a form of passive immunity (see Ch. 10), augmenting the placental transfer of IgG to the fetus. The baby's own immune system is further stimulated by factors in the milk. Breastfed babies have superior responses to vaccination programmes and have higher IgA in their saliva, nasal secretions and urine (Prentice 1987, Prentice et al 1987).

IgA is stable at low pH and resistant to proteolytic enzymes so it survives in the gastrointestinal tract. IgA has an important role in the defence against infection, slowing bacterial and viral invasion of the mucosa. It adheres to the gastric mucosa and prevents adhesion of microorganisms. IgA promotes closure of the gut and so decreases its permeability to allergens such as cow's milk β-lactoglobulin and serum bovine albumin.

### *Binding proteins*

Lactoferrin is an iron-binding protein that facilitates the absorption of iron from milk. In binding iron, it reduces the amount of free iron available for microorganisms in the gut, thus inhibiting the growth of certain pathogenic bacteria. It is suggested that lactoferrin in breast milk helps to reduce the incidence of gastrointestinal tract infections. Excess free iron is associated with increased bacterial pathogens in the gut. These bacteria have a high iron requirement and can cause gut damage and microhaemorrhages, which themselves can lead to iron-deficient anaemia.

### *Other protective properties*

Breast milk contains high levels of lysozyme, which is protective against gram-positive bacteria and viruses. Lactose and bifidus factor stimulating the growth of lactobacilli promote an acidic environment, which is protective. Fibronectin, which is present in high concentrations in human milk, is a non-specific opsonin (see Ch. 10) that increases phagocytosis of bacteria. Milk also contains other protective factors (Table 16.4).

### *Immune cells*

Milk is not sterile but contains about $4 \times 10^9$ cells per litre including lymphocytes from maternal Peyer's patches and scavenger macrophages and neutrophils. Levels of cells are particularly high in the colostrum.

## Formula feeds

In Western countries, where dairy farming is established, cow's milk is modified and processed into the formula feeds, which are the basis of bottle feeding. Human children in other cultures are reared on buffalo, goat, horse, camel and yak milk. Mammalian milks may be quantitatively similar but the quality is variable, being species specific.

Cow's milk is supplemented with carbohydrate, either lactose or maltodextrin, which dilutes the higher mineral and protein content. Cow's milk fat (which has a high commercial value as butter and cream) is substituted with vegetable/butter fat blends. This increases the absorption efficiency; unabsorbed fat decreases the energy content, lowers calcium absorption and produces steatorrhoea.

For whey-dominant formulas, demineralized whey (which is expensive) is blended with skimmed milk to increase the whey : casein ratio and decrease the electrolyte content. The profit margin of whey-dominant formulas is lower than casein-dominant formulas. Casein-dominant formulas are marketed for the 'hungrier baby' and, although the energy content is constant, are considered to be a progressive step in feeding. Mothers often demonstrate a strong brand loyalty when choosing formula milk.

Trace minerals and vitamins are added in line with legal limits. Packaging of formula feed is important. Anaerobic storage and copper supplementation help to reduce fatty acid oxidation. Scoop and granule size are carefully designed to optimize precision in reconstitution.

## Weaning

Weaning can be defined as the progressive transition from milk to a normal family diet. Before 4 months, it is considered unnecessary being associated with increased incidence of diarrhoea and interference with the maintenance of breastfeeding (the nutritional value of the complement is usually lower than breast milk). An increase in dietary cereals and vegetables tends to affect the absorption of iron, which can be delicately balanced in younger infants. By 6 months, many babies will require complementary feeding and will have sufficiently developed to cope with it. Deciduous teeth erupt at about 6 months. Incisors, which cut food, are the first teeth to appear followed by molars at about 12 months, which allow grinding of food.

Determination of the appropriate time to introduce foods other than milk is not just by age but should also take into consideration the food available, conditions to prepare it, the growth velocity and the neuromuscular development of the infant. It is not clear which pattern of growth is optimal. Growth charts are based on weight and height data from clinical surveillance. Ethnicity and both environmental and genetic factors affect growth. Practically, the high weight velocity, which is seen in the first 3 months of life, is not related to overfeeding. The deceleration of growth after 3 months is not in itself an indicator to wean. Early weaning is associated with an increased number of respiratory symptoms (Forsyth et al 1993).

By 6 months, normal physiological development can support the introduction of alternative foods. The baby is able to hold its head erect and can control the movement of its hands to mouth. The tongue extrusion reflex is waning and can be overcome. Indeed, it is suggested that there is a critical window for introducing solid food and if it is not done within this

**Table 16.4** *Protective factors in milk*

| Factor | Function |
|---|---|
| Cells | |
| B lymphocytes | Produce antibodies against specific microbes |
| T lymphocytes | Kill infected cells |
| Macrophages | Produce lysoszyme and activate parts of the immune system |
| Neutrophils | Phagocytose bacteria |
| Lacto bifidus factor | Promotes an acidic environment favourable for the growth of *Lactobacillus bifidus* and inhibits the growth of pathogenic microorganisms |
| Immunoglobulins (Antibodies IgA, IgG, IgM, IgD and IgE) | Active against specific organisms i.e. poliomyelitis, salmonella |
| Immunoglobulin A (IgA) | Lines the gut to discourage adhesion of pathogenic microorganisms and limits allergen entry |
| Lactoferrin | Decreases iron available by binding to iron for bacterial growth<br>Acts as a bacteriostatic agent |
| Lysozymes<br>Lactoperioxidase<br>Complement | Act in a non-specific way by damaging the cell walls of microorganisms |
| Lipids | Inhibit growth of staphylococcus and viruses by disrupting cell membranes |
| Fibronectin | Promotes macrophage activity and aids repair to damaged gut tissue |
| $\gamma$-interferon | Promotes activity of immune cells |
| Mucins | Adhere to microorganisms inhibiting attachment to the gut wall |
| Oligosaccharides | Inhibit attachment of microorganisms to mucosal surfaces |
| Bile salt-stimulated lipase | Acts as an antiprotozoal |
| Bile salt-stimulated lipase<br>Lipoprotein lipase $\alpha$-amylase | Promote fat and protein digestion |
| $\alpha_1$-antitrypsin<br>$\alpha_1$-antichymotrypsin | Prevent breakdown of protective factors |
| Epidermal growth factor | Promotes maturation of the gut wall |
| Binding proteins<br>$B_{12}$-binding protein<br>Lactoferrin<br>Transferrin<br>Folate-binding protein<br>Somatomedin C | Increase absorption of nutrients and limit availability of nutrients utilized by bacteria |

window the baby tends to develop a preference for liquid feeds and may become a child with feeding problems. The kidneys are mature enough to cope with a solute load.

Weaning is an important biological and social learning process as well as offering foods of higher nutrient and energy density than milk. Exposing different tastes to children has already begun in feeding. Compounds ingested by the mother are transported into the milk (Mennella 1995). This may present an important learning experience not received by bottle-fed babies.

## Key points

- The physiological unit of the mammary gland is the alveolus. Prolactin, from the anterior pituitary, stimulates milk production from the alveolar cells. Oxytocin, from the posterior pituitary, stimulates contraction of the myoepithelial cells lining the alveoli and the ducts, resulting in milk ejection or 'let-down'.
- Prolactin secretion slowly reaches a peak following stimulation at the nipple. Secretion is pulsatile and circadian and is controlled by the abrogation of tonic inhibition from dopamine produced by the hypothalamus. Prolactin inhibits ovulation thus suppressing fertility.
- Oxytocin release is stimulated by nipple stimulation and by thinking about or hearing the baby. Secretion of oxytocin immediately follows stimulation and can be inhibited by stress.
- The effects of prolactin are locally controlled by the production of FIL in the milk. Increased concentrations of FIL suppress the response to prolactin thus inhibiting milk production. This is important in mammary gland involution when breastfeeding is curtailed.
- Lactating women appear to have increased efficiency of energy utilization. The nutritional composition of the milk is not affected greatly by maternal diet unless the mother is extremely undernourished; however, concerns have been expressed about effects on maternal calcium balance and the tendency to develop obesity. Breastfeeding is associated with a reduced risk of maternal breast and ovarian cancer.
- Human milk provides optimal nutrition for the human neonate, which has immature renal, hepatic and gastrointestinal functions and a rapidly developing nervous system. Breastfed babies have a lower incidence of infection.
- Colostrum is the early secretion from the breast; it provides important anti-infective properties and promotes favourable colonization of the gut.
- Protein requirements are relatively low as the human neonate has a relatively slow growth rate. Human milk has a high concentration of whey proteins and non-protein nitrogen components, which include growth factors. The amino acid composition of human milk protein compensates for the neonate's limited ability to convert essential amino acids to non-essential amino acids; the net protein utilization of human milk is high.
- Fat is the main energy source in milk and the most variable constituent. The proportion of fat is higher in hindmilk. The fatty acid composition of human milk allows optimum absorption. Human milk fat is rich in polyunsaturated fatty acids required for development of the brain and nervous system.
- Lactose is the major carbohydrate of milk; it provides energy, aids absorption of other nutrients and promotes an environment favourable to beneficial microorganisms.
- Human milk has important immunological properties and is associated with a lower incidence of infections and a persistently more responsive immune system in breastfed babies.

### Application to practice

It is consistently shown that breastfeeding is influential in the reduction of many disease states and thus should be encouraged. The midwife is uniquely placed to influence the overall health of the nation.

Knowledge of lactation and the benefits are important if the midwife is to promote breastfeeding in practice.

## Annotated further reading

Akre J 1991 Infant feeding: the physiological basis. WHO, Geneva

*Physiological aspects of breastfeeding are explained clearly and precisely within this text which relates the composition of breast milk to the nutritional and developmental needs of the neonate.*

Black R F, Jarman L, Simpson J B 1998 The science of breastfeeding. Jones & Bartlett, Toronto

*Module 3 of the Lactation Specialist Self-Study series which is based on the competencies published by the International Lactation Consultant Association. This volume covers anatomy and physiology in relation to lactation and infant feeding, nutritive and non-nutritive components of human*

*milk, maternal nutritional requirements and practical considerations.*

Darby M K, Loughead J L 1996 Neonatal nutritional requirements and formula composition: a review. Journal of gynaecology and neonatal nursing 25:209–217
*This article reviews the composition of human and artificial milks in relation to the nutritional requirements of the neonate.*

Fomon S J 1993 Nutrition of normal infants. C V Mosby, St Louis
*Reference textbook targeted at practitioners which covers the growth and nutrition of normal, full-term infants in industrialized countries.*

Jelliffe D B, Jelliffe E F P 1979 Human milk in the modern world: psychosocial, nutritional and economic significance. Oxford University Press, Oxford
*A broad consideration of a range of issues associated with breastmilk feeding including composition of human milk and economic impact of not breastfeeding.*

Palmer G 1993 The politics of breastfeeding. Pandora, London
*Discusses social, historic and economic factors affecting a woman's decision to breastfeed and the implications of the type of infant feeding method.*

Riordan J, Auerbach K G 1993 Breast feeding and human lactation, 2nd edn. Jones & Bartlett, London
*A comprehensive text on breastfeeding aimed at midwives, breastfeeding consultants, antenatal teachers, dieticians and nutritionists. Covers cultural aspects, anatomy and physiology, breastfeeding education and practical considerations such as breast pumps, donor milk and breastfeeding the ill child.*

Rogers I S 1997 Relactation. Early Human Development 49:S75–S81
*This article discusses the possibility of re-establishing lactation in certain situations and includes information on promoting lactation in women who have never been pregnant.*

Wharton B 1997 Nutrition in infancy. British Nutrition Foundation, London
*A British Nutrition Foundation briefing paper produced after a conference about the nutritional requirements of infants; a concise, authoritative and easy to read report summarizing and reviewing current knowledge.*

Worthington-Roberts B, Williams S R 1996 Nutrition in pregnancy and lactation, 6th edn. C V Mosby, St Louis
*A comprehensive textbook about nutritional needs before and during pregnancy and during lactation. Includes practical information on assessing nutritional risk and counselling and supporting breastfeeding mothers.*

## References


Adlercreutz H 1995 Phytoestrogens—epidemiology and a possible role in cancer protection. Environmental Health Perspectives 103:103–112

Anderson A N, Schioler V 1982 Influence of breastfeeding patterns on pituitary–ovarian axis of women in an industrialised community. American Journal of Obstetrics and Gynecology 143:673–677

Bayley T M, Alasmi M, Thorkelson T et al 1998 Influence of formula versus breast milk on cholesterol synthesis rates in four-month-old infants. Pediatric Research 44:60–67

Ben-Jonathan N, Laudon M, Garris P A 1991 Novel aspects of posterior pituitary function: regulation of prolactin secretion. Frontiers in Neuroendocrinology 12:231–277

Britton H 1993 Mother–infant interaction: relationship to early infant nutrition and feeding. In: Suskind R M, Lewinter-Suskind L (eds) Textbook of pediatric nutrition. Raven Press, New York, pp 43–48

Broadhurst C L, Cunnane S C, Crawford M A 1998 Rift Valley lake fish and shellfish provided brain-specific nutrition for early Homo. British Journal of Nutrition 79:3–21

Carlson S E 1985 Human milk non-protein nitrogen: occurrence and possible functions. Advances in Pediatrics 32:43–63

Chang S-J 1990 Antimicrobial proteins of maternal and cord sera and human milk in relation to maternal nutritional status. American Journal of Clinical Nutrition 51:183–187

Crawford M A 1993 The role of essential fatty acids in neural development: implications for perinatal nutrition. American Journal of Clinical Nutrition 57(suppl):S703–S710

Dewey K G 1997 Energy and protein requirements during lactation. Annual Review of Nutrition 17:19–36

Ebrahim G J 1990 The scientific contribution of breast feeding research. Maternal Child Health March:92–93

Emmett P M, Rogers I S 1997 Properties of human milk and their relationship with maternal nutrition. Early Human Development 49:S7–S28.

Forsyth J S, Ogston S A, Clark A, Florey C du V, Howie P W 1993 Relationship between early introduction of solid food to infants and their weight and illnesses during the first two years of life. British Medical Journal 306:1572–1576

Golding J 1997 Unnatural constituents of breast milk—medication, lifestyle, pollutants, viruses. Early Human Development 49:S29–S43.

Golding J, Emmett P M, Rogers I S 1997 Does breast feeding have any impact on non-infectious, non-allergic disorders? Early Human Development 49:S131–S142

Gray R H, Campbell O M, Zacur H A, Labbok M H, MacRae S L 1987 Postpartum return of ovarian activity in nonbreastfeeding women monitored by urinary assays. Journal of Clinical Endocrinology and Metabolism 64:645–650

Hartmann P, Sherriff J, Kent J 1995 Maternal nutrition and the regulation of milk synthesis. Proceedings of the Nutrition Society 54:379–389

Howie P W, McNeilly A S 1982 Effect of breastfeeding patterns on human birth intervals. Journal of Reproduction and Fertility 63:545–551

Howie P W, McNeilly A S, McArdle T, Smart L, Houston M 1980 The relationship between suckling-induced prolactin response and lactogenesis. Journal of Clinical Endocrinology and Metabolism 50:670–673

Illingworth P J, Jung R T, Howie P W, Leslie P, Isles T E 1986 Diminution in energy expenditure during lactation. British Medical Journal 292:437–442

Jackson A A, Golden M H N 1978 The human rumen. Lancet 1978:764–767

Johnston J M, Amico J A 1986 A prospective longitudinal study of the release of oxytocin and prolactin in response to infant suckling in long term lactation. Journal of Clinical Endocrinology and Metabolism 62:653–657

Karjalainen J, Martin J M, Knip M et al 1992 A bovine albumin peptide as a possible trigger of insulin-dependent diabetes mellitus. New England Journal of Medicine 327:302–307

Koppe J G 1995 Nutrition and breast-feeding. European Journal of Obstetrics, Gynecology and Reprodutive Biology 61:73–78

Lane P A, Hathaway W E 1985 Vitamin K in infancy. Journal of Pediatrics 106:351–359

Lonnerdal B 1985 Dietary factors affecting trace element bioavailability from human milk, cow's milk and infant formulae. Progress in Food and Nutrition Science 9:36–62

Lucas A, Cole T J 1990 Breast milk and neonatal necrotising enterocolitis. Lancet 336:1519–1523

Lucas A, Ewing G, Roberts S B, Coward W A 1987 How much energy does the breast fed infant consume and expend? British Medical Journal 295:75–77

Lucas A, Morley R, Cole T J, Lister G, Leeson-Payne C 1992 Breast milk and subsequent intelligence quotient in children born preterm. Lancet 339:261–264

McNeilly A S, Robinson I C A F, Houston M J, Howie P W 1983 Release of oxytocin and prolactin in response to suckling. British Medical Journal 286:257–259

McVeagh P, Miller J B 1997 Human milk oligosaccharides: only the breast. Journal of Paediatrics and Child Health 33:281–286

Martin R H, Glass M R, Chapman C, Wilson G D, Woods K L 1980 Human α-lactalbumin and hormonal factors in pregnancy and lactation. Clinics in Endocrinology 13:223–230

Mennella J A 1995 Mother's milk: a medium for early flavor experiences. Journal of Human Lactation 11:39–45

Menella J A, Beauchamp G K 1991 The transfer of alcohol to human milk: effects on flavor and the infant's behavior. New England Journal of Medicine 325:981–985

Monte C S, Johnston C S, Roll L E 1994 Bovine serum albumin detected in infant formula is a possible trigger for insulin dependence diabetes mellitus. Journal of the American Dietetic Association 94:314–316

Ohlin A, Rossner S 1996 Factors related to body weight changes during and after pregnancy: the Stockholm pregnancy and weight development study. Obesity Research 4:271–276

Ojofeitimi E O, Elegbe I A 1982 The effect of early initiation of colostrum feeding on proliferation of intestinal bacteria in neonates. Clinics in Pediatrics 21:39–42

Peaker M 1989 Evolutionary strategies in lactation: nutritional implications. Proceedings of the Nutrition Society 48:53–57

Pisacane A, Impagliazzo N, Russo M et al 1994 Breast feeding and multiple sclerosis. British Medical Journal 308:1411–1412

Pond C (ed) 1992 Reproductive Physiology. Open University, Milton Keynes, pp 197, 200

Porter T E, Grandy D, Bunzow J, Wiles C D, Civelli O, Frawley L S 1994 Evidence that stimulatory dopamine receptors may be involved in the regulation of prolactin secretion. Endocrinology 134:1263–1268

Prentice A 1987 Breast feeding increases concentration of IgA in infants' urine. Archives of Disease in Childhood 62:792–795

Prentice A M, Prentice A 1995 Evolutionary and environmental influences on human lactation. Proceedings of the Nutrition Society 54:391–400

Prentice A, Ewing G, Roberts S B et al 1987 The nutritional role of breast-milk IgA and lactoferrin. Acta Paediatrica Scandinavica 76:592–598

Rogan W J, Gladen B C, McKinney J D et al 1987 Polychlorinated biphenyls (PCBs) and dichlorodiphenyl dichloroethane (DDE) in human milk: effects on growth, morbidity and duration of lactation. American Journal of Public Health 77:1294–1297

Rogers I S 1997 Lactation and fertility. Early Human Development 49(suppl):S185–S190

Sanders T A B, Ellis F R, Dickerson J W T 1978 Studies of vegans: the fatty acid composition of plasma choline-phosphoglycerides, erythrocytes, adipose tissue, breastmilk and some indicators of susceptibility to ischemic heart disease in vegans and omnivore controls. American Journal of Clinical Nutrition 31:805–813

Schreiner R L, Brady M S, Franken E A, Stevens D C, Lemons J A, Gresham E L 1979 Increased incidence of lacto bezoars in low birth weight infants. American Journal of Disease in Childhood 133:936–940

Sowers M 1996 Pregnancy and lactation as risk factors for subsequent bone loss and osteoporosis. Journal of Bone Mineral Research 11:1052–1060

Tram T H, Miller J C B, McNeil Y, McVeagh P 1997 Sialic acid content of infant saliva: comparison of breast fed with formula fed infants. Archives of Disease in Childhood 77:315–318

Turgeon-O'Brien H, Lachapelle D, Gagnon P F, Larocque I, Mahen-Robert L F 1996 Nutritive and non-nutritive suckling habits. Journal of Dentistry for Children 63:321–327

Van de Perre P 1995 Postnatal transmission of human immunodeficiency virus type 1: the breast-feeding dilemma. American Journal of Obstetrics and Gynecology 173:483–487

Wharton B A, Balmer S E, Scott P H 1994 Faecal flora in the newborn: effect of lactoferrin and related nutrients. Advances in Experimental Medicine and Biology 357:91–98

Wilde C J, Prentice A, Peaker M 1995 Breast-feeding: matching supply with demand in human lactation. Proceedings of the Nutrition Society 54:401–406

Williams G L, McVey W R, Hunter J F 1993 Mammary somatosensory pathways are not required for suckling-mediated inhibition of luteinizing hormone secretion and delay of ovulation in cows. Biology of Reproduction 49:1328–1337

Woodward A, Grgurinovich N, Ryan P 1986 Breast feeding and smoking hygiene: major influenences on cotinine in urine of smokers' infants. Journal of Epidemiology and Community Health 40(3):309–315

Woolridge M W 1996 Breastfeeding: physiology into practice. In: Davies D P (ed) Nutrition in child health. RCOP, London, pp 13–31

Woolridge M W, Fisher C 1988 Colic, 'overfeeding', and symptoms of lactose malabsorption in the breast-fed baby: a possible artefact of feed management? Lancet ii:382–384

# Glossary

**Aerobic metabolism** The production of ATP requiring oxygen.

**Aetiology** The cause of.

**Afferent** Conducting or leading towards a target or centre.

**Agonist** A substance that interacts with a receptor molecule that initiates the same response as the hormone/transmitter usually binding to that site.

**Aliphatic** An organic compound that contains carbon atoms arranged in a chain rather than a ring formation.

**Alkalosis** An increase above that within the normal pH range of the body.

**Allograph** Implanted tissue that is of different genetic origin to the donor.

**Alopecia** The loss of body and scalp hair.

**Amoeboid** Appearing and behaving like the large single-celled organism called an amoeba.

**Amplitude** The difference between the highest and lowest measurement within a regular cycle.

**Anabolic metabolism** The synthesis of biological compounds involving the expenditure of energy.

**Anaerobic metabolism** The production of ATP in the absence of oxygen.

**Anastomose** The joining up of two tubes, vessels, etc., ensuring that the lumen remains patent between them.

**Androsperm** A sperm carrying a Y chromosome.

**Aneuploidy** Presence of an abnormal number of chromosomes.

**Angiogenesis** The formation of new blood vessels.

**Anisogamy** The existence of different forms of gametes related to sexual dimorphism.

**Antagonist** A substance that blocks receptor sites and then inhibits any further responses.

**Anteflexed** Curved inwards.

**Anteverted** Folded over.

**Antibody (immunoglobulin)** A 'Y'-shaped molecule that combines with an antigen (foreign protein) as part of the immune response, synthesized by white blood cells.

**Antigen** A molecule that initiates the immune response found within foreign tissue.

**Antral** A cavity within the body.

**Apoptosis** The genetic programming resulting in the death of a cell.

**Aquatic** Pertaining to an underwater environment.

**Arborize** To grow in a branch-like formation.

**Asynclitism** To be tilted laterally on either side of the anterior/posterior mid plane.

**Atresia** The abnormal narrowing or closure of the lumen in a tube or vessel.

**Atretic** Having the characteristics of or pertaining to atresia; without an opening.

**Atrophy** Decreased functioning due to hypoplasia with increasing age.

**Attenuated** Modified to have less of an effect than normal.

**Bactericidal** Containing substances that can kill bacteria.

**Bacteriostatic** Containing substances that inhibit the reproduction of bacteria.

**Basal metabolic rate** The amount of energy expenditure required for the maintenance of essential body function only.
**Behaviour** The study of how organisms interact within the environment.
**Biosynthesis** The manufacture of body tissues and substances.
**Breech** Pertaining to the fetal rump.
**Carotenoid** Naturally occurring fat-soluble pigments that colour plants red, yellow, orange or brown.
**Catabolic metabolism** The breakdown of compounds requiring the expenditure of energy.
**Cephalic** Pertaining to the fetal head.
**Chemoattractant** A substance that acts as an attractant.
**Chemostasis** The maintenance of a chemical balance.
**Chorioamnionitis** Infection of the chorion and amnion during pregnancy.
**Circadian** About one day.
**Clonal expansion** The ability of white blood cells to duplicate rapidly as part of the immune response.
**Codominant** Expression of both of two differing alleles in the phenotype when present in the genotype.
**Coitus** The act of sexual intercourse.
**Colloidal** A protein suspended in a liquid.
**Contraception** Prevention of pregnancy by intervention.
**Cortex** The outer tissue layer or part of a structure.
**Cranial** Pertaining to the skull.
**Cyanosis** The bluish appearance of body tissues in situations of hypoxia.
**Cyclical** Repeated on a regular basis.
**Cytoplasm** The intercellular tissue contained within the cell membrane.
**Decidualization** The formation of the decidua of pregnancy.
**Deletion** The loss of part of a chromosome.
**Dermatome** Area of skin supplied by a single spinal nerve; derived from segmental development during embryonic stage.
**Desquamation** The loss of the outer layers of a continuously growing squamous tissue.
**Detumescence** The resolution of the inflammatory response.
**Diapedesis** The passage of blood cells through the blood vessel wall into the surrounding tissue.
**Diastolic** The period of relaxation of the ventricles of the heart.
**Dichrotic** A notch observed on the downstroke of the arterial pressure waveform that indicates the closure of the aortic valve.
**Differentiation** The division of cells resulting in the daughter cells becoming different owing to the activation of particular genes.
**Dimorphism** The existence of an organism in distinct forms such as male and female.
**Diploid** The normal number of paired chromosomes.
**Discoid** Disc-like.
**Dorsal** Pertaining to the back.
**Dysgenesis** Abnormal formation.
**Dyspnoea** Difficulty in breathing.
**Ectopic pregnancy** Implantation occurs outside the uterine cavity, usually in a uterine tube.
**Efferent** Carrying away from a centre (e.g. a blood vessel or nerve).
**Endocytosis** The process by which substances are transported into the cell within envelopes formed out of the outer cell membrane.
**Endogenous** Pertaining to the internal physiological environment.
**Entrained** Reset by an external factor.
**Enzyme** A protein that is able to speed up a chemical reaction without being structurally altered by the process itself.
**Epitopes** A cluster of antigens that evoke an immune response.
**Ergometrine** A drug derived from alkaloids of ergot that causes a sustained, strong contraction of the myometrium.
**Erythropoietin** A hormone produced chiefly by the kidneys (in the adult) and by the liver (in the fetus) that initiates red blood cell production.
**Eugenics** The science aimed at producing the perfect individual.
**Euploidic** Contains the normal number of chromosomes.
**Evolution** The study of genetic variation and change within generations of populations.
**Exogenous** Pertaining to the external environment.
**Extended** Tilted away from.
**Flexed** Tilted towards.
**Follicle** Tissue structure that is fluid filled.
**Free radical** An oxygen molecule containing an unpaired electron.
**Gametogenesis** The formation of gametes.

**Gastrulation** The formation of the inner layers of the embryo by cell migration in a process of invagination.
**Gene manipulation** The science of artificially adding or removing genes to effect a change within an individual.
**Gene pool** The total number of genes within a population.
**Genome** The total number of genes within a single organism.
**Gluconeogenesis** The synthesis of glucose from non-carbohydrate sources.
**Glycolytic** The breakdown of glucose.
**Graft rejection** The rejection of donor tissue by the recipient's immune system.
**Gynosperm** A sperm carrying a X chromosome.
**Haemoptysis** The presence of blood in sputum.
**Half-life** The time taken for the reduction by half of the quantity present.
**Haploid** Half of the normal chromosomal number (containing only one chromosome from the normal paired chromosomes).
**Hermaphrodism** The presence of male and female sex organs within the same individual.
**Heterozygous** Alleles at a particular locus of paired chromosomes each coding for a different phenotype.
**Hirsutism** The presence of excess body hair.
**Homeothermic** A warm-blooded animal (sometimes referred to as endothermic).
**Homozygous** Alleles at a particular locus of paired chromosomes both coding for the same phenotype.
**Hydrolytic** Dissolving in water.
**Hyperaemia** An excessive quantity of blood.
**Hyper/hypoglycaemia** Abnormally high/low level of glucose within the blood.
**Hyperprolactinaemia** Abnormally raised levels of the hormone prolactin.
**Hyperventilation** Overbreathing resulting in alkalosis.
**Imprinting** A behaviour pattern initiated by specific stimulation of a neural pathway that cannot be further influenced once it has occurred.
**Incompatible** Not tolerated and so initiating the immune response.
**Inherent** Having a genetic basis, hereditary, innate.
**Innate** Present from birth, congenital, e.g. a behaviour pattern that is not learnt but instinctive.
**Invaginate** To fold inwards to form a pouch.
**Inversion** The translocation of a portion of a chromosome comprising an upside-down switch.
**Ischaemia** The death of tissues due to a reduction or loss of the blood supply.
**Keratinized** Containing the protein keratin.
**Ketotic** Detectable amounts of ketone bodies present indicating the metabolism of fats is occurring.
**Lipophilic** Having an affinity for fat.
**Luteolysis** The degradation of the corpus luteum.
**Macromolecules** Large organic compounds.
**Macrosomic** Larger than normal body size.
**Maturation** The achievement of full function following a period of growth and/or development.
**Medulla** The central tissue layer or part of a structure.
**Menarche** The commencement of the menstrual cycles.
**Menopause** The cessation of the menstrual cycles.
**Menses** The period of shedding of the endometrium during the menstrual cycle.
**Mentum** Pertaining to the fetal chin.
**Methylation** The addition of a methyl compound $-CH_3$ to a compound.
**Micturition** The voiding of urine.
**Mitogen** A substance that initiates the process of mitosis.
**Morphogenesis** The formation of body structure.
**Morphology** The development of form and size.
**Necrotic** The bacterial decomposition of dead tissue.
**Neurolation** The embryonic formation of the neural tube from the neural plate.
**Neuronal** Pertaining to the nervous system.
**Neurotransmitter** A chemical that crosses a synaptic gap to initiate an action potential in the receiving neuron.
**Nidation** The process of implantation of the blastocyst into the uterine endometrium.
**Nocturia** The need to void urine frequently at night.
**Nomenclature** Terminology describing systematic naming.
**Occiput** A bone at the posterior lower part of the skull.
**Oedema** Excess fluid in the extracellular compartments.
**Opsonization** The process by which bacteria and other cells are made susceptible to phagocytosis.
**Oxidative** The combination of oxygen with other molecules.
**Pathogen** A foreign organism that causes harm.

**Penile** Pertaining to the penis.
**Perfusion** The blood flow.
**Peristaltic** Coordinated contraction of smooth muscle around the lumen of a tube or vessel that facilitates the unidirectional movement of the contents within the lumen.
**Phagocytic** The ingestion of foreign material by phagocytes.
**Phosphorylation** The addition of an organic phosphate group to a molecule (often activating an enzyme).
**Photoperiod** The period of natural daylight exposure.
**Placebo** An inert/harmless substance that has no pharmacological effect, used in double-blind trials in comparison with drugs to assess their clinical effectiveness.
**Placentation** The formation of the fetal and maternal components of the placenta.
**Placentomes** A lobe of the placenta.
**Poikilothermic** A cold-blooded animal (sometimes referred to as exothermic).
**Polycythaemic** An abnormally high number of red blood cells.
**Polysperm** Fertilization by more than one sperm.
**Postprandial** The period following the consumption of a meal.
**Preantral** Before the antral phase.
**Precursor** A substance that is altered into another substance.
**Primordial** Existing from the beginning.
**Proliferative** The ability to increase quickly in numbers.
**Prophylaxis** Treatment aimed at prevention rather than cure.
**Pseudopodia** A temporary protrusion in the cell membrane.
**Psychogenic** The development of the mind.
**Pulsatile** Released episodically rather than continuously.
**Pyrexia** An abnormally high body temperature.
**Rate limiting** A process that proceeds in relation to the amount of precursor available.
**Receptor** A molecule that combines with a chemical signal that initiates a response within the cell.
**Reticulocyte** An immature red blood cell.
**Sacrum** The bony vestigial remains of the prehensile tail that forms the posterior part of the pelvis.
**Senescence** Old age.
**Septum (pl. septa)** A structure that divides the body or body area/organ.
**Sinciput** Pertaining to the fetal forehead.
**Sinusoids** An irregularly shaped blood vessel.
**Specific gravity** The relative density of a fluid in relation to pure water.
**Sphincter** A ring of muscle that can occlude a tube or vessel when contracted.
**Steroidogenesis** The production of steroid hormones.
**Stroma** The structural framework of a cell or organ.
**Syncytium** A mass of cells in which the cellular membranes have broken down forming a continuous mass.
**Syntocinon** A synthetic analogue of naturally occurring oxytocin used in obstetrics as a pharmacological method of augmenting uterine contractions via a controlled intravenous infusion.
**Tactile** Pertaining to touch.
**Teratogen** A chemical that interferes with the formation of the embryo.
**Thermostasis** The maintenance of a constant body temperature.
**Totipotent** A cell that has the capability of dividing to form a complete new individual.
**Transcription** The process of synthesizing mRNA from a DNA template.
**Translation** The process of forming an amino acid chain from a coded sequence of mRNA bases.
**Transudation** Blood plasma that collects within the interstitial space.
**Unicellular** Made up of one cell.
**Vascularization** The growth of blood vessels into tissue.
**Vascularized** Perfused with blood vessels.
**Vasoactive** Has an effect on vascular smooth muscle.
**Vasoconstriction** Contraction of smooth muscle within the blood vessels.
**Vasodilation** Relaxation of the smooth muscle within blood vessels.
**Ventral** Pertaining to the front.
**Vestigial** A physical characteristic (structure) in evolutionary decline—i.e. remaining present but no longer necessary for survival.
**Villus (pl. villi)** A finger-like projection from a membrane surface.
**Volatile** Evaporates at ambient temperatures.
**Zygote** A totipotent cell formed from the fusion of two gametes.

# Index